Hormones in Blood

Hormones in Blood

THIRD EDITION

Volume 3

Edited by

C. H. GRAY
*Division of Clinical Chemistry,
Clinical Research Centre, Harrow,
Middlesex, UK*

V. H. T. JAMES
*Department of Chemical Pathology,
St. Mary's Hospital Medical School,
London, UK*

1979

ACADEMIC PRESS

LONDON · NEW YORK · SAN FRANCISCO
A Subsidiary of Harcourt Brace Jovanovich, Publishers

ACADEMIC PRESS INC. (LONDON) LTD.
24/28 Oval Road
London NW1

United States Edition published by
ACADEMIC PRESS INC.
111 Fifth Avenue
New York, New York 10003

British Library Cataloguing in Publication Data
Hormones in blood. – 3rd ed.
Vol. 3
1. Hormones   2. Blood
I. Gray, Charles Horace   II. James, Vivian
Hector Thomas
612'.405   QP571   78–73882
ISBN 0-12-296203-6

Printed in Great Britain by
Page Bros. (Norwich) Ltd.
Mile Cross Lane, Norwich.

Contributors to Volume 3

D. R. BANGHAM, *National Institute for Biological Standards and Control, Holly Hill, Hampstead, London NW3 6RB, UK.*

J. P. COGHLAN, *Howard Florey Institute of Experimental Physiology and Medicine, University of Melbourne, Parkville, Victoria 3052, Australia.*

K. FOTHERBY, *Department of Steroid Biochemistry, Royal Postgraduate Medical School, Hammersmith Hospital, Du Cane Road, London W12 0HS, UK.*

RAYMOND GREEN, *106 Harley Street, London W1N 1 AF, UK.*

MITHAL GREEN, *Department of Chemical Pathology, St. Bartholomew's Hospital, West Smithfield, London EC1A 7BE, UK.*

I. A. HUGHES, *Tenovus Institute for Cancer Research, The Welsh National School of Medicine, The Heath, Cardiff CF4 4XX, UK.*

J. LANDON, *Department of Chemical Pathology, St. Bartholomew's Hospital, West Smithfield, London EC1A 7BE, UK.*

BRENDA J. LECKIE, *MRC Blood Pressure Unit, Western Infirmary, University of Glasgow, Glasgow G11 6NT, UK.*

C. K. LIM, *Division of Clinical Chemistry, Clinical Research Centre, Harrow, Middlesex HA1 3UJ, UK.*

P. J. LOWRY, *Department of Chemical Pathology, St. Bartholomew's Hospital, West Smithfield, London EC1A 7BE, UK.*

J. A. MILLAR, *MRC Blood Pressure Unit, Western Infirmary, University of Glasgow, Glasgow G11 6NT, UK.*

J. J. MORTON, *MRC Blood Pressure Unit, Western Infirmary, University of Glasgow, Glasgow G11 6NT, UK.*

M. A. F. MURRAY, *Department of Chemical Pathology, St. Mary's Hospital Medical School, London W2 1PG, UK.*

M. POURFARZANEH, *Department of Chemical Pathology, St. Bartholomew's Hospital, West Smithfield, London EC1A 7BE, UK.*

G. READ, *Tenovus Institute for Cancer Research, The Welsh National School of Medicine, The Heath, Cardiff CF4 4XX, UK.*

M. J. REED, *Department of Chemical Pathology, St. Mary's Hospital Medical School, London W2 1PG, UK.*

LESLEY H. REES, *Department of Chemical Endocrinology, St. Bartholomew's Hospital, West Smithfield, London EC1A 7BE, UK.*

DIANA RIAD-FAHMY, *Institute for Cancer Research, The Welsh National School of Medicine, The Heath, Cardiff CF4 4XX, UK.*

D. SCOGGINS, *Howard Florey Institute of Experimental Physiology and Medicine, University of Melbourne, Parkville, Victoria 3052, Australia.*

P. F. SEMPLE, *MRC Blood Pressure Unit, Western Infirmary, University of Glasgow, Glasgow G11 6NT, UK.*

K. D. R. SETCHELL, *Division of Clinical Chemistry, Clinical Research Centre, Harrow, Middlesex HA1 3UJ, UK.*

D. S. SMITH, *Department of Chemical Pathology, St. Bartholomew's Hospital, West Smithfield, London EC1A 7BE, UK.*

H. J. VAN DER MOLEN, *Department of Biochemistry (Division of Chemical Endocrinology), Medical Faculty, Erasmus University, Rotterdam, The Netherlands.*

A. VERMEULEN, *Department of Endocrinology and Metabolic Diseases, Academic Hospital, University of Ghent, B-9000 Ghent, Belgium.*

M. WINTOUR, *Howard Florey Institute of Experimental Physiology and Medicine, University of Melbourne, Parkville, Victoria 3052, Australia.*

Preface

When the second edition of "Hormones in Blood" was published in 1967, endocrinology had reached a stage when new methodology had opened up our knowledge of the normal levels in blood of those hormones and metabolites known at that time. During the 11 years which have elapsed since then not only have methods of hormone analysis advanced mainly towards greater precision and accuracy but well established hormones have been shown to be heterogeneous, prohormones and new hormones have been identified, and much has been learned of control mechanisms, interaction and synergism between hormones, metabolic pathways as well as of the details of the molecular basis of action. During this period the rate of the development of the subject of endocrinology has accelerated so much that at no time did it seem opportune to attempt to bring out a new and up-dated edition, even allowing for the publisher's agreement to publish if possible within six months of receipt of manuscripts.

At present, endocrinology has reached a stage for taking stock of its position. The value and limitations of radioimmunoassay (RIA) have been recognised, competitive protein binding and receptor assays have been developed, the latter especially has combined the sensitivity of RIA with a specificity which approximates with rather less discrepancy to biological activity; there is ever increasing development of sensitive biological assays using isolated or culture cells and even intracellular membranes. These new methods have been so rigidly characterised for the hormones being analysed, there is no special chapter devoted to them as there was in 1967 for gas-liquid chromatography (GLC) gel filtration, thin-layer chromatography, immuno-assay, and spectrophotometry. However, three general techniques, high pressure liquid chromatography, non-isotopic immunoassay and gas-liquid chromatography-mass spectrometry have warranted separate chapters, the first because despite its great resolving power it has not yet been widely used with hormones, even with the polypeptides for which it is specially suited; with the development of more sensitive detectors it will inevitably be found to have many applications. The second will ultimately replace RIA by a method less demanding of expensive equipment, although the disagreement between international bodies concerned with standardisation in enzyme assays suggest that the widespread application of enzyme-immunoassay may have to be delayed. The combination of GLC with mass spectrometry has mostly been of value in the detailed analyses of urinary steriods, but Dr Smythe in his new chapter on serotonin has no doubt that it is only the expense of the equipment which prevents its wide use.

The third edition of "Hormones in Blood" has other new chapters, two on gastro-intestinal peptides; one on vitamin D because it is the precursor of the true hormone 1,25-dihydroxycholecalciferol, which, with parathyroid hormone play so important a role in calcium metabolism, a chapter on somatomedin and one on erythropoietin. Dr Schally and his colleague have reviewed the enormous changes brought about by the identification, synthesis, mode of action and practical application of what in 1967 were only known as hypothalamic releasing and inhibiting factors.

We have given much thought as to whether the prostaglandins should be regarded as hormones and have decided that they are, because they function as chemical messengers and are carried in the blood to remote target organs as well as targets within the cells or structures in which they are synthesised. The field has expanded enormously since their discovery, and the recognition of the various prostaglandins and their precursors and metabolites has been more than usually dependent on the development of more sensitive and specific forms of analysis, especially with the now widely appreciated heterogeneity of the peptide hormones. The editors hope that there will be some cross-fertilisation of ideas and that some of the experimental techniques may prove to be of value in endocrinology.

The acceptance of SI units by some countries and not others has presented a problem. Where possible we have provided all concentrations in SI units along with traditional units. To avoid enlarging tables undesirably we have provided conversion factors. When early work is described in which methods had not been properly established (e.g. with the steroids and smaller poly-peptides) traditional units alone have been given; more recent results obtained when methods and standard preparations were available have been presented in both systems of units.

The symbols and abbreviations which have been used are those which are generally accepted in current scientific publications. We have in addition used u for international units and, unless otherwise stated, $\pm$ refers to the s.e.m. All temperatures are in °C (Celcius).

We are grateful to those authors who complied so splendidly with the request for prompt ·delivery of their manuscripts, as well as to those who relieved our anxiety by producing their manuscripts better late than never. As some contributors were unable to meet our deadline and did not conform to our stated requirements, rather than delay publication we decided not to return these chapters for revision, which accounts for a few of the chapters being less comprehensive than we would have liked. Our thanks are also due to Miss Nancy Blamey for all the help she gave us during preparation of this publication, and to Miss Helen Wortham of Academic Press who has been so patient with us, especially in respect of some late changes we required.

C. H. GRAY and V. H. T. JAMES   *August, 1979*

Standards for Hormones

D. R. BANGHAM

Almost all assays to estimate the concentration of a hormone are comparative assays, in which the test sample is compared with a measured quantity of a reference preparation of the hormone. For hormones such as steroids and peptides of a few residues, any preparation of the pure chemical may be suitable for this purpose providing it complies with precise specifications of identity and purity. But for hormones of more complex structure (such as glycoproteins or peptides of more than say 20 residues) that cannot be completely characterised by chemical and physical means alone, it is necessary to use suitably prepared reference materials. Moreover, in order to be able to correlate results obtained using them, it is necessary to relate such reference materials ultimately in terms of a single preparation, which has recognised international status. It is for this purpose that a service of international biological standards and reference materials has been provided since 1925. This service is administered under the aegis of the Expert Committee on Biological Standardisation of the World Health Organization; and the following list includes those International Standards and International Reference Preparations of hormones as well as other reference preparations currently distributed from the National Institute for Biological Standards and Control.

Certain hormones, such as thyrotrophin (TSH), follicle stimulating hormone (FSH), luteinising hormone (LH) and human chorionic gonadotrophin (hCG), are particularly complex, e.g. they appear to consist of heterogenous mixtures of slightly dissimilar glycoproteins. In these instances, and until there is general and sustained agreement on its exact chemical structure, a hormone is identified by the biological response that it elicits; since it is the standard that is used as the yardstick with which to measure that activity, it is thus the material used in the standard that helps to "define" that hormone. It is essential that such a standard is thoroughly characterised by chemical, physical and biological procedures to obtain information on its identity, purity, activity, stability and suitability to serve as a standard for use with various assay methods. Such evidence is a prerequisite for the establishment of each WHO International Reference Material and is summarised in the report on each standard, which is usually published (see list of standards). Guidance on how to prepare, ampoule and characterise international, national and laboratory standards has been published (Annex 4, 29th Report of WHO ECBS, 1978).

The introduction of radioimmunoassays, hormone receptor assays and other protein binding assays highlighted many fundamental problems of standardisation in hormone assays. While a hormone is identified as that (form of a) molecule that directly elicits the characteristic biological response that defines it, many problems arise from the lack of—or inappropriate— specificity of many protein-binding assay systems for a single "form" of a hormone. Thus a sample of biological fluid or a tissue extract may contain precursor forms and metabolised fragments of the hormone, or artefactually altered forms caused by *in vitro* handling. Other hormones such as TSH, LH, FSH and HCG are naturally heterogeneous, that is they exist as populations of slightly dissimilar molecules.

The problems for standards arising from such diversity of molecular forms has been discussed in detail (Bangham and Cotes, 1974; 26th Report of WHO ECBS, 1975). The subject is currently under active consideration by special committees of WHO, the International Federation of Clinical Chemistry, the International Society of Endocrinology and the International Atomic Energy Agency.

Meanwhile new international preparations consisting where possible of the most highly purified preparations of hormones are established each year and are listed in successive reports of the ECBS of WHO.

BIOLOGICAL STANDARDS AND REFERENCE MATERIALS

The following reference materials are available to scientists in limited quantities for use as standards to define units of biological activity or as reference materials for binding assays. Some of these preparations have been provided and characterised as a result of international collaboration; some of them have been designated British or International Standards or Reference Preparations. They are not for administration to man.

Ampoules of these preparations, together with relevant information, are issued in response to written application from the scientist concerned, stating the purpose for which the material is required, addressed to:

> National Institute for Biological Standards and Control,
> Holly Hill, Hampstead, London NW3 6RB, UK.

REFERENCES

Bangham, D. R. and Cotes, P. M. (1974). Standardization and standards. *Br. med. Bull.* **30**, 12.

26th Report of WHO Expert Committee on Biological Standardization (1975). WHO Tech. Rep. Ser. No. 565.

29th Report of WHO Expert Committee on Biological Standardization (1978). WHO Tech. Rep. Ser. No. 626.

30th Report of WHO Expert Committee on Biological Standardization (1979). WHO Tech. Rep. Ser. (in press).

Standard	Ampoule code No.	Defined activity	Approximate composition of ampoule contents	Other information
1st IS for glucagon, porcine, for bioassay	69/194	1·49 u/amp	1·5 mg glucagon, 5 mg lactose, 0·24 mg sodium chloride	*Acta endocr., Copenh.* **77**, 705, 1974; *J. biol. Stand.* **3**, 263, 1975
1st IRP of glucagon, porcine, for immunoassay	69/194	1·49 u/amp	1·5 mg glucagon, 5 mg lactose, 0·24 mg sodium chloride	*J. biol. Stand.* **3**, 263, 1975; *Acta endocr., Copenh.* **77**, 705, 1974.
4th IS for insulin, bovine and porcine, for bioassay	58/6	24·0 u/mg	100 mg crystals, 42% porcine insulin, 58% bovine insulin	*Bull. Wld Hlth Org* **20**, 1209, 1959; *Diabetologia* **11**, 581, 1975
1st IRP of insulin, human, for immunoassay	66/304	3·0 u/amp	130 µg insulin, 5 mg sucrose	WHO/BS/74.1084
Insulin C-peptide for immunoassay	76/561	2·5 nm/amp	10 µg synthetic human insulin C-peptide analogue, 50 µg human albumin	synthetic (64-formyllysine) human proinsulin 31-65 WHO/BS/78. 1223
2nd IS for chorionic gonado-trophin, human, for biossay	61/6	5,300 u/amp	2 mg chorionic gonadotrophin, 5 mg lactose	*Bull. Wld Hlth Org.* **31**, 111, 1964
1st IRP of chorionic gonado-trophin, human, for immunoassay	75/537	650 u/amp	70 µg chorionic gonadotrophin, 5 mg human albumin	*Bull. Wld Hlth Org.* **54**, 463, 1976
1st IRP of α-subunit of chorionic gonadotrophin, human, for immunoassay	75/569	70 u/amp	70 µg chorionic gonadotrophin α-subunit, 5 mg human albumin	*Bull. Wld Hlth Org.* **54**, 463, 1975
1st IRP of β-subunit of chorionic gonadotrophin, human, for immunoassay	75/551	70 u/amp	70 µg chorionic gonadotrophin β-subunit, 5 mg human albumin	*Bull. Wld Hlth Org.* **54**, 463, 1975

Standard	Ampoule code No.	Defined activity	Approximate composition of ampoule contents	Other information
1st IRP for FSH/LH, human, pituitary, for bioassay	69/104	FSH 10 u/amp LH 25 u/amp	0·5 mg FSH/LH, lactose 1·25 mg	*J. clin. Endocr. Metab.* **36**, 647, 1973
1st IRP of LH, human pituitary, for immunoassay	68/40	77 u/amp	11·6 µg LH, 5 mg lactose, 1 mg human albumin, 1 mg sodium chloride	*Acta endocr., Copenh.* **88**, 250, 1978
IS FSH/LH, human, urinary, for bioassay	70/45	FSH-54 u/amp LH-46 u/amp	1 mg human post-menopausal urine extract, 5 mg lactose	*Acta endocr., Copenh.* **83**, 700, 1976
Gonadorelin	77/596	38 nm/amp	36 nmoles synthetic gonadorelin, 2·5 mg lactose, 0·5 mg human albumin	ovine sequence WHO/BS/78. 1219
Angiotensin I (Asp Isoleu[5])	71/328	9 µg/amp nominal	9 µg synthetic angiotensin I, 2 mg mannitol	*Clin. Sci. mol. Med.* **48**, 135.S, 1978
Angiotensin II (Asp Ileu[5])	70/302	24 µg/amp nominal	24 µg synthetic angiotensin II, 2 mg mannitol	*Clin. Sci. mol. Med.* **48**, 135.S, 1978
1st IRP of renin, human, for bioassay	68/356	0·1 u/amp	0·27 mg renal extract, 5 mg lactose, phosphate buffer	*Clin. Sci. mol. Med.* **48**, 135.S, 1978
IRP calcitonin, human, for bioassay	70/234	1·0 u/amp	10 µg synthetic calcitonin of sequence found in tumours, 5 mg mannitol	WHO/BS/78. 1229
1st IRP of calcitonin, porcine, for bioassay	70/306	1·0 u/amp	10 µg purified extract, 5 mg mannitol	WHO/BS/74. 1077
1st IRP of calcitonin, salmon, for bioassay	72/158	80 u/amp	20 µg synthetic salmon calcitonin I, 2 mg mannitol	WHO/BS/74. 1077

Preparation	Code	Unit	Contents	Reference
1st IRP of parathyroid hormone, bovine, for bioassay	67/342	200 u/amp	0·6 mg gland extract, 5 mg lactose	WHO/BS/74. 1078
1st IRP of parathyroid hormone, bovine, for immunoassay	71/324	2·0 u/amp	1 μg purified extract, 200 μg human albumin, 1 mg lactose	WHO/BS/74. 1078
Parathyroid hormone, human, for immunoassay	75/549	0·25 u/amp	250 ng extract of human adenomata, 250 μg human albumin, 1·25 mg lactose	
3rd IS for corticotrophin (ACTH), porcine, for bioassay. International Working Standard	59/16	5·0 u/amp	50 μg pituitary extract, 5 mg lactose	Bull. Wld Hlth Org. 27, 395, 1962
	various	5·0 u/amp		
Corticotrophin human	74/555		11·6 μg corticotrophin, 5 mg human albumin, 2·5 mg mannitol	WHO/BS/78. 1233
2nd IRP of erythropoietin, human, urinary, for bioassay	67/343	10 u/amp	2 mg urinary extract containing erythropoietin, 3 mg sodium chloride	Bull. Wld Hlth Org. 47, 99, 1972
Gastrin I, human (G-17)	68/439	12 u/amp	12·6 μg synthetic gastrin as hexamonium salt, 5 mg lactose, phosphate buffer	
Gastrin II, porcine (G-17)	66/138	10 u/amp	10 μg gastrin II, 5 mg sucrose, phosphate buffer	
2nd IS for serum gonadotrophin, equine, for bioassay	62/1	1600 u/amp	0·8 mg extract, 5 mg lactose	Bull. Wld Hlth Org. 35, 761, 1966
2nd IS for prolactin, ovine, for bioassay	57/8	22 u/mg	10 mg extract	Bull. Wld Hlth Org. 29, 721, 1963

Standard	Ampoule code No.	Defined activity	Approximate composition of ampoule contents	Other information
IRP prolactin, human, for immunoassay	75/504	0.650 u/amp	20 μg extract, 1 mg human albumin, 5 mg lactose	*J. Endocr.* **80**, 157, 1979
IRP of placental lactogen, human, for immunoassay	73/545	0·850 mu/amp	850 μg placental lactogen, 5 mg mannitol	*Br. J. Obstet. Gynaec.* **85**, 451, 1978
1st IS for growth hormone, bovine, for bioassay	55/1	1·0 u/mg	30 mg purified growth hormone	WHO/BS/77.1156
1st IRP of growth hormone, human, for immunoassay	66/217	0·35 u/amp	175 μg growth hormone, 5 mg sucrose, phosphate buffer	
1st IS for thyrotrophin, bovine, for bioassay	53/11	13·5 u/mg	1 part pituitary extract, 19 parts lactose	*Bull. Wld Hlth Org.* **13**, 917, 1955
1st IRP of TSH, human, for immunoassay	68/38	147 u/amp	46·2 μg TSH extract, 5 mg lactose, 1 mg human albumin	
4th IS oxytocin for bioassay	76/575	12·5 u/amp	24 μg synthetic oxytocin acetate, 5 mg human albumin, citric acid	WHO/BS/78. 1227
1st IS arginine vasopressin for bioassay	77/501	8·2 u/amp	20 μg synthetic arginine vasopressin, 5 mg human citric acid	WHO/BS/78. 1231
1st IS lysine vasopressin	77/512	7·7 u/amp	30 μg synthectic lysine vasopressin acetate, 5 mg human albumin, citric acid	WHO/BS/78. 1230

Contents of Volume 3

I. Non-isotopic Immunoassay of Hormones in Blood
J. LANDON, MITHAL HASSAN, M. POURFARZANEH and D. S. SMITH

II. High Performance Liquid Chromatography
C. K. LIM

III. Gas Chromatography–Mass Spectrometry
K. D. R. SETCHELL

IV. Adrenocorticotrophin and Lipotrophin
LESLEY H. REES and P. J. LOWRY

V. Corticosteroids
DIANA RIAD-FAHMY, G. READ and I. A. HUGHES

VI. The Oestrogens
M. J. REED and M. A. F. MURRAY

VII. The Androgens
A. VERMEULEN

VIII. Progesterone. I. Physico-chemical and Biochemical Aspects
H. J. VAN DER MOLEN

IX. Progesterone. II. Clinical Aspects
K. FOTHERBY

X. Aldosterone
J. P. COGHLAN, B. A. SCOGGINS and E. M. WINTOUR

XI. The Renin–Angiotensin System
BRENDA J. LECKIE, J. A. MILLAR, J. J. MORTON and P. F. SEMPLE

XII. Endocrinology in Clinical Medicine
RAYMOND GREEN .

Contents of Volume 1

Contents of Volume 2

I. Non-isotopic Immunoassay of Hormones in Blood

J. LANDON, MITHAL HASSAN,
M. POURFARZANEH and D. S. SMITH

INTRODUCTION

As the name implies, an immunoassay is an analytical procedure based on the use of an antibody, while the term non-isotopic immunoassay (NIIA) denotes that none of the reactants is labelled with a radioisotope. This chapter will classify the place of immunoassays with regard to other analytical techniques; suggest an appropriate terminology; discuss some of the existing NIIA procedures and consider their general advantages and disadvantages as compared with radioimmunoassay (RIA) for the determination of hormones and their binding proteins in biological fluids. Finally a personal view will be given as to the present role of NIIA in endocrinology.

Analytical procedures can be classified into three broad categories (Chard, 1978), namely biological techniques (also termed bioassays), those based on physical and/or chemical methods and others that depend upon the non-covalent binding of one reactant by another (Table 1). The term binding assays is employed to cover the latter, which comprise a variety of methods that depend upon the specific reaction between a ligand and a binding protein and which obey the law of mass action:

$$L + BP \underset{k_2}{\overset{k_1}{\rightleftharpoons}} L:BP$$

(free fraction)   (bound fraction)

where L represents the ligand, BP the binding protein and $L:BP$ the bound complex. At equilibrium, some of the free reactants will be combining, with a rate constant k_1, to form more of the complex, while some of the complex will be dissociating, with a rate constant k_2, to give free ligand and binding protein. Such assays can be subdivided into immunoassays (in which the binding protein is a specific antibody and the ligand an antigen), receptor binding protein assays (in which the receptor protein is usually extracted from the target organ of the particular hormone) and circulating binding protein assays employing a naturally occurring plasma protein—such as thyroxine binding globulin (TBG) for the assay of thyroxine (T_4) and transcortin for the assay of cortisol or progesterone.

Immunoassays are by far the most common form of binding assay employed in endocrinology (Ekins, 1976a). This is because antibodies can be raised against an immense range of hormones; they display marked structural specificity; the high affinity with which antibodies bind their appropriate antigen enables great sensitivity to be achieved and, indeed, sets the ultimate sensitivity that can be attained; and, finally, they can be employed either to determine the concentration of a hormone or, as discussed briefly in the next section, to detect the presence of antibodies.

It should be noted that estimates of hormone concentration which are based on the biological activity or function of the hormone may differ significantly from estimates using an immunoassay. This is because the latter are structural assays which, indeed, assess only part of the hormone's structure—termed the antigenic determinant. In the case of a peptide or protein hormone the antigenic determinant (that part of the molecule bound by the antibody) comprises only some four to six amino acids and most RIA will determine any circulating prohormone, the hormone itself and any

Table 1

A general classification of assays employed in endocrinology with especial reference to binding assays.

Analytical techniques

Bioassays   Binding assays   Physical/chemical assays

For binding protein   For ligand

   (i)   Employing antibodies as binding protein (immunoassay)
   (ii)   Employing receptor proteins
   (iii)   Employing natural circulating binding proteins

⟵————— Assess function —————⟶   ⟵————— Assess structure —————⟶

fragments of the hormone which contain the antigenic determinant. In contrast, bioassays will usually determine only the hormone itself. An elegant example of bioassay–immunoassay dissociation follows cleavage of the S–S ring of oxytocin or arginine vasopressin, which causes a complete loss of biological activity but does not affect most RIA results.

It follows from the above that hormone values obtained by bioassay may be lower than those determined by RIA. Since endocrinologists are generally concerned with the ability of a hormone to exert its biological effects it also follows that, at least for peptide hormones, bioassays must remain the reference method in endocrinology against which all others should be assessed. Furthermore, the cytochemical group of bioassays, introduced by Chayen et al. (1972), are more sensitive than RIA and can, for example, detect plasma levels of adrenocorticotrophin as low as 20 fg/ml and be applied to heelprick samples from neonates (Holdaway et al., 1973). Physical and chemical methods (like immunoassays) depend upon the structure of the hormone to be determined, such as the need for a hydroxyl group in the 11 position of the steroid nucleus in the fluorimetric assay for cortisol described by Mattingly (1962). Some of the techniques, including gas chromatography—mass spectroscopy are both more specific and sensitive than RIA. For example one such method can routinely measure 50 fg of prostaglandin $F_{2\alpha}$ with a precision of $\pm 10\%$ (Wilson et al., 1976). However, none of these assays approach the practicality and wide application of RIA and related analytical techniques.

A. GENERAL CLASSIFICATION OF IMMUNOASSAY PROCEDURES

Immunoassays are commonly considered as techniques for the detection and quantitation of antigens. However, as stated earlier, they can be used to determine the presence of antibodies. Indeed, the pioneer work of Berson and his colleagues in RIA followed their use of ^{131}I-labelled insulin to demonstrate circulating antibodies in patients treated with insulin (Berson et al., 1956). A similar approach was later adopted to show that the failure of several dwarfed children to maintain their response to early preparations of relatively impure human growth hormone (hGH) was due to antibody production (Parker et al., 1964: Prader et al., 1964). Such assays are also being employed to enable the rapid detection of antibodies against other hormones (including porcine and salmon calcitonin, arginine vasopressin and adrenocorticotrophin (Landon et al., 1967) and against other proteins of interest to endocrinologists (such as human antibodies to thyroglobulin (Nye et al., 1978)). For reasons of space, they will not be discussed further.

Immunoassays for the detection and quantitation of antigen can be categorised into those in which no labelled reactant is required, those employing labelled antigen and others in which specific antibodies are labelled (Table 2).

Table 2
A general classification of immunoassays employed in endocrinology.

For the detection of antibodies
For the quantitation of antigens (including hormones)
    Employing no labelled reactant
    Employing labelled antigen (including radioimmunoassay)
        With a separation step
        With no separation step
    Employing labelled antibodies (including immunoradiometric assays)
        Single site
        Two site sandwich techniques

---

1. Non-labelled Immunoassays

There are several immunoassay techniques which do not require the use of a labelled reactant (Ritchie, 1975). One group depends on the precipitin line which forms in a gel support when a protein antigen comes into contact with its specific antibody. These include qualitative procedures (such as immunoelectrophoresis and that described by Ouchterlony) and quantitative techniques (including radial immunodiffusion and rocket electroimmuno-diffusion). For example, the rocket system described by Laurell has been employed to assay serum TBG levels. Several hundred samples can be run in a working week, with a coefficient of variation less than 5% (Bradwell et al., 1976). A similar approach has been adopted for the assay of human placental lactogen (hPL) in serum during the third trimester of pregnancy.

Manual and automated assays have also been developed for many of the plasma proteins in which the formation of antigen:antibody complexes is detected by the increase in light scattering produced. Recent developments in this general area include a kinetic approach and the use of a laser beam as the light source. Although further advances can be expected as the result of improved instrumentation it is difficult to envisage the extensive application of non-labelled immunoassay systems, despite their relative simplicity, in endocrinology—other than for the quantitation of various carrier proteins, such as TBG, sex hormone binding globulin (SHBG) and transcortin.

The main reason for their limitations with regard to the assay of hormones is the need to form very large antigen:antibody complexes for these to be detectable. Thus they are applicable only to the assay of proteins (since hapten:antibody complexes do not form a precipitin line or scatter light) and high concentrations of such proteins must be present, which limits their sensitivity to the µmol/l or upper nmol/l range. These non-labelled immuno-assays also employ relatively high concentrations of monospecific antisera; are not, unless a kinetic end-point or blank measurement is made, suitable for very turbid or haemolysed samples and, finally, may give spurious results in the presence of antigen excess—due to the prozone phenomenon.

2. Immunoassays Employing Labelled Antigen

The development of the first RIA, for insulin, by Yalow and Berson (1960) has proved to be an important milestone in endocrinology with its need for specific, sensitive, precise and practical analytical techniques. Thus, use of antigen labelled with an isotope has enabled the assay of haptens (such as the steroid and thyroid hormones) as well as proteins; resulted in a million-fold increase in sensitivity; removed the need for monospecific antisera and markedly reduced the concentration of antisera required; overcame the problem of antigen excess and enabled the assay of haemolysed and turbid samples by both manual and automated procedures. In the same year Ekins had recognised the wider implications of binding assays and developed techniques for both serum T_4 (Ekins, 1960) and vitamin B_{12} (Barakat and Ekins, 1961) employing circulating carrier proteins. His use of the general term "saturation analysis" and, more recently, "limited reagent methods" was to indicate that the concentration of binding protein must be insufficient to bind all the ligand (Ekins, 1976). The labelled antigen is employed as a tracer to enable determination of the distribution of total antigen between the antibody bound and unbound (free) fractions. If the amounts of labelled reactant and of antiserum are kept constant then the percentage of the counts present in the bound fraction will be inversely related to the initial amount of unlabelled ligand in the standards or samples being assayed.

The dominant reactant in all immunoassays for antigens is the antibody since it is this which, in large part, determines both the specificity and ultimate sensitivity that can be achieved—the latter, as mentioned earlier, depending on the affinity with which the antibody binds the antigen. The labelled antigen is employed only as a tracer and any label would be suitable provided its determination is relatively simple and sufficiently sensitive for the purpose to which the assay will be applied; there are no significant problems with other materials present in the sample; means are available to link the label to the antigen and the antibody does not distinguish significantly between labelled and unlabelled antigen (Landon, 1977). It is not surprising, therefore, that many different materials have been employed for labelling purposes, in addition to gamma- and beta-emitting isotopes. These will be considered individually in a later section.

3. Immunoassays Employing Labelled Antibodies

Miles and Hales (1968) introduced a new type of immunoassay which they termed *immunoradiometric analysis* (IRMA), based on the use of isotopically labelled specific antibodies. Such antibodies were prepared by affinity chromatography on columns containing the antigen covalently linked to a support, radioiodinated on the column (to prevent introduction of isotope into their binding sites) and then eluted for use. In an assay, standards or unknown samples are incubated with an excess of labelled antibody and, after equilibrium has been attained, the unused labelled antibody is removed by affinity chromatography and the bound fraction counted. They employed the technique successfully both for the assay of insulin and human growth hormone (Miles and Hales, 1968a, b, c).

IRMA differs markedly from RIA as an analytical technique (Table 3).

Table 3

Differences between radioimmunoassay and immunoradiometric analysis.

IRMA	RIA
$Ag + Ab^* \rightleftharpoons Ag{:}Ab^*$	$Ag + Ag^* + Ab \rightleftharpoons Ag{:}Ab{:}Ag^*$
Two reactants	Three reactants
Employs labelled antibody	Employs labelled antigen
Separate bound and free antibodies	Separate bound and free antigens
Counts in bound fraction directly related to initial concentration of antigen	Counts in bound fraction inversely related to initial concentration of antigen
Reagent excess technique, therefore:	Limited reagent technique, therefore:
(i) rapid	(i) slow
(ii) pipetting accuracy not critical	(ii) pipetting accuracy critical
No problems in labelling antibodies	May have problems in labelling some antigens
Labelled antibodies have long shelf-life	Some labelled antigens have short shelf-life
Can employ only high affinity antibodies with improved sensitivity	Employ both high and low affinity antibodies

In the standard procedure only two, not three, reactants are required and, of course, antibody as opposed to antigen is labelled. Since excessive amounts of labelled antibody are added to ensure that all the hormone is bound, IRMA can be defined as a "reagent excess" procedure as distinct from the "limited reagent" techniques described above. It is necessary to separate the antibody (as opposed to the antigen) in the bound form from that in the free fraction and, finally, the counts in the bound fraction are related directly to the total amount of antigen present, in contrast to the inverse relationship characteristic of RIA. These differences offer several advantages in favour of IRMA. The labelled antibodies are, in general, more stable than labelled antigens and are relatively easy to prepare—whereas difficulties may arise in iodinating haptens, fragile antigens or peptides lacking tyrosine or histidine residues (Rodbard and Weiss, 1973). Use of a reagent excess shortens the time necessary to reach equilibrium (which depends on the concentrations of the various reactants) and, since it is possible to employ only the high affinity antibodies in an antiserum, there is a potential (though seldom realised) gain in sensitivity. However, considerable expertise is required to prepare the immunoadsorbants and labelled antibodies and IRMA is more wasteful of antisera than RIA.

In addition to conventional IRMA, sandwich techniques have been developed for the assay of large molecules with more than one antigenic determinant—an approach pioneered by Wide *et al.* (1967) and shown to be suitable for the assay of such hormones as human growth hormone (Addison and Hales, 1971) and follicle stimulating hormone (Readhead *et al.*, 1973).

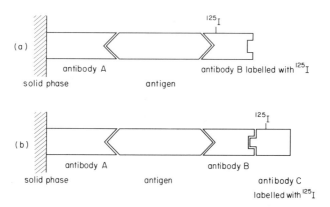

Fig. 1(a). Representation of a sandwich immunoradiometric assay for an antigen with two antigenic determinants. Antibody A, attached to a solid phase, is directed against one determinant and antibody B, which is labelled with ^{125}I, is directed against the other. (**b**) The principle of sandwich immunoradiometric assays employing a common label is similar to the above except that antibody A, in addition to being directed against a different antigenic determinant than antibody B, is from a different species. For example, antibody A may be raised in a sheep and antibody B in a rabbit, in which case a third antibody (C), labelled with ^{125}I, would be added, which is directed against rabbit immunoglobulins.

The standard or sample is first incubated with an excess of an antibody covalently linked to an insoluble support and directed against one antigenic determinant. After careful washing, excess of a second, isotopically labelled antibody directed against another part of the molecule is added (Fig. 1(a)) and, after further washes, the counts present in the bound fraction can be determined and will be related directly to the amount of antigen added. Such sandwich techniques have the advantage of improved specificity, since fragments of a hormone containing only one of the antigenic determinants will not affect the result. Subsequently, Beck and Hales (1975) further modified sandwich assays for HGH, insulin, glucagon and parathyroid hormone (PTH) by adding an excess of an isotopically labelled second antibody. This has the merit that, for example, labelled goat anti-rabbit gamma globulin sera can be used for all assays based on a rabbit first antibody (Figl 1(b)).

B. TYPES OF NON-ISOTOPIC LABEL EMPLOYED

The number of different materials that have been employed to label the antigen or antibody for immunoassay procedures is increasing rapidly and includes gamma- and beta-emitting isotopes, free radicals, enzymes, co-enzymes and enzyme inhibitors, viruses, proteins, fluorescent and chemiluminescent molecules, red blood cells, latex and other particles. Considerable confusion is inevitable unless a terminology is employed that, for example, clearly distinguishes whether what is being referred to is an RIA for an enzyme (Landon *et al.*, 1977) or an immunoassay employing an enzyme as the label (Engvall and Perlmann, 1971).

Any terminology should have regard to the names suggested by the originators, to the suitability of any likely acronym and, in particular, to the principles involved. Thus the term radioimmunoassay and its acronym RIA is excellent in that it signifies that a radioisotope is employed and that the assay is based on an immunological reaction. It is suggested that NIIA in which the antigen is labelled other than isotopically should follow this convention, for example enzymoimmunoassay (EIA), fluoroimmunoassay (FIA) and viroimmunoassay (VIA). The term immunoradiometric analysis and its acronym IRMA is also well known and well suited for immunoassays employing specific antibodies labelled with an isotope. Thus it would seem correct to employ similar terms for NIIA such as immunoenzymometric assays (IEMA) and immunofluorometric assays (IFMA) involving the use of specific antibodies labelled with enzymes and with fluorogenic molecules respectively. This will ensure that the type of label is instantly recognisable while its placement after that part of the name reflecting the binding protein should be confined to immunoassays employing labelled antibodies (in contrast to its placement before, which should be confined to assays using labelled antigens).

Two other terms commonly employed in NIIA require definition, namely heterogeneous and homogeneous. All immunoassays employing a labelled antigen involve the series of steps:

(i)   addition of sample (or standard), labelled antigen and appropriate dilution of antiserum,

(ii) incubation until equilibrium is achieved (other than with some automated systems),

(iii) separation of antibody-bound and free antigen,

(iv) end-point detection of the label in the antibody-bound and/or free fraction,

(v)   calculation of results.

Of these, only two—the separation step and the method of end-point detection—may vary depending on the label. Rubenstein, Schneider and Ullman (1972) suggested the term homogeneous for those immunoassays that do not require separation of the antibody-bound and free fractions prior to end-point detection, to distinguish them from those, including RIA, in which separation is essential and for which they suggested the name heterogeneous. A classification of NIIA employing labelled antigen, based on whether or not a separation procedure is required, is given in Table 4.

Table 4

Classification of immunoassays employing labelled antigen.

Requiring a separation step—heterogeneous (such as RIA and ELISA)
Not requiring a separation step—homogeneous
    Due to antibody binding changing the nature of the signal (such as FRAT)
    Due to antibody binding decreasing the signal
      —direct quenching (EMIT)
      —excitation transfer (applicable only to FIA)
    Due to antibody binding increasing the signal
      —enhancement
      —indirect quenching
      —polarisation fluorescence (applicable only to FIA)

It is perhaps surprising that the first homogeneous NIIA was described in 1953, several years before the introduction of RIA (Stavitsky and Arquilla, 1953). Thus Arquilla and Stavitsky (1956) employed insulin labelled with erythrocytes to detect the presence of antibodies in diabetics treated with insulin and to assay nanogram amounts of insulin in buffer. Following incubation, complement (in the form of guinea-pig serum) was added and caused lysis of erythrocytes in the bound but not in the free fraction, the resultant release of haemoglobin into the supernatant being quantitated spectrophotometrically. The assay was not sufficiently sensitive to detect insulin in biological fluids and little further attention appears to have been given to homogeneous NIIA until the development of a spin immunoassay procedure (Leute et al., 1972). They employed morphine labelled with a free radical and determined the change in electron spin resonance that followed antibody binding for the detection of morphine in urine, which they termed the Free Radical Assay Technique (FRAT).

Most work relating to NIIA has been based on the use of enzymes or fluorescent molecules for labelling and it is with these types that the remainder of this chapter will be mainly concerned.

1. Enzymes

(a) Immunoassays employing enzyme-labelled antigen

Reasons for the emphasis given to enzyme labelling include the prior application of this approach in histochemistry and cytochemistry; the wide availability and relative inexpensiveness of many enzymes and of manual and automated systems for their assay; the prolonged shelf life of the labelled products which can be measured in years; freedom from any radiation hazard during labelling; and a potential sensitivity, specificity and applicability similar to RIA.

The first essential is to develop methods for covalently binding an enzyme to an antigen or antibody, without significantly impairing either the enzyme's activity or antigen–antibody binding. This seldom poses a problem to the skilled chemist and a wide variety of enzymes (including acetylcholinesterase, alkaline phosphatase, malate dehydrogenase, egg white lysozyme, horse-radish peroxidase and β-galactosidase) and of coupling procedures (including the use of glutaraldehyde, carbodiimide, toluene diisocyanate and mixed anhydride methods) have proved suitable for the preparation of the labelled reactant. EIA have already been introduced for an extensive range of proteins and haptens in biological fluids, including many hormones, and the subject has been discussed in detail in two recent reviews (Scharpe et al., 1976; Wisdom, 1976).

(1) Enzymoimmunoassays requiring a separation step. These are similar to RIA other than that a different end-point detection system is required. An enzyme also differs from a radioisotope in terms of its size so that there is less difference between the bound and free fractions with regard to molecular weight and charge (Landon et al., 1975). In general, this lack of difference limits the separation procedures that can be applied in an EIA to those based on addition of second antibody or to solid phase systems in which the

first antibody is absorbed onto, or covalently bound to, an insoluble matrix or to a combination of the two, such as the Double Antibody Solid Phase (DASP) system.

The separation step in an EIA can serve a second important function, namely to separate the exogenous enzyme being employed as the label from any endogenous enzymes in the sample which have similar biological effects or from any other constituents in the sample, such as enzyme inhibitors, which could effect the signal. Indeed, as discussed later, it is only if such background influences are removed that the sensitivity of present-day EIA, based on the amplification which is inherent in all enzyme–substrate reactions, can approach that of RIA.

The first heterogeneous EIA were developed independently by two groups. Thus Engvall and Perlmann (1971) described an assay for rabbit IgG, using alkaline phosphatase labelled rabbit IgG as tracer, while van Weeman and Schuurs (1971a, b) introduced EIA for oestradiol—17β and oestriol. These assays were termed Enzyme Linked Immunosorbent Assays (ELISA). Since this time heterogeneous EIA have been established for a wide range of

Table 5

Some available enzymoimmunoassays for hormones.

Hormone	References
Oestradiol—17β	van Weeman and Schuurs (1971a)
Oestriol	van Weeman and Schuurs (1971a)
Total oestrogens	Bosch et al. (1975)
Testosterone	Bosch et al. (1978)
Progesterone	Dray et al. (1975); Joyce et al. (1977)
Cortisol	Comoglio and Celada (1976)
Thyroxine[a]	Ullman et al. (1975)
Thyroid stimulating hormone	Miyai et al. (1976)
Human chorionic gonadotrophin	van Weeman and Schuurs (1971b); van der Waart and Schuurs (1976)
Human placental lactogen	Bosch et al. (1975)
Pregnancy associated α macroglobulin	Stimson and Sinclair (1974)
Insulin	Miedema et al. (1972); Ishikawa (1973); Kato et al. (1975); Kleinhammer et al. (1976); Kitagawa and Aikawa (1976)

[a]Homogeneous assay, all others heterogeneous.

many other haptens and proteins. Indeed diagnostic EIA kits are now commercially available for human placental lactogen (hPL), total oestrogens, insulin, T_4 and triiodothyronine (T_3).

Such assays have a specificity similar to RIA, which is inherent in all analytical techniques involving use of an antibody. It appears applicable to all steroid, thyroid, protein and glycoprotein hormones (Table 5). Furthermore, the ability of heterogeneous EIA to determine serum levels of thyroid stimulating hormone (TSH), which lie in the low pmol/l range, shows that the same sensitivity can be attained as by RIA. It is important to appreciate that no NIIA can achieve a greater sensitivity than RIA. Thus the sensitivity of any immunoassay is ultimately set by the affinity with which the antibody binds the antigen. Use of a gamma-emitting isotope to label an antigen, or antibody, enables this sensitivity to be obtained. In an EIA the ability to attain this maximum inherent sensitivity depends on such factors as the molar ratio of enzyme to hormone; the catalytic number of the enzyme; the reaction employed to assess enzymatic activity; the time the enzyme: substrate reaction is allowed to proceed; and the detection system employed. In general enzymatic reactions with a fluorimetric end-point will enable greater sensitivity than colorimetric procedures.

In our experience of a heterogeneous EIA for hPL, employing hPL labelled with alkaline phosphatase as the tracer, such assays are somewhat more complex, take longer to perform and are slightly less precise than RIA — due to the increased number of centrifugation and wash steps required together with the longer duration and poorer precision of determining enzymatic activity as opposed to radioactivity. Nonetheless such assays have immediate application in the developing world and in countries with severe legal restrictions on the use of radioisotopes, while there are clinical situations (though few in endocrinology) in which precision is not very important. In the latter context, for example, heterogeneous EIA has much to offer in such plus/minus situations as the detection of Australian antigen in blood (Wolters et al., 1976). Furthermore, simpler separation procedures, such as the use of antibodies adsorbed to tubes, as in an EIA kit for testosterone, improves their practicality.

(2) *Enzymoimmunoassays not requiring a separation step.* Virtually all work relating to homogeneous EIA has originated from the Syva Corporation who have developed a number of innovative approaches to NIIA.

(i) *Quenching EIA.* In this category are EIA in which the antibody in the bound fraction can be considered (possibly naively) to sterically hinder the reaction between the substrate and the enzyme's active site (Fig. 2). Thus only the free fraction retains full enzymatic activity. Such assays were initially developed to detect drugs of abuse (such as opiates, barbiturates, amphetamines, methadone and the metabolites of cocaine) in urine and employed lysozyme for labelling. This analytical approach, which initially proved unsuitable for serum samples because of an unacceptable background, was termed an Enzyme Multiplied Immunossay Technique and given the acronym EMIT (Schneider et al., 1973).

B

Subsequently the Syva group successfully developed a range of homogeneous quenching EIA suitable for the measurement of serum levels of antiepileptic drugs (including phenytoin, phenobarbital, primidone, carba-

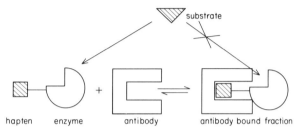

Fig. 2. Representation of a direct quenching enzymoimmunoassay in which the enzyme activity in the bound fraction is impaired due to the antibody sterically hindering the reaction between the enzyme and its substrate.

mazepine and ethosuximide). Glucose-6-phosphate dehydrogenase, of bacterial origin, was employed as label and the need for a cofactor (NAD) in addition to the substrate enhanced the potential for steric hindrance in the bound fraction. The assays take only minutes to perform, require less than 10µl of serum and achieve a coefficient of variation of less than 10%. Assays of this type have also been introduced for theophylline and a variety of cardioactive drugs, including digoxin.

Work is in progress to develop a tri-iodothyronine (T_3) uptake test and to introduce homogeneous EIA kits for cortisol, oestriol and T_3. Since circulating levels of these three hormones are equivalent to or greater than those of digoxin, success can be anticipated.

(ii) *Enhancement EIA.* In direct contrast to quenching EIA, other assays exist of the enhancement type in which antibody binding potentiates the activity of the enzyme employed to label the antigen (Fig. 3). This has had

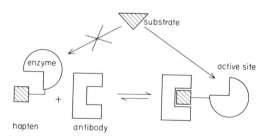

Fig. 3. Representation of an enhancement enzymoimuunoassay in which the enzyme activity in the bound fraction is enhanced following antibody binding.

its main impact in the thyroid field with the introduction of homogeneous EIA for T_4 of the enhancement type suitable for both manual (Ullman *et al.*, 1975) and automated (Galen and Forman, 1977) use. The tracer is a thyroxine derivative covalently linked to malate dehydrogenase, of beef or pork heart origin, such that the enzyme has little activity. However, there is a marked increase in enzymatic activity following addition of antibodies raised against T_4, enabling the assay of T_4 employing only 50μl of serum with results that correlate well with those of RIA.

Avoidance of a separation step in all homogeneous systems simplifies the assay, reduces the level of technical expertise required and improves precision to help compensate for the time taken and imprecision caused by the need to measure enzymatic activity. However, there are problems with achieving a sensitivity adequate for the many hormones which circulate in the pmol/l range. Thus the lower the concentration of antigen to be determined (i) the lower must be the concentration of enzyme labelled antigen employed and, therefore, the longer must the enzyme:substrate reaction be allowed to proceed in order to give an adequate signal and (ii) the larger must be the volume of biological fluid employed in the assay, with the resultant danger of significant background effects. The two homogeneous systems discussed above have the additional disadvantage, as compared with heterogeneous EIA or RIA, of not being suitable for the assay of proteins—because the distance between the sites of the antigenic determinants and of enzyme attachment will usually be so great that antibody binding will not affect enzymatic activity. Indirect quenching procedures of the type described in the FIA section may well be appropriate but, to our knowledge, have only been briefly studied in relation to EIA (Ullman, 1978).

(b) Immunoassays employing enzyme-labelled antibodies

Immunoenzymometric assays (IEMA), similar to the IRMA discussed earlier, have been developed (van Weeman and Schuurs, 1974; Maiolini *et al.*, 1975). The general applicability of this approach has been studied using hPL as a model, antibodies to hPL labelled with horse-radish peroxidase (by means of periodate oxidation) as the tracer and an automated or a manual method for the determination of enzymatic activity (Barbour, 1976). Problems were encountered when assaying serum samples and determining enzymatic activity in the supernatant, due to the presence of endogeneous peroxidases, especially in slightly haemolysed samples. Success was achieved when the enzymatic activity of the free labelled antibody fraction was determined—because, in the separation step using hPL covalently bound to a solid phase, this fraction is precipitated and can be washed free from endogeneous sample contamination as in heterogeneous EIA. However, this greatly prolonged the analytical time and the results were not sufficiently precise (coefficient of variation, 12%) for monitoring feto-placental function.

IEMA of the sandwich type have also been introduced for large molecules, such as rat and human α-fetoprotein (Belanger et al., 1973; Maiolini and Masseyeff, 1975), with more than one antigenic determinant.

All current assays employing enzyme labelled antibodies are of the heterogeneous type and there seems little opportunity of avoiding a separation step to compensate for the greater imprecision and time taken to determine enzymatic as opposed to isotopic activity. As with IRMA, the expertise necessary to isolate and label specific antibodies probably explains the limited number of publications relating to IEMA as compared with EIA.

2. Fluorescent Molecules

(a) Immunoassays employing antigens labelled with a fluorogenic molecule

The use of fluorogenic compounds as alternatives to isotopes for the labelling of reactants in immunoassay has several advantages. Fluorimetry is a well established technique with an extensive theoretical and practical base. This fortunate situation has arisen because, during the last three decades, semi-quantitative immunofluorescence techniques (usually involving fluorescense microscopy) have found wide application in the detection of antigens and antibodies in biological materials while, more recently, Dandliker et al. (1964, 1970) have employed antigens labelled with fluorophores in fluorescense polarisation studies of antigen:antibody reactions.

Many fluorogenic compounds are available, with fluorescein occupying a dominant position as the fluorophore of choice for labelling in FIA. Thus fluorescein (and fluorescein-labelled reactants) has a high quantum yield of fluorescence, approaching the maximum possible quantum yield of one (Goldman, 1968); fluorescein (and fluorescein-labelled reagents) has a useful absorption spectrum which extends up to about 500 nm, enabling excitation by a variety of light sources; the green fluorescence lies within the efficient wave-length response region of most photomultipliers; fluorescein and fluorescein-labelled reagents show no significant photolability under conditions of normal fluorimetry; they have a low temperature coefficient of fluorescence (Feuerstein and Selleck, 1963) so that the effects of ambient temperature fluctuations on signal intensity are negligible; the labelled products have a practically indefinite shelf life (Watson et al., 1976; Smith, 1977); the fluorescein group is hydrophilic, thereby increasing the water solubility of labelled materials; and the time between excitation and emission (the fluorescence lifetime) of 4–5 nsec is appropriate for the measurement of fluorescence polarisation—the basis of the polarisation FIA to be discussed later.

Fluorescein labelling of proteins or of any molecules with a primary or secondary amino group is easily carried out by reaction with fluorescein isothiocyanate. When the species to be labelled has no amino group, other synthetic methods are available. For example, coupling at the carbonyl group of an oestrogen has been achieved by carbodiimide condensation with fluorescein amine (Dandliker et al., 1977). When no suitable reactive group is available it may be possible to label a structurally-related molecule. Thus α,α-diphenylglycine labelled with fluorescein isothiocyanate gave a labelled product suitable for the development of an FIA for phenytoin (McGregor et al., 1978).

Because of the versatility of the fluorescence technique, a large variety of methods have been developed of which some, at the present time, have only been shown to be feasible in principle. All these methods will be considered briefly in the following sections.

(1) *Fluoroimmunoassays requiring a separation step.* These are similar to RIA and, because of the relatively small molecular weight of fluorescein (as compared with an enzyme), most of the separation procedures suitable for RIA are also applicable to a heterogeneous FIA—such as precipitation of the bound fraction with neutral salts or polyethylene glycol.

One of the first assays of this type was for human gamma globulin (Tengerdy, 1965). Our group has developed heterogeneous FIA for determining serum gentamicin levels, using an ammonium sulphate separation step and measurement of the free fraction of the fluorescein-labelled antibiotic in the supernatent (Shaw et al., 1977a); serum phenytoin levels, using a sodium sulphate separation step, followed by measurement of either the free fraction (in the supernatant) or the bound fraction (in the precipitate) after it had been redissolved in NaOH (Kamel et al., 1978); and levels of human albumin in serum, urine and cerebrospinal fluid (Nargessi et al., 1978a) and of human immunoglobin G (Nargessi, unpublished observations). In the heterogeneous FIA for specific proteins, antibodies are covalently linked to magnetisable particles, thereby enabling virtually instantaneous separation by a magnet and avoiding time-consuming centrifugation (Nye et al., 1976). Heterogeneous FIA have also been established for the assay of serum levels of total T_4 (Fig. 4) using either antibodies bound to magnetisable particles or neutral salt precipitation. Assays of this type are also being developed for oestriol levels in pregnancy, the bile acids and cortisol.

(2) *Fluoroimmunoassays not requiring a separation step.* As with EIA, these can be subdivided into those in which antibody binding decreases fluorescence and the signal is given by the free fraction (including quenching FIA, release FIA and fluorescent excitation transfer immunoassay) and others in which the signal is from the bound fraction (enhancement FIA, indirect quenching FIA and polarisation FIA).

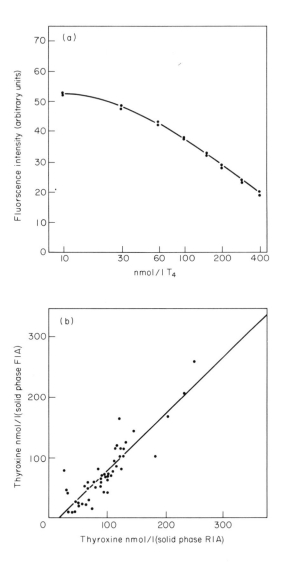

Fig. 4(a). A standard curve for a heterogeneous fluoroimmunoassay of thyroxine. Standards, thyroxine labelled with fluorescein and an appropriate dilution of anti-serum covalently bound to magnetisable particles are allowed to attain equilibrium. The bound fraction is precipitated by means of a magnet and the supernatant (containing the free fraction) aspirated. Methanol/ammonia is then added to the precipitate and fluorescence determined. (**b**) A comparison of thyroxine values obtained for 49 serum samples by means of a radioimmunoassay and the fluoroimmunoassay discussed above ($r = 0.877$).

(i) *Quenching FIA*. A quenching FIA has been developed for the assay of serum levels of gentamicin (Shaw *et al.*, 1977b), and for two other aminoglycosides (amikacin and tobramycin), which exploits the observation that the fluorescence of fluorescein-labelled gentamicin is partially quenched when bound by antibody. Measurement of the extent of quenching serves as the basis of one of the simplest immunoassay methods yet devised. A sample diluter is used to add 20µl of sample (or standard) and 2ml of a solution of fluorescein labelled gentamicin into a disposable cuvette and a reading taken. Antiserum is then added and, a few minutes later, a second reading enables the degree of quenching to be determined. The potential of the method for simple automation has been realised using a continuous-flow system employing standard Auto-Analyzer modules and results on patient samples correlate closely with those by microbiological assay (Shaw *et al.*, 1976).

(ii) *Fluorescent excitation transfer FIA*. This novel approach, introduced by the Syva Corporation (Ullman *et al.*, 1976), involves the use of one reactant labelled with fluorescein (F) as donor, and a second labelled with rhodamine (R) which acts as an acceptor—because of its overlap with the emission of fluorescein. In one form, the reaction can be represented as follows:

$$Ag - F + Ab - R \rightleftharpoons Ag - F:Ab - R$$

Upon excitation at the appropriate wavelength the free fraction will give a signal, but the proximity of the fluorescein and rhodamine in the bound fraction results in up to 70% fluorescence quenching, due to energy transfer to the acceptor molecule by a dipole-dipole resonance mechanism. This is, in effect, equivalent to a direct quenching FIA, and has been applied to the assay of morphine and would probably be applicable only to haptens. A further adaptation, in which highly purified antibodies are labelled with fluorescein and with rhodamine, is considered later.

(iii) *Release FIA*. Another type of homogeneous FIA, introduced by Burd *et al.* (1977a), involves the use of a non-fluorescent labelled antigen which releases a fluorophore when split by an appropriate hydrolytic enzyme. Steric hindrance by the antibody in the bound fraction inhibits the action of the enzyme so that only the free fraction contributes to the signal. A practical assay for determining serum levels of gentamicin has been described (Burd *et al.*, 1977b) but limitations to the general application of this approach may prove to be the considerable chemical expertise required for the design and synthesis of suitable labelled antigens.

(iv) *Enhancement FIA*. FIA based on enhancement of the fluorescence of labelled antigen upon antibody binding, equivalent to enhancement EIA, is also possible. In one study (Smith, 1977), fluorescein-labelled T_4 was found to give an abnormally low fluorescence yield—probably due to intra-molecular quenching of the fluorophore by the iodine-containing thyroxine moiety. A 4 fold increase in fluorescence was caused by antibody binding (presumably by inhibiting the quenching effect) and served as the basis of an FIA.

(v) *Indirect quenching FIA*. The three techniques described above are applicable only to the assay of haptens and, for example, antibody binding of a protein labelled with a fluorophore rarely results in any significant change in fluorescence intensity (Dandliker *et al.*, 1970)—probably because of the distance between the antigenic determinant and site of label attachment

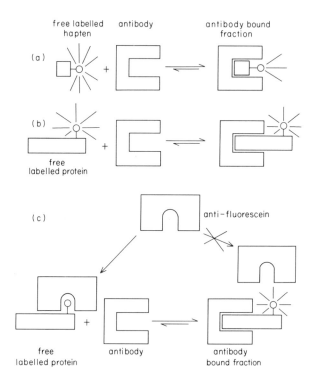

Fig. 5(a). Representation of a direct quenching fluoroimmunoassay for a hapten in which antibody binding is associated with a marked decrease in fluorescence. **(b)** Representation of why direct quenching fluoroimmunoassays are not applicable to large molecules, such as proteins, because the distance between the antigenic determinant and the site of attachment of the label is such that antibody binding does not influence fluorescence. **(c)** Representation of an indirect quenching fluoro-immunoassay in which an antiserum to fluorescein is added to (b). This binds to and completely quenches the fluorescein in the free fraction but does not bind to the label in the bound fraction because of steric hindrance by the first antibody.

(Fig. 5(b)). Nonetheless, it has proved possible to develop homogeneous FIA for proteins based on an indirect approach which makes use of the fact that binding of fluorescein itself (Lopatin and Voss, 1971; Portman *et al.*, 1975) and of fluorescein-labelled species (Levison *et al.*, 1970; Voss *et al.*, 1976) by antifluorescein sera causes virtually complete quenching of fluorescence. Fortunately the fluorescein group is a potently immunogenic hapten (Blakeslee, 1976) and it is relatively easy to raise suitable antisera.

Sample (or standard), labelled antigen and antibody are incubated and, after equilibrium has been attained, an excess of the anti-fluorescein sera is added. This immediately binds to, and quenches, the fluorescence of the free fraction but, because of steric hindrance effects by the first antibody, is unable to bind the fluorescein label in the bound fraction (Fig. 5(c)) which continues to fluoresce. Indirect quenching FIA have been developed for human albumin (Nargessi *et al.*, 1978b), immunoglobin G and placental lactogen (Nargessi *et al.*, 1978c). As mentioned in the section on EIA, this homogeneous indirect quenching approach should be applicable to labels other than fluorescein. Thus, for example, enzymes are excellent immunogens (Landon *et al.*, 1977) and anti-enzyme sera often inhibit enzymatic activity.

(*vi*) *Polarisation FIA*. This technique was described independently by two groups (Dandliker *et al.*, 1973; Spencer *et al.*, 1973). If a solution of fluorescent molecules is excited with polarised light, the polarisation of the emitted light will depend on the extent of random Brownian rotation of the molecules which occur during the life time of their excited state (4–5 nsec in the case of fluorescein labelled molecules). The smaller the labelled antigen the faster will be their random rotation, reflected by a low signal. Binding by the large antibody molecule is equivalent to an increase in effective size and results in a greatly enhanced signal.

The principle of polarisation FIA has been demonstrated in assay systems for human chorionic gonadotrophin (Dandliker *et al.*, 1973), for insulin (Spencer *et al.*, 1973), for oestradiol-17β (Dandliker *et al.*, 1977) and for hPL (Crookall-Greening and Smith, unpublished observations). However, its use for the assay of biological fluids and practical clinical applicability has only been demonstrated for determination of serum levels of gentamicin (Watson *et al.*, 1976) and phenytoin (McGregor *et al.*, 1978). The technique has also been applied for the study of antibodies to insulin (Spencer *et al.*, 1973), conalbumin (Tengerdy, 1967) and penicillin (Dandliker *et al.*, 1965) by measurement of the increase in fluorescence polarisation employing fluoro-phore-labelled antigens.

Polarisation FIA is simple, quick and precise, however, it has some major disadvantages. The first, and most important obstacle to its wider use is the lack of availability of convenient, relatively inexpensive, specially con-structed polarisation fluorimeters capable of providing a direct readout.

Second is the sensitivity, limited to the μmol/l and upper nmol/l range with respect to antigens in biological samples and, finally, is a lack of applicability to antigens with a molecular weight above about 20,000 because it depends upon the detection of a marked increase of effective size following antibody binding.

(b) *Immunoassays employing antibodies labelled with a fluorogenic molecule*

Early immunofluorometric assays (IFMA) were based on the precipitin reaction and separation of the bound complex from excess unreacted labelled antibody by centrifugation (Head, 1962; Tengerdy, 1963) or filtration (Neurath, 1965). Techniques have also been developed in which the binding of labelled antibodies onto antigens attached to the surface of paper discs is assessed by a fluorimeter designed to measure surface fluorescence (Toussaint and Anderson, 1965) and in which agarose beads and microfluorimetry are employed (Capel, 1974; Knapp and Ploem, 1974; Deelder and Ploem, 1974). In the latter, it has proved possible to determine the fluorescence signal from individual beads and average the signal from several beads for quantitative purposes. However, the complexity of the microfluorimetric equipment poses a major limitation.

Most recent work relating to IFMA has involved use of the sandwich approach. Excess antibody attached to a solid phase is first used to bind all the antigen from the sample. After washing, fluorescent-labelled antibody is added in excess and that bound to the solid phase, via the antigen, gives a direct measurement of the amount of antigen. Quantitation can be achieved after elution of the labelled antibodies from the solid phase as in an assay for human IgG (Aalberse, 1973). Alternatively, techniques have been developed that permit direct fluorimetry of bound fluorescent antibody on the solid phase. One approach, employed for the determination of serum levels of human complement components C3 and C4 (Burgett *et al.*, 1977a, b) employs a polyacrylamide bead solid support. However, by far the most extensively used is the commercial FIAX/StiQ system comprising a fluorimeter especially designed to measure fluorescence on the surface of the StiQ samplers— individual antigen-binding discs designed to facilitate the several incubation and washing steps required in assays of this type. Initially assays were established for serum levels of human immunoglobulins G, A and M (Kameda *et al.*, 1976) and have since been developed for several other proteins and adapted for competitive FIA for gentamicin and T_4.

All the labelled antibody techniques described in this chapter have required a separation step; however, Ullman *et al.* (1976) have successfully developed an homogeneous IFMA based on fluorescent excitation transfer for large antigens, such as proteins, with more than one antigenic determinant. Thus, one population of highly specific antibodies directed against human

IgG was labelled with fluorescein (F) and another population with rhodamine (R). When an excess of both were added to the sample,

$$Ag + Ab - R + Ab - F \rightleftharpoons Ab - R:Ag:Ab - F$$

only the free fractions fluoresced fully, quenching in the bound fraction resulting from energy transfer from the donor (F) to the acceptor (R). This differs from the excitation transfer FIA described earlier in that only labelled antibodies and not labelled antigen is employed.

Spatially selective excitation of the fluorescence provides another means of avoiding the separation step. Light undergoing total internal reflection at the quartz side of a quartz–water interface penetrates into the aqueous medium to a depth of only a few hundred nanometers. Thus if antigen is attached directly (or indirectly via an antibody) to the quartz surface and then fluorescent-labelled antibody is added to the aqueous medium, that bound to the antigen may be excited by light of suitable wavelength—while unreacted labelled antibody will not encounter the exciting light and will not, therefore, fluoresce. A helium–cadmium laser has been employed to demonstrate the feasibility of this approach (Kronick and Little, 1975).

3. Bacteriophages

The term bacteriophage is applied to a virus that has bacteria as its host. Typically such viruses comprise a head (consisting of a protein membrane enclosing a central core of DNA), tail fibres for fixation to the bacterial capsule and a contractile sheath to enable injection of their DNA through the bacterial cell wall. Following injection, the DNA rapidly replicates to form as many as 200 new viruses and, within 30 minutes, the bacterial capsule bursts to release its contents including the new viruses which then immediately infect adjacent bacteria. This process can be visualised by inoculating an agar plate covered by a layer of *Escherichia coli* with a small number of appropriate bacteriophages. Each of these will cause the sequential destruction of several thousand bacteria and give rise to a small area of translucency, a plaque—with the number of plaques being related to the number of viruses in the initial inoculum.

It had long been known that antibodies to bacteriophages could be detected with extreme sensitivity by their ability to inhibit viral infectivity. Haimovich and Sela (1966) extended this approach by reacting the bacterio-phage T4B (whose host is *E. coli* B) with *N*-carboxy-DL alanine anhydride and showing that phage activity was inhibited by rabbit antisera directed against the hapten. Independently, Mäkelä (1966) had performed similar studies using 3-iodo-4-hydroxy-5-nitrophenyl acetic acid coupled to two other phages, T2 and T7. Although designed to enable detection of minute concentrations of antibodies for single cell studies, it was noted that addition of the hapten or of hapten analogues in amounts as little as 100 pg could, by competing for antibodies, enable the viral activity of hapten:bacteriophage conjugates to be retained—thereby leading the way for the development of homogeneous viroimmunoassays (VIA). Work in which bacteriophages were conjugated to the antibody fragment (Fab') of appropriate antisera, by Taussig (1969), provides the basis for immunovirometric assays.

One of the first applications of a VIA was for the assay of the octapeptide, angiotensin II (Hurwitz *et al.*, 1970). Rabbit anti-angiotensin II serum (diluted to yield a 90–95% in activation of angiotensin–phage conjugate) was incubated with a series of angiotension II standards. Angiotensin II covalently linked to bacteriophage (T4) by means of glutaraldehyde was then added and, after a further period of incubation, phage activity determined. A sensitivity of about 10 pg/ml was achieved in buffer but the assay was not applied to biological fluids. Similar assays have been developed for the two plant hormones indole-3-acetic acid and gibberellic acid (Fuchs *et al.*, 1971).

Such assays have several advantages including a shelf life of the labelled reactant measured in years, avoidance of the need to separate the bound and free fractions and a sensitivity comparable to RIA. However, the literature relating to VIA is relatively limited as compared with that concerning EIA—probably because of the difficulties experienced in successfully coupling antigen to bacteriophage, the complexity of end-point detection and the likelihood that factors present in biological samples, other than the antigen to be determined, may influence phage activity.

Successful labelling requires that antigen be located primarily on phage tail fibres (since only then does antibody binding inactive the bacteriophage); that the antigenic determinants of the antigen remain exposed and that sufficient phage survive the conjugation reaction to retain adequate bacterial infectivity. Although up to 80% survival of phage has been reported (Hurwitz *et al.*, 1970) it is not uncommon for 99% of the bacteriophages to become inactivated during labelling. An end-point based on plaque counting is obviously time consuming and costly, but a recent development in the Nichols Institute (Nichols, personal communication) may overcome this. Thus rather than determining the number of plaque forming units, the amounts of bacterial β-galactosidease released during virally-induced bacterial eruption is quantitated colorimetrically after addition of a suitable substrate. This approach has been applied in the development of a VIA for human thyrocalcitonin with a sensitivity of 30 pg/ml. Nonetheless, the time taken for sufficient bacteria to be infected and release the enzyme is in excess of an hour.

4. Other Non-isotopic Labels

(a) Proteins

The limitations of non-labelled immunoassays in endocrinology have been outlined earlier. Thus, for example, only large antigen:antibody aggregates form a precipitin line or scatter light and such aggregates are found only when the antigen is a protein (with several antigen determinants) and is present in high concentration. However, such techniques can be applied to the assay of haptens, provided hapten conjugated to protein is employed as label. Thus Cambiaso et al. (1974a, b) described automated immunoprecipitation techniques for the assay of DNP-lysine (with a sensitivity of 1 ng/ml) and of progesterone (with a sensitivity of 10 ng/ml), although difficulties were experienced in applying such a procedure to serum when, for example, the presence of rheumatoid factor or Clq may influence the results obtained.

(b) Metals

Recently metalloimmunoassays have been described (Cais et al., 1977) employing metal atoms, in the form of their organometallic or co-ordination complexes, for labelling haptens and larger antigens. These assays are of the heterogeneous type and, after separation of the antibody bound and free fractions, the amount of metal present in one or other is determined by suitable methods—such as emission absorption, fluorescence spectrometry or neutron inactivation. Among the haptens studied were oestrone, oestradiol-17β, oestriol, cannabis and barbiturate while bovine serum albumin was employed as a protein model. It does not seem likely that such assays will be of relevance to endocrinology, in the near future, because of the lack of sensitivity (2–50 ng/ml) and complexity of available end-point detection systems.

(c) Chemiluminescence and bioluminescence

Chemiluminescence is associated with certain chemical reactions that result in the emission of photons of light. One of the best known and efficient reactions of this type is the oxidation of luminol (5-amino-2,3'-dihydro-phthalazine-1,4-dione) by, for example, hydrogen peroxide in the presence of a catalyst. Bioluminescence refers to chemiluminescent reactions that involve a biological reactant. The best known of these, the luciferin–luciferase system, was discovered nearly a century ago by Dubois. Sources of the various luciferins (the substrates) and luciferases (the enzymes) include the firefly, some bacteria (such as Photobacterium fischerii) and certain jellyfish.

In the firefly system:

luciferase + luciferin + ATP + Mg^{++} ———→ luciferase:luciferin:AMP

luciferase:luciferin:AMP + O_2 ———→ oxyluciferin + AMP + CO_2 + H_2O

and emission of light with a λ_{max} of 562 nm.

The reagents are all commercially available, appropriate instrumentation exists and such systems are exquisitively sensitive because of the ease and precision of determining very low levels of light emission. Thus, the luciferase–luciferin reaction can be employed to determine less than 10^{-13}M ATP (Hercules and Sheehan, 1978) and the ATP content of a single bacterium (Seitz and Neary, 1974). However, we were unable to label antigens with luminol (or its derivatives) and still retain chemiluminescent activity, while neither luciferase or luciferin have yet been bound successfully to an antigen or antibody. Even if achieved, labelling with luciferase would provide only a further example of EIA and IEMA and would be likely to have many inherent problems—especially with regard to reagent purity.

The only practical assay to date, involving chemiluminescence, is an EIA for staphylococcal enteroxin B employing antigen labelled with peroxidase, antibodies covalently linked to a solid phase and end-point detection of the bound fraction by the enzyme catalysing the oxidation of pyrogallol by hydrogen peroxide (Velan and Halmann, 1978).

(d) Cofactors

The use of cofactors would seem an attractive alternative to enzyme labelling especially since it would be anticipated that the antibody in the bound fraction would be more likely to sterically hinder the approach of both substrate and enzyme than, as in most EIA, of the substrate alone. Schroeder *et al.* (1976) successfully labelled biotin and dinitrofluorobenzene with an NAD analogue and developed a homogeneous assay employing a bioluminescent end-point. This group (Carrico *et al.*, 1976) were also successful in preparing ATP labelled antigens as the basis of a homogeneous assay.

We have also successfully coupled NAD to various ligands. However, it is a formidable chemical task that significantly decreases cofactor activity. Of more importance, cofactors are present in all biological fluids and even in the distilled water (probably as a result of prior bacterial contamination) which made homogeneous assays of a sensitivity appropriate for hormone measurement impractical. As heterogeneous assays, such techniques would not appear to offer any advantages over EIA and, in all probability, would have some additional disadvantages.

(e) Particles

Reference has already been made to early work by Arquilla and Stavitsky (1956) which involved the use of insulin labelled with red blood cells. Many other examples of immunoassays employing RBC as the label exist including for example, a haemagglutination—inhibition assay for the detection of morphine (Adler and Leu, 1971). Large numbers of tests have also been developed in which antigens or antibodies are labelled with latex particles with the end-point being the visual determination of latex agglutination. Among the most common are pregnancy tests employing particles coated with antisera to hCG which agglutinate in the presence of hCG in a urinary sample. Kits of this type are available commercially for a wide range of antibodies (including anti-thyroglobulin and anti-microsomal) and antigens (such as fibrin degradation products, several plasma proteins and some viral and bacterial antigens). Indeed, the number of samples currently assayed by this means may well approach that by RIA.

Such techniques are usually qualitative rather than quantitative, however, the availability of instruments to count platelets and other blood cells has made possible the recent introduction of sensitive, quantitative *particle counting immunoassays* (PACIA)—based on the reduction of the total number of particles when they are agglutinated. In its simplest form, for the assay of large molecules with several antigenic determinants, latex particles of some 0·8 micron size are coated with antiserum and, after incubation, the number of single particles remaining will be inversely proportional to the amount of antigen present in the sample.

For the assay of haptens with only a single antigenic determinant the technique must be modified slightly. For example, in the assay of T_4, macromolecules of dextran to which have been linked several T_4 molecules (the T_4 conjugate) are incubated with the antibody coated latex particles and the sample (or standard). In the absence of T_4 several of the latex particles will become bound to the T_4 conjugate and the number of single particles will be small. In the presence of increasing levels of T_4, which will block binding sites on the antibody coated latex particles so that they no longer agglutinate with the T_4 conjugate, the number of single particles will increase proportionally.

Sensitivities of a few nmol/l were achieved for both hPL and α-fetoprotein by the first procedure and of about 10 nmol/l for T_4 by the inhibition technique. Coefficients of variation ranged from 2–10% and both manual and automated assays were developed (Cambiaso et al., 1977). Specialised and hence expensive equipment is necessary and problems were encountered initially with some samples due to latex particle agglutination by rheumatoid factor or Clq. However, these are being successfully overcome by prior treatment of the samples and a modification of the procedures using the F(ab′)$_2$ fragments (Limet et al., 1979). Furthermore, new approaches to PACIA are enabling even greater sensitivity to be achieved.

C. COMPARISON OF THE ADVANTAGES AND DISADVANTAGES OF ISOTOPIC AND NON-ISOTOPIC LABELLING IN IMMUNOASSAY

The future role of NIIA in endocrinology will depend upon their advantages and disadvantages as compared with immunoassay employing an isotopically labelled reactant. Thus any alternatives to RIA and IRMA must be equally practical, employ as simple and efficient a detection system and enable the appropriate specificity, sensitivity, accuracy and precision to be achieved.

All manual immunoassays, irrespective of the label employed, have much in common including the need for standards, quality control samples and antisera; the addition of the reactants in a set order, usually in µl amounts; a period of incubation until equilibrium is reached—that depends, in large part, on the concentration of the reactants and may vary from minutes (for compounds present in the µmol/l range) to several days (for compounds in the low pmol/l range); and the calculation of results. It must be stressed, since there have been claims to the contrary (Leute *et al.*, 1972b), that the time taken to attain equilibrium in an immunoassay is not influenced by the label employed (although, as discussed below, the time required for end-point detection may vary substantially). The specificity will also be similar since this is dependant predominantly on the antiserum used.

The relative merits of the various alternative labels with respect to other aspects of an immunoassay are discussed below, while a balanced summary of the relative merits of isotopes and enzymes for labelling purposes has recently been published by Ekins (1976).

1. Preparation and Stability of Labelled Reactant

Much of the early success of RIA can be attributed to the development, by Greenwood *et al.* (1963), of an efficient and simple means for radioiodinating peptides and proteins containing tyrosine and/or histidine residues. Many other procedures have since been introduced for labelling steroids, thyroid hormones and other haptens as well as alternative techniques for labelling protein and glycoprotein hormones. Reactants labelled with gamma-emitting isotopes, in particular ^{125}I, are being employed increasingly for clinical purposes in preference to those labelled with a beta-emitting isotope, such as ^{3}H or [14]C. This is because of the much shorter counting times required and the avoidance of the need for liquid scintillant and of applying corrections for quenching or chemiluminescence. Excellent methods also exist for the labelling of haptens and proteins with enzymes and with fluorescent molecules, in part because of the prior use of such labelled products in other fields such as histopathology.

Few problems exist with regard to labelling with latex particles, erythrocytes or free radicals. However, there are two types of alternative label, namely phages and some chemiluminescent molecules, where the actual labelling poses major difficulties. Thus there are problems in retaining the viability of bacteriophages during the labelling procedure while chemiluminescent molecules, such as luminol, may fail to react after their conjugation to other molecules.

Considerable concern is often expressed about the radiation hazards associated with RIA and IRMA. Thus isotopes can be absorbed through the skin while volatile ^{125}I can be released into the atmosphere (Bogdanove and Strash, 1975) and inhaled. It is essential to distinguish clearly between the risk of performing a radioiodination and of carrying out an actual RIA or IRMA. In the former, one or two millicuries of ^{125}I are commonly employed with the need for proper facilities and precautions. However, performing an RIA involves the use of only about 0·1 µCi of ^{125}I and there are no risks provided simple rules are obeyed—such as not using a mouth pipette or eating or smoking in the laboratory. The Radiochemical Centre, Amersham, has demonstrated that the rate of release of volatile ^{125}I during the course of an assay is less than 1% and that it is impossible for a laboratory worker, irrespective of the number of RIA performed, to inhale more than a miniscule percentage of the maximum permitted dose.

The prolonged shelf life, measured in years, is a major advantage of reactants labelled with enzymes, fluorescent molecules and various other alternatives as compared to those labelled with a gamma-emitting isotope. Thus the latter have a relatively limited shelf life due to the short half life of such isotopes (about 60 days in the case of ^{125}I) and the rapid degradation of some labelled antigens. The use of new and gentler radioiodination procedures together with the availability of purer and more stable antigens and antibodies is helping to improve the situation. Thus isotopically labelled antigens can now normally be used for at least 12 weeks while radioiodinated antibodies can be employed for up to six months. Nonetheless, the short shelf life of antigens labelled with a gamma-emitting isotope poses considerable problems for commercial kit producers since it necessitates frequent radioiodinations and markedly increases the cost of production, quality control and distribution.

2. Need for a Separation Step

RIA and IRMA require a separation step prior to isotope counting because it is impossible to distinguish between the radioactivity in the bound and free fractions. A variety of separation procedures have been developed, which depend upon chemical, physical or immunological differences (Ratcliffe, 1974). However, the separation step is one of the main sources of imprecision in a manual RIA; requires considerable work and technical expertise; adds to the time taken to complete an assay if centrifugation and multiple washes are necessary; and, finally, has posed problems in the development of fully automated RIA systems.

It is not surprising, therefore, that those NIIA which do not require a separation step are simpler, take less time to perform, and are potentially more precise provided end-point detection is also simple, quick, sensitive and precise. Unfortunately when sensitivity is required, as it often is in hormone measurement, homogeneous EIA, FIA and VIA may be affected significantly by endogeneous materials present in the sample which may either increase or decrease the signal. Indeed, under such circumstances, it may be necessary to reintroduce a separation step to remove such endogeneous materials. Furthermore, such a step appears to be a requisite of virtually all assays employing labelled antibodies, irrespective of the label used, since the act of binding seldom influences the signal.

3. End-point Detection

It would seem logical first to consider the criteria on which the ideal end-point detection system would be based and then assess how these criteria are met when the various labels, previously discussed, are employed. Some suggested criteria are: cost, speed and simplicity of detection technique; cost and availability of appropriate instrumentation; precision, accuracy and sensitivity of end-point detection: dependent on signal to background ratio; no influence of biological samples on end-point detection; ability to check; non-hazardous; and suitable for automation. A personal assessment of how well RIA, EIA and FIA meet these criteria is presented in Table 6.

The use of detection systems for reactants labelled with gamma-emitting isotopes offers many advantages. Relatively inexpensive manual and automated gamma counters are widely available and becoming increasingly so; such counters are very efficient (greater than 70% efficiency when ^{125}I is being counted); it is difficult to envisage a simpler method of end-point detection than the introduction of the sample into the well of a sodium iodide crystal; counting precision obeys known physical laws such that, when 10,000 counts are collected, the coefficient of variation is only 1% for repeated counts on the same sample; and the time taken to generate 10,000 counts is short (usually 10–120 sec) with the high specific activity ^{125}I-labelled reactants commonly employed. Of particular importance in endocrinology, the use of isotopically labelled reactants enables attainment of the maximum

Table 6

A comparison of end-point detection systems[a].

	Radio-immunoassay[b]	Enzymo-immunoassay	Fluoro-immunoassay
Precision	9	5	10
Sensitivity	10	heterogeneous 10	heterogeneous 6
		homogeneous 4	homogeneous 4
Speed	8	5	10
Simplicity	9	5	10
Ability to check	10	2	10
Non-hazardous	2	10	10
Availability of instrumentation	7	10	5
Influence of biological samples	10	heterogeneous 9	heterogeneous 9
		homogeneous 5	homogeneous 5

[a]Based on an arbitrary maximum score of 10. The values given are solely the personal view of the authors. It is appreciated that others might give very different scores and that new advances may lead to a total re-evaluation.

[b]Employing a gamma-emitting isotope. Assays using a beta-emitting isotope would receive a lower score with regard to speed (5), simplicity (5), availability of instrumentation (3) and influence of biological samples (7).

sensitivity set by the affinity of the antibody while biological samples do not affect the number of counts recorded nor are samples themselves radioactive so that they do not contribute an endogenous background signal.

From the standpoint of end-point detection, instruments for determining enzyme activity are the most widely available of all; no hazards are involved and heterogeneous EIA can attain maximum sensitivity. However, the additional step of determining enzyme activity prolongs the assay, makes it more complex and increases imprecision; the amplification made possible by use of an enzyme to attain sensitivity will also magnify an error; it is difficult to check a value; a change in temperature of less than 1° greatly influences enzymatic activity; and, of especial importance as noted earlier, biological samples may contain enzymes with similar biological effects and factors, such as enzyme inhibitors or haemolysis, may affect the result.

End-point detection systems for FIA offer a surprising number of advantages. Manual and flow-through fluorimeters are not very expensive and are efficient; introduction of the sample is easy and the result is available within seconds; precision of measurement is excellent (with coefficients of variation less than 0·2%); results are not significantly affected by normal changes in ambient temperature; there are no hazards and rechecking poses no problem. However, fluorimeters are not widely available and, at their present stage of development, FIA are relatively insensitive covering only the μmol/l and upper nmol/l range—in part due to other compounds present in samples (such as bilirubin) which cause a variable background.

4. Legislation

Most countries base their legislation concerning the use and disposal of radioisotopes upon the recommendations of the International Commission on Radiation Protection. However, wide differences exist in the inter-pretation of these regulations. The aim should be to enable maximum use of clinically valuable *in vitro* procedures while safeguarding the health of laboratory staff and the general public against the dangers. Since, as dis-cussed earlier, there is no significant hazard involved in determining hormone levels by RIA or IRMA it might be expected that no significant legislation problems would exist.

Such is the fortunate situation that exists in the United Kingdom and United States while, in West Germany and despite very detailed regulations, the only problems concern the disposal of solid radioactive waste and the requirement to keep extremely careful records. However, in some countries (including France) legislation has been so framed as to prohibit all but a few centres from performing RIA—with consequent difficulties in the practice of endocrinology. It might also be expected that in other countries, especially Japan, there may be emotive problems in employing radioisotopes.

No such problems exist with the majority of non-isotopic labels (although it is possible that difficulties might arise if viruses were to be employed extensively for labelling). Thus it is certain that in countries with very restrictive legislation or a strong emotive bias against the use of isotopes that increasing use will be made of some forms of NIIA in endocrinology irrespective of their merits and demerits as compared with RIA.

5. Automation

There are several factors which suggest the need for fully automated immuno-assay systems (Landon *et al.*, 1975) and indicate that their introduction may have the same profound impact as did the Auto-Analyser in clinical chemistry. These include the rapidly increasing demand for existing assays (such as for T_4 and TSH in screening programmes to detect neonatal hypothyroidism); the application of immunoassay to a rapidly increasing range of compounds in such diverse fields as pharmacology (Landon and Moffat, 1976), oncology (Bagshawe, 1974), microbiology and parasitology (Voller *et al.*, 1976), and haematology (Newmark and Gordon, 1974) as well as in endocrinology; and the need to improve precision and reduce costs (by such means as reducing reagent volumes and removing the need for running duplicates). Such systems may also significantly shorten assay time. Thus, in a manual immuno-assay it is essential to attain equilibrium because of the impossibility of keeping the time between reagent addition and the separation step constant. In automated systems, particularly those of the continuous flow-type, accurate timing is simple and disequilibrium assays can be employed.

Much recent work has related to automating RIA, and developments have reflected closely those seen previously in routine clinical chemistry. Thus, following the introduction of partially automated equipment, fully automated procedures are being introduced which can be divided into discrete and continuous-flow systems (Table 7). The main problem concerned the

Table 7

Some available automated radioimmunoassay systems.

Name	Separation procedure	References
Continuous flow		
	Second antibody/filtration	Pollard et al. (1965)
	Second antibody/filtration	Bagshawe et al. (1967)
	Second antibody/sedimentation	Johnson et al. (1972)
	Antibodies attached to RBC/sedimentation	Lunar (1975)
Gammaflow (Squibb)	Column of Dowex and charcoal	Brooker et al. (1976)
ARIA II (Becton Dickinson)	Reusable immobilised antibodies	Reese and Johnson (1978)
Star (Technicon)	Antibodies linked to magnetisable particles	Forrest (1977)
Southmead System	Immobilised antibodies/filtration	Ismail et al. (1978)
Discrete		
Centria (Union Carbide)	Centrifugation through Sephadex G25 columns	Lo and Ertingshausen (1976)
Concept 4 (Micro Medic)	Antibody coated tubes	Painter and Hasler (1976)
Pace 4 (Picker)	Second antibody/filtration	Bagshawe (1975)
Ismatec	Second antibody/filtration	Marschner et al. (1975)

separation step. This has been overcome in a number of ingenious ways in-cluding the use of antibodies covalently linked to magnetisable particles and a magnetic field (Forrest, 1977) and of magnetisable charcoal (Dawes and

Gardner, 1978). Such automated assays are proving of considerable value in endocrinology (Nye *et al.*, 1978).

Similar approaches are certain to occur with those techniques, such as heterogeneous EIA, which require a separation step. Indeed, a generation of fully automated immunoassay systems can be envisaged in which several different end-point detectors can be employed depending on the particular assay. However, the development of fully automated equipment is particularly easy for those immunoassays that do not require separation of the bound and free fractions. Thus automated immunoprecipitation procedures have been introduced, by Technicon, for large numbers of specific plasma proteins and several references have been made, during the course of this chapter, to automated FIA and EIA. Development in the field of automated particle counting immunoassays (PACIA) are of especial interest in endocrinology because of their potential sensitivity and precision. Nonetheless, in the immediate future, it seems certain that most automated immunoassays for hormones will enjoy an isotopically labelled reactant—since many large commercial companies are making a major investment in this area.

D. CONCLUSIONS ON THE ROLE OF NON-ISOTOPIC IMMUNOASSAYS IN ENDOCRINOLOGY

The immense impact that RIA has had in endocrinology reflects its specificity, sensitivity, precision, practicality and wide applicability. It is possible that the availability of fully automated RIA will have a further impact by decreasing individual sample assay costs and enabling virtually unlimited sample numbers to be handled. Current NIIA share this specificity (which is a function of the antibody), wide applicability (which reflects the ease of raising antibodies against a vast range of molecular species) and potential for automation. However, problems may arise with regard to sensitivity, precision and practicality.

To date, of the commonly employed NIIA, only the heterogeneous EIA can attain a sensitivity equivalent to that of RIA. Homogeneous EIA and all forms of FIA are currently limited to the assay of compounds which circulate at concentrations in the $\mu mol/l$ or $nmol/l$ range and, even then, difficulties may be encountered at low $nmol/l$ levels. As shown in Table 8, most hormones circulate in the low $pmol/l$ range, well below the present sensitivity. It is of interest that the majority of hormones lying in the $nmol/l$ range are either those associated with pregnancy (oestriol and HPL) or others which circulate largely bound to carrier proteins (such as T_4 and T_3), free levels of which lie in the $pmol/l$ range.

These low levels are in sharp contrast to those of drugs. Thus alcohol at

Table 8

Approximate circulating levels of a variety of naturally occurring compounds.

	mmol/l		μmol/l
Sodium	140	Albumin	600
Chloride	105	Urate	250
Bicarbonate	30	Phenylalanine	125
Glucose	5	Immunoglobulin G	90
Urea	4	Ammonia	30
Cholesterol	4	Iron	20
Calcium	2·5	Bilirubin (total)	10
Triglycerides (fasting)	1	Immunoglobulin M	1
	nmol/l		pmol/l
Oestriol (late pregnancy)	600	Aldosterone	180
Thyroxine binding globulin	500	Insulin	120
Cortisol	400	Parathyroid hormone	100
Placental lactogen	300	Growth hormone	50
Thyroxine (total)	125	Luteinising hormone	10
Corticosterone	20	Triiodothyronine (free)	10
Triiodothyronine	2	Adrenocorticotrophin	10
Prolactin	1	Thyroid stimulating hormone	5
Oestradiol 17β (women)	1	Angiotensin 11	4
Progesterone	1	Oxytocin	1
		Arginine vasopressin	1

twice the permitted driving level has the third highest blood concentration of any compound, at about 40 mmol/l, while therapeutic levels of lithium and salicylates are also in the mmol/l range. The majority of drugs for which homogeneous EIA and FIA have been developed circulate in the μmol/l range, about one million times higher than many hormones. Digoxin is an exception in this respect since its therapeutic levels lie in the low nmol/l range.

Despite their potential sensitivity, heterogeneous EIA must remain technically more complex and less precise than RIA for the reasons considered in the earlier section relating to end-point detection. Even the manual homogeneous EIA for T_4 is more complex and takes longer to perform than many of its RIA counterparts.

It is helpful in drawing conclusions concerning the possible role of NIIA in endocrinology to also consider briefly their undoubted value in other areas of clinical practice:

(i) NIIA is playing an increasingly important role in detecting the presence of antibodies against a wide range of parasites, bacteria, viruses and other organisms. Examples include the screening of pregnant women for the presence of IgM and IgG antibodies to *Rubella* and the use of EIA with a simple visual end-point in the developing world. Similar procedures would be of value in endocrinology for the detection of, for example, circulating antibodies to the thyroglobin or thyroid microsomal antigens; but this is a relatively limited requirement.

(ii) NIIA has an extensive and valuable role in detecting the presence of antigens such as Australian antigen. Thus there are many medical situations of the plus/minus type for which precision is unimportant. The detection of human chorionic gonadotrophin or the β-subunit provides such an example, and NIIA (with antibodies covalently bound to erythrocytes or latex particles) are already used extensively. However, in endocrinology, it is usually important to make quantitative measurements of hormone levels, rather than to detect them.

(iii) NIIA have a much less important role in the exact quantitation of antigens and especially hormones. Indeed, in the context of endocrinology, the role of NIIA in their present stage of development may well be limited to the following: (a) the developing world, which does not have easy access to gamma counters, and in which the relative instability of reactants labelled with a gamma-emitting isotope may cause problems; (b) countries with legal restrictions on the use of isotopes, or an emotive bias against their use. Under such circumstances it is acceptable for laboratory staff to perform technically more complex, time consuming and imprecise analytical procedures; (c) hormones and carrier proteins which circulate in the μmol/l and high nmol/l range and for which homogeneous techniques exist. Immunoassays not employing labelled reactant are sufficiently sensitive for some carrier proteins, including TBG. Homogeneous EIA and FIA have proved suitable for the assays of serum levels of total T_4 and assays for oestriol and cortisol should not pose a problem. However, it is not yet certain if the practicality and precision of such assays will be such that they replace conventional RIA.

Thus we conclude (and we believe our experience with both RIA and NIIA prevents uninformed bias) that the predominant use of isotopically labelled reagents will continue in endocrinology (and in some other areas, such as the assay of tumour-associated antigens) during the next decade, and that RIA and NIIA will have complementary rather than exclusive roles. We believe that NIIA will prove of immense value in many medical fields other than endocrinology, for example therapeutic drug monitoring and microbiology. We also conclude (though here we would admit to bias) that FIA will prove more practical than EIA for quantitative determinations, while the latter will dominate in plus/minus and in third world situations. Finally, it seems too early to forecast the impact of other alternative labels, but the use of particle counting immunoassay will be followed with especial interest.

REFERENCES

Aalberse, R. C. (1973). *Clin. chim. Acta*, **48**, 109.

Addison, G. M. and Hales, C. N. (1971). *Horm. Metab. Res.* **3**, 59.

Adler, F. L. and Lau, C. T. (1971). *J. Immunol.* **106**, 1684.

Arquilla, E. R. and Stavitsky, A. B. (1956). *J. clin. Invest.* **35**, 458.

Bagshawe, K. D., Harris, F. W. and Orr, A. H. (1967). *In* "Automation in Analytical Chemistry", Vol. 2, p. 53. Technicon Symposia, Mediad, New York.

Bagshawe, K. D. (1974). *Br. med. Bull.* **30**, 68.

Bagshawe, K. D. (1975). *Lab. Pract.* **24**, 573.

Barakat, R. M. and Ekins, R. P. (1961). *Lancet*, **ii**, 25.

Barbour, H. M. (1976), *J. immunol. Methods*, **11**, 15.

Beck, P. and Hales, C. N. (1975). *Biochem. J.* **145**, 607.

Belanger, L., Sylvestre, C. and Dufour, D. (1973). *Clin. chim. Acta*, **48**, 15.

Berson, S. A., Yalow, R. S., Baumann, A., Rothschild, M. A., Newerly, K. (1956). *J. clin. Invest.* **35**, 170.

Blakeslee, D. (1976). *J. immunol. Methods*, **12**, 19.

Bogdanove, E. M. and Strash, A. M. (1975). *Nature, Lond.* **257**, 426.

Bosch, A. M. G., van Heli, H., Brands, J. (1975). *Clin. Chem.* **21**, 1009.

Bosch, A. M. G. (1978). *Anal. Chem.* **290**, 98.

Bradwell, A. R., Burnett, D., Ramsden, D. B., Burr, W. A., Prince, H. P. and Hoffenberg, R. (1976). *Clin. chim. Acta*, **71**, 501.

Brooker, G., Terasaki, W. L. and Price, M. G. (1976). *Science*, **194**, 270.

Burd, J. F., Carrico, R. J., Fetter, M. C., Buckler, R. T., Johnson, R. D., Boguslaski R. C. and Christner, J. E. (1977a). *Anal. Biochem.* **77**, 56.

Burd, J. F., Wong, R. C., Feeney, J. E., Carrico, R. J. and Boguslaski, R. C. (1977b). *Clin. Chem.* **23**, 1402.

Burgett, M. W., Fairfield, S. J. and Monthony, J. F. (1977a). *Clin. chim. Acta*, **78**, 277.

Burgett, M. W., Fairfield, S. J. and Monthony, J. F. (1977b). *J. immunol. Methods*, **16**, 211.

Cais, M., Dani, S., Edden, Y., Gandolfi, O., Horn, M., Issacs, E. E., Josephy, Y., Saar, Y., Slovin, E., and Snarsky, L. (1977). *Nature, Lond.* **270**, 534.

Cambiaso, C. L., Masson, P. L. and Heremans, J. F. (1974a). *J. immunol. Methods*, **5**, 153.

Cambiaso, C. L., Riccomi, H. A., Masson, P. L. and Heremans, J. F. (1974b). *J. immunol. Methods*, **5**, 293.

Cambiaso, C. L., Leek, A. E., de Steenwinkel, F., Billen, J. and Masson, P. L. (1977). *J. immunol. Methods*, **18**, 33.

Capel, P. J. A. (1974). *J. immunol. Methods*, **5**, 295.

Carrico, J. R., Yeung, K. K., Schroeder, H. R., Boguslaski, R. C., Buckler, R. T. and Christner, J. E. (1976). *Anal. Biochem.* **76**, 95.

Chard, T. (1978). *In* "An Introduction to Radioimmunoassay and Related Techniques" (T. S. Work and E. Work, eds). Biochemical Press, Elsevier, North Holland.

Chayen, J., Loveridge, N. and Daly, J. R. (1972). *Clin. Endocr.* **1**, 219.
Dandliker, W. B., Schapiro, H. C., Meduski, J. W., Alonso, R., Feigen, G. A. and Hamrick, J. R. (1964). *Immunochemistry*, **1**, 165.
Dandliker, W. B., Halbert, S. P., Florin, M. C., Alonso, R. and Schapiro, H. C. (1965). *J. exp. Med.* **122**, 1029.
Dandliker, W. B. and de Saussure, V. A. (1970). *Immunochemistry*, **7**, 799.
Dandliker, W. B., Kelly, R. J., Dandliker, J., Farquhar, J. and Levin, J. (1973). *Immunochemistry*, **10**, 219.
Dandliker, W. B., Hicks, A. N., Levison, S. A. and Brawn, R. J. (1977). *Biochem. biophys. Res. Commun.* **74**, 538.
Dawes, C. and Gardner, J. (1978). *Clin. chim.* Acta, **86**, 353.
Deelder, A. M., and Ploem, J. S. (1974). *J. immunol. Methods*, **4**, 239.
Dray, F., Andrieu, J. M. and Renaud, R. (1975). *Biochim. biophys. Acta*, **403**, 131.
Ekins, R. P. (1960). *Clin. chim. Acta*, **5**, 453.
Ekins, R. P. (1976). *Lancet*, **ii**, 176.
Ekins, R. P. (1976a). *In* "Hormone Assays and Their Clinical Application" (J. A. Loraine and E. T. Bell, eds), p. 1. Churchill Livingstone, London.
Engvall, E. and Perlmann, P. (1971). Immunochemistry, **8**, 871.
Ertingshausen, G., Shapiro, S. I., Green, G. and Zborowski, G. (1975). *Clin. Chem.* **21**, 1305.
Feuerstein, D. L. and Selleck, R. E. E. (1963). *J. san. Eng. Div. A.S.C.E.* **89**, 1.
Forrest, G. C. (1977). *Ann. clin. Biochem.* **14**, 1.
Fuchs, S., Haimovich, J. and Fuchs, Y. (1971). *Eur. J. Biochem.* **18**, 384.
Galen, R. S. and Forman, D. (1977). *Clin. Chem.* **23**, 119.
Goldman, M. (1968). "Fluorescent Antibody Methods." Academic Press, New York and London.
Greenwood, F. C., Hunter, W. M. and Glover, J. S. (1963). *Biochem. J.* **89**, 114.
Haimovich, J. and Sela, M. (1966). *J. immunol.* **97**, 338.
Head, W. F. (1962). *J. pharm. Sci.* **51**, 662.
Hercules, D. M. and Sheehan, T. L. (1978). *Anal. Chem.* **50**, 22.
Holdaway, I. M., Rees, L. H. and Landon, J. (1973). *Lancet*, **ii**, 1170.
Hurwitz, E., Dietrich, F. M. and Sela, M. (1970). *Eur. J. Biochem.* **17**, 273.
Ishikawa, E. (1973). *J. Biochem.* **73**, 1319.
Ismail, A. A. A., West, P. M. and Goldie, D. J. (1978). *Clin. Chem.* **24**, 571.
Johnson, H., Brann, B. E., Ritchie, R. F. and Graves, J. (1972). *In* "Automation in Analytical Chemistry", Vol. 2. p. 69. Technicon Symposia, Mediad, New York.
Joyce, S. (1977). Steroids, **29**, 761.
Kameda, N., Harte, R. A. and Deindoerfer, F. H. (1976). *Clin. Chem.* **22**, 1200.
Kamel, R. S., McGregor, A. R., Landon, J. and Smith, D. S. (1978). *Clin. chim. Acta*, **89**, 93.
Kato, K., Hamaguchi, Y., Fukui, H. and Ishikawa, E. (1975). *J. Biochem.* **78**, 235.
Kitagawa, T. and Aikawa, T. (1976). *J. Biochem.* **79**, 233.
Kleinhammer, G., Lenz, H., Linke, R. and Gruber, W. (1976). *Z. anal. Chem.* **279**, 145.
Knapp, W. and Ploem. J. S. (1974). *J. immunol. Methods*, **5**, 259.
Kronick, M. N. and Little, W. A. (1975). *J. immunol. Methods*, **8**, 235.
Landon, J., Friedman, M. and Greenwood, F. C. (1967). *Lancet*, **i**, 652.
Landon, J., Rees, L. and Nye, L. (1975). *Br. J. hosp. Equip.* **1**, 29.
Landon, J., Crookall, J. and McGregor, A. (1975). *In* "Steroid Immunoassay" (E. H. D. Cammeron, S. G. Hiller and K. Griffiths, eds). Alpha-Omega, Cardiff.

Landon, J. and Moffat, A. C. (1976). *Analyst*, **101**, 225.

Landon, J. (1977). *Nature, Lond.* **268**, 483.

Landon, J., Carney, J. and Langley, D. (1977). *Ann. clin. Biochem.* **14**, 90.

Leute, R. K., Ullman, E. F., Goldstein, A. and Herzenberg, L. A. (1972a). *Nature New Biol.* **236**, 93.

Leute, R. K., Ullman, E. F. and Goldstein, A. (1972b). *J. Am. med. Assoc.* **221**, 1231.

Levison, S. A., Kierszenbaum, F. and Dandliker, W. B. (1970). *Biochemistry*, **9**, 322.

Limet, J. N., Moussebois, C. H., Cambiaso, C. L., Vaerman, J. P. and Masson, P. L. (1979). (In press.)

Lo, D. H. and Ertingshausen, G. (1976). *Clin. Chem.* **22**, 1165.

Lopatin, D. E. and Voss, E. W. (1971). *Biochemistry*, **10**, 208.

Lunar, S. J. (1975). *Anal. Biochem.* **65**, 355.

Maiolini, R., Ferrua, B. and Masseyeff, R. (1975). *J. immunol. Methods*, **6**, 355.

Maiolini, R. and Masseyeff, R. (1975). *J. immunol. Methods*, **8**, 223.

Mäkelä, O. (1966). *Immunology*, **10**, 81.

Marschner, I., Erhardt, F., Henner, J. and Scriba, P. C. (1975). *Z. klin. Chem. klin. Biochem.* **13**, 481.

Mattingly, D. (1962). *J. clin Pathol.* **15**, 374.

McGregor, A., Grookall-Greening, J. D., Landon, J. and Smith, D. S. (1978). *Clin. chim. Acta*, **83**, 161.

Miedema, K., Boelhouwer, J. and Otten, J. W. (1972). *Clin. chim. Acta*, **40**, 187.

Miles, L. E. M. and Hales, C. N. (1968a). *Nature, Lond.* **219**, 186.

Miles, L. E. M. and Hales, C. N. (1968b). *Biochem. J.* **108**, 611.

Miles, L. E. M. and Hales, C. N. (1968c). *Lancet*, **ii**, 492.

Miyai, K., Ishibashi, K. and Kumahara, Y. (1976). *Clin. chim. Acta*, **67**, 263.

Nargessi, R. D., Landon, J., Pourfarzaneh, M. and Smith, D. S. (1978a). *Clin. chim. Acta.* **89**, 455.

Nargessi, R. D., Landon, J. and Smith, D. S. (1978b). *Clin. chim. Acta.* **89**, 461.

Nargessi, R. D., Landon, J. and Smith, D. S. (1978c). *J. immunol. Methods*, **26**, 307.

Neurath, A. R. (1965). *Z. Naturf.* **206**, 974.

Newmark, P. A. and Gordan, Y. B. (1974). *Br. med. Bull.* **30**, 86.

Nye, L., Forrest, G. C., Greenwood, H., Gardner, J. S., Jay, R., Roberts, J. R. and Landon, J. (1976). *Clin. chim. Acta*, **69**, 387.

Nye, L., Anderson, M. J., Dawes, C., Landon, J. and Forrest, G. C. (1978). *Clin. chim. Acta*, **87**, 307.

Painter, K. and Hasler, M. J. (1976). *Clin. Chem.* **22**, 1164.

Parker, M. L., Mariz, I. K., Daughaday, W. H. (1964). *J. clin. Endocr.* **24**, 994.

Pollard, A. and Waldron, C. B. (1966). *In* "Automation in Analytical Chemistry", Vol. 1, p. 49. Technicon Symposia, Mediad, New York.

Portman, A. J., Levison, S. A. and Dandliker, W. B. (1975). *Immunochemistry*, **12**, 461.

Prader, A., Wagner, H., Szeky, J., Illig, R., Touber, J. L., Maingay, D. (1964). *Lancet*, **ii**, 378.

Ratcliffe, J. G. (1974). *Br. med. Bull.* **30**, 32.

Readhead, C., Addison, G. M., Hales, C. N. and Lehmann, H. (1973). *J. Endoc.* **39**, 313.

Reese, M. G. and Johnson, L. R. (1978). *Clin. Chem.* **24**, 342.

Ritchie, R. F. (1975). *Fed. Proc.* **34**, 2139..

Rodbard, D. and Weiss, G. H. (1973). *Anal. Biochem.* **52**, 10.

Rubenstein, K. E., Schneider, R. S. and Ullman, E. F. (1972). *Biochem. biophys. Res. Comm.* **47**, 846.

Scharpe, S. L., Cooreman, W. M., Bloome, W. J. and Lackeman, G. M. (1976). *Clin. Chem.* **22**, 733.

Schneider, R. S., Lindquist, P., Wong, E. T., Rubenstein, K. E. and Ullman, E. F. (1973). *Clin. Chem.* **19**, 821.

Schroeder, H. R., Carrico, R. J., Boguslaski, R. C. and Christner, J. E. (1976). *Anal. Biochem.* **72**, 283.

Seitz, W. R. and Neary, M. P. (1974). *Anal. Chem.* **46**, 188.

Shaw, E. J., Watson, R. A. A. and Smith, D. S. (1977a). *Eur. J. Drug metab. Pharmacokin*, **4**, 191.

Shaw, E. J., Watson, R. A. A., Landon, J. and Smith, D. S. (1977b). *J. clin. Path.* **30**, 526.

Shaw, E. J., Watson, R. A. A. and Smith, D. S. (1976). *In* "Rapid Methods and Automation in Microbiology" (H. H. Johnston and S. W. B. Newsom, eds), p. 78. Learned Information, Oxford.

Smith, D. S. (1977). *FEBS Lett.* **77**, 25.

Spencer, R. D., Toledo, F. B., Williams, B. T. and Yoss, N. L. (1973). *Clin. Chem.* **19**, 838.

Stavitsky, A. B. and Arquilla, E. R. (1953). *Fed. Proc.* **12**, 461.

Stimson, W. and Sinclair, J. (1974). *FEBS Lett.* **47**, 190.

Taussig, M. J. (1970). *Immunology*, **18**, 323.

Tengerdy, R. P. (1963). *Anal. Chem.* **35**, 1084.

Tengerdy, R. P. (1965). *J. Lab. clin. Med.* **65**, 859.

Tengerdy, R. P. (1967). *J. Lab. clin. Med.* **70**, 707.

Toussaint, A. J. and Anderson, R. I. (1965). *Appl. Microbiol.* **13**, 552.

Ullman, E. F., Blackemore, J., Leute, R. K., Eimstad, W. and Jaklitsch, A. (1975). *Clin. Chem.* **21**, 1011.

Ullman, E. F., Schwarzberg, M. and Rubenstein, K. E. (1976). *J. biol. Chem.* **251**, 4172.

Ullman, E. F. (1978). *Clin. Chem.* **24**, 973.

van Weeman, B. K. and Schuurs, A. H. W. M. (1971a). *FEBS Lett.* **15**, 232.

van Weeman, B. K. and Schuurs, A. H. W. M. (1971b). *FEBS Lett.* **24**, 77.

van Weeman, B. K. and Schuurs, A. H. W. M. (1974). *FEBS Lett.* **43**, 215.

Velan, B. and Halmann, M. (1978). *Immunochemistry*, **15**, 331.

Voller, A., Bidwell, D. E. and Bartlett, A. (1976). *In* "Manual of Clinical Immunology (N. Rose and H. Feldman, eds), p. 506. American Society for Microbiology.

Voss, E. W., Eschenfeldt, W. and Root, R. T. (1976). *Immunochemistry*, **13**, 447.

Watson, R. A. A., Landon, J., Shaw, E. J. and Smith, D. S. (1976). *Clin. chim. Acta*, **73**, 51.

Wide, L., Bennich, H. and Johansson, S. G. O. (1967). *Lancet*, **ii**, 1105.

Wilson, B. W., Snedden, W. and Parker, R. B. (1976). *Adv. mass Spec. biochem. Med.* **11**, 487.

Wisdom, G. B. (1976). *Clin. Chem.* **22**, 1243.

Wolters, G., Kuijpers, L., Kacaki, J. and Schuurs, A. (1976). *J. clin. Path.* **29**, 873.

Yalow, R. S. and Berson, S. A. (1960). *J. clin. Invest.* **39**, 1157.

II. High Performance Liquid Chromatography

C. K. LIM

INTRODUCTION

High performance liquid chromatography (HPLC) permits separation, detection and estimation with great efficiency of substances insufficiently stable for gas–liquid chromatography (GLC) without the need for transformation into a volatile derivative. Its theoretical efficiency is equalled only by the capillary GLC column. GLC has great sensitivity when used with appropriate detectors but the usual necessity of preparing a volatile derivative suggests that when equally sensitive detectors are available for HPLC, this technique will be more widely used than GLC and the existence of many unsuspected isomers of hormones and their metabolites may well be demonstrated. At present GLC has the great advantage that it can be linked on-line with the mass spectrometer (MS), while HPLC-MS is still essentially at the development stage.

The high resolving power of HPLC and its applicability without derivatisation suggest that its wide use in endocrinology is almost certain whether linked on-line or not with a mass spectrometer.

A. BASIC EQUIPMENT

An HPLC system consists of a reservoir (or reservoirs for gradient elution), a filter, a high pressure pump, a column with an injection unit through which samples are injected into the top of the column, and a suitable detector.

1. Pumps

Pumps are either gas displacement or mechanical with pulse suppression. Many commercial pumps are available and it is important to ensure reliability, freedom from pulsation, and accurately controllable constant flow rate. The requirements for the basic parts of an HPLC system have been reviewed by McNair and Chandler (1976) who also listed the features and specifications of instruments supplied by various manufacturers.

2. Injectors

Sample injection may be by septum or by loop or valves. Minimum band spreading is obtained with on column injection through a septum (Smuts, Solms, Von Niekerk and Pretorius, 1969; Henry, 1971), which, however, has disadvantages compared with a loop or valve in requiring regular replacement, leakage at high pressure and blockage due to septum particles falling on to the column inlet. Sample loop or valve also allow more precise sample injection in quantitative analysis.

3. Detectors

Detectors usually depend on refractivity (of no value with gradient elution) or visible and/or ultraviolet spectrometry, preferably with variable wavelength, although the major mercury emission line at 254 nm is of such high energy that this may be used for the detection of many substances with an absorption maximum considerably removed from this wavelength. Fluorimetric and electrochemical detection (Kissinger, Lawrence, Riggin, Pachla and Wenke, 1974; Fleet and Little, 1974; Kissinger, 1977; Bollet, Oliva and Caude, 1978) are also widely used while flame ionisation (Scott and Lawrence, 1969; Privett and Erdahl, 1978), electron capture (Willmott and Dolphin, 1974), spray impact (Mowery and Juvet, 1974), catalytic (Nachtmann, Knapp and Spitzy, 1978), photochemical (Twitchett, Williams and Moffat, 1978) and photodiode array (Dessy, Nunn, Titus and Reynolds, 1976; Milano, Lam and Grushka, 1976; Milano and Grushka, 1977; Milano, Lam, Savonis, Pautler, Pav and Grushka, 1978) detectors are either available or in course of development. Apart from such detectors, separate fractions may be collected and analysed by any of the conventional detection methods such as colorimetry, competitive protein-binding (Butler, Fantl and Lim, 1976), radioimmuno- or immunoassay (Mee and Smith, 1976; Twitchett, Gorvin, Moffat, Williams and Sullivan, 1976). On-line post-column reaction systems can also be used in combination with spectrophotometry, fluorimetry (Udenfriend, Stein, Bohlen, Dairman, Leingruber and Weizele, 1972; Roth and Hampai, 1973; Katz and Pitt, 1972; Muusze and Huber, 1974; van der Wal and Huber, 1977b) or electrochemical detection (Takata and Muto, 1973) to improve sensitivity and specificity.

A potentially important detector for HPLC is the mass spectrometer. Although HPLC-MS systems are now commercially available their applications are still limited. One such interface introduced the HPLC effluent into the mass spectrometer via a moving endless thin ribbon (McFadden, 1977). A liquid chromatography–chemical ionisation quadrupole system has been developed (Arpino, Colin and Guiochon, 1977) and the use of laser vaporisation and molecular beam techniques for rapid heating and reducing contact of a non-volatile solute with solid surfaces has been described (McAdams, Blakley and Vestal, 1977).

B. COLUMN PACKINGS

The practical aspects of HPLC theory have been admirably reviewed by Knox (1977) who describes the derivation of column efficiency in terms of reduced plate height. He also defines the requirements for optimum performance in terms of the infinite diameter principle. To prevent wall effects HPLC columns must have a particular relationship between length and diameter. With current HPLC systems which use 8 μl flow cell and 10–20 μl injections a minimum of 5 mm in ID and 100 mm in length is required for highest column performance.

Column packings of particle size ranging from 5–40 μm diameter are either pellicular consisting of a thin porous outer layer on a solid glass bead or are totally porous. Analytical separations are best performed with pellicular packings which equilibrate at a moderate rate but have a low sample capacity, while in preparative separations, large particle porous packings are used because of the high sample capacity although they equilibrate more slowly. Microparticulate packings (5–10 μm) which equilibrate rapidly and have high sample capacity, are of general use; pellicular packings are mainly used as guard or pre-columns for preliminary sample clean up.

HPLC packings, extensively reviewed by Majors (1977a) may be classified as adsorption (liquid–solid), partition (liquid-liquid and bonded phase), ion-exchange, molecular size or steric exclusion (gel permeation). Some examples of the more commonly used bonded phase column packings make use of:

(i) Alkylamines, especially aminopropylsilane acting as normal phase, or weak anion exchange;

(ii) octadecylsilanes (ODS) for reverse phase or for ion-pairs (see below);

(iii) cyanopropylsilane for reverse-phase or normal phase and of intermediate polarity;

(iv) tetra-alkylamino ($-N^+R_3$) and sulphonic acid (SO_3^-) groups bonded to silica for anion or cation exchanges respectively.

(v) silica gel bonded in various ways for gel permeation or molecular size (steric) exclusion chromatography;

(vi) specially designed packing, e.g. μ-Bondapak-carbohydrate are specially suitable for separating carbohydrates, sugars and other polyhydroxy compounds, and μ-Bondapak-fatty acid for fatty acid analysis.

Bonded phase packings of these types will continue to be developed for specific analyses. However, unlike GLC, the mobile phase in HPLC is an important parameter in developing a separation. By adjusting the chemical composition of the mobile phase, a wide variety of compounds can be separated using the same bonded phase column. This will probably tend to limit the needs for numerous bonded phase packings.

1. Adsorption

Adsorption packings may be acidic, such as silica or florisil, and selectively adsorb basic solutes, e.g. those bearing amino groups. Basic adsorption packings, such as alumina, retain acidic components such as phenols. Such packings are used for unionised compounds soluble in organic solvents of molecular weight 100–2000 which are eluted in order of increasing polarity (Snyder, 1968; Snyder and Kirkland, 1974); they have been of value in separating isomeric substances differing in their stereochemistry or containing different functional groups or different numbers of functional groups. The comparative performances of spherical and angular silica and alumina in the 1–10 μm size range have been studied by Unger, Messer and Krebs (1978).

2. Partition

The earlier partition packings consisted of a liquid layer coated on solid particles but are usually unstable because of gradual bleeding of the stationary phase; most partition columns now consist of an organic stationary phase, chemically bonded to a solid supporting material usually silica. According to the polarity of the stationary phase, partition packings may be normal phase (polar stationary phase, non-polar mobile phase) or reverse-phase (non-polar stationary phase, polar mobile phase).

Partition chromatography may be used for compounds which are capable of being distributed between the stationary and mobile phases. Since the degree of retention of a compound in the column is primarily a function of the distribution coefficient, compounds of widely different absolute solubility may be chromatographed under similar conditions.

Reverse-phase chromatography is one of the most widely used forms of HPLC techniques because of its versatility and simplicity. The theory and practice of reverse-phase HPLC has been reviewed (Horvath and Melander, 1977; Colin and Guiochon, 1977). A comparison of chromatographic behaviours (Hemetsberger, Maasfed and Ricken, 1976) and analytical properties (Colin, Ward and Guiochon, 1978) of different types of reverse-phase packings have been described.

3. Ion-exchange

Ionisable compounds are best separated in the fully ionised form by either ion-exchange or ion-pair chromatography. Resolution is influenced by pH of the eluent which affects selectivity and ionic strength which influences total retention.

Apart from the commonly used tetra-alkylamino and sulphonic acid types of bonded phase ion-exchange silica, a new class of bonded exchangers obtained by reacting vinylmethoxysilane with silica have been made and evaluated (Lefevre, Divry, Caude and Rosset, 1975; Gareil, Heritier, Caude and Rosset, 1976; Caude and Rosset, 1977). A bonded phase anion-exchanger made by reacting aminopropyltriethyloxysilane with silica was reported to be good for carbohydrate separation (Schwarzenbad, 1976). The properties and chromatographic behaviours of chemically bonded ion-exchangers have been studied by Asmus, Low and Novotny (1976a; 1976b).

4. Steric Exclusion

Steric exclusion chromatography is a useful screening technique for a sample of unknown composition or as a prefractionation technique for other HPLC modes. Steric exclusion chromatography has been reviewed (Vivilecchia, Lightbody, Thimot and Quinn, 1977; Gaylor and James, 1978) and its application to small molecule separation has also been discussed (Krishen, 1977).

C. SOLVENT SELECTION

The choice of a solvent system for separation obviously depends on separation technique, i.e. adsorption, partition, ion-exchange and ion-pair or steric exclusion, employed. Solvents are chosen to provide adequate resolution with convenient retention times.

The retention characteristics of compounds in HPLC depend not only on the column packings (stationary phase) but also the chemical composition of the mobile phase. Selectivity is determined by the interactions between solute–solvent, solute–stationary phase and solvent–stationary phase. The ability to manipulate these parameters allows the development and optimisation of HPLC separations. The general subject of phase systems and solvent effects in adsorption, partition and ion-exchange chromatography has been described by Unger (1975).

1. Adsorption

In adsorption chromatography, solutes and solvents compete for adsorption sites on the surface of the solid. Mobile phases in adsorption chromatography are typically binary systems of a non-polar major component such as heptane or dichloromethane and a polar minor component (modifying solvent). The modifiers, commonly alcohols, acetonitrile, dimethylsulphoxide or water, do not normally exceed 5% (v/v) of the solvent system and are partly adsorbed on the column support and therefore alter its activity. By varying the amount of modifier, the retention power of the column can be controlled. The most commonly used solvent-pairs for adsorption chromatography are n-heptane:isopropanol and dichloromethane:ethanol. Ternary mixtures such as hexane:dichloromethane:methanol and dichloromethane:ethanol:water have also been widely used.

When a solvent system containing water is used, the water content of the mobile and of stationary phases has to be strictly controlled (Boehme and Engelhardt, 1977; Thomas, Brun and Bounine, 1977) as the capacity factors and selectivity of the different solutes are influenced by a slight change of water content (Engelhardt, 1977; Thomas, Caude, Brun and Bounine, 1977). The effects and influence of mobile phase composition on silica were studied by Golkiewicz (1976), Saunders (1977), Siouffi, Guillemonat and Guiochon (1977) and Paanakker, Kraak and Poppe (1978).

The systematic design of binary solvent systems for adsorption chromatography on silica gel has been studied using the retention behaviour of steroids (Hara, Fuju, Hirasawa and Miyamoto, 1978). The nature of solute–solvent interaction on the silica gel surface has been examined by Scott and Kucera (1978).

2. Partition

In partition chromatography, the mobile phases are again usually binary systems in which the compound to be separated is sparingly soluble in the primary solvent, retention being modified by addition of a good solvent for the sample. Optimum resolution is obtained when the correct balance of the two solvents is used, excess modifying solvent will cause too rapid elution and excess primary solvent too much retention. Typical solvent pairs for normal phase partition chromatography are hexane–dichloromethane or chloroform or dichloromethane–methanol. For reverse-phase, an aqueous based solvent system is used, usually water mixed with acetonitrile or methanol. Weak acids and bases can be separated by reverse-phase and ion-suppression, i.e. elution with basic eluents for basic and acid eluents for acids; the tailing or broadening of peaks due to the tendency of weak acids or bases to dissociate when performing reverse-phase partition chromatography can therefore often be corrected by adding a small quantity of acetic acid or ammonia solution to suppress ionisation of the compounds being separated.

The roles and effects of solvents in reverse-phase chromatography have been studied by Locke (1974), Karger, Gant, Hartkopf and Weiner (1976), Tanaka and Thornton (1977), Horvath, Melander and Molnar (1976), Horvath and Melander (1977), and Horvath, Melander and Molnar (1977).

3. Ion-exchange

Modern bonded phase ion-exchange chromatography probably involves adsorption and partition, as well as true ion-exchange, since the retention of a sample often cannot be explained by the ion-exchange mechanism alone, making the chromatographic behaviour difficult to predict. The most commonly used solvent systems are acetate and phosphate buffers between the pH limits in which a bonded ion-exchange silica column is stable (*ca* 2·4–7·9).

4. Ion-pair

Ion-pair chromatography combines ion-exchange and partition chromatography and it is especially useful for separating ionisable organic compounds. It allows simultaneous separation of acids, bases and neutral compounds, an advantage over ion-exchange chromatography. In normal phase ion-pair chromatography (Crommen, Fransson and Schill, 1977; Knox and Jurand, 1976; Persson and Lagerstrom, 1976; Terweij-Groen and Kraak, 1977) the solute ions are distributed between a non-polar organic mobile phase and a polar hydrophobic stationary liquid phase on a suitable matrix. The stationary phase carries a counter-ion (usually perchlorate) for bases, and a quaternary amine for acids.

In reverse-phase ion-pair chromatography (Wittmer, Nuessle and Haney, 1975; Knox and Laird, 1976; Wahlund and Lund, 1976) a permanently bonded non-polar stationary phase, normally ODS is used, the mobile phase usually containing not more than 0·005 M counter-ion, often long chain alkyl sulphonates, acetyl trimethylammonium or tetrabutylammonium ion. The retention of a solute is affected by the concentration of the ion-pairing reagent (Knox and Laird, 1976) and maximum retention is obtained when an optimum concentration of the counter-ion is used. The practical aspects of reverse-phase ion-pair chromatography have been reviewed by Gloor and Johnson (1977).

5. Steric Exclusion

Solvent selection is easier in steric exclusion chromatography since only a single solvent in which to dissolve and run the sample is used. Modern bonded phase steric exclusion packings are compatible with both organic and aqueous solvents.

D. GRADIENT ELUTION

In liquid-chromatography the retention of samples greatly depends on the composition of the solvent system. In the applications of HPLC to the separation of complex mixtures, especially those containing widely dissimilar components or polarities, it is necessary to change the composition of the mobile phase in order to elute all of the components present in the sample satisfactorily from the column. In these cases gradient elution may be applied. The rational selection of an optimum gradient in reverse-phase liquid-chromatography has been discussed (Schoenmakers, Billiet, Tijssen and Galan, 1978). Gradient elution, however, is inconvenient when repetitive analysis is required because of the long time for equilibration after each run.

In gradient elution, the mixing of two different solvents, especially those of different viscosities, may cause concentration instabilities and oscillations (Helmer, 1977) and care must be taken against false peaks in an ultraviolet detector produced by rapid changes in solvent composition (Jandera, Janderova and Churacek, 1975; Berek, Bleha and Pevna, 1976).

E. COLUMN SWITCHING

An alternative to gradient elution is the column switching technique (Huber, Van der Linden, Ecker and Oreans, 1973; Huber and Vodenik, 1976; Huber and Eisenbeiss, 1978) in which part of the chromatogram from the first column is diverted before detection to a second column by means of a switching valve for further resolution. The second column is often one with higher resolving power or having a high loading of stationary phase or surface area to increase the capacity although columns of entirely different packing materials have been used (Johnson, Gloor and Majors, 1978). The schematic diagram of column switching system is shown:

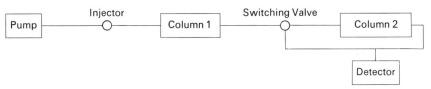

Column switching has the advantages over gradient elution in that it is cheaper and usually operates with a mobile phase of constant composition and is thus compatible with all types of HPLC detectors. The analysis time is also shorter as no re-equilibration of column is required and the strongly retained solutes travel only along a short length of column.

F. COLUMN PACKING TECHNIQUES

Pellicular and large particle size packings (30–40 µm) can be dry packed. Special packing techniques, however, are required for microparticulates, the most widely used being the slurry method. The density of the suspending solvent may be slightly less than that of the packing (balanced density) or much less (non-balanced density). Typical balanced density slurry solvents are tetrabromoethane (Majors, 1972), tetrachloroethylene (Cassidy, Legal and Frei, 1974) and diiodomethane (Strubert, 1973). For non-balanced density packing, carbon tetrachloride (Coq, Gonnett and Rocca, 1975; Webber and McKerrell, 1976), methanol (Webber and McKerrell, 1976; Bather and Gray, 1976), acetone (Cox, Luscombe, Slucutt, Sudgen and Upfield, 1976), isopropanol (Chang, Gooding and Regnier, 1976b), dioxane-methanol (Linder, Keller and Frei, 1976), tetrahydrofuran-water (Little, Dale, Ord and Marten, 1977) and chloroform-methanol (Kirkland and Antle, 1977) had been used. Upward slurry packing has been found to be advantageous (Bristow, Brittain, Riley and Williamson, 1977) and other techniques have also been investigated (Bar, Caude and Rosset, 1976; Linder, Keller and Frei, 1976; Martin and Guiochon, 1977; Keller, Erni, Linder and Frei, 1977). In the slurry method of column packing a high pressure, high flow rate pump must be used to transfer the slurry from the reservoir into the column to prevent sedimentation and to fill the column rapidly. The general subject of column packing techniques has been reviewed (Majors, 1977b; Martin and Guiochon, 1977; Bristow, 1976).

G. SAMPLE PREPARATION

The analysis of hormones and their metabolites in blood often presents technical difficulties. Small sample size and the presence of substances that interfere with the analysis are the two major problems. A good sample preparation procedure not only minimises quantitative errors but also prolongs the life of the column. Soluble protein, present in large quantities in human serum or plasma, must be removed before analysis by HPLC. The following methods have been used.

1. Ultrafiltration

This is done by centrifugation in a membrane cone or by filtration under pressure using an ultrafiltration cell. This method removes proteins but not other interfering substances.

2. Precipitation

Protein precipitation can be effected by trichloroacetic acid, perchloric acid, ammonium sulphate, alcohols, chloroform, acetone, heavy metals or heat followed by filtration or centrifugation. These methods, however, may not remove proteins completely and coprecipitation of the substance to be estimated with proteins is also a problem.

3. Solvent Extraction

Hormones which have a favourable partition coefficient can be selectively extracted with organic solvents. For compounds which are insoluble in organic solvents derivatives which are soluble in organic solvents can be prepared before solvent extraction. However, derivatisation often leads to loss of materials which is already present in small quantities and multiple products may be formed. For ionic compounds ion-pair formation followed by solvent extraction can be useful.

4. Column Chromatography

Selective adsorption of hormones on to silica, alumina, Amberlite XAD and ion-exchange resins, are useful for compounds that are poorly soluble in organic solvents. Ion-exchange resins are particularly useful when ionic compounds are analysed. They not only allow sample concentration on the column but also effect a partial sample clean-up. Anion-exchange resin can thus be used to remove proteins, neutral and cationic compounds and cation-exchange resin removes proteins, neutral and anionic compounds. However, this method may need an extra concentration step.

5. Pre-column

In addition to the above methods of sample preparation a pre-column is often used to protect the analytical column from irreversible adsorption or blockage. Pre-columns are usually 5 mm in length and are packed with materials similar to that used in the analytical column. However, pellicular packings which are cheaper and can be dry packed are used to protect microparticulate analytical columns. It is sometimes necessary to inject plasma or serum directly because the compound to be analysed is unstable or because there is no effective sample preparation procedures. In these cases the use of a pre-column is essential.

H. APPLICATION OF HPLC IN HORMONE ANALYSIS

Apart from the polypeptide hormones the majority of hormones and their metabolites have been analysed by HPLC; catecholamine and steroids have been extensively studied. For hormones which cannot be detected by any of the common HPLC detectors described above, e.g. prostaglandins and steroids with no ultraviolet absorbance, pre-column derivation (Ross, 1977; Masanobu and Keihei, 1977; Frei, 1977) with introduction of ultraviolet absorbing or fluorescent groups followed by ultraviolet or fluorimetric detection, is often used.

1. Catecholamines

The most promising method of analysing catecholamines and their metabolites seemed to be bonded-phase cation-exchange or ion-pair chromatography with electrochemical detection. Improved resolution of catecholamines and their metabolites can be obtained using the ion-pair technique with the electrochemical detector providing sensitive and specific detection. Recent work on the HPLC separation of catecholamines and their metabolites is summarised in Table 1.

2. Iodine-containing Hormones

Little has been done in the application of HPLC to the analysis of iodine-containing hormones. Detection and sample preparation are the two major problems. The thyroid hormones tend to adhere strongly to glass and other solids especially when present in low concentrations. This makes extraction from serum difficult. Although it may be possible to detect serum levels of thyroxine (T_4) with an ultraviolet detector, the detection of triiodothyronine (T_3) and reversed-triiodothyronine (rT_3) require detectors of higher sensitivity. Karger, Su, Marchese and Persson (1974) reported the separation of mixtures of pure thyroid hormones by normal phase ion-pair chromatography using n-butanol-dichloromethane (15:85 v/v) as the mobile phase and silica supporting 40% by weight of 0.2 M $HClO_4$–0.8 M $NaClO_4$ as the stationary phase. Nachtman, Knapp and Spitzy (1978) determined plasma T_4 and T_3 by reverse-phase chromatography using water-acetonitrile (5:2) with 1% of acetic acid as the eluent. A post-column catalytic detection system was used and sub-nanogram of the hormones could be detected. The hormones can also be separated by reverse-phase ion-pair chromatography (Fig. 1).

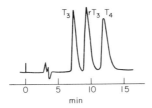

Fig. 1. Separation of T_3, rT_3 and T_4. Conditions: column, partisil—10 ODS; solvent, 0·005M pentane sulphonic acid—acetonitrile (65:35 v/v); detection, UV 230 nm; flow rate, 1 ml/min.

3. Peptide Hormones

The possibility of analysing peptide hormones is well illustrated by a number of recent publications on the use of HPLC for the separation of polypeptides and proteins. Small peptides were easily separable by reverse-phase chromatography using either acetonitrile–water or methanol–water as the eluents (Hansen, Greibrokk, Currie, Nils-Gunner Johansson and Folkers, 1977; Hancock, Bishop and Hearn, 1976), while polypeptides usually require the presence of a buffer or surfactant for satisfactory resolution (Krummen and Frei, 1977; Molnar and Horvath, 1977). Moench and Dehnen (1977, 1978) developed a gradient system for the separation of polypeptides and proteins of mw <450,000 on an ODS column using 0·05 M KH_2PO_4-2-methoxyethanol (95:5, pH 2) and isopropanol-2-methoxyethanol (95:5, pH 2) as the elution mixtures. The separation of eight model proteins, including insulin, were demonstrated. New polar bonded phases, the glycophases, which have a combination of high permeability and mechanical rigidity, have been developed and shown to be useful for the separation of proteins (Regnier and Noel, 1976; Chang, Noel and Regnier, 1976; Chang, Gooding and Regnier, 1976a, b).

4. Prostaglandins

The analysis of prostaglandins have already been discussed (see Vol 2, Ch. VI). To overcome detection problems most workers separated prostaglandins as their p-nitrophenacyl esters with strong ultraviolet absorption (Morozowich and Douglas, 1975; Fitzpatrick, 1976; Merritt and Bronson, 1976,

Table 1

HPLC of catecholamines.

Compounds	Stationary phase	Mobile phase	Detector	References
Dopamine, noradrenaline	Cation exchange	$0.1M$ $HClO_4$: $0.01M$ $NaHSO_3$	Electrochemical	Refshauge, Kissinger, Dreiling, Blank, Freeman and Adams (1974)
Dopamine	Cation exchange	$0.01M$ H_2SO_4 : $0.04M$ Na_2SO_4	Electrochemical	Riggin, Alcorn and Kissinger (1976)
Dopamine, noradrenaline, 6-hydroxydopamine	Cation exchange	$0.1M$ $HClO_4$	Dual electrochemical	Blank (1976)
Dopamine, noradrenaline	Cation exchange (pellicular)	Acetate-citrate buffer pH 5.2	Electrochemical	Keller, Oke, Mefford and Adams (1976)
Dopamine, serotonin	Cation exchange	Acetate-citrate buffer pH 5.1	Electrochemical	Sasa and Blank (1977)
Dopamine, noradrenaline	Reverse-phase ODS (reverse-phase ion-pair chromatography)	Phosphate-citrate buffer + sodium octylsulphate, pH 3.25	Electrochemical	Kissinger, Bruntlett, Davis, Felice, Riggin and Shoup (1977)
Catecholamines and metabolites	Cation exchange	$0.1M$ $HClO_4$	Electrochemical	Borchardt, Hegazi and Schowen (1978)
Catecholamines and metabolites	Reverse-phase ODS	Phosphate buffer	Ultraviolet	Molnar and Horvath (1976)
Catecholamines and metabolites	Reverse-phase ODS/ TMS (reverse-phase ion-pair)	$CH_3CN:H_2O:H_2SO_4$ + sodium dodecane sulphonic acid $CH_3CN:H_2O:H_2SO_4$ + sodium lauryl sulphate	Ultraviolet	Jurand (1976)

Compound	Column/Phase	Mobile phase	Detection	Reference
Catecholamine and metabolites	Alumina (adsorption) / Silica (loaded with 0·1M $HClO_4$ and 0·9M $NaClO_4$ for normal phase ion-pair chromatography)	Butanol:acetic acid:water butanol acetic acid:diethylether:water / Butanol:methylene chloride	Ultraviolet	Knox and Jurand (1976).
Dopamine, noradrenaline	Reverse-phase ODS	Acetic acid (0·17M)	Ultraviolet	Mell and Gustafson (1977)
Adrenaline	Cation exchange	0·05M KH_2SO_4, pH 4·5	Ultraviolet	Fu and Sibley (1977)
Adrenaline, noradrenaline, dopamine	Cation exchange	Ammonium phosphate containing 1% acetonitrile, pH 8·5	Ultraviolet	Klaniecki, Corder, McDonald and Feldman (1977)
Noradrenaline (O-phthalaldehyde derivative prepared)	Reverse-phase ODS	Methanol:0·08M acetic acid (50:50)	Ultraviolet fluoroscent	Mell and Dasler (1978)
Dopamine, adrenaline, noradrenaline	Cation exchange Reverse-phase ODS	Formate buffer	Post column reactor and fluorescent	Schwedt (1977a; 1977b; 1977c)
Dopamine, adrenaline, noradrenaline (dansyl derivatives prepared)	Silica Reverse-phase ODS	Ethyl acetate:cyclohexane (3:2) Acetonitrile:water (65:35) Methanol:water (72:28)	Fluorescent	Schwedt and Busseman (1977)
Dopamine, noradrenaline (fluorescamine derivatives prepared)	TSK gel 160 (glycol-type gel)	Methanol:0·5M Tris-hydrochloric acid buffer (pH 8·0) containing 10 μg/ml EDTA and 20 μg/ml ascorbic acid	Fluorescent	Imai, Tsukamoto and Tamura (1977)

Table 2

HPLC of steroids.

Compounds	Stationary phase	Mobile phase	Detector	References
Cortisol	Bonded silica-nucleosil NO_2	CH_2Cl_2:iso-PrOH:H_2O (97·5:2·3:0·2)	Ultraviolet	Van Den Berg, Mol, Deelder and Thijssen (1977)
Corticosteroids	Permaphase ETH	Hexane:chloroform linear gradient	Radioimmunoassay	Saito, Hashita, Miyamoto and Takeda (1977)
Cortisol	Silica	MeOH:H_2O:EtOH:CH_2Cl_2 (5:12:20:963)	Ultraviolet	Matsuzawa, Kato, Masahiko, Sekiguetu and Ishiguro (1977)
Cortisol	Silica	1·5% MeOH and 0·2% H_2O in $CHCl_3$	Ultraviolet	Schwedt, Bussemas and Lippmann (1977)
Corticosteroids	Silica	HOAc:EtOH:CH_2Cl_2:hexane (0·2:3·5:20:66·3)	Ultraviolet	Loo and Jordan (1977)
Corticosteroids	Reverse-phase ODS	Acetonitrile:water, methanol: water, solvent programming	Ultraviolet	Tymes (1977)
Aldosterone	Silica	1·5% methanol in chloroform half saturated with water	Ultraviolet	De Vries, Popp-Snijder, De Kieviet and Akkerman-Faber (1977)
Androgens Oestrogens	Silica Reverse-phase ODS	Chloroform:isooctane (6:4) Acetonitrile:water 4:6)	Ultraviolet	Satyaswaroop, Lopez de la Osa and Gurpide (1977)
Prednisolone	Silica	0·2% HOAc:6% EtOH:30% CH_2Cl_2 in hexane	Ultraviolet	Loo, Butterfield, Moffatt and Jordan (1977)

Application	Stationary phase	Mobile phase	Detection	Reference
18-Hydroxydeoxy-corticosterone, corticosterone	Bondapak phenyl/porasil B	Acetonitrile:water (30:70)	Ultraviolet	Chan, Moreland, Hum and Birmingham (1977)
General, most steroids	Silica Reverse-phase ODS	n-Hexane:ethyl acetate; n-hexane:diethyl ether; n-hexane:isopropanol Methanol:water; acetonitrile:water	Ultraviolet and refractiometer	Hara and Hayashi (1977)
Oestrone, oestradiol oestriol	Silica Reverse-phase ODS	5% ethanol in n-hexane Methanol:0.1% ammonium carbonate (55:45)	Ultraviolet	Dolphin and Pergande (1977).
17-Ketosteroids, sulphates and glucuronides	Reverse-phase (ODS)	Methanol:water (49.4:50.6)	Refractometer	Lafosse, Keravis and Durand (1976)
Free and conjugated steroid hormones	Reverse-phase ODS	Methanol:water	Refractometer and ultraviolet	Keravis, Lafosse and Durand (1977)
Oestrogen sulphates	Silica loaded with 0.1M tetra-ethylammonium	Dichloromethane:pentanol (9:1)	Ultraviolet	Fransson, Wahlund, Johansson and Schill (1976)
Oestrogen sulphates and glucuronides	Anion-exchange cellulose-diatomite: anion-exchange cellulose	0.025M perchlorate + 0.01M phosphate; 0.025M perchlorate + 0.0125M phosphate	Ultraviolet	Van der Wal and Huber (1977a; 1977b)
Oestrogen sulphate and glucuronides	Comparative study of a wide range of stationary phases		Ultraviolet	Van der Wal and Huber (1978)

1977) on silica or reverse-phase (ODS) columns. Fitzpatrick, Wynalda and Kaiser (1977) also described the use of p-nitrobenzyloximes of prostaglandin esters for ultraviolet detection. Silver ion-loaded cation exchange resin has been used to improve resolution of closely related prostaglandins (Merritt and Bronson, 1976, 1977).

5. Steroids

HPLC has been widely used for the analysis of steroids particularly those which absorb ultraviolet light. Recent publications on HPLC separation of steroid hormones and their conjugates are summarised in Table 2.

CONCLUSION

The literature reviewed here is that thought to be most useful in the application of HPLC to hormone analysis. Although the detection of some hormones in blood is still a problem, sensitive detectors for specific groups of hormones are available, e.g. electrochemical detector for catecholamine and catalytic detection for iodine-containing hormones. Detection systems suitable for other hormones will undoubtedly be developed and these, with modern high efficiency columns, will greatly extend the application of HPLC to hormone research.

ACKNOWLEDGEMENTS

I thank Professor C. H. Gray, Dr F. L. Mitchell and Dr S. S. Brown for helpful discussion and encouragement.

REFERENCES

Arpino, P. J., Colin, H. and Guiochon, G. (1977). 25th Ann. Conf. Mass Spec. All. Top., Washington DC, p. 377.
Asmus, P. A., Low, C. E. and Novotny, H. (1976a). *J. Chromat.* **119**, 25.
Asmus, P. A., Low, C. E. and Novotny, H. (1976b). *J. Chromat.* **123**, 109.
Bar, D., Cause, M. and Rosset, R. (1976). *Analusis*, **4**, 108.
Bather, J. M. and Gray, R. A. C. (1976). *J. Chromat.* **122**, 159.
Berek, D., Bleha, T. and Pevna, Z. (1976). *J. chromat. Sci.* **14**, 560.
Blank, C. L. (1976). *J. Chromat.* **117**, 35.
Boehme, W. and Engelhardt, H. (1977). *J. Chromat.* **133**, 67.

Bollet, C., Olivia, P. and Caude, M. (1978). *J. Chromat.* **149**, 625.
Borchardt, R. T., Hegazi, M. F. and Schowen, R. L. (1978). *J. Chromat.* **152**, 255.
Bristow, P. A. (1976). Lig. Chromatogr. in Practice, hetp, Handforth, U.K., p. 32.
Bristow, P. A., Brittain, P. N., Riley, C. M. and Williamson, B. F. (1977). *J. Chromat.* **131**, 57.
Butler, J., Fantl, V. and Lim, C. K. (1976). *In* "High Pressure Liquid Chromatography in Clinical Chemistry" (P. F. Dixon, C. H. Gray, C. K. Lim and M. S. Stoll, eds), p. 59. Academic Press, London and New York.
Cassidy, R. M., Legal, D. S. and Frei, R. W. (1974). *Anal. Chem.* **46**, 340.
Caude, M. and Rosset, R. (1977). *J. chromat. Sci.* **15**, 405.
Chan, T. H., Moreland, M., Hum, W. T. and Birmingham, M. K. (1977). *J. Steroid Biochem.* **8**, 243.
Chang, S. H., Noel, R. and Regnier, F. E. (1976). *Anal. Chem.* **48**, 1839.
Chang, S. H., Gooding, K. M. and Regnier, F. E. (1976a). *J. Chromat.* **120**, 321.
Chang, S. H., Gooding, K. M. and Regnier, F. E. (1976b). *J. Chromat.* **125**, 103.
Colin, H. and Guiochon, G. (1977). *J. Chromat.* **141**, 289.
Colin, H., Ward, N. and Guiochon, G. (1978). *J. Chromat.* **149**, 169.
Coq, B., Gonnett, C. and Rocca, J. L. (1975). *J. Chromat.* **106**, 249.
Cox, G. B., Luscombe, C. R., Slucutt, M. J., Sudgen, K. and Upfield, J. W. (1976). *J. Chromat.* **117**, 269.
Crommen, J., Fransson, B. and Schill, G. (1977). *J. Chromat.* **142**, 283.
Dessy, R. E., Nunn, W. G., Titus, C. A. and Reynolds, W. R. (1976). *J. chromat. Sci.* **14**, 195.
De Vries, C. P., Popp-Snijders, C., De Kieviet, W. and Akkerman-Faber, A. C. (1977). *J. Chromat.* **143**, 624.
Dolphin, R. J. and Pergande, P. J. (1977). *J. Chromat.* **143**, 267.
Engelhardt, H. (1977). *J. chromat. Sci.* **15**, 380.
Fitzpatrick, F. A. (1976). *Anal. Chem.* **48**, 499.
Fitzpatrick, F. A., Wynalda, M. A. and Kaiser, D. G. (1977). *Anal. Chem.* **49**, 1032.
Fleet, B. and Little, C. J. (1974). *J. chromat. Sci.* **12**, 747.
Fransson, B., Wahlund, K. G., Johansson, J. M. and Schill, G. (1976). *J. Chromat.* **125**, 327.
Frei, R. W. (1977). *Res. Dev.* **28**, 42.
Fu, C. C. and Sibley, M. J. (1977). *J. pharm. Sci.* **66**, 425.
Gariel, P., Heritier, A., Caude, M. and Rosset, R. (1976). *Analusis*, **4**, 71.
Gaylor, V. F. and James, H. L. (1978), *Anal Chem.* **50**, 29R.
Gloor, R. and Johnson, E. L. (1977). *J. chromat. Sci.* **15**, 413.
Golkiewicz, W. (1976). *Chromatographia*, **9**, 113.
Hancock, W. S., Bishop, C. A. and Hearn, M. T. W. (1976). *FEBS Lett.* **72**, 139.
Hansen, J. J., Greibrokk, T., Currie, B. L., Nils-Gunnar Johansson, K. and Falkers, K. (1977). *J. Chromat.* **135**, 155.
Hara, S., Fuju, Y., Hirasawa, M. and Miyamoto, S. (1978). *J. Chromat.* **149**, 143.
Hara, S. and Hayashi, S. (1977). *J. Chromat.* **142**, 689.
Helmer, J. C. (1977). *Anal. Chem.* **48**, 1741.
Hemetsberger, H., Maasfed, W. and Ricken, H. (1976). *Chromatographia*, **7**, 303.
Henry, R. A. (1971). *In* "Modern Practice of Liquid Chromatography" (J. J. Kirklands, eds), Ch 2. Wiley-Interscience, New York.
Horvath, C., Melander, W. and Molnar, I. (1976). *J. Chromat.* **125**, 129.
Horvath, C. and Melander, W. (1977). *J. chromat. Sci.* **15**, 393.
Horvath, C., Melander, W. and Molnar, I. (1977). *Anal. Chem.* **49**, 142.

Huber, J. F. K. and Eisenbeiss, F. (1978). *J. Chromat.* **149**, 127.

Huber, J. F. K., van der Linden, R., Ecker, E. and Oreans, M. (1973). *J. Chromat.* **83**, 267.

Huber, J. F. K. and Vodenik, R. (1976). *J. Chromat.* **122**, 331.

Imai, K., Tsukamoto, M. and Tamura, Z. (1977). *J. Chromat.* **137**, 357.

Jandera, P., Janderova, M. and Churacek, J. (1975). *J. Chromat.* **115**, 9.

Johnson, E. L., Gloor, R. and Majors, R. E. (1978). *J. Chromat.* **149**, 571.

Jurand, J. (1976). *In* "High Pressure Liquid Chromatography in Clinical Chemistry" (P. F. Dixon, C. H. Gray, C. K. Lim and M. S. Stoll, eds,), p. 125. Academic Press, London and New York.

Karger, B. L., Gant, J. R., Hartkopf, A. and Weiner, P. H. (1976). *J. Chromat.* **128**, 65.

Karger, B. L., Su, S. C., Marchese, S. and Persson, B. A. (1974). *J. chromat. Sci* **12**, 678.

Katz, S. and Pitt, Jr. W. W. (1972). *Anal. Lett.* **5**, 177.

Keller, H. P., Erni, F., Linder, H. R. and Frei, R. W. (1977). *Anal. Chem.* **49**, 1958.

Keller, R., Oke, A., Mefford, I. and Adams, R. N. (1976). *Life Sci.* **19**, 995.

Keravis, G., Lafosse, M. and Durand, M. H. (1977). *Chromatographia*, **10**, 678.

Kirkland, J. J. and Antle, P. E. (1977). *J. chromat. Sci.* **15**, 137.

Kissinger, P. T. (1977). *Anal. Chem.* **49**, 447A

Kissinger, P. T., Bruntlett, C. S., Davis, G. C., Felice, L. J., Riggin, R. M. and Shoup, R. E. (1977). *Clin. Chem.* **23**, 1449.

Kissinger, P. T., Lawrence, J. F., Riggin, R. M., Pachla, L. A. and Wenke, D. C. (1974). *Clin. Chem.* **20**, 992.

Klaniecki, T. S., Corder, C. N., McDonald, R. H. Jr. and Feldman, J. A. (1977). *J. Lab. clin. Med.* **90**, 604.

Knox, J. H. (1977). *J. chromat. Sci.* **15**, 352.

Knox, J. H. and Jurand, J. (1976). *J. Chromat.* **125**, 89.

Knox, J. H. and Laird, G. R. (1976). *J. Chromat.* **122**, 17.

Krishen, A. (1977). *J. chromat. Sci.* **15**, 434.

Krummen, K. and Frei, R. W. (1977). *J. Chromat.* **132**, 429.

Lafosse, M., Keravis, G. and Durand, M. H. (1976). *J. Chromat.* **118**, 283.

Lefevre, J. P., Divry, A., Caude, M. and Rosset, R. (1975). *Analusis*, **3**, 533.

Linder, H. R., Keller, H. P. and Frei, R. W. (1976). *J. chromat. Sci.* **14**, 234.

Little, C. J., Dale, A. D., Ord, D. A. and Marten, T. R. (1977). *Anal. Chem.* **49**, 1311.

Locke, D. C. (1974). *J. chromat. Sci.* **12**, 433.

Loo, J. C. K., Butterfield, A. G., Moffatt, J. and Jordan, N. (1977). *J. Chromat.* **143**, 275.

Loo, J. C. K. and Jordan, N. (1977). *J. Chromat.* **143**, 314.

Majors, R. E. (1972). *Anal. Chem.* **44**, 1722.

Majors, R. E. (1977a). *J. chromat. Sci.* **15**, 334.

Majors, R. E. (1977b). *J. Ass. Off. anal. Chem.* **60**, 186.

Martin, M. and Guiochon, G. (1977). *Chromatographia*, **10**, 194.

Masanobu, M. and Keihei, U. (1977). *Kagaku no Ryoiki*, **31**, 27.

Matsuzawa, T., Kato, M., Sekiguchi, M. and Ishiguro, I. (1977). *Rinsho Kagaku*, **5**, 239.

McAdams, M. J., Blakley, C. R. and Vestal, M. L. (1977). 25th Ann. Conf. Mass Spec. All. Top. Washington DC., p. 376.

McFadden, W. F. (1977). U.S. Patent 4055981, 1 Nov. 1977, Appl. 664058, 4 March 1976, 4pp.

McNair, H. M. and Chandler, C. D. (1976). *J. chromat. Sci.* **14**, 477.
Mee, T. J. X. and Smith, J. A. (1976). *In* "High Pressure Liquid Chromatography in Clinical Chemistry" (P. F. Dixon, C. H. Gray, C. K. Lim and M. S. Stoll, eds), p. 119. Academic Press, London and New York.
Mell, L. D. and Dasler, A. R. (1978). *J. liq. Chromat.* **1**, 261.
Mell, L. D. and Gustafson, A. H. (1977). *Clin. Chem.* **23**, 473.
Merritt, M. V. and Bronson, G. E. (1976). *Anal. Chem.* **48**, 1851.
Merritt, M. V. and Bronson, G. E. (1977). *Anal. Biochem.* **80**, 392.
Milano, M. J. and Grushka, E. (1977). *J. Chromat.* **133**, 352.
Milano, M. J., Lam, S. and Grushka, E. (1976). *J. Chromat.* **125**, 315.
Milano, M. J., Lam, S., Savonis, M., Pautler, D. B., Pav, J. W. and Grushka, E. (1978). *J. Chromat.* **149**, 599.
Moench, W. and Dehnen, W. (1977). *J. Chromat.* **140**, 260.
Moench, W. and Dehnen, W. (1978). *J. Chromat.* **147**, 415.
Molnar, I. and Horvath, C. (1976). *Clin. Chem.* **22**, 1497.
Molnar, I. and Horvath, C. (1977). *J. Chromat.* **142**, 623.
Morozowich, W. and Douglas, S. L. (1975). *Prostaglandins*, **10**, 19.
Mowery, Jr., R. A. and Juvet, Jr., R. S. (1974). *J. chromat. Sci.* **12**, 687.
Muusze, R. G. and Huber, J. F. K. (1974). *J. chromat. Sci.* **12**, 779.
Nachtmann, F., Knapp, G. and Spitzy, H. (1978). *J. Chromat.* **149**, 693.
Paanakker, J. E., Kraak, J. C. and Poppe, H. (1978). *J. Chromat.* **149**, 111.
Persson, B. A. and Lagerstrom, P. O. (1976). *J. Chromat.* **122**, 305.
Privett, O. S. and Erdalt, W. L. (1978). *Anal. Biochem.* **84**, 449.
Refshauge, C., Kissinger, P. T., Dreiling, R., Blank, L., Freeman, R. and Adams, R. N. (1974). *Life. Sci.* **14**, 311.
Regnier, F. E. and Noel, R. (1976). *J. chromat. Sci.* **14**, 316.
Riggin, R. M., Alcorn, R. L. and Kissinger, P. T. (1976). *Clin. Chem.* **22**, 782.
Ross, M. S. F. (1977). *J. Chromat.* **141**, 107.
Roth, M. and Hampai, A. (1973). *J. Chromat.* **83**, 353.
Saito, Z., Hashiba, T., Miyamoto, M. and Takeda, R. (1977). *Nippon Naibumpi Gakkai Zasshi*, **53**, 765.
Sasa, S. and Blank, L. C. (1977). *Anal. Chem.* **49**, 354.
Satyaswaroop, P. G., Lopez de la Osa, E. and Gurpide, E. (1977). *Steroids*, **30**, 139.
Saunders, D. L. (1977). *J. chromat. Sci.* **15**, 372.
Schoenmakers, P. J., Billiet, H. A. H., Tijssen, R. and de Galan, L. (1978). *J. Chromat* **149**, 519.
Schwarzenbach, R. (1976). *J. Chromat.* **117**, 206.
Schwedt, G. (1977a). *Chromatographia*, **10**, 92.
Schwedt, G. (1977b). *J. Chromat.* **143**, 463.
Schwedt, G. (1977c). *Anal. chim. Acta*, **92**, 337.
Schwedt, G. and Bussemas, H. H. (1977). *Fresenius Z. anal. Chem.* **283**, 23.
Schwedt, G., Bussemas, H. H. and Lippmann, C. (1977). *J. Chromat.* **143**, 259.
Scott, R. P. W. and Kucera, P. (1978). *J. Chromat.* **149**, 93.
Scott, R. P. W. and Lawrence, J. G. (1969). *J. chromat. Sci.* **7**, 65.
Siouffi, A. M., Guillemonat, A. and Guiochon, G. (1977). *J. Chromat.* **137**, 35.
Smuts, T. W., Solms, D. J., Von Niekerk, F. A. and Pretorius, V. (1969). *J. chromat. Sci.* **7**, 24.
Snyder, L. R. (1968). "Principles of Adsorption Chromatography." Marcel Dekker, New York.

Snyder, L. R. and Kirkland, J. J. (1974). "Modern Liquid Chroma ography", p. 69. Wiley-Interscience, New York.

Strubert, W. (1973). *Chromatographia*, **6**, 50.

Takata, Y. and Muto, G. (1973). *Anal. Chem.* **45**, 1864.

Tanaka, N. and Thornton, E. R. (1977). *J. Am. chem. Soc.* **99**, 7300.

Terweij-Groen, C. P. and Kraak, J. C. (1977). *J. Chromat.* **138**, 245.

Thomas, J.-P., Brun, A. and Bounine, J.-P. (1977). *J. Chromat.* **139**, 21.

Thomas, J.-P., Caude, M., Brun, A. and Bounine, J.-P. (1977). *Analusis*, **5**, 205.

Twitchett, P. J., Gorvin, A. E. P., Moffat, A. C., Williams, P. L. and Sullivan, A. T. (1976). *In* "High Pressure Liquid Chromatography in Clinical Chemistry" (P. F. Dixon, C. H. Gray, C. K. Lim and M. S. Stoll, eds), p. 201. Academic Press, London and New York.

Twitchett, P. J., Williams, P. L. and Moffat, A. C. (1978). *J. Chromat.* **149**, 683.

Tymes, N. W. (1977). *J. chromat. Sci.* **15**, 151.

Udenfriend, S., Stein, S., Bohlen, P., Dairman, W., Leingruber, W. and Weigele, M. (1972). *Science*, **178**, 871.

Unger, K. (1975). *Fresenius Z. anal. Chem.* **277**, 311.

Unger, K., Messer, W. and Krebs, K. F. (1978). *J. Chromat.* **149**, 1.

Van den Berg, J. H. M., Mol, C. R., Deelder, R. S. and Thijssen, J. H. H. (1977). *Clin. chim. Acta*, **78**. 165.

Van der Wal, Sj. and Huber, J. F. K. (1977a). *J. Chromat.* **135**, 287.

Van der Wal, Sj. and Huber, J. F. K. (1977b). *J. Chromat.* **135**, 305.

Van der Wal, Sj. and Huber, J. F. K. (1978). *J. Chromat.* **149**, 431.

Vivilecchia, R. V., Lightbody, B. G., Thimot, N. Z. and Quinn, H. M. (1977). *J. chromat. Sci.* **15**, 413.

Wahlund, K. G. and Lund, U. (1976). *J. Chromat.* **122**, 269.

Webber, T. J. N. and McKerrell, E. H. (1976). *J. Chromat.* **122**, 243.

Willmott, F. W. and Dolphin, R. J. (1974). *J. chromat. Sci.* **12**, 695.

Wittmer, D. P., Nuessle, N. O. and Haney, W. G. (1975). *Anal. Chem.* **46**, 1422.

III. Gas Chromatography – Mass Spectrometry

K. D. R. SETCHELL

INTRODUCTION

The rapid progress in radioimmunological and related techniques for measuring hormones has masked developments in mass spectrometry. While it is difficult to compete with such procedures in terms of sample turnover and cost effectiveness, gas chromatography–mass spectrometry should be considered as an important complementary technique offering high sensitivity and greater specificity.

Recent developments in instrumentation have led to an appreciation of the potential of the technique in the qualitative and quantitative analysis of complex mixtures of components in biological samples. Important major advances have included the application of open-tubular glass capillary columns with extremely high chromatographic resolving power, the use of less energetic forms of ionisation, the application of computers to the acquisition and processing of mass spectral data and the development of selected ion monitoring techniques. These will be discussed in detail in the light of their application to hormones in blood.

A. GAS CHROMATOGRAPHY

The principles and techniques of gas chromatography (GC) have been well described in many reviews (e.g. Brooks and Zabkiewicz, 1967; Ettre and Zlatkis, 1967; Krugers, 1968; Littlewood, 1970). This chapter will therefore deal only with recent developments in gas chromatography appropriate to combined gas chromatography–mass spectrometry (GC–MS); developments in GC detectors will not be discussed since the mass spectrometer functions as a sensitive and specific detector, while gas chromatography separates and purifies components in mixtures.

1. Gas Chromatography Columns

Rapid developments in recent years in column technology have led to great improvements in the chromatographic resolving power of the technique. Three basic types of columns are currently in use—packed columns, micro-packed columns and open-tubular columns.

(a) Packed columns

These were first introduced by Martin and James (1952) and have the advantage that any type of support material can be used which can be coated or impregnated with a variety of stationary liquid phases prior to packing. Column sizes are normally ca. 1·3 m × 4 mm i.d. Columns can easily be prepared in a reproducible manner and relatively large samples can be chromatographed.

The efficiency of separation of a chromatography column is dependent on the number of theoretical plates (N). For packed columns N is ca. 3000–5000 compared with 100,000–250,000 plates for capillary columns. The Trenzahl value (TZ) is a more useful parameter (Kaiser, 1962) which indicates the separating power of the column and is given by the number of peaks which can be completely resolved between two members of a homologous series, using isothermal conditions. n-Alkanes, C_{24}–C_{28} (Kaiser, 1962) or C_{11}–C_{12} (Grob and Grob, 1977) are commonly employed and the TZ value for a good capillary column is ca 50.

(b) Packed capillary and micropacked columns

Halasz (1968) introduced packed capillary columns which were prepared from conventional packed columns by heating and drawing into a capillary tube. This technique limited the type of stationary phase that could be used to those stable at high temperature; this type of column therefore had limited applications. A method was later described for the preparation of micropacked columns (Cramers, Rijks and Bocek, 1971). These columns of ca 14 m $\times$ 0·8 mm i.d. were packed under pressure with commercially available packing materials which were sieved to provide small particles ($< 20\,\mu$). Total efficiencies of 15,500 theoretical plates per column were attained and a comparison of their performance against open-tubular capillary columns was reported (Cramers $et\ al.$, 1971).

(c) Open-tubular capillary columns

This type of column was first introduced by Golay (1958) and in spite of the numerous examples from other workers which demonstrated their potential in resolving complex mixtures of organic compounds, subsequent progress in their application was slow. Technical problems in the preparation of reproducible and thermostable capillary columns have now largely been overcome and their current extensive use suggests they may soon supersede conventional packed columns in gas chromatography. A typical example of a gas chromatographic analysis of a multicomponent urinary steroid extract using a packed column and a wall coated open-tubular glass capillary column is compared in Fig. 1.

Capillary columns which range in length from 20–100 m $\times$ 0·3–0·6 mm i.d. and separation efficiencies of up to 250,000 theoretical plates/column, have been made from various tubing materials, but currently glass is the most widely used and because of its low catalytic properties is therefore most suited to the analysis of small amounts of labile compounds in biological systems.

Two types of open-tubular capillary columns are currently in use: wall coated open-tubular columns and support coated open-tubular columns.

(1) Wall coated open tubular (WCOT) glass capillary columns. The WCOT

capillary column, in which the stationary phase is coated on the inside of the column leaving a central channel for the mobile phase, was introduced by Golay (1958). The preparation of WCOT glass capillary columns which has been described in detail by Grob (1965, 1968), Tesařík and Novotný (1968), Bouche and Verzele (1968), Novotný, Blomberg and Bartle (1970), Novotný and Zlatkis (1971), Ilkova and Mistryukov (1971), Rutten and Luyten (1972), Alexandre and Rutten (1973), Alexandre, Garzó and Páyli (1974), Novotný and Bartle (1974a, b), Schomburg, Husmann and Weeke (1974). Roeraade (1975), Grob and Grob (1976), and Marshall and Parker (1976), comprises a number of stages:

(i) Drawing of glass capillaries. Several commercially manufactured glass drawing machines are available which operate on the general principles first described by Desty, Haresnape and Whyman (1960). Capillaries of desired length and internal diameter can be prepared in either Pyrex or soda glass.

(ii) Pretreatment of glass surface. This is essential since it is necessary both to deactivate the glass and to produce a surface which during coating will promote the spreading of a uniform film of the stationary phase. A number of methods have been employed to achieve these goals. Surface carbonisation (Grob, 1975) led to the deposition of a fine layer of carbon on the glass surface. Etching the surface with gaseous hydrogen chloride or hydrogen fluoride to produce the formation of crystals on the surface of the glass, was first described by Novotný and Tesařík (1968) and Tesařík and Novotný (1968), and later used effectively by others (Alexandre and Rutten, 1973, 1974; Alexandre et al., 1974). Aqueous alkali (NaOH, NH₃) or acid (HCl, HF) have also been used but shown to be less effective than gaseous treatment. Recently Grob and Grob (1976) reported a technique for promoting the formation of barium carbonate crystals on the glass surface. This treatment, which has advantages over the etching methods, can be performed with any type of glass and provides a means of preparing glass capillary columns for coating with a variety of stationary phases.

The methods described above lead to an increase in the roughness of the glass surface which assists spreading of the stationary phase. Selective monomolecular layers chemically bonded to the glass surface may be used, though at present not widely (Novotný and Grohmann, 1973; Bartle and Novotný, 1974), to increase the "wettability" or "critical surface tension" of the glass (Zisman, 1964).

(iii) Deactivation. It is essential to reduce the activity of reactive silanol groups and metal oxides in glass. Commonly employed procedures include silanisation (Novotný and Tesařík, 1968; Novotný and Bartle, 1970), the use of surface active agents such as benzyltriphenylphosphonium chloride (Metcalfe and Martin, 1967; Grob, 1968; Malec, 1971; Rutten and Luyten, 1972) and coating by thin films of polymers (Aue, Hastings and Kapila, 1973;

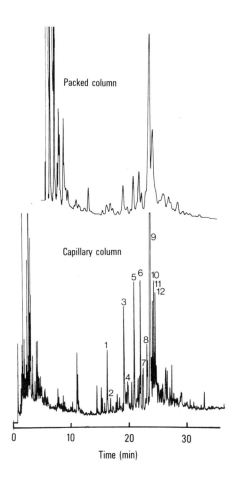

Fig. 1. The gas chromatographic separation of steroids excreted in the urine of the adult female owl monkey (*Aotus trivirgatus*) is compared when the analysis was performed on a conventional packed column and a wall coated open-tubular (WCOT) glass capillary column. The packed column analysis was carried out using a Varian Aerograph 2700 gas chromatograph housing a glass column (3 m × 0·4 cm) packed with 3% Silicone OV-1 on Chromasorb W and temperature programming from 200–270° with increments of 2°/min. The capillary column analysis was performed by a Becker 409 gas chromatograph housing a 25 m column coated with silicone OV-1. Samples were introduced via an automatic solid injection system. Helium was the carrier gas and the flow rate through the column was *ca* 2 ml/min. Temperature programmed operation from 180–260° in increments of 2·5°/min was used. The principal steroids are indicated as follows: 1—androsterone, 2—aetiocholanolone, 3—oestrone, 4—oestradiol-17β, 5—17-hydroxypregnanolone, 6—androstane-3,16, 17-triol, 7—pregnanediol, 8—pregnanetriol, 9—6β-hydroxypregnanolone, 10—pregnenediol, 11, 12—16-hydroxypregnanolone isomers (Setchell and Bonney, 1979).

Hastings, Augl, Kapila and Aue, 1973; Grob and Grob, 1976). In addition to deactivating the surface such procedures aid in increasing the "wettability" of the glass.

(iv) Coating. A *dynamic* method was originally described by Dijkstra and DeGoey (1958); the stationary phase, dissolved in a suitable solvent, is slowly passed through the column. The solvent is evaporated leaving a thin film of stationary phase on the wall, the thickness being mainly dependent upon the solute and its concentration, surface tension and rate of flow (Tesařik and Nečasová, 1972; Bartle, 1973; Bartle and Novotný, 1974). The thickness of the liquid film has been shown to be an important factor in dictating the behaviour of the column (Grob and Grob, 1978). The introduction of a small plug of mercury following the solution improved the reproducibility of the procedure (Schomburg, *et al.*, 1974).

A *static* method of coating was described by Bouche and Verzele (1968); the column is filled with a solution of the stationary phase, sealed at one end and reduced pressure applied to the other end and the solvent evaporated leaving a deposit of the stationary phase on the surface of the glass.

Although the *dynamic* method is faster than the *static* coating procedure, there is no apparent difference in the quality of columns produced.

(2) *Support coated open-tubular glass capillary columns.* First introduced by Kaiser (1968) and later exploited successfully by German, Pfaffenberger, Thenot, Horning and Horning (1973), Blummer (1973), Nikelly and Blummer (1974), Schulte and Acker (1974), an alternative method of preparing open-tubular glass capillary columns involves coating the capillary wall with a finely powdered support material, usually silanised silica particles (Silanox), that is capable of retaining the stationary phase. The technique which initially proved suitable only for apolar stationary phases was modified to enable the preparation of polar columns (Van Hout, Szafranek, Pfaffenberger and Horning, 1974; Deelder, Ramaekers, Van den Berg and Wetzels, 1976; McKeag and Hougen, 1977). The procedure can be used with any type of glass but because thicker films of stationary phase are formed the resolving power of this type of column is relatively lower than that of wall coated open-tubular glass capillary columns. However, their greater capacity and ease of preparation has resulted in their wide use.

2. Practical Aspects of Gas Chromatography using Glass Capillary Columns

Only a few instruments are at present manufactured specially for capillary column chromatography; although this will certainly alter in the future. Almost all conventional gas chromatographs can, however, be modified, simply by altering the connections of the capillary column to the GC inlet and detector and the mechanism of sample introduction (Novotný and Zlatkis, 1971; Schomburg et al., 1974; Grob, 1975; Kaiser and Reider, 1975; Hartigan and Ettre, 1976).

The two general methods for connecting to capillary columns involve (i) straightening each end of the glass capillary column and inserting these directly into the inlet and into the detector using silicone rubber seals or Swagelock fittings, or (ii) using a short length of glass-lined metal capillary tubing with a piece of heat "shrink" Teflon tubing (less satisfactory due to the limited temperature tolerance of Teflon and its tendency to leak) or preferably a Swagelock fitting. Direct insertion of the capillary column ends has the advantages that the dead volume, particularly in the GC detector, is minimal and the integrity of the column is retained. This method of connection is more difficult.

3. Sample Introduction

The capacity of open-tubular glass capillary columns (ca 500 ng) is considerably lower than that of conventional packed columns and this presents a technical problem of introducing small amounts of sample onto the column.

The problem was initially overcome by the injection of excessive amounts of sample and the use of splitters which would allow as little as 1% of the sample onto the column while the remainder escaped to atmosphere; this was unsatisfactory for quantitative analysis. Discrimination between compounds of different molecular weight occurs due to their different volatilities and non-uniform splitting can take place. Furthermore, the analysis of trace substances in complex mixtures requires much larger samples. An early injection technique employed a short pre-column packed with conventional GC packing or silanised glass beads and controlled split ratios which concentrated the compounds while the solvent passed to the atmosphere (German and Horning, 1973).

Direct injection (splitless) onto the stationary phase has been recognised as the only satisfactory method of sample introduction (Desty, 1965) and methods for splitless injection have been described (Cramers and Van Kessel, 1968; Groenendijk and Van Kemenade, 1969; Grob and Grob, 1969a, b, 1972) based upon trapping the sample on the capillary column, which is cooled during injection and subsequently heated to the operating temperature.

Sample introduction via vaporisation in an injection zone, although not essential, is commonplace and the disadvantages in quantitative analysis have been indicated by Verzele, Verstappe, Sandra, van Luchene and Vuye (1972) and Grob and Grob (1978). Most injection devices incorporate the undesirable feature of a rubber septum at the injection point. Problems

arising from the septum include adsorption of the sample, constant release
of volatile plasticizers which create "ghost" peaks and the deposition of
minute particles of rubber, cut by the syringe needle, into the injection zone
or onto the top of the column. In spite of the incorporation of septum
flushing devices these problems are not overcome. Recently Grob and
Grob (1978) described an injector which functioned without a septum and
allowed the introduction of up to several microlitres of sample onto the
capillary column without prior vaporisation, thereby overcoming many of
the disadvantages associated with conventional injection techniques.

Solid injectors have been particularly useful with high boiling point
compounds, e.g. steroids, and which are relatively stable when dried. A
variety of all-glass solid injectors are available based upon the principles
described by Van den Berg and Cox (1972). The liquid sample is carefully
injected onto the tip of a glass needle and the carrier gas diverted to vaporise
the solvent to atmosphere. When the sample is dry the needle is lowered
into the heated injection zone near the top of the capillary column where
volatilisation occurs.

Although numerous sample introduction techniques have been designed,
the choice of which to employ will depend largely upon the type of sample
to be analysed.

4. The Gas Chromatograph-Mass Spectrometer Interface

For mass spectrometric analysis, it is necessary to vaporise the sample in the
low pressure environment of the ion-source of the instrument. The gas chromatograph offers an ideal route for sample introduction, but technical problems of the pressure difference between the gas chromatograph (atmospheric
pressure) and the mass spectrometer (1.33×10^{-5} kPa) delayed its coupling
with the mass spectrometer. The first separators were designed which inter-
faced the GC with the MS (Ryhage, 1964; Watson and Biemann, 1964) and
which subsequently led to successful combined GC–MS.

The separator removes the excess carrier gas passing from the GC column,
developing a pressure-gradient between the GC and the MS, and enriching
the solute before entering the ion-source. Since the introduction of the
original two-stage jet orifice separator of Ryhage, numerous developments
have improved the GC–MS interface (Watson, 1969, 1972).

The coupling of capillary GC columns to the mass spectrometer was
complicated by the lower carrier gas flow rate (1–2 ml/min) compared with
that of conventional packed columns (30–50 ml/min). Two main procedures
have been employed to overcome this difficulty; (i) direct coupling of the
capillary column to the ion source via a platinum resistance capillary
(Schultze and Kaiser, 1971; Grob and Jaeggi, 1973; Maume and Luyten,

1973; Neuner-Jehle, Etzweiler and Zarske, 1974; Eyem, 1975; Thome and Young, 1976); (ii) the use of carrier gas added at the end of the column to act as scavenger, producing a flow rate equivalent to that for a packed column, permitting the use of the conventional separator. A single stage jet separator has also been described by Ryhage (1965) as a suitable interface for a capillary column and recently an adjustable jet separator was employed (Ryhage, 1973).

It is generally accepted that the direct coupling method is better since it prevents peak broadening and losses that may occur in the separator, but a high pumping capacity is necessary to maintain the vacuum in the ion source.

5. Deactivation of Gas Chromatography-Mass Spectrometry Systems

The adsorption and decomposition of compounds on gas chromatography columns and other parts of the GC–MS system are important factors affecting the sensitivity and precision of measurements. With conventional packed columns, the support material is often the major cause of adsorption and standard techniques such as the use of silanised diatomite support material reduce or minimise these effects (Horning, Maddock, Anthony and Van den Heuvel, 1963; Van den Heuvel and Horning. 1964; Supina, Henley and Kruppa, 1966; Ottenstein, 1968; Simmonds and Lovelock, 1976). Where a single compound is to be analysed, pre-treatment and conditioning of the column with that compound is a useful means of improving sensitivity. Wilson, Snedden, Tham and Willoughby (1976) detected fg levels of prostaglandins using such a procedure. Alternative methods of minimising these effects are the use of carefully selected derivatives or the addition of a stable isotope-labelled carrier in excess.

With glass capillary columns losses of compounds in the injection system, the GC–MS interface and the connecting devices are usually greater than effects due to the column. Metal surfaces should be avoided where possible and glass connections thoroughly deactivated by silanisation. Axelson (1977) investigated the factors affecting the loss of steroid derivatives in GC and GC–MS systems with open-tubular glass capillary columns. Coating of metal surfaces, including the separator jets, with water glass (sodium silicate solution) followed by treatment with benzyltriphenylphosphonium chloride was an effective means of deactivating the system.

6. Derivatisation

The requirement of volatility is a prime requisite for GC–MS analysis. Due to the relatively high molecular weight or the presence of numerous polar

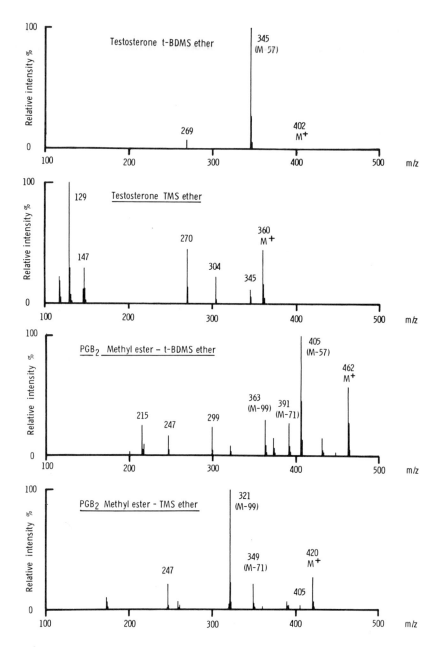

Fig. 2. Representative mass spectra of *tert*-butyldimethylsilyl (t-BDMS) ether and trimethylsilyl (TMS) ether derivatives are compared for a steroid (testosterone) and a prostaglandin (PGB₂-methyl ester).

functional groups, many hormones are non-volatile and/or thermally unstable and unsuited to gas chromatography. Chemical derivatisation will often be necessary to render a compound suitable for GC–MS analysis. In addition to increasing volatility, derivatisation often stabilises the molecule, improves chromatographic behaviour and minimises adsorption. More important, in GC–MS, derivatisation aids structural characterisation by directing fragmentation in the molecule so as to provide information on the number, type and position of functional groups (see below). The choice of derivative will largely be influenced by the type of analysis performed. For example, in qualitative analysis the derivative chosen should provide as much information as possible by producing a large number of fragment ions in the mass spectrum. In quantitative analysis, improved precision and sensitivity will be achieved if little fragmentation occurs and a large proportion of the total ionisation resides in one or few ions which are monitored. The differences between the *tert*-butyldimethylsilyl (t-BDMS) ether derivative (Corey and Venkateswarlu, 1972) and the trimethylsilyl (TMS) ether derivative readily illustrate this point (Fig. 2). The t-BDMS ether derivatives of steroids (Phillipou, Bigham and Seamark, 1975; Kelly and Taylor, 1976) and prostaglandins (Watson and Sweetman, 1974; Kelly and Taylor, 1976; Brash and Baillie, 1978) frequently give rise to extremely simple electron impact mass spectra compared with respective TMS ether derivatives. Whilst in many instances little structural information can be gained from their mass spectra, the increased abundance of fragments at higher mass (a particular feature being the prominent fragment arising from loss of 57 mass units from the molecule due to the tertiary butyl group) would make the use of these derivatives in quantitative selected ion detection GC–MS superior.

Many different derivatives can be prepared of functional groups (Cummins, 1971; Zweig and Sherma, 1972; Drozd, 1975; Brooks, Edmonds, Gaskell and Smith, 1978) and those most commonly employed for GC–MS analysis of hormones are seen in Table 1. A useful handbook of derivatives for chromatography has been published by Blau and King (1978).

B. MASS SPECTROMETRY

1. Principles

The basic requirement for mass spectrometry is volatilisation of the sample, which immediately imposes a limitation on the type of compound that can be analysed. A second restriction is that the maximum mass of an ion which can be recorded by most instruments is 1000, although some more powerful instruments can analyse compounds of molecular weights up to 3000. With hormones, except the polypeptides, these factors do not limit the use of the

Table 1

Table of selected ion monitoring GC–MS methods for hormones and their metabolites.

Compound	Mass spectro-metry[a]	Derivative[b]	Internal standard[c]	Ions m/z monitored[a]	References
STEROIDS					
Testosterone	LR-ei	TMS	[4-^{14}C]-Testosterone	432/434	Björkhem et al. (1975b)
Testosterone	LR-ei	HFB	[4-^{14}C]-Testosterone	680/682	Siekmann et al. (1972); Siekmann (1974); Breuer and Siekmann (1975)
Testosterone	LR-ei	BDMS	[d$_4$]-Testosterone	438/442	Chapman and Bailey (1974)
Testosterone	LR-ei	HFB-acetate	4-Methyl-19-nortestosterone	526	Dehennin et al. (1974a, b)
Testosterone	LR-ei	MO-TMS	[4-^{14}C]-Testosterone	389/391	Jeannine, Bournot, Maume and Maume (1978)
Testosterone	LR-ei	t-BDMS	19-Nortestosterone	345/331	Seamark, Phillipou and McIntosh (1977)
Testosterone	LR-ei	TFA	[1,2,6,7-^{3}H$_4$]-Testosterone	480/486	Vestergaarde, Saybergh and Mowat (1975)
Testosterone	HR-ei	TMS	No internal standard	360-248	Millington (1975)
Testosterone	HR-ei	t-BDMS	5β-Dihydro-epitestosterone	347-240	Gaskell and Pike (1978)

Compound	Method	Derivative	Internal standard	m/z	Reference
5α-Dihydrotestosterone	LR-ei[a]	t-BDMS	No internal standard	347 → 271	Gaskell and Millington (1978)
5α-Dihydrotestosterone	LR-ei	HFB	[4-^{14}C]-5α-Dihydro-testosterone	682/686	Siekmann et al. (1976a)
Progesterone	LR-ei	HFB	[4-^{14}C]-Progesterone	510/512	Björkhem et al. (1975a)
Progesterone	LR-ei	HFB	4-Ethylandrostenedione	510	Dehennin et al. (1974a, b)
Progesterone	LR-ei	TFA	19-Norandrostenedione	382/368	Seamark et al. (1977)
18-Hydroxyprogesterone	LR-ei	MO-TMS	MO-[d_{18}]-TMS derivative	517/535	Prost and Maume (1974a)
Cortisol	LR-ei	MO-TMS	[4-^{14}C]-Cortisol	605/607	Björkhem et al. (1974)
Cortisol	LR-ei	MO-TMS	[1,2-^{3}H$_2$]-Cortisol	605/609	Siekmann (1974); Breuer and Siekmann (1975)
Corticosterone	LR-ei	Persilyl	[1,2-^{3}H$_2$]-Corticosterone	634/638	Siekmann et al. (1976b)
18-Hydroxycorticosterone	LR-ei	MO-TMS	MO-[d_{27}]-TMS derivative	605/632	Prost and Maume (1974a, b)
18-Hydroxy-DOC	LR-ei	MO-TMS	MO-[d_{18}]-TMS derivative	517/535	Prost and Maume (1974a, b)
Aldosterone	LR-ei	HFB	1,2-[^{3}H$_2$]-Aldosterone	538/452	Siekmann (1974); Breuer and Siekmann (1975); Siekmann et al. (1976b)
Dehydroepiandrosterone	LR-ei	t-BDMS	19-Nor testosterone	345/331	Seamark et al. (1977)
Dehydroepiandrosterone	HR-ei	TMS	No internal standard	360·248	Millington (1975)

Compound	Mass spectrometry[a]	Derivative[b]	Internal standard[c]	Ions m/z monitored[a]	References
Oestrone	LR-ei	TMS	[d$_9$]-TMS derivative	342/351	Adlercreutz et al. (1974c)
Oestrone	LR-ei	t-BDMS	19-Nor testosterone	327/331	Seamark et al. (1977)
Oestrone	LR-ei	TMS	6,7-[d$_2$]-Oestrone	342/344	Siekmann (1974)
Oestradiol-17β	LR-ei	t-BDMS	19-Nor testosterone	433/331	Seamark et al. (1977)
Oestradiol-17β	LR-ei	TMS	[d$_{18}$]-TMS derivative	416/424	Adlercreutz et al. (1974c)
Oestradiol-17β	LR-ei	HFB	4-[^{14}C]-Oestradiol-17β	664/666	Siekmann et al. (1973)
Oestradiol-17β	HR-ei	TMS	No internal standard	416-257	Millington (1975)
Oestriol	LR-ei	TMS	[d$_{27}$]-TMS derivative	504/531	Adlercreutz, Nylander and Hunnemann (1974a)
Oestriol	LR-ei	TFA	4-[^{14}C]-Oestriol	576/578	Siekmann et al. (1978)
2-Methoxyoestrone	LR-ei		[d$_9$]-TMS derivative	[M$^+$]	Adlercreutz et al. (1974c)
15-Hydroxyoestrone			[d$_{18}$]-TMS derivative		
16$\alpha(\beta)$-Hydroxyoestrone			[d$_{18}$]-TMS derivative		
Oestradi 1-17α		TMS	[d$_{18}$]-TMS derivative		

16-oxo-Oestradiol-17β	LR-ei	TMS	$[d_{18}]$-TMS derivative	$[M^+]$	Adlercreutz *et al.* (1974c)
16-Epioestriol	LR-ei	TMS	$[d_{27}]$-TMS derivative	$[M^+]$	Adlercreutz *et al.* (1974c)
17-Epioestriol	LR-ei	TMS	$[d_{27}]$-TMS derivative	$[M^+]$	Adlercreutz *et al.* (1974c)
THYROID HORMONES					
Tyroxine (T_4)	LR-ei	TMS	No internal standard	218	Heki, Noto, Hosojima, Takahashi and Murata (1976)
3,3,5′-Triiodothyronine (T_3)	LR-ei	HFB-Me ester	No internal standard	844	Petersen and Vouros (1977)
3,3′,5-Triiodothyronine (rT_3)	LR-ei	TMS	No internal standard	218	Heki *et al.* (1976)
3,3′,5-Triiodothyronine (rT_3)	LR-ei	HFB-Me ester	No internal standard	844	Petersen and Vouros (1977)
3,3′,5,5′-Tetraiodothyro-acetic acid	LR-ei	Dimethyl	3,3′,5,5′-Tetraiodothyro-propionic acid	776/790	Crossley *et al.* (1978)
3,3′,5,5′-Tetraiodothyro-formic acid	LR-ei	TMS-Me ester	No internal standard	834/820	Ramsden *et al.* (1974)
PROSTAGLANDINS[f]					
$PGF_{2\alpha}$	LR-ei	Butyl boronate-TMS-Me ester	$[d_4]$-$PGF_{2\alpha}$	435/439	Kelly (1972, 1974)
$PGF_{2\alpha}$	LR-ei	Acetyl-Me ester	$[d_4, {}^3H_2]$-$PGF_{2\alpha}$	314/318	Axen *et al.* (1971); Gréen *et al.* (1973)

Compound	Mass spectrometry[a]	Derivative[b]	Internal standard[c]	Ions m/z monitored[d]	References
$PGF_{2\alpha}$	LR-ei	Acetyl-Me ester	$[^3H_2]$-$PGF_{2\alpha}$	314/318	Hammarström, Hamberg, Samuelsson, Duell, Stawiski and Voorhees (1975)
$PGF_{2\alpha}$	LR-ei	TMS-Me ester	ω-Trinor-16-cyclohexyl-$PGF_{2\alpha}$	423	Cory, Lascelles, Millard, Snedden and Wilson (1976)
$PGF_{2\alpha}$	LR-ei	TMS-Me ester	No internal standard	423	Wilson et al. (1976)
$PGF_{2\alpha}$	LR-ei	TMS-Me ester	$[d_4]$-$PGF_{2\alpha}$	423/427	Sweetman, Watson, Carr, Oates and Frolich (1973)
$PGF_{2\alpha}$	LR-ei	MO-t-BDMS-Me ester	$[d_4]$-$PGF_{2\alpha}$	653/657	Kelly (1977)
15-Keto-dihydro-$PGF_{2\alpha}$	LR-ei	Acetyl-Me ester	$[d_4, ^3H_2]$-15-keto-dihydro-$PGF_{2\alpha}$	332/336	Gréen et al. (1973)
Dihydro-$PGF_{2\alpha}$	LR-ei	Acetyl-Me ester	$[d_4, ^3H_2]$-Dihydro-$PGF_{2\alpha}$	316/320	Gréen et al. (1973)
$PGF_{1\alpha}$	LR-ei	MO-Acetyl-Me ester	$[d_6]$-$PGF_{1\alpha}$	316/321	Goldyne and Hammarström (1978)
PGE_1	LR-ei	MO-Me ester	$[d_3]$-MO-Me ester derivative	470/473	Samuelsson et al. (1970)
PGE_1	LR-ei	MO-Acetyl-Me ester	$[d_6]$-PGE_1	330/335	Goldyne and Hammarström

Compound	MS	Derivative	Internal standard	m/z	Reference
PGE$_2$	LR-ei	MO-Acetyl-Me ester	MO-[d$_6$]-Acetyl-Me ester derivative	419/422	Watson (1971)
PGE$_2$	LR-ei	MO-Acetyl-Me ester	[d$_4$,^{3}H$_2$]-PGE$_2$	419/423	Axen et al. (1971); Gréen et al. (1973)
PGE$_2$	LR-ei	MO-Acetyl-Me ester	[^{3}H$_2$]-PGE$_2$	419/423	Hammarström et al. (1975)
PGE$_2$	LR-ei	TMS-Me ester	No internal standard	421	Wilson et al. (1976)
PGE$_2$	LR-ei	MO-t-BDMS-Me ester	[d$_4$]-PGE$_2$	666/670	Kelly (1977)
15-Keto-dihydro-PGE$_2$	LR-ei	MO-Acetyl-Me ester	[d$_4$,^{3}H$_2$]-15-Keto-dihydro-PGE$_2$	375/379	Samuelsson and Gréen (1974)
PGA$_2$	LR-ei	TMS-Me ester	[d$_4$,^{3}H$_2$]-PGA$_2$	349/353	Gréen and Steffenrund (1976)
PGA$_2$	LR-ci	TMS-Me ester	[d$_4$]-PGA$_2$	349/353	Frolich, Sweetman, Carr, Hollifield and Oates (1975)
Thromboxane B$_2$	LR-ei	TMS-Me ester	[d$_8$]-Thromboxane B$_2$	256/264	Hamberg and Samuelsson (1974b); Hamberg (1976)
Thromboxane B$_2$	LR-ei	t-BDMS-Me ester	No internal standard	669	Smith, Harland and Brooks (1977)
Thromboxane B$_2$	LR-ei	TMS-Me ester	No internal standard	301	Smith et al. (1977)
BIOGENIC AMINES					
Adrenaline	LR-ei	PFP	α-Methylnoradrenaline	176/190	Costa et al. (1972); Koslow (1973)
Adrenaline	LR-ei	TFA	Synephrine	140/140:328	Wang, Imai, Yoshioka and Tamura (1975a)

Compound	Mass spectrometry[a]	Derivative[b]	Internal standard[c]	Ions m/z monitored[a]	References
Noradrenaline	LR-ei	PFP	α-Methylnoradrenaline	190/190	Koslow et al. (1972, 1974); Costa et al. (1972); Cattabeni, Koslow and Costa (1972b); Koslow (1973)
Noradrenaline	LR-ci	PFP	No internal standard	590	Miyazaki et al. (1974)
Dopamine	LR-ei	PFP	α-Methyldopamine	428/442	Koslow et al. (1972, 1974); Costa et al. (1972); Cattabeni, Koslow and Costa (1972b); Koslow (1973)
Dopamine	LR-ei	PFB-TMS	2-Amino-2-phenylpropanol	267/298	Lhugenot and Maume (1974)
Dopamine	LR-ei	TFA	d_4-Dopamine	328/331	Curtius et al. (1974)
Dopamine	LR-ei	TFA	Synephrine	328/140:328	Wang et al. (1975a)
Dopamine	LR-ci	PFP	No internal standard	592	Miyazaki et al. (1974)
6-Hydroxydopamine	LR-ei	TFA	Isopreterenol	440	Curtius et al. (1974)
6-Hydroxydopamine	LR-ci	PFP	No internal standard	608	Miyazaki et al. (1974)
Octopamine	LR-ei	PFB-TMS	2-Amino-2-phenylpropanol	267/298	Lhugenot and Maume (1974)
Normetanephrine	LR-ei	PFB-TMS	2-Amino-2-phenylpropanol	297/298	Lhugenot and Maume (1974)

Compound	Method	Derivative	Internal standard	m/z	Reference
Normetanephrine	LR-ei	TFA	Phenylephrine	358/342	Wang, Yoshika, Imai and Tamura (1975b)
Metanephrine	LR-ei	TFA	Phenylephrine	358/342	Wang et al. (1975b)
Homovanillic acid (HVA)	LR-ei	HFB	[d₂]-homovanillic acid	392/394	Sedvall et al. (1974); Fri, Wiesel and Sedvall (1974a)
Homovanillic acid (HVA)	LR-ei	HFB-Me ester	HFB-[d₃]-Me ester derivative	392/395	Sjöquist and Änggård (1972); Änggård et al. (1973); Dailey and Änggård (1973)
Homovanillic acid (HVA)	LR-ei	ME ester-TMS	iso-Homovanillic acid	209	Narasimhachari (1974)
Homovanillic acid (HVA)	LR-ei	PFP	[d₂]-Homovanillic acid	460/462	Fri, Wiesel and Sedvall (1974b)
Homovanillic acid (HVA)	LR-ei	HFB-Me ester	[d₅]-Homovanillic acid	392/397	Bertilsson and Palmér (1973); Sjöquist, Lindström and Änggård (1973)
Homovanillic acid (HVA)	LR-ei	TFA	[d₃]-Homovanillic acid	292/295	Gordon, Oliver, Black and Kopin (1974)
Homovanillic acid (HVA)	LR-ei	PFP-Me ester	[d₃]-Homovanillic acid	283/286	Muskiet, Fremouw-Ottevangers, Meulen, Wolthers and de Vries (1978a)
Iso-homovanillic acid	LR-ei	HFB-Me ester	—	332:392	Bertilsson and Palmér (1973)
4-Hydroxy-3-methoxy-phenylglycol (HMPG)	LR-ei	TFA	[d₂]-HMPG	472/474	Bertilsson (1973)

Compound	Mass spectrometry[a]	Derivative[b]	Internal standard[c]	Ions m/z monitored[a]	References
4-Hydroxy-3-methoxy-phenylglycol (HMPG)	LR-ei	PFP	Tryptophol	311:458/289	Karoum, Lefèvre, Bigelow and Costa (1973)
4-Hydroxy-3-methoxy-phenylglycol (HMPG)	LR-ei	TFA	[d$_3$]-HMPG	472/475	Sjöquist, Lindström and Änggård (1975)
4-Hydroxy-3-methoxy-phenylglycol (HMPG)	LR-ei	PFP	[d$_3$]-HMPG	311:458/ 314:461	Karoum, Gillin, Wyatt and Costa (1975)
4-Hydroxy-3-methoxy-phenylglycol (HMPG)	LR-ei	PFP	No internal standard	458:662	Zambotti et al. (1975)
4-Hydroxy-3-methoxy-phenylglycol (HMPG)	LR-ei	TFA	[d$_3$]-HMPG	345/348	Gordon et al. (1974)
4-Hydroxy-3-methoxy-phenylglycol (HMPG)	LR-ei	PFP	VMA-methyl ester	445	Braestrup (1973)
4-Hydroxy-3-methoxy-phenylglycol (HMPG)	LR-ei	Acetyl-TFA	[d$_3$]-HMPG	249:376/ 252:379	Takahashi et al. (1977)
4-Hydroxy-3-methoxy-phenylglycol (HMPG)	LR-ei	TFA	[d$_3$]-HMPG-sulphate	358/360	Murray et al. (1977)
4-Hydroxy-3-methoxy-phenylglycol (HMPG)	LR-ei	PFP-Me ester	[d$_5$]-HMPG	445/448	Muskiet et al. (1978b)
4-Hydroxy-3-methoxy-phenylethanol (HMPE)	LR-ei	PFP	Tryptophol	296/289	Karoum et al. (1973)
4-Hydroxy-3-methoxy-phenylethanol (HMPE)	LR-ei	PFP	[d$_2$]-HMPE	269:460/ 297:462	Karoum et al. (1975)

Compound	Method	Derivative	Internal standard	Ions	Reference
4-Hydroxy-3-methoxy-phenylethanol (HMPE)	LR-ei	TFA	[d$_5$]-HMPE	312/319	Muskiet et al. (1978a)
Vanilmandellic acid (VMA)	LR-ei	TFA	[d$_3$]-VMA	345/348	Gordon et al. (1974)
Vanilmandellic acid (VMA)	LR-ei	PFP-Me ester	[d$_3$]-VMA	417:445/420:448	Karoum et al. (1975)
Vanilmandellic acid (VMA)	LR-ei	PFP-Me ester	[d$_3$]-VMA	445/448	Takahashi et al. (1977); Muskiet et al. (1978b)
5-Hydroxyindoleacetic acid (5-HIAA)	LR-ei	PFP	[d$_2$]-5-HIAA	438/440	Fri et al. (1974b)
5-Hydroxyindoleacetic acid (5-HIAA)	LR-ei	HFB-Me ester	[d$_2$]-5-HIAA	538/540	Bertilsson et al. (1972)
5-Hydroxyindoleacetic acid (5-HIAA)	LR-ei	PFP	[d$_2$]-5-HIAA	615/607	Beck et al. (1977)
Indole-3-acetic acid	LR-ei	HFB-Me ester	5-Methyl-indole-acetic acid	326/340	Bertilsson and Palmér (1972)
5-Hydroxytryptamine (5-HT)	LR-ei	PFP	No internal standard	438	Koslow et al. (1974)
5-Hydroxytryptamine (5-HT)	LR-ei	PFP	[d$_4$]-5-Hydroxytryptamine	451/454	Beck et al. (1977)
5-Hydroxytryptamine (5-HT)	LR-ei	PFP	α-Methyl-5-HT	451/465	Cattabeni et al. (1972a); Koslow and Green (1973)
5-Hydroxytryptamine (5-HT)	LR-ei	HFB	No internal standard	144:538:551	DoAmaral (1973)
N-Acetyl-5-HT	LR-ei	PFP	N-Acetyltryptamine	492/330	Cattabeni et al. (1972, 1973)
5-Methoxytryptamine	LR-ei	PFP	α-Methyl-5-HT	306/465	Cattabeni et al. (1972, 1973); Koslow (1974)

Compound	Mass spectrometry[a]	Derivative[b]	Internal standard[c]	Ions (m/z) monitored[d]	References
5-Methoxytryptamine	LR-ei	TFA	Phenylephrine	246/245	Wang et al. (1975)
5-Hydroxytryptophol (5-HTOL)	LR-ei	PFP	[d$_4$]-5-HTOL	305:469/ 308:473	Takahashi et al. (1978)
5-Hydroxytryptophol (5-HTOL)	LR-ei	PFP	5-Fluoro-α-methyltryptamine	305/321	Curtius et al. (1975)
5-Hydroxytryptophol (5-HTOL)	LR-ei	PFP	[d$_2$]-5-HTOL	451/440	Beck et al. (1977)
5-Methoxytryptophol	LR-ei	PFP	5-Fluoro-α-methyltryptamine	319/321	Curtius et al. (1975)
Melatonin	LR-ei	TMS	ω-N-n-Hexanoyl-5-methoxy-tryptamine	232	Wilson et al. (1977)
Melatonin	LR-ei	PFP	N-Acetyltryptamine	360/330	Cattabeni et al. (1972a)
Melatonin	LR-ei	PFP	[d$_3$]-Melatonin	360/363	Kennaway, Frith, Phillipou, Matthews and Seamark (1977)
Melatonin	LR-ei[g]	PFP	[d$_4$]-N-Acetyl-5-methoxy-tryptamine	320/323	Lewy and Markey (1978)

Mass spectrometric conditions employed are indicated by:

[a] LR—low resolution; HR—high resolution; ei—electron impact ionisation; ci—chemical ionisation.
[b] The following abbreviations are used: TMS—trimethylsilyl ether; HFB—heptafluorobutyrate; t-BDMS—tert—butyldimethylsilyl ether; TFA—trifluoroacetate; MO—methyloxime; Me—methyl ester; PFP—pentafluoropropionate; PFB—perfluorobenzylimine.
[c] Where internal standards incorporate deuterium these are shown by the abbreviation [d$_x$] where the subscript denotes the number of atoms incorporated.
[d] The ions monitored for the analyte and the internal standard are indicated, e.g. 432/434 implies that m/z 432 was used to monitor the analyte and m/z 434 the internal standard. Where the ion is common to both, a single value is quoted. Where several ions are employed these are indicated.
[e] Metastable peak monitoring.

technique since most hormones are of relatively small molecular weight and are either volatile or a suitable derivative can be prepared to render them volatile. The two basic types of mass spectrometers commonly employed are the magnetic sector instrument and the quadrupole.

(a) Magnetic sector instrument

The principles of mass spectrometry using a magnetic sector instrument (Beynon, 1960; Biemann, 1962; Waller, 1972) will be described only briefly and a schematic representation of the general principle is shown in Fig. 3. Once the sample has been volatilised and introduced into the high vacuum environment (1.33×10^{-5} kP) of the ion source of the instrument, the molecules are ionised and the positively charged ions generated by this process are then focused into an ion beam and accelerated, by way of an applied negative potential, into a magnetic field. On entering the magnetic field an ion will be deflected, the radius of its path being related to the mass/charge (m/z, referred also by m/e) ratio according to the equation:

$$m/z = \frac{H^2 r^2}{2V}$$

where H = magnetic field, V = accelerating voltage, and r = radius of ion path.

If the magnetic field and the accelerating voltage are constant the degree of deflection of any ion will be dependent upon its mass, i.e. ions of low mass will be deflected to a greater extent than those of high mass. This phenomenon provides a means of dispersing the ion beam into a spectrum of ions according to their m/z ratio. By continuously varying either the magnetic field or the accelerating voltage the ions impinging at the detector can be focused through detector slits and their abundance measured.

The ability to separate ions of different mass, which is largely governed by the differences in kinetic energy of ions of the same m/z value and the width of the source and detector slits, is termed the resolving power (R) and can be expressed by the equation $R = M/\Delta m$ (where Δm is the difference between two masses M_1 and M_2. The separation of ions of nominal mass is referred to as low resolution. High resolution is employed where accurate mass measurements are required and while resolving powers of up to 100,000 can be attained, in practice ca 10,000 is generally sufficient for most purposes.

(b) Quadrupole instrument

The quadrupole mass spectrometer is a non-magnetic field instrument, so named because it consists of four parallel rods arranged symmetrically

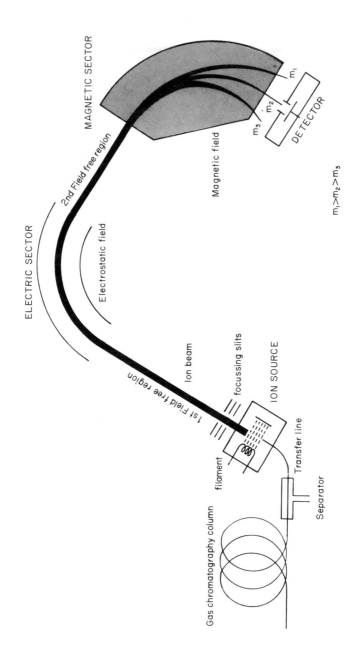

Fig. 3. A schematic representation of the layout and principles of a double focusing, magnetic sector mass spectrometer.

between the ion source and the detector. Positively charged ions generated in the ion source are accelerated into the quadrupole region and become influenced by a combination of direct current (d.c.) and oscillating radio frequency potentials applied between the. rods. The trajectories are complex and for an ion to reach the detector it must traverse the quadrupole region without colliding with the rods (Fig. 4). The principles involved in this type of instrument have been described by Dawson and Whetton (1969, 1971). Limitations of this type of instrument are the limited mass range and the lower sensitivities at high mass compared with the magnetic sector instrument, but they are particularly suitable for use in the selected ion monitoring mode (see below) and their relative lower cost has contributed to their widespread use (Jenden and Cho, 1973; Falkner, Sweetman and Watson, 1975).

2. Methods of Ionisation

(a) Electron impact ionisation

A beam of electrons is generated by passing a 50–100 µA current through a fine wire filament. The filament acts as a cathode and the fine electron beam is drawn towards an anode at an angle of 90° to the ion beam. The ionisation of a molecule, i.e. to produce the molecular ion (M^+), requires the energy of the bombarding electrons to be ca 10 eV. As the electron energy is increased by 5–10 eV above this threshold, considerable fragmentation of the molecular ion occurs by internal bond cleavage. The degree of fragmentation increases with increasing electron energy and reaches a plateau at well below 70 eV, the usual operating energy. The degree of fragmentation can thus be controlled by the energy of the bombarding electrons. When high energy is employed, maximum structural information can be gained from the large amount of fragmentation of the molecule.

(b) Chemical ionisation

Chemical ionisation GC–MS which provides a less energetic ionisation of the sample is a relatively recent development but its potential is rapidly being realised. The principles of chemical ionisation have been described in detail elsewhere (Field, 1968; Arsenault, 1972) and general applications have been reviewed recently (Hatch and Munsun, 1977; Munsun, 1977). Chemical ionisation occurs when the vaporised sample is reacted with reactant ions generated from the electron impact ionisation of a reagent gas in a high source pressure (1.33×10^{12} kPa). Many different reagent gases have been employed, for example, hydrogen, methane, propane, isobutane, ammonia, water and methanol, but often the reagent gas employed also acts as the carrier gas for the gas chromatography. Ionisation of sample molecules is induced by proton transfer from, or hydrogen abstraction by, the ionised reagent gas thereby giving rise to a quasi-molecular ion $(M \pm 1)^+$. The amount of energy transferred to the sample molecules by this process is low

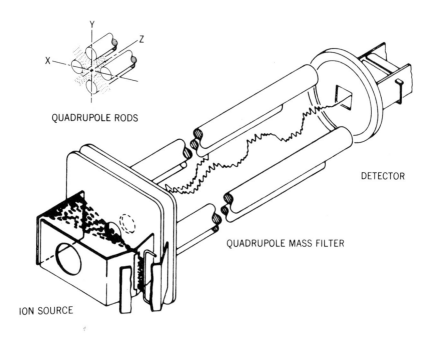

Fig. 4. A schematic representation of a quadrupole mass spectrometer. The complex ion trajectories are indicated and the insert illustrates the spacial arrangement of the four rods (reprinted from Watson, 1972, with the permission of Wiley-Interscience, New York).

compared with electron impact ionisation and as a result a typical chemical ionisation mass spectrum shows a prominent quasi-molecular ion (which, due to its greater stability, is often the most prominent ion) and very few fragment ions. Under these circumstances a great deal of structural information is lost compared with the electron impact mass spectrum but this feature can be useful in quantitative analysis since it may lead to increased sensitivity in selected ion monitoring (see later).

(c) Other ionisation procedures

Other ionisation procedures can be employed in mass spectrometry (Wilson, 1977), although these are not all applicable in GC–MS. Field ionisation and field desorption provide a useful method of analysing, by mass spectrometry, compounds which are highly polar, non-volatile or are thermally unstable (Schulten and Beckley, 1972; Derrick, 1977; Schulten, 1978). The technique has been used to advantage in the direct quantitative analysis of a number of steroid glucuronide conjugates (Adlercreutz, Soltmann and Tikkanen, 1974b) and biogenic amines (Wood, Mak and Hobb, 1976).

3. Ion Detection Recording

The detection of positive ions is commonly carried out using an electron multiplier which depends on secondary electron emission to effect an amplification of the signal received. This type of detector has a very rapid response and high sensitivity, factors which are essential when fast scan rates and weak ion currents are encountered.

The output from the electrical detector is amplified and can be monitored by an oscillographic recorder, or recorded in a semi-permanent manner on UV sensitive paper. Some instruments calibrate the ion recordings by providing simultaneous mass marker recordings. Where this is not possible the interpretation of the spectrum is often time-consuming, especially when a large number of scans have to be analysed.

With the adaptation of computers to GC–MS instrumentation, it is possible to acquire, process and store a large number of scans. A simple computer can be employed to calibrate and assign mass units to each ion current recorded, to subtract background peaks and to present the mass spectra graphically in a normalised form. Rapid progress has been made in the application of computers to the processing of mass spectrometric data.

An interesting detection system used in certain high resolution mass spectrometers is the photographic plate. Ten to 30 high resolution spectra may be recorded in a format comprising vertical lines for each ion. The plate is calibrated using standards which yield ions of accurately known mass so that the relative positions of the unknown lines in the spectrum can be measured accurately using a microdensitometer and exact masses assigned. The technique will measure to less than 1 millimass unit and thus the exact elemental composition of all ions can be determined.

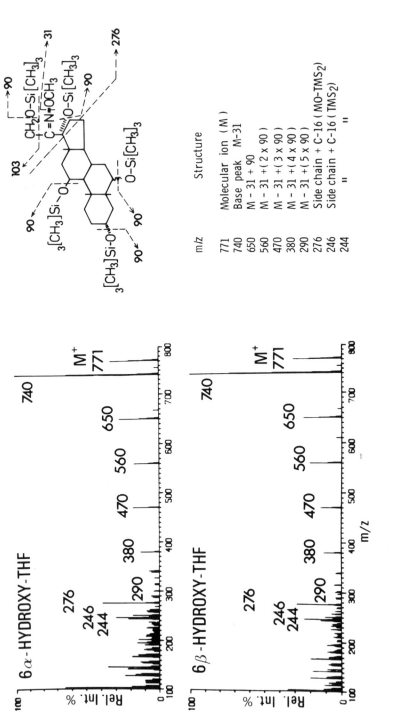

m/z	Structure
771	Molecular ion (M)
740	Base peak M-31
650	M − 31 + 90
560	M − 31 + (2 × 90)
470	M − 31 + (3 × 90)
380	M − 31 + (4 × 90)
290	M − 31 + (5 × 90)
276	Side chain + C-16 (MO-TMS₂)
246	Side chain + C-16 (TMS₂)
244	=

Fig. 5. The complete electron impact ionisation (70 eV) mass spectra of the methyloxime-trimethylsilyl ether derivative of 6α-hydroxy-THF (3α,6α,11β,17α,21-pentahydroxy-5β-pregnan-20-one) and 6β-hydroxy-THF (3α,6β,11β,17α,21-pentahydroxy-5β-pregnan-20-one). The structurally significant ions in the spectra and the fragmentation mechanism by which these ions arise are indicated.

4. Characteristics of the Mass Spectrum

The mass spectrum has a number of characteristic features which provide useful information about the structure of the original molecule and to illustrate these, the mass spectra of the methyloxime-trimethysilyl (MO-TMS) ether derivative of two isomers of the recently identified steroid $3\alpha,6,11\beta,17\alpha,$-21-pentahydroxy-5$\beta$-pregnan-20-one (6-hydroxy-THF; Setchell, Axelson, Sjövall and Gontscharow, 1976b; Setchell, Axelson, Sjövall, Morgan and Kirk, 1978a), is shown in Fig. 5.

(i) The molecular weight of a compound can generally be determined provided a sufficient number of molecular ions (M^+) remain intact during their ionisation, acceleration through the magnetic field and collection at the detector. The time taken for this process is approximately 2×10^{-5} sec. When high energy ionisation procedures are employed as in electron impact ionisation, the molecular ion is often so unstable that it is absent or its relative abundance very low. In the example shown the molecular ion of both isomers is present and indicates the molecular weight of the compounds to be 771. When less energetic ionisation procedures are employed, e.g. chemical ionisation, the relative intensity of the molecular ion in the mass spectrum can be enhanced and these more recently developed techniques have considerable potential for molecular weight determinations.

(ii) The mass spectrum of a compound is unique and because it can be reproduced under specified conditions provides a means for identifying the structure of a particular compound. In the example shown, the most abundant ion (referred to as the base peak and expressed as 100% relative intensity) is at m/z 740 and is formed by the loss of 31 mass units from the molecular ion due to the loss of the C-20 methyloxime derivative. The presence of five derivatised hydroxyl groups is indicated by the prominent ions at m/z 650, 560, 470, 380 and 290 which arise out of the stepwise loss of 5×90 mass units from the base peak. The ions at m/z 244, 246 and 276 formed by cleavage of the side chain, together with carbon atom C-16, are characteristic ions in the mass spectra of all corticosteroids possessing a dihydroxyacetone side chain. The fragmentation pattern therefore provides important information on the number, type and often the position of any functional groups in the parent molecule. Exceptions to this rule are stereoisomers (as shown in the example) which often provide identical mass spectra and in these instances it may be necessary to use additional techniques to allow the accurate elucidation of the stereochemistry. When gas chromatography is coupled with mass spectrometry the chromatographic retention volumes generally provide sufficient information to enable the stereochemistry of the compound to be determined.

(iii) The abundance of the ions generated is directly related to the total ionisation of the molecule and to the mass of sample ionised and provides the basis of methods for quantitative analysis.

5. Repetitive Scanning Techniques

The repetitive acquisition of mass spectral data was first described by Hites and Biemann (1968). This mode of operation allows a continuous qualitative and quantitative analysis of components eluted from the gas chromatography column. The method which is invaluable to multicomponent analysis, involves the rapid scanning at frequent intervals, of the entire mass range, during the elution of components from the GC column. Using a magnetic sector instrument, depending upon the mass range scanned and the resetting time of the instrument, each scan will take several seconds (although more rapid scans, 100 μs, can be achieved with quadrupole instruments) and therefore in a single 30 min gas chromatographic analysis up to 300 individual mass spectra may be accumulated. A computer for the acquisition and interpretation of the large amount of data generated by this mode of operation is essential and systems have been described in the literature for quantitative and qualitative analysis (Hites and Biemann, 1970; Reimendal and Sjövall, 1971, 1972, 1973; Burlingame and Johanson, 1972; Biemann, 1972a; Nau and Biemann, 1973).

(a) Qualitative analysis

The repetitive scanning mode has a number of advantages. The data stored on file are a record of the variation in intensity of all ion currents and therefore the complete mass spectrum of each component in the GC profile can be examined individually if required. Manual examination of the data is extremely tedious and time consuming but rapid examination of the data using the computer can reveal almost all of the components in a complex mixture. By selecting certain ion current (m/z) values it is possible to identify general or specific structures typical of the compounds under investigation. Figure 6 shows computer reconstructed ion current chromatograms obtained from the repetitive scanning of the GC eluent of the methyloxime-trimethylsilyl ether derivatives of steroids excreted as glucuronide conjugates in the urine of a normal subject. An advantage of this type of analysis is the ability to resolve components which have identical gas chromatographic retention times. For example, the derivatives of β-cortolone and β-cortol which are not resolved even using wall coated open-tubular glass capillary columns, can be easily identified from the ion current chromatograms when the individual m/z values for each steroid are plotted (Fig. 6). This type of approach can be employed to achieve a relatively unbiased analysis. A selection of m/z values typical of methyloxime-trimethylsilyl ether and trimethylsilyl ether derivatives of steroid structures has been published by Setchell, Almé, Axelson and Sjövall (1976a) and using this type of approach 108 different steroid conjugates were identified from normal human urine.

(b) Quantitative analysis

Quantitative determination of compounds can be achieved from data acquired from repetitive scanning analyses by measurement of the area of the peaks recorded for specific ion current chromatograms. By the addition of a suitable internal standard to known amounts of the reference compound it is possible to relate the area for an ion current chromatogram obtained in any sample to that obtained for the reference material using the internal standard to correct for different amounts injected into the instrument. The linear relationship between mass and area for different ion current (m/z) chromatograms has been reported for progesterone and a number of its metabolites (Axelson, Schumacher and Sjövall, 1974). This type of quantitative analysis has been used effectively by Sjövall's group (Reimendal and Sjövall, 1972) who have demonstrated coefficients of variation of between 3–10% for synthetic steroid mixtures, with detection limits as low as 1 ng.

One of the major drawbacks of this technique is its relatively low sensitivity compared with the selected ion monitoring (see later) of only a few m/z values. However, it is the only satisfactory means of obtaining specific qualitative and quantitative information of multicomponent samples. A compromise between the two methods of operation can be achieved by the repetitive scanning of a limited mass range, e.g. 3–10 mass units using magnetic or accelerating voltage scanning. By this technique improvements in the sensitivity of 100–300 fold can be attained (Reimendal and Sjövall, 1972; Baczynskyi, Duchamp, Zieserl and Axén, 1973). This type of procedure is useful in qualitative and quantitative studies of the metabolic fate of compounds labelled with stable-isotope atoms since it readily allows the simultaneous detection of closely related molecular species differing only in the number of stable labelled atoms incorporated and thereby avoids errors that may occur due to isotope separation effects (Axelson, Cronholm, Curstedt, Reimendal and Sjövall, 1974).

(c) Library searching

There has been a continuing and increasing use of computer data systems coupled to GC–MS instruments. With the trend more and more towards increased automation, computerised library search methods for the identi-

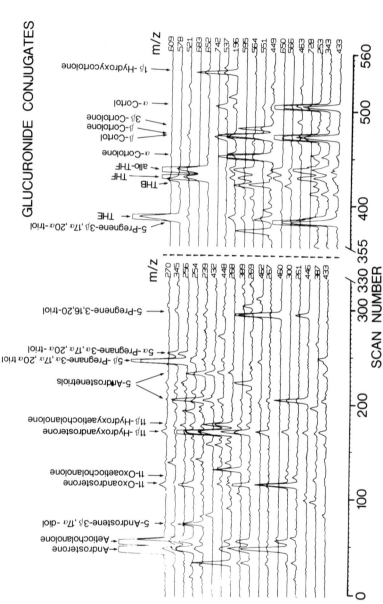

Fig. 6. Computer reconstructed profiles of ion current (m/z) chromatograms obtained during the repetitive magnetic scanning (10 spectra/min) GC–MS analysis of TMS ether and MO–TMS ether derivatives of steroids present as glucuronide conjugates in normal adult urine. Gas chromatography was performed on a 25 m open tubular glass capillary column coated with Silicone OV-1. Temperature programmed operation from 235–275° with increments of 0·6°/min was carried out following an isothermal period of 23 min. Two series of ion current chromatograms characteristic of structurally significant fragments or molecular ions of steroids having retention times of less than and greater than 1·5 that of 5α-cholestane are presented. Details of the structure indicated by the m/z values selected have been reported (Setchell *et al.*, 1976a). Some of the principal steroids are indicated; the criteria for their occurrence being a coincidence in the peaking of two or more ion current chromatograms characteristic in the mass spectrum of the steroid. This method of analysis allows the identification of compounds which cannot be resolved

fication of mass spectra have rapidly developed and been reviewed (Ward, 1971, 1973; Ridley, 1972; Heller, 1974; Naegeli and Clerc, 1974; Mellon, 1975, 1977). Several general approaches have been used in library search methods. The simplest procedure matches the unknown spectrum against reference spectra stored in a library file and gives an indication of the degree of similarity to suggested structures. To minimise computer search time, spectra are usually stored in a reduced format, where three or less of the most intense ions in each group of 14 ions are recorded (Hertz, Hites and Biemann, 1971; Bell, 1972; Grotch, 1973; Heller, Fales and Milne, 1973), although some systems also include ions of particularly high structural significance (Venkataraghavan, Kwok, Pesyna and McLafferty, 1973). Additional details such as nuclear magnetic resonance or infra red spectroscopy data have also been included to increase the certainty of computer prediction of structures (Clerc, Erni, Jost, Meili, Naegeli and Schwarzenbach, 1973).

More sophisticated methods examine each spectrum and look for fragmentation patterns characteristic of known structures in much the same way as manual interpretation. Others simulate mass spectral fragmentation patterns. These types of programme were described by Biemann, Cone, Webster and Arsenault (1966) and Senn and McLafferty (1966) as an aid to peptide sequencing.

The inclusion of a gas chromatographic retention index reduces the computer search time and aids the identification of isomeric forms of compounds giving essentially identical mass spectral data. In these methods, standards, often n-alkanes, are injected with the sample. The computer recognises the positions of the standards from given m/z values and relates those to the positions of unknown spectra (Nau and Biemann, 1974; Sweeley, Young, Holland and Gates, 1974).

In spite of the large number of library search systems described the inherent disadvantage of relying entirely upon the computer for interpretation is the limited number of reference spectra that are contained in most libraries. However, several international mass spectral data retrieval systems now operate with which the analyst can communicate with a large central library via a telephone line (Heller, Fales, Milne, Feldman, Daly, Maxwell and McCormick, 1973; Carhart, Johnson, Smith, Buchanan, Dromey and Lederberg, 1975).

A novel technique has been described by Jellum, Helland, Eldjard, Markwardt and Marhöfer (1975) whereby the mass spectra recorded during a repetitive scanning analysis of a pathological sample is compared against a library file of pre-recorded spectra from a sample from normal subjects. The computer is then used to determine the presence or absence of ions in the sample and thus for differences between the two profiles. The system so far has only been applied to the detection of abnormalities in organic acid metabolism, but could be applied to the screening of disorders in hormone metabolism.

6. Selected Ion Monitoring

This technique first described by Henneberg (1961) and applied by Sweeley, Elliott, Fries and Ryhage (1966) and Hammer, Holmstedt and Ryhage (1968) has also been referred to as selected ion detection, single or multiple ion monitoring and more commonly mass fragmentography. This latter terminology is not ideal since in many instances the ion being recorded is a molecular ion (M^+) and not a fragment ion as the name would imply.

By selecting a single ion from the mass spectrum and measuring its intensity it becomes possible to increase greatly the sensitivity of the GC–MS technique and afford a means of quantifying the compound, since the signal carried by an ion current is proportional to the mass of sample ionised. It is this principle that is employed in selected ion monitoring (SIM). Figure 7 shows an example of the simultaneous SIM recordings for the molecular ions of the di-TMS ether derivatives of oestradiol-17β (m/z 416) and [$^2H_4$]-oestradiol-17β (m/z 420). The responses obtained from 0, 66, 132, 198 and 264 fmols (0, 18, 36, 54 and 72 pg respectively) of oestradiol-17β which were added to a constant amount (ca 200 pg) of the tetradeuterated analogue (used to correct for differences in the amounts injected on column) shows a linear relationship and illustrates the high sensitivity of the selected ion monitoring technique.

When the instrument is operated at low resolution and a single ion is monitored, it is extremely important to utilise the GC retention index of the compound for identification. Additionally it is possible to simultaneously monitor more than one ion characteristic of the compound (referred to as multiple ion monitoring) and in these circumstances the specificity of the technique is increased.

The simultaneous monitoring of more than one ion provides a basis for stable isotope dilution analysis and considerably increases the specificity of the SIM technique (see later). In this case a single ion characteristic of the analyte is monitored together with the corresponding ion for the internal standard which will have a higher mass according to the number of stable isotope atoms in the molecule or fragment monitored (Fig. 7).

In practice the technique requires that the mass spectrometer be focused to detect only the ion current of the masses to be monitored. This is generally achieved by fixing the magnetic field to focus the ion current of lowest mass, then by adjusting the accelerating voltage it is possible to focus ions of higher mass. During the analysis an accelerating voltage alternator is used to switch continuously between the pre-adjusted accelerating voltages and an ion current recording produced for each selected mass. Technical problems due to the finite time necessary to switch between voltages and the range of switching, which is usually 20–30% of that of the lowest mass, impose limitations on the precision and sensitivity of the technique. Furthermore a high stability in the magnetic field and other parameters is essential for satisfactory precision and in many instruments the control of many parameters is now performed by computer.

An alternative method for operation is to use a constant accelerating voltage and to switch the magnetic field but while this mode of operation will overcome the limited mass range of accelerating voltage switching, the sensitivity which can be achieved is reduced due to the slower switching rates.

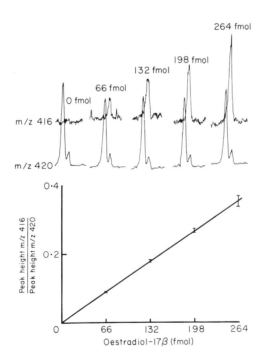

Fig. 7. Typical recordings obtained from the simultaneous selected ion monitoring of the molecular ions for oestradiol-17β (m/z 416) and [$^2H_4$]-oestradiol-17β (m/z 420). Different amounts of oestradiol-17β are added to a constant amount (ca 700 fmol) of the deuterated oestradiol-17β which acts as an internal standard. The peak height of the responses m/z 416/m/z 420 plotted against the amount of oestradiol-17β yields a linear calibration graph which can be used in quantitative analysis.

The quadrupole instrument is widely employed for SIM since it is capable of very fast switching rates and has no limitation in the mass range of switching. The application of this instrument to SIM has been reviewed (Falkner et al., 1975).

The most important advantage of the SIM mode of operation is its extremely high sensitivity (Fig. 7), which is of the order of 1000 times that of flame ionisation detection-gas chromatography or repetitive magnetic scanning methods of GC–MS and in some instances detection limits may be in the femtogram region. The sensitivity which can be attained is influenced by:

(i) The gas-chromatographic characteristics of the compound.

(ii) Number of ions monitored; the sensitivity and precision decreases with the increasing number of ions monitored.

(iii) The ionisation process used and the proportion of the total ion current carried by the ions monitored. Chemical ionisation provides a useful means of attaining high specificity (since the quasi-molecular ion can often be monitored) and high sensitivity (because the fewer ions generated carry higher proportions of the total ionisation).

(iv) Interference from impurities or related compounds co-eluting with the compound measured may give rise to ions of similar mass. The presence of background ions arising out of column "bleed" will also affect the sensitivity, although this problem is less when capillary columns are employed. This general problem can be overcome by single ion monitoring at high resolution and sample preparation can thus be kept to a minimum (Millington, 1973; Gaskell and Pike, 1978).

The most widespread application of SIM is in quantitative analysis and a number of reviews have emphasised the high accuracy and precision of the technique for clinical chemistry and endocrinology (Breuer and Siekmann, 1975; Björkhem, Blomstrand, Lantto, Svensson and Ohmann, 1976; Adlercreutz, Härkönen and Järvenpää, 1978).

To enable quantitation the response obtained for the selected ion is measured relative to that of an ion of an internal standard, the choice of which is a critical factor in the attainment of high precision, sensitivity and accuracy. The internal standard should be closely related in structure, chemical properties and gas chromatographic behaviour to the analyte, especially when pre-instrumental stages such as extraction, purification and derivatisation are performed. Homologous and analogous compounds have been used for internal standards in SIM.

(i) Homologues. These have been employed in many methods, e.g. 19-nor-derivatives of steroids for the measurement of progesterone, testosterone and androstenedione (Dehennin, Reiffsteck and Schöller, 1974a, b). The catecholamines, noradrenaline and dopamine in brain tissue has been measured with the methyl homologues, α-methylnoradrenaline and α-methyl-dopamine as internal standards (Koslow, Cattabeni and Costa, 1972). A homologue is less satisfactory than an analogue but is often used when a single ion is monitored and it becomes necessary to separate the internal standard from the analyte during gas chromatography. The major disadvantages of homologues are the differences in chemical and chromatographic properties which preclude accurate correction for losses or errors in the pre-instrumental procedures. Millard (1977) has discussed some of the factors relating to the choice of internal standards and compared homologues with analogues.

(ii) Analogues. The most desirable analogues are stable-isotope labelled forms of the analyte but the prohibitive costs, availability and the difficulty in synthesising such compounds have severely limited their application. However, there has recently been an exponential growth in the application of stable-isotope labelled compounds for quantitative and metabolic studies (Klein and Klein, 1978a, b).

(a) Stable-isotope dilution analysis

The use of stable-isotope labelled internal standards forms the basis of the method of stable-isotope dilution analysis. The stable-isotope labelled standard is added to the sample and thus compensates for losses during the extraction, isolation and purification procedures, differences in the yields during the derivatisation and when added in excess can be used to minimise the losses due to adsorption on the GC column ("carrier" effect). Known amounts of the analyte are added to a constant amount of internal standard and the ratio of the peak height of the ion current recordings for the analyte/internal standard calculated from which a calibration curve is constructed (see Fig. 7).

The important requirements of a stable-isotope labelled standard are therefore:

(i) The stable-labelled atoms are incorporated in that part of the molecule which is selected for monitoring and that they are chemically stable during any pre-instrumental procedures. One of the earliest examples of the use of stable-isotope labelled analogues is that of Samuelsson, Hamberg and Sweeley (1970) who described a method for the measurement of the prostaglandin PGE_1 as its methyl ester-methyloxime-TMS-ether derivative in which the internal standard employed was the trideuterated-methyloxime derivative. The disadvantage of the procedure was the inability to account for losses during the sample preparation since the derivatisation of sample and of internal standard are performed separately before their co-injection on the GC column. Similar comments apply to an elegant technique for the determination of eleven oestrogens in plasma, bile and urine using the deuterated labelled trimethylsilyl ether derivatives of five oestrogens as standards (Adlercreutz, Tikkanen and Hunneman, 1974c).

(ii) The isotopic enrichment should be high to minimise the relative amount of the natural isotopic species (non-labelled compound) present in the stable-isotope labelled compound, factors which will affect the precision and sensitivity of the assay. The requirement of a high chemical purity is not necessarily a critical factor provided any impurities present do not give rise to ions which interfere with those recorded.

(iii) The number of stable-isotope labelled atoms incorporated into the molecule should be sufficient to minimise interference that will arise from the natural isotopic species present in the analyte. The incorporation of at least three atoms per molecule are usually necessary but if this number is too large the internal standard and the analyte may be resolved during gas chromatography. This "isotope effect" is more enhanced when open-tubular capillary columns are employed and it may sometimes be advantageous to employ packed columns for SIM, particularly when the sample to be analysed is relatively pure.

Due to the prohibitive costs of many stable isotope labelled compounds radioactive labelled analogues, e.g. [^{14}C]- and [^{3}H]-labelled steroids have been used for internal standards in assays described for progesterone (Björkhem, Blomstrand and Lantto, 1975a), testosterone (Siekmann, Martin and Breuer, 1972; Siekmann, 1974; Björkhem, Lantto and Svensson, 1975b; Breuer and Siekmann, 1975), 5-dihydrotestosterone (Siekmann, Martin, Siekmann and Breuer, 1976a), cortisol (Björkhem, Blomstrand, Lantto, Löf and Svensson, 1974; Siekmann, 1974), aldosterone (Siekmann, 1974) and oestradiol-17β (Siekmann, Siekmann and Breuer, 1978).

C. APPLICATIONS OF GC–MS TO HORMONE ANALYSIS IN BLOOD

In hormone analysis GC–MS has been most used for the steroid hormones and prostaglandins. Application to the biogenic amines is rapidly increasing and a way being opened towards the greater understanding of brain chemistry in normal and in abnormal subjects. The application of GC–MS to the thyroid hormones and peptide hormones has been limited by the instability, involatility and with the latter, the large molecular weight of these hormones.

The number of publications describing GC–MS to studies on hormones is vast and the following outlines some of the recent work as well as work of historical importance.

1. Steroid Hormones

Some of the earliest applications were in the validation of GC techniques for steroids where the specificity was established from mass spectrometric analysis of the GC effluent by comparison against reference compounds (Sjövall and Vihko, 1965; Sjövall, Sjövall, Maddock and Horning, 1966; Sjövall and Vihko, 1966a).

The structural elucidation of many previously unidentified steroids has been made possible by GC–MS and detailed studies have identified steroids in umbilical cord blood (Laatikainen, Peltonen and Nylander, 1973), plasma (Sjövall and Vihko, 1966b, 1968; Jänne, Vihko, Sjövall and Sjövall, 1969; Hellström, Sjövall and Vihko, 1969) and in plasma from pregnant women (Sjövall, Sjövall and Vihko, 1968; Sjövall, 1970a,b; Baillie, Anderson, Sjövall and Sjövall, 1976a).

Much of the steroid work by Sjövall's group has centred on the use of GC–MS in studying the metabolism of steroid sulphate conjugates (Sjövall and Vihko, 1968; Baillie, Sjövall and Sjövall, 1975b, 1976b), the effects of ethanol administration on plasma steroid sulphates (Cronholm and Sjövall, 1968, 1970; Cronholm, Sjövall and Sjövall, 1969) and on alterations in steroid metabolism during intrahepatic cholestasis of pregnancy (Sjövall and Sjövall, 1970).

Steroid sulphate conjugates which are not suitable for direct GC–MS analysis have been determined as free steroids after their separation into groups of conjugates by liquid-gel chromatography and enzymatic/solvolytic cleavage of the sulphate moiety. Groups of steroid conjugates have been separated by systems based on Sephadex LH-20 (Sjövall and Vihko, 1968) and more recently lipophilic ion exchange gels (Sjövall, 1975; Setchell et al., 1976a; Setchell, Taylor, Adlercreutz, Axelson and Sjövall, 1979).

Mass spectrometry can determine the position of a sulphate group in the steroid molecule. Free hydroxyl groups are first protected by acetylation and after solvolytic hydrolysis of the sulphate group(s) the TMS ether derivative is prepared of the freed hydroxyl group(s). The mass spectrometric fragmentation patterns for the mixed acetate-TMS ether derivatives are sufficiently specific to enable positions of the original sulphate moiety to be located. Cronholm (1969) published a series of spectra for sulphate conjugates of 5-androstenediols, androstanediols and 5-pregnenediols, illustrating this application of mass spectrometry to the analysis of steroid sulphates in human plasma.

The GC–MS analysis of steroid glucuronides without prior enzymatic hydrolysis has been investigated by Thompson (1976) who prepared premethylated derivatives of oestrogen glucuronides. Similarly the n-propyl ester O-trimethylsilyl ether derivatives of oestrogen conjugates have been investigated (Miyazaki, Ishibashi, Itoh, Morishita, Sudo and Nambara, 1976), and preliminary data from the analysis of urine samples indicate that such methods may prove useful, but it is doubtful if this direct approach to the analysis of glucuronide conjugates, particularly of the polar neutral steroids in plasma, will be successful.

Sjövall and Sjövall (1968) identified in pregnancy plasma the mono-sulphate conjugate of 5α-pregnane-3α,20α,21-triol in concentrations greater than 20 µg/100 ml and reported this steroid to be present in much higher concentrations in patients with pruritis during pregnancy. This work showed how the combined use of gas chromatographic retention data and differences in the fragmentation patterns of mass spectra can be used to differentiate configurational differences in closely related structures. For example, the stereochemistry of the 3α-hydroxyl group in 5α-pregnane-3α,20α,21-triol was confirmed from the mass spectrum of the TMS ether derivative of the aldehyde which gave a base peak for the fragment of mass $[M^+\text{-}15]$ formed by the loss of a methyl function while the analogous 3β-hydroxy steroids gave a base peak at $[M^+\text{-}90]$ due to loss of trimethylsilanoxy group (Sjövall and Sjövall, 1968).

A further example of the specificity of mass spectrometric fragmentation patterns was shown by Allen, Thomas, Brooks and Knight (1969) who demonstrated how the stereochemistry of the hydrogen at position C-5 could be accurately determined using GC–MS in all 3,6-dioxygenated steroids when the methyloxime derivative was prepared. This particular approach was used to provide definitive evidence for the position of the C-6 hydroxyl in the recently identified steroid 6α-hydroxy-THF (Setchell *et al.*, 1976b, 1978a).

Stable-isotope dilution GC–MS analysis, because of its specificity has been the technique of choice for the development of definitive and reference methods for numerous analytes (Cali, Mandel and Young, 1972) and in recent years attention has focused on the steroid hormones (Breuer and Siekmann, 1975; Björkhem *et al.*, 1976). Many analyses yield results of high precision but not of a comparable accuracy. Radioimmunoassays frequently yield higher values than GC–MS analyses (Onikki and Adlercreutz, 1973; Wilson, John, Groom, Pierrepoint and Griffiths, 1977; Dehennin *et al.*, 1974b; Björkhem *et al.*, 1975a, b; Millington, Golder, Cowley, Landon, Roberts, Butt and Griffiths, 1976; Setchell *et al.*, 1979).

Many SIM analyses for steroids using low or high resolution with either single or multiple ion monitoring have recently been published (Table 1), and many would be satisfactory as reference techniques.

A potentially exciting area which has recently been investigated for quantitative analysis is that of the selected monitoring of metastable ions.

A metastable ion is formed from a decomposition of an ion in the field-free region (Fig. 3) during its passage from the ion source to the magnetic sector, and can be represented by the equation:

$$[m_1^+] \longrightarrow [m_2^+] + [\text{neutral fragment}]$$

The metastable ion $[m_2^+]$ is formed with loss of energy and is focused at lower mass than an ion of mass m_2 produced in the ion source. In double focusing instruments, by linked scanning of the magnetic and the electrostatic sector voltage a spectrum of all metastable ions derived from an ion $[m_1^+]$ can be recorded (Boyd and Beynon, 1977; Millington and Smith, 1977). By applying this linked scanning procedure the occurrence of a metastable ion can be detected and recorded continuously. Gaskell and Millington (1978a, b) have utilised this facility in the quantitative analysis of 5α-dihydrotestosterone as the t-butyldimethylsilyl ether derivative. The metastable ion formed in the transition of $[M-57]^+ \to [(M-57)-76)^+$ was monitored and a detection limit of 20 pg attained. Depending upon the type of compound, this approach to SIM potentially offers considerably increased specificity and sensitivity compared with low resolution SIM and an alternative to high resolution GC–MS which has been employed as a means of improving specificity in quantitative analysis using SIM (Millington, 1975; Gaskell and Pike, 1978).

Classical methods of investigating metabolic pathways have involved the administration of radioactive compounds as tracers but for ethical reasons the administration of such compounds is prohibited by many centres, in studies on pregnant women or newborn infants. When alternative tracers labelled with stable-isotopes are utilised, GC–MS provides a powerful tool for investigating metabolism during pregnancy. Apart from providing general pharmacokinetic data such as pool sizes, secretion rates and half-lives, when stable-isotopes are incorporated into the molecule, depending upon their position, additional information can be gained on the fate of the parent molecule and on the positions in the molecule of specific metabolic reactions. The potential of this approach to elucidating metabolic pathways is evident from the work of Baillie et al. (1975b, 1976a, b) who investigated the origin of the steroid 5α-pregnane-3α,20α,21-triol-3-sulphate previously identified in the plasma of pregnant women (Sjövall and Sjövall, 1968). These workers administered to pregnant women the deuterated steroid 3α-hydroxy-5α-[3α,11,11-²H₃]-pregnan-20-one (Baillie, Sjövall and Hertz, 1975a) and demonstrated active metabolism of sulphated steroid, with reduction at C-20 and 21-hydroxylation yielding the 5α-pregnane-3α,20α,21-triol-3-sulphate. The findings provide evidence for the source of the elevated concentrations of this steroid in patients with intrahepatic cholestasis in pregnancy since it has previously been demonstrated that these patients have high concentrations of the precursor (Sjövall and Sjövall, 1970). Similar studies have also been performed with other deuterated analogues of sulphated pregnane derivatives, notably 3β-hydroxy-5α-pregnan-20-one-3-sulphate, 5α-pregnane-3β,20α-diol-3-sulphate and 5α-pregnane-3β,20α-diol-sulphate. The studies demonstrated that these compounds are metabolised directly without prior cleavage of the sulphate group and that this occurred in the maternal rather than the foetal compartment (Baillie et al., 1976b). The production rate for six $C_{21}O_2$ steroid sulphates was ca 80 mg/day indicating that the conversion of progesterone to sulphated pregnane metabolites constitutes a major metabolic pathway during pregnancy (Baillie et al., 1976b).

The multicomponent analysis of steroids using repetitive scanning GC–MS has been less frequently employed compared with selected ion detection methods, probably because of the requirement for a computer system to handle the data acquired. Furthermore, due to the limited sensitivity of this approach, a greater emphasis is needed on pre-instrumental steps of sample concentration and removal of interfering contaminants.

The neutral polymer resin Amberlite XAD-2 which has proved so useful for urinary steroid analysis (Bradlow, 1968) has been shown to give a quantitative extraction of steroids from plasma when used at 64° (Axelson and Sjövall, 1974). Lipophilic gels have been developed for the purification and isolation of steroids before GC–MS analysis. Sephadex LH-20 has been used for the separation of conjugates of neutral steroids (Sjövall and Vihko, 1968) and of oestrogens (Tikkanen and Adlercreutz, 1970). Recently, lipophilic ion exchange gels (Ellingboe, Almé and Nyström, 1970; Almé and Nyström, 1971; Sjövall, 1975; Setchell et al., 1976a; Axelson and Sjövall, 1977) permitted separation of conjugated steroids into groups. The anion exchange gel, diethylaminohydroxypropyl Sephadex LH-20 (DEAP-LH-20) provides a useful method for the separation of free steroids from conjugated steroids, the latter being retained by this gel (Setchell et al., 1976a). The multi-component analysis of steroids in maternal and cord plasma of nine patients with placental sulphatase deficiency has been reported. Analysis of the monosulphate conjugate fraction isolated by chromatography on DEAP-LH-20 provided a means of pre-natal diagnosis of this disorder Taylor and Shackleton, 1979). Recently a method for the group separation of oestrogen conjugates including the A-ring and D-ring glucuronides has been reported (Setchell et al., 1979). With the weaker anion exchange gel, triethylaminohydroxypropyl Sephadex LH-20 (TEAP-LH-20) unconjugated neutral steroids and phenolic steroids have been separated and the analysis of unconjugated steroids in plasma from pregnant women described (Axelson and Sjövall, 1977). The lipophilic cation exchange gel sulphoethyl Sephadex LH-20 (SE-LH-20, Setchell et al., 1976a) permits selective isolation from plasma of 3-oxo-4-ene steroids; these are converted to their oximes, retained on the cation exchange gel by interaction with the positive charge on the oxime, and eluted with methanol:pyridine (20:1, v/v). Sufficient purification and concentration is obtained to allow the equivalent of 1–2 ml of plasma to be loaded on a glass capillary column and analysed by repetitive scanning GC–MS techniques (Axelson and Sjövall, 1976).

2. Thyroid Hormones

The thyroid hormones have proved difficult to analyse by GC–MS due to their polar nature, relative involatility and low concentrations in serum (thyroxine, T_4, ca 100 nmol/l, 3,3,5'-triiodothyronine, T_3, ca 2–3 nmol/l). Radioimmunoassay and other indirect methods have largely been used to determine levels of thyroid hormones. Relatively little is known of their metabolism, but tetraiodothyroacetic acid and diiodotyrosine are present in serum (Nelson, Weiss, Lewis, Wilcox and Palmer, 1974; Ramsden, Raw and Hoffenberg, 1975; Crossley, Ramsden and Hoffenberg, 1978) and with the possibility that other analogues may be present, Lawson, Ramsden, Raw and Hoffenberg (1974) investigated the mass spectrometric fragmentation patterns of trimethylsilyl ether derivatives of thyroxine and 16 related compounds to assess their properties for quantitative analysis. At levels below 500 ng per injection all derivatives were adsorbed strongly and a more suitable derivative for quantitative use is the N,O-heptafluorobutyrate-methyl ester (Petersen and Vouros, 1977). The electron impact mass spectrum of this derivative exhibits a well defined molecular ion and predominant ions of high mass, and using capillary column GC–MS, SIM detection limits were reported to be in the sub-picogram level for rT_3 (3,3'5'-triiodothyronine) and 100 pg for T_3, the differences being attributed to the carrier effect of the trideutereo-methyl ester of rT_3 which was added to the sample before gas chromatography but not employed in quantitation. The determination of 3,3',5,5'-tetra-iodothyroacetic acid in human serum using SIM has recently been described (Crossley et al., 1978). The 3,3',5,5'-tetra-iodothyropropionate homologue was used as the internal standard and the molecular ion at m/z 776 for the analyte and m/z 790 for internal standard were monitored. The detection limits of the method were equivalent to 50 ng/l and euthyroid concentrations of 60–125 ng/l are lower than in previous reports.

3. Peptide Hormones

At present quantitative analysis of peptide hormones is not possible by GC–MS, but considerable effort has recently been devoted to the qualitative analysis of peptides in general, by sequencing techniques (Biemann, 1972b;

Morris and Dell, 1975; Arpino and McLafferty, 1976; Nau, 1976a; Falter, 1977). Due to problems of involatility and high molecular weight, these large molecules can be analysed only after degradation to small fragments. Biemann and coworkers (Nau, Kelly and Biemann, 1973; Hudson and Biemann, 1976; Kelly, Nau, Förster and Biemann, 1975; Nau, Förster, Kelly and Biemann, 1975; Nau, 1976a, b, 1978; Nau & Biemann, 1976a, b, c) have developed general procedures for the sequencing of peptides and polypeptides. Selective enzymic or chemical cleavage reduces the peptide to a mixture of di-, tri- and tetrapeptides and after acetylation and esterification they are converted to the corresponding polyaminoalcohols and analysed by GC–MS after derivatisation. The TMS ether derivatives are very volatile and show excellent gas chromatographic characteristics while their electron impact mass spectra exhibit easily interpretable and informative fragmentation patterns (Kelly et al., 1975). The trifluoroacetyl-methyl ester (Weygand, Prox, Jorgensen, Axen and Kirchner, 1963), pentafluoropropionyl-methyl ester (Caprioli, Siefert and Sutherland, 1973) and heptafluorobutyryl-methyl ester (Anderson, 1967) have also been used. Biemann's group used computer analysis of the data recorded from repetitive scanning of the GC effluent and by this approach the structure of the entire peptide was elucidated by matching the overlapping sequences in the peptide fragments (Nau et al., 1975; Kelly et al., 1975; Nau and Biemann, 1976c).

An alternative approach to sequencing utilises the enzyme dipeptidylaminopeptidase (McDonald, Callahan and Ellis, 1972) which cleaves a dipeptide from the free-NH_2 terminal of a polypeptide. By stepwise enzymatic hydrolysis of the polypeptide and analysis of the dipeptide units the structure of the parent molecule is determined (Ovchinnikov and Kiryushkin, 1972; Förster, Kelly, Nau and Biemann, 1972; Caprioli et al., 1973).

Chemical ionisation mass spectrometry has been used as an alternative to electron impact ionisation mass spectrometry for peptide sequencing (Gray, Wojcik and Futrell, 1970; Kiryushkin, Fales, Axenrod, Gilbert and Milne, 1971; Baldwin and McLafferty, 1973; Bowen and Field, 1973; Mudgett, Bowen, Field and Kindt, 1975, 1977; Arpino and McLafferty, 1976) but much of the work has involved the direct introduction of the sample into the mass spectrometer. The first 34 amino acid residues of human parathyroid hormone were sequenced using chemical ionisation mass spectrometry of the phenylthiohydantoin derivatives of the products of Edman degradation (Fales, Nagai, Milne, Brewer, Bronzert and Pisano, 1971). Similarly, as the trimethylsilyl ether derivatives, the structure of luteinising hormone releasing hormone (LHRH) was elucidated (Burgus, Butcher, Amoss, Ling, Monahan, Rivier, Fellows, Blackwell, Vale and Guillemin, 1972).

Open-tubular capillary column GC–MS has been used for the analysis of oligopeptides of up to five amino acid residues as the N-acyl-O,N-permethylated derivatives (Priddle, Rose and Offord, 1977).

At present, although GC–MS offers little serious challenge to radio-immunoassay and related methods in quantitative analysis it will continue to be of value in the structural elucidation of peptide hormones.

4. Prostaglandins

Because of their very low concentrations in blood, the prostaglandins have posed challenging problems to the analyst. The role of GC–MS in the structural elucidation and quantification of prostaglandins has been reviewed by Falkner et al. (1975) and Crain, Desiderio and McCloskey (1975).

GC–MS in the SIM mode has provided a specific and sensitive technique which because of the ease and rapidity with which assays can be developed, has been extensively exploited in the understanding of prostaglandin bio-synthesis and metabolism. The first isotope dilution SIM techniques to be described for prostaglandins were by Gréen and Samuelsson (1967), Samuelsson et al. (1970), Samuelsson, Granström, Gréen and Hamberg (1971) and Watson (1971). These early methods used tri-deuterated-methyl-oxime derivatives as internal standards and excessive adsorption of this derivative was avoided by the addition of up to a 1000 fold excess of un-labelled compound to produce a "carrier" effect for the endogenous prosta-glandins. Using this type of isotopic internal standard, no allowance for pre-instrumental errors was made and the sensitivity of the method was limited because the ions suitable for monitoring (i.e. those containing the three deuterium atoms) represented as little as 1% of the total ionisation. In spite of the limitations of the methodology, PGE_2 concentrations in blood were measured and reported to be 700 pg/ml (Samuelsson et al., 1971).

The preparation of the first deuterated prostaglandin analogues, 3,3,4,4-$[^2H_4]$-PGE_2 and 3,3,4,4-$[^2H_4]$-$PGE_{2\alpha}$ (Axen, Gréen, Horlin and Samuels-son, 1971; Gréen, Granström, Samuelsson and Axen, 1973) led to con-siderable improvements in sensitivity, accuracy and precision of SIM methods for PGE_2 (Axen et al., 1971) and $PGF_{2\alpha}$ (Gréen, 1972). Con-centrations of PGE_2 and $PGF_{2\alpha}$ in blood were determined to be less than 100 pg/ml and 150 pg/ml respectively using these procedures and were suppressed to insignificant levels after aspirin administration (Gréen, 1972; Gréen et al., 1973).

The PG_1-series, although present in smaller amounts, exhibit a greater biological activity than the PG_2-series (Peery, Johnson and Pastan, 1971; Maganiello and Vaughan, 1972) and Goldyne and Hammerström (1978) described the measurement of PGE_1 and $PGF_{1\alpha}$. Argentation thin layer chromatography of the methyl ester derivative was used to separate these prostaglandins from both the respective two-series analogues and the isomeric metabolites, 13,14-dihydro-PGE_2 and 13,14-dihydro-$PGF_{2\alpha}$ which otherwise caused interference in the GC–MS assay.

A method for the determination of PGA_2 in plasma using a mixed stable isotope-labelled and radioactive-labelled internal standard (3,3,4,4-[$^2H_4$]-17,18-[$^3H_2$])-PGA_2 was described by Gréen and Steffenrud (1976). The concentration of this prostaglandin in 10 normal subjects ranged from 5–10 pg/ml, approximately the detection limit of the method. These results are not in agreement with the higher levels found when RIA was used for assay (Zusman, Caldwell and Speroff, 1972; Jaffe, Behrman and Parker, 1973; Pletka and Hickler, 1974) and the theory that this prostaglandin functioned as a circulating hormone.

Sweetman, Frölich and Watson (1973) described an alternative approach to the determination of the PGE-series which were converted in high yield to either the PGA or PGB series. The methyl ester-trimethylsilyl ether derivative chosen provided sufficient sensitivity to exclude the need for excess standard as a carrier, because the mass spectrum is characterised by little fragmentation and most of the ionisation is carried by a few ions.

The basic principles of the SIM assay developed for prostaglandins are similar—the differences between individual methods is often attributed to the choice of derivative for gas chromatography–mass spectrometry. The commonly employed derivatives for prostaglandins are apparent from Table 1 and these have also been described by Salmon and Flowers (1979) in Vol. 2. The use of the t-butyldimethylsilyl ether derivative has recently been described for prostaglandin assays (Watson and Sweetman, 1974; Kelly and Taylor, 1976; Kelly, 1977) and the mass spectrometric characteristics of this type of derivative have been compared with those of the TMS ether derivative for a number of prostaglandins (Brash and Baillie, 1978).

Basal levels of most of the circulating prostaglandins are near the detection limits of the GC–MS methods and many workers have preferred to measure specific metabolites, present in much greater amounts, and which are considered to reflect the production rate of the primary prostaglandin. SIM isotope dilution assays have been reported for 9α,11α-dihydroxy-15-keto-prost-5-enoic acid (Gréen and Granström, 1973), 7α,11-dihydroxy-5-keto-tetranorprost-9-enoic acid (Oates, Sweetman, Gréen and Samuelsson, 1976), 7α-hydroxy-5,11-diketo-tetranorprostane-1,16-dioic acid (Hamberg, 1972, 1973, 1974; Seyberth, Sweetman, Frölich and Oates, 1976), 5α,7α-dihydroxy-11-keto-tetranorprostane-1,16-dioic acid (Brash, Baillie, Clare and Draffan, 1976). Clinical disorders with overproduction of prostaglandin E_2 have been identified by a quantitative stable isotope dilution mass spectrometric assay for PGE_2 and the major urinary metabolite 7α-hydroxy-5,11-diketo-tetranorprostane-1,16-dioic acid (Oates, Seyberth, Frölich, Sweetman and Watson, 1973). In hypercalcaemia associated with certain tumours elevated levels of the metabolite are excreted in the urine (Seyberth, Segre, Morgan, Sweetman, Potts and Oates, 1975), while in Bartter's syndrome there is associated increased urinary excretion of PGE_2 (Bartter, Gill, Frölich, Bowden, Hollifeld, Radfar, Keiser, Oates, Seyberth and Taylor, 1976).

The application of GC–MS to the structural elucidation of many prostaglandins has proved invaluable and much of this work has been pioneered by Samuelsson and Hamberg. The mass spectrometric fragmentations induced during electron impact ionisation have been reviewed by Crain et al. (1975), together with a comprehensive list of published mass spectra.

The isolation and identification of the prostaglandin endoperoxides by Hamberg and Samuelsson (1973) and Hamberg, Svensson, Wakabayashi and Samuelsson (1974) was important in understanding the pathway of prostaglandin biosynthesis from arachidonic acid. The first two endoperoxides, 15-hydroxyperoxy-9α,11α-peroxide-prosta-5,13-dienoic acid (PGG_2) and 15-hydroxy-9α,11α-peroxide-prosta-5,13-dienoic (PGH_2) were isolated after a brief incubation of arachidonic acid with the microsomal fraction of the sheep vesicular gland. Their identification was established by indirect methods, using GC–MS to characterise the products formed after mild reduction, dehydration and isomerisation and demonstrated for the first time that the introduction of the oxygen function at C-15 of prostaglandins occurs by a dioxygenase (cyclo-oxygenase) reaction (Hamberg et al., 1974). The endoperoxides are potent in inducing rapid irreversible aggregation of human blood platelets and PGG_2 was essential for normal platelet haemostasis (Malmsten, Hamberg, Svensson and Samuelsson, 1975).

The potential of GC–MS in structural elucidation is evident by the ever-increasing number of prostaglandin structures which are being identified. After the identification of endoperoxides, specific metabolites of these compounds were identified from which a new group of compounds, the thromboxanes, were discovered (Hamberg, Svensson and Samuelsson, 1975). Thromboxane B_2, previously called PHD,[8-(1-hydroxy-3-oxo-propyl)-9,12L]-dihydroxy-5,10-heptadecadienoic acid (Hamberg and Samuelsson, 1974a) which is biologically inactive is derived from PGG_2 by the incorporation of one molecule of water. Recently an unstable intermediate (37°, $T_{\frac{1}{2}} = 32$ sec) was isolated by trapping into methanol the products formed after a 30 sec incubation of human blood platelets with arachidonic acid. Mass spectrometric analysis of the methyl ester-trimethylsilyl ether derivative showed its structure to be similar to Thromboxane B_2 but lacking the hemiacetal group and possessing an oxane ring and it was referred to as Thromboxane A_2. This intermediate was shown to be potent at inducing irreversible platelet aggregation (Hamberg et al., 1975).

In spite of the advances in open-tubular glass capillary column technology

E

we have yet to see a widespread breakthrough in their application to prostaglandin analysis, although preliminary data have been reported (Maclouf,
Rigaud, Durand and Chebroux, 1976; Rigaud, Chebroux, Durand, Maclouf
and Mandani, 1976). Fitzpatrick (1978) recently described the separation of
24 prostaglandin analogues using a 25 m open-tubular glass capillary
column coated with silicone OV-1. The samples were introduced by an
all-glass solid injection system (Van den Berg and Cox, 1972) and the
complete separation of prostaglandin methyl ester-TMS ether, methyl ester-
MO-TMS ether and methyl ester-butyloxime derivatives was described. A
large separation was found between the *syn*- and *anti*-isomers of the oxime
derivatives and while this may be of advantage in characterising certain
prostaglandins, the great differences between the mass spectrometric fragmentation patterns for the *syn*- and *anti*- forms of some structures, e.g. PGE_1-
methyl ester-MO-TMS ether (Gréen, 1969) make this phenomenon less
desirable in quantitative analysis by GC–MS. Furthermore with an ever-
increasing number of prostaglandin metabolites being identified, multicomponent analyses are considerably simplified by derivatives which yield
single components during gas chromatography. The qualitative reproducibility and high sensitivity attainable with open-tubular capillary
columns may, however, ensure their future application in the GC–MS
analysis of prostaglandins.

5. Biogenic Amines

GC–MS, especially the SIM mode, offers considerable advantages in
sensitivity, specificity and flexibility over conventional and radioimmunological methods for the determination of the biogenic amines and their
metabolites (Table 1), and has opened the way for a greater understanding
of their role in many physiological and pathological processes.

Koslow, Cattabeni and Costa (1972) using the pentafluoropropionate
derivative (Karoum, Cattabeni, Costa and Ruthven, 1972) developed one of
the first SIM methods for the measurement of noradrenaline and dopamine
in brain tissue; the sensitivity was about 10 fmol. For noradrenaline the ion
at low mass, m/z 176, corresponding to the fragment $[CH_2NHCOC_2F_5]^+$
and for dopamine m/z 428 resulting from the loss of the fragment
$[NHCOC_2F_5]^+$ were used. The internal standards were the α-methyl
homologues and the analogous fragments which were monitored had a
difference of 14 mass units. The catecholamine content of specific areas of
rat brain was measured (Koslow and Schlumpf, 1974; Koslow, Racagni and
Costa, 1974) and while a general qualitative agreement with histochemical
observations on the location of catecholamines in discrete nuclei was found,
GC–MS provided additional quantitative data.

With a combination of SIM and radiochemistry, using [^{3}H]-tyrosine, Costa, Green, Koslow, LeFevre, Revuelta and Wang (1972) found the turnover rate of noradrenaline and dopamine in rat heart ventricles to be 0·69 and 0·78 nmol/g/hr respectively.

Most early SIM methods for catecholamines illustrated the potential of this technique for neuroendocrinology but like the early prostaglandin and steroid methods, were probably inaccurate due to the internal standards employed. The introduction of compounds labelled with stable isotopes as internal standards has significantly improved the accuracy of these SIM techniques.

Several stable isotope labelled catecholamines and their precursors for use in SIM methods were synthesised by Lindström, Sjöquist and Änggård (1974). Curtius, Wolfensberger, Steinmann, Redweik and Siegfried (1974) used tetra-deuterated dopamine as an internal standard for the measurement of dopamine in brain biopsies from patients with phenylketonuria in an attempt to ascertain the role of catecholamines in the pathogenesis of the neurological symptoms and the mental retardation that occurs in these patients. The dopamine concentration in the caudate nucleus was reduced, as was urinary dopamine excretion, which may therefore be a useful indication of brain dopamine production. Sedvall, Bjerkenstedt, Swahn, Wiesel and Wode-Helgodt (1977) have reviewed the application of SIM to the study of dopamine metabolism and described methods for the analysis of dopamine and its metabolites and applications to the study of human brain tissue and cerebrospinal fluid (CSF) from normal and psychotic patients.

Chemical ionisation GC–MS is often more sensitive than electron impact ionisation for SIM methods. Miyazaki, Hashimoto, Iwanaga and Kubodera (1974) have shown that for noradrenaline the sensitivity of CI–GC–MS using isobutane as reagent gas and monitoring the ion m/z 590 was ça 10 times greater than with electron impact ionisation and quantification of as little as 1 pg was possible. The mass spectra of this class of compound using CI are considerably less complex than those obtained by electron impact ionisation.

Homovanillic acid (3-hydroxy-4-methoxyphenylacetic acid) is the major metabolite of dopamine and decreased levels found in patients with depression and the increasing use of l-dopa in the treatment of Parkinson's disease have led to the development of many methods for its measurement (Table 1).

Iso-homovanillic acid was used as an internal standard for a SIM assay of homovanillic acid (Narasimhachari, 1974) but since this isomer is present in human CSF at levels of ca 2% that of homovanillic acid, samples were assayed with and without the addition of the internal standard, demonstrating one disadvantage of using a nomologue as an internal standard.

Sedvell, Fyrö, Nybäck, Wiesel and Wode-Helgodt (1974) used a SIM method to assess changes in homovanillic acid concentrations in CSF from schizophrenic patients during their treatment with neuroleptic drugs. While clinical doses of the drugs chlorpromazine, haloperidol and thioridazine elevated the level of homovanillic acid in CSF, the relationship to therapeutic outcome was obscure.

An important application for GC–MS is the study of catecholamine turnover; stable isotopically labelled compounds and GC–MS provide an important alternative to radioactive compounds for such metabolic studies (Änggård, Sjöquist and Lewander, 1978). Änggård, Lewander and Sjöquist (1974) determined total body turnover (3·8 mol/hr), the size of the peripheral body pool (3·4 mol) the half-life in plasma (0·66 hr) and the urinary excretion rate (1·7 mol/hr) for homovanillic acid after administration of penta-deuterated homovanillic acid to healthy men. Plasma concentrations of endogenous and penta-deuterated homovanillic acid were determined by SIM using di-deuterated homovanillic acid as an internal standard. The study showed that homovanillic acid is eliminated by mechanisms other than by renal clearance since the rate of formation of homovanillic acid exceeded its rate of urinary excretion.

The formation of dopamine from tyrosine requires the enzyme tyrosine-3-hydroxylase (EC 1.10.3.1), molecular oxygen and a reduced pteridine cofactor. To study the quantitative turnover of dopamine in brain (Mayevesky, Sjöquist, Fri, Samuel and Sedvall, 1973) exposed rats to an $^{18}O_2$ enriched atmosphere and measured the rates of formation of the specific metabolite, homovanillic acid in brain tissue. By measuring the ions at mass m/z 392 corresponding to the molecular ion of the methyl ester-HFB derivative of homovanillic acid and m/z 394, one atom of ^{18}O was shown to be incorporated into each molecule. Measurement of the fragment ions in the mass spectrum confirmed the site of incorporation of ^{18}O to be at the C-3 position. When the animals were injected with $H_2^{18}O$, there was no significant incorporation of ^{18}O atoms into homovanillic acid. This work provided definitive *in vivo* evidence for the atmospheric origin of the oxygen at the C-3 position in the enzymatic hydroxylation step in the biosynthesis of dopamine from tyrosine.

In repeating similar experiments, Neff, Galli and Costa (1977) questioned the validity of using $^{18}O_2$ to determine dopamine turnover. Monitoring by GC–MS, the ions corresponding to the molecular ion [M$^+$], the [M + 2] and [M + 4] ions of the PFP derivative of dopamine and the hexafluoro-isopropyl-PFP derivative of homovanillic acid they demonstrated that two atoms of ^{18}O were incorporated into dopamine and concluded that incorporation also occurred in the step phenylalanine to tyrosine. This was confirmed by the identification of ^{18}O-tyrosine in significant amounts. These findings indicate the complexity of the kinetics of dopamine formation and while experiments of this type might offer a more direct method of estimating brain catecholamine turnover, since molecular oxygen can freely enter the brain via the blood stream, their potential value for the diagnosis and treatment of disorders of the CNS in man, however, remains to be seen.

4-Hydroxy-3-methoxyphenylglycol (HMPG), one of the main metabolites of noradrenaline may be estimated by many GC–MS methods (Table 1). The suggestion that sulphate conjugation of HMPG takes place in the brain while HMPG-glucuronide is formed elsewhere in the body, prompted the development of methods for the separate determination of free and conjugated HMPG. Bertilsson (1973) used liquid–liquid partition and enzymatic hydrolysis to isolate free and conjugated HMPG, and by SIM demonstrated a predominance of the conjugated form of this metabolite in CSF. Recently, Murray, Baillie and Davies (1977) used Sephadex LH-20 to isolate specifically HMPG-sulphate from urine. As an alternative to enzymatic or acid hydrolysis of HMPG-sulphate, used by most workers, the mild conditions employed in the preparation of the trifluoroacetate derivative for GC–MS were sufficient to hydrolyse the conjugate (Murray et al., 1977). Similarly, the simultaneous hydrolysis and derivatisation using butanol saturated with HCl has been used effectively in the preparation of derivatives for GC–MS of sulphate-conjugated metabolites of the anti-hypertensive drug α-methyldopa (Setchell, Lawson, Jones and Cummings, 1977; Setchell, Lawson and Cummings, 1978b) and this type of procedure may prove useful in the analysis of conjugated metabolites of biogenic amines.

The potential clinical value of GC–MS in the determination of catechol-amine metabolites in amniotic fluid for the differential diagnosis of congenital neuroblastoma and maternal pheochromocytoma has been discussed by Muskiet, Jeuring, Nagel, de Bruyn and Wolthers (1978b). Free and conjugated HMPG in addition to homovanillic acid and 3-methoxy-4-hydroxyphenylmandelic acid (VMA) have been measured by SIM techniques in amniotic fluid obtained by amniocentesis (Muskiet et al., 1978). In early pregnancy (weeks 15–17) the concentrations were similar to those in serum of normal adults (Änggård, Sjöquist, Fyrö and Sedvall, 1973; Takahashi, Godse, Warsh and Stancer, 1977) and their finding of an increase in concentration of free HMPG with gestational age corroborated the earlier observation of Zambotti, Blau, King, Campbell and Stuart (1975). HMPG is excreted in increased amounts in patients with neuroblastoma and an overproduction of catecholamines and their metabolites by a foetal neuro-blastoma has been reported (Voute, Wadman and van Putten, 1970).

The finding that depression and antidepressant and psychotomimetic drugs affect the metabolism of the indole 5-hydroxytryptamine (serotonin) has led to the utilisation of GC–MS for the measurement of this and other putative neuro-transmitters of the indole structure. Cattabeni, Koslow and Costa (1972a) described a method for the measurement of the indole alkylamines 5-hydroxytryptamine, 5-methoxytryptamine, N-acetyl-5-hydroxytryptamine and melatonin using SIM of the pentafluoropropionate derivatives. Estimates of these indoles in pineal gland tissue were reported. Green, Koslow and Costa (1973) demonstrated the presence of 5-methoxytryptamine in the rat hypothalamus which had previously been reported to be present only in the pineal gland and suggested that this indole might be a neuro-transmitter (Koslow, 1974).

5-Hydroxyindole-3-acetic acid, the main metabolite of 5-hydroxytryptamine, has been used as an index of brain metabolism of the latter and SIM methods have been developed (Bertilsson, Atkinson, Althaus, Härfast, Lindgren and Holmstedt, 1972; Swahn, Sandgarde, Wiesel and Sedvall, 1976; Beck, Wiesel and Sedvall, 1977) and used in studies on patients with depression (Åsberg, Bertilsson, Tuck, Cronholm and Sjöquist, 1973).

Most of the GC–MS applications in biogenic amine research have been in the development and application of sensitive and relatively specific methods for their measurement using SIM. Due to the extremely low concentrations of these compounds their positive identification has relied upon multiple ion detection in which the molecular ion (M^+) and a number of relatively specific fragment ions are monitored simultaneously. Characterisation depends upon a coincidence in peaking of these ions at the same gas-chromatographic retention time as the authentic compound and on relative responses of the ion-current chromatograms in agreement with those for the authentic compound.

Melatonin which is secreted by the pineal gland has been shown to play a role in chronobiology, pituitary function, the neuroendocrine–reproductive axis (Axelrod, 1974; Cardinali, 1974; Reiter, 1976; Reiter and Vaughan, 1977) and be implicated in the pathogenesis of schizophrenia. This hormone is formed from 5-hydroxytryptamine by the action of the enzyme hydroxy-indole-O-methyl transferase and it was chemically characterised from extracts of bovine pineal glands (Lerner, Case, Takahasi, Lee and Mori, 1958; Lerner, Case and Heinzelman, 1959); Smith, Mullen, Silman, Snedden and Wilson (1976) proved unequivocally by GC–MS its presence in plasma and CSF. The mass spectrum of the TMS ether derivative was compared with that of an authentic standard of melatonin. High resolution GC–MS analysis of the intense fragments m/z 232 and 245 gave accurate mass measurements identical with those of the authentic melatonin standard, and these fragments were subsequently employed in a SIM assay for melatonin (Wilson, Sneddon, Silman, Smith and Mullen, 1977).

There is a growing interest in the antigonadal activity of a number of indoles, other than melatonin, which are of pineal gland origin (Reiter and Vaughan, 1977). The neutral indoles, 5-hydroxytryptophol and 5-methoxytryptophol, have from animal experiments, been implicated in the inhibition of LH and FSH respectively but possibly due to the difficulties of assaying these indoles, data available are limited. GC–MS methods for the estimation of these compounds have been described (Curtius, Wolfensberger, Redweik, Leimbacher, Maibach and Isler, 1975; Takahashi, Godse, Naqvi, Warsh and Stancer, 1978) and applied to their measurement in human CSF. The application of similar GC–MS methods with their high sensitivity and specificity has advantages over RIA methods and could prove useful in the evaluation of the role of these indoles in the human reproductive cycle.

D. FUTURE TRENDS IN GAS CHROMATOGRAPHY-MASS SPECTROMETRY

Despite the improvement in gas chromatographic separations with the advent of open-tubular glass capillary columns, their application to date has been restricted largely to gas chromatography. Now that many of the problems of interfacing this type of column to the mass spectrometer are overcome, wider application in the combined GC–MS technique can be expected.

The use of the SIM mode for assays of specific compounds is widespread, but severely underuses many of the features of large mass spectrometers, and in recognition of this, it is to be hoped that manufacturers will develop smaller, relatively less expensive instruments dedicated principally to this type of routine analysis. Effort has been devoted to improving the reliability and ease of operation of GC–MS instruments by way of computer controlling many of the parameters, and features are being designed to allow for completely automated instruments.

An increasing use of chemical ionisation, particularly with the SIM mode seems inevitable, to provide the necessary sensitivity for many hormone assays. Recently, negative ion mass spectrometry (for review see Jennings, 1977) has been developed which may provide the necessary enhancement of sensitivity if incorporated in small instruments. Hunt, Stafford, Crow and Russell (1976) described the technique of pulsed positive ion-negative ion chemical ionisation which facilitates the simultaneous recording of positive and negative ion CI mass spectra, a feature with obvious potential in structural elucidation studies. Using SIM, results have shown that negative ion CI offers an increase in sensitivity of 100–1000 fold compared with positive ion CI and the detection of as little as 30 amol (30×10^{-18} mol) of dopamine as the pentafluorobenzylimine-TMS ether derivative was demonstrated (Hunt and Crow, 1978) thereby illustrating its obvious advantages in trace compound analysis. One of the first applications of negative ion chemical ionisation in the hormone field is that of Lewy and Markey (1978) in which a SIM assay for melatonin in plasma is described and the results compared with previous published data for this hormone.

The exploitation of this new methodology is at present hampered by the inability of conventional GC–MS instruments to detect negative ions; a modification of the ion source and ion detection system is necessary; and the success of the technique depends upon the use of derivatives with good electron capture properties. The potential of this technique having been demonstrated, its future growth in biomedical research is ensured.

The analysis of metastable ions is an exciting area offering considerable potential to qualitative and quantitative GC–MS studies; it will be of interest to follow its future development.

Further developments in mass spectrometry are actively proceeding, with the sensitivity, specificity, practicability and versatility of the technique being rapidly extended. The future application of GC–MS to the hormone field promises to be exciting and rewarding.

REFERENCES

Adlercreutz, H., Härkönen, M. and Järvenpää, P. (1978). In "Quantitative Mass Spectrometry in Life Sciences" (A. P. de Leenheer, R. R. Roncucci and C. Van Peteghem, eds), Vol. II, p 119. Elsevier Publishing Co., Amsterdam.

Adlercreutz, H., Nylander, P. and Hunneman, D. H. (1974a). *Biomed. Mass Spectrom.* **1**, 332.

Adlercreutz, H., Soltmann, B. and Tikkanen, M. J. (1974b). *J. steroid Biochem.* **5**, 163.

Adlercreutz, H., Tikkanen, M. J. and Hunneman, D. H. (1974c). *J. steroid Biochem.* **5**, 211.

Alexander, G., Garzó, G. and Pályi, G. (1974). *J. Chromat.* **91**, 25.

Alexander, G. and Rutten, G. A. F. N. (1973). *Chromatographia*, **6**, 231.

Alexander, G. and Rutten, G. A. F. N. (1974). *J. Chromat.* **99**, 81.

Allen, J. G., Thomas, G. H., Brooks, C. J. W. and Knight, B. A. (1969). *Steroids*, **13**, 133.

Almé, B. Nyström, E. (1971). *J. Chromat.* **59**, 45.

Andersson, B. A. (1967). *Acta chem. Scand.* **21**, 2906.

Änggård, E., Lewander, T. and Sjöquist, B. (1974). *Life Sci.* **15**, 111.

Änggård, E., Sjöquist, B., Fryö, B. and Sedvall, G. (1973). *Eur. J. Pharm.* **24**, 37.

Änggård, E., Sjöquist, B. and Lewander, T. (1978). In "Stable Isotopes—Applications in Pharmacology, Toxicology and Clinical Research" (T. A. Baillie, ed.), p. 235. Macmillan, London.

Arpino, P. J. and McLafferty, F. W. (1976). In "Determination of Organic Structures of Physical Methods" (F. C. Nachod, J. J. Zuckerman and E. W. Randall, eds), Vol. 6, p. 1. Academic Press, New York and London.

Arsenault, G. P. (1972). In "Biomedical Applications of Mass Spectrometry" (G. R.

Waller, ed), p. 817. Wiley-Interscience, New York.

Åsberg, M., Bertilsson, L., Tuck, D., Cronholm, B. and Sjöquist, F. (1973). *Clin. Pharm. Therapeut.* 14, 277.

Aue, W. A., Hastings, C. R. and Kapila, S. (1973). *J. Chromat.* 77, 299.

Axelrod, J. (1974). *Science*, 184, 1341.

Axelson, M. (1977). *J. steroid Biochem.* 8, 693.

Axelson, M., Cronholm, T., Curstedt, T., Reimendal, R. and Sjövall, J. (1974). *Chromatographia*, 7, 502.

Axelson, M., Schumacher, G. and Sjövall, J. (1974). *J. chromat. Sci.* 12, 535.

Axelson, M. and Sjövall, J. (1974). *J. steroid Biochem.* 5, 733.

Axelson, M. and Sjövall, J. (1976). *J. Chromat.* 126, 705.

Axelson, M. and Sjövall, J. (1977). *J. steroid Biochem.* 8, 683.

Axén, U., Gréen, K., Horlin, D. and Samuelsson, B. (1971). *Biochem. biophys. Res. Commun.* 45, 519.

Baczynskyi, L., Duchamp, D. J., Zieserl, J. F. Jr. and Axén, U. (1973). *Anal. Chem.* 45, 479.

Baillie, T. A., Anderson, R. A., Sjövall, K. and Sjövall, J. (1976a). *J. steroid Biochem.* 7, 203.

Baillie, T. A., Sjövall, J. and Herz, J. E. (1975a). *Steroids*, 26, 438.

Baillie, T. A., Sjövall, J. and Sjövall, K. (1975b). *FEBS Lett.* 60, 145.

Baillie, T. A., Sjövall, K. and Sjövall, J. (1976b). *In* "Proceedings 2nd International Conference on Stable Isotopes" (E. R. Klein and P. D. Klein, eds), p. 367. Nat. Tech. Inf. Ser., US Dep. Commerce.

Baldwin, M. A. and McLafferty, F. W. (1973). *Org. Mass Spectrom.* 7, 1111.

Bartle, K. D. (1973). *Anal. Chem.* 45, 1831.

Bartle, K. D. and Novotný, M. (1974). *J. Chromat.* 94, 35.

Bartter, F. C., Gill, J. R., Frölich, J. C., Bowden, R. E., Hollifield, J. W., Radfar, N., Keiser, H. R., Oates, J. A., Seyberth, H. W. and Taylor, A. A. (1976). *Trans. Assoc. Am. Phys.* 89, 77.

Beck, O., Wiesel, F. A. and Sedvall, G. (1977). *J. Chromat.* 134, 407.

Bell, N. W. (1972). Proc. 20th Ann. Conf. Mass Spectrom. Allied Topics, p. 353. Dallas, Texas.

Bertilsson, L. (1973). *J. Chromat.* 87, 147.

Bertilsson, L., Atkinson, Jr. A. J., Althaus, J. R., Härfast, A., Lindgren, J.-E. and Holmstedt, B. (1972). *Anal. Chem.* 44, 1434.

Bertilsson, L. and Palmér, L. (1972). *Science*, 177, 74.

Bertilsson, L. and Palmér, L. (1973). *Life Sci.* 13, 859.

Beynon, J. H. (1960). "Mass Spectrometry and its Applications to Organic Chemistry." Elsevier, Amsterdam.

Biemann, K. (1962). "Mass Spectrometry, Applications to Organic Chemistry." McGraw-Hill, New York.

Biemann, K. (1972a). *In* "Applications of Computer Techniques in Chemical Research" (P. Hepple, ed.), p. 5. Institute of Petroleum, London.

Biemann, K. (1972b). *In* "Biochemical Applications of Mass Spectrometry" (G. R. Waller, ed.), p. 405. Wiley-Interscience, New York.

Biemann, K., Cone, C., Webster, B. R. and Arsenault, C. P. (1966). *J. Am. chem. Soc.* 88, 5598.

Björkhem, I., Blomstrand, R. and Lantto, O. (1975a). *Clin chim. Acta*, 65, 343.

Björkhem, I., Blomstrand, R. Lantto, O., Löf, A. and Svensson, L. (1974). *Clin. chim. Acta*, 56, 241.

118   K. D. R. SETCHELL

Björkhem, I., Blomstrand, R., Lantto, O., Svensson, L. and Öhman, G. (1976). *Clin. Chem.* **22**, 1789.
Björkhem, I., Lantto, O. and Svensson, L. (1975b). *Clin. chim. Acta,* **60**, 59.
Blau, K. and King, G. (1978), "Handbook of Derivatives for Chromatography." Heyden and Son Ltd., London.
Blumer, M. (1973). *Anal. Chem.* **45**, 980.
Bouche, J. and Verzele, M. (1968). *J. gas Chromat.* **6**, 501.
Bowen, D. V. and Field, F. H. (1973). *Int. J. pept. prot. Res.* **5**, 435.
Boyd, R. K. and Beynon, J. H. (1977). *Org. mass. Spectrom.* **12**, 163.
Bradlow, H. L. (1968). *Steroids,* **11**, 265.
Braestrup, C. (1973). *Anal. Biochem.* **55**, 420.
Brash, A. R. and Baillie, T. A. (1978). *Biomed. mass. Spectrom.* **5**, 346.
Brash, A. R., Baillie, T. A., Clare, R. A. and Draffan, G. H. (1976). *Biochem. Med.* **16**, 77.
Breuer, H. and Siekman, L. (1975). *J. steroid Biochem.* **6**, 685.
Brooks, C. J. W., Edmonds, C. G., Gaskell, S. J. and Smith, A. G. (1978). *Chem. Phys. Lipids,* **21**, 403.
Brooks, C. J. W. and Zabkiewicz, J. A. (1967). *In* "Hormones in Blood" (C. H. Gray and A. L. Bacharach, eds), Vol. 2, p. 51. Academic Press, London and New York.
Burgus, R., Butcher, M., Amoss, M., Ling, N., Monahan, M. Rivier, G., Fellows, R., Blackwell, R., Vale, W. and Guillemin, R. (1972). *Proc. natn. Acad. Sci. USA,* **69**, 278.
Burlingame, A. L. and Johanson, G. A. (1972). *Anal. Chem.* **44**, 337R.
Cali, J. P., Mandel, J. and Young, D. S. (1972). *Nat. Bur. Stand. Spec. Publ.* **36**, 260.
Caprioli, R. M., Seifert, W. E. and Sunderland, D. E. (1973). *Biochem. biophys. Res. Commun.* **55**, 67.
Cardinali, D. P. (1974). *In* "Current Topics in Experimental Endocrinology" (V. H. T. James and L. Martini, eds), Vol. 2, p. 107. Academic Press, New York and London.
Carhart, R. E., Johnson, S. M., Smith, D. H., Buchanan, B. G., Dromey, R. G. and Lederberg, J. (1975). *In* "Computer Networking and Chemistry" (P. Lykos, ed.) p. 192. ACS Symp. Ser. 19, American Chemical Society, Washington, DC.
Cattabeni, F., Koslow, S. H. and Costa, E. (1972a). *Science,* **178**, 166.
Cattabeni, F., Koslow, S. H. and Costa, E. (1972b). *Adv. Biochem. Psychopharm.* **6**, 37.
Chapman, J. R. and Bailey, E. (1974). *J. Chromat.* **89**, 215.
Clerc, J. T., Erni, F., Jost, C., Meili, T., Naegeli, D. and Schwarzenbach, R. (1973). *Z. Anal. Chem.* **264**, 192.
Corey, E. J. and Venkateswarlu, A. (1972). *J. Am. chem. Soc.* **94**, 3190.
Cory, H. T., Lascelles, P. T., Millard, B. J., Snedden, W. and Wilson, B. W. (1976). *Biomed. mass Spectrom.* **3**, 117.
Costa, E., Green, A. R., Koslow, S. H., LeFevre, F., Revuelta, A. V. and Wang, C. (1972). *Pharm. Rev.* **24**, 167.
Crain, P. F., Desiderio, D. M. and McCloskey, J. A. (1975). *Meth. Enzymol.* **35B**, 359.
Cramers, C. A., Rijks, J. A. and Bocek, P. (1971). *Clin. chim. Acta,* **34**, 159.
Cramers, C. A. and Van Kessel, M. M. (1968). *J. gas Chromat.* **6**, 577.
Cronholm, T. (1969). *Steroids,* **14**, 285.
Cronholm, T. and Sjövall, J. (1968). *Biochem. biophys. Acta,* **152**, 233.
Cronholm, T. and Sjövall, J. (1970). *Eur. J. Biochem.* **13**, 124.
Cronholm, T., Sjövall, J. and Sjövall, K. (1969). *Steroids,* **13**, 671.

Crossley, D. N., Ramsden, D. B. and Hoffenberg, R. (1978). *In* "Quantitative Mass Spectrometry in Life Sciences" (A. P. de Leenheer, R. R. Roncucci and C. van Peteghem, eds), Vol. II, p. 219. Elsevier, Amsterdam.

Cummins, L. M. (1971). *In* "Recent Advances in Gas Chromatography" (I. I. Domsky and J. A. Perry, eds), p. 313. Marcel Dekker, New York.

Curtius, H. Ch., Wolfensberger, M., Redweik, U., Leimbacher, W., Maibach, R. A. and Isler, W. (1975). *J. Chromat.* **112**, 523.

Curtius, H. Ch., Wolfensberger, M., Steinmann, B., Redweik, U. and Siegfried, J. (1974). *J. Chromat.* **99**, 529.

Dailey, J. W. and Änggård, E. (1973). *Biochem. Pharm.* **22**, 2591.

Dawson, P. D. and Whetten, N. R. (1969). *Adv. Electronics Electron. Phys.* **27**, 59.

Dawson, P. D. and Whetten, N. R. (1971). *In* "Dynamic Mass Spectrometry" (D. Price, ed), p. 1. Heyden and Son. Ltd., London.

Deelder, R. S., Ramaekers, J. J. M., Van den Berg, J. H. M. and Wetzels, M. L. (1976). *J. Chromat.* **119**, 99.

Dehennin, L., Reiffsteck, A. and Schöller, R. (1974a). *J. steroid Biochem.* **5**, 81.

Dehennin, L., Reiffsteck, A. and Schöller, R. (1974b). *J. steroid Biochem.* **5**, 767.

Derrick, P. J. (1977). *In* "Mass Spectrometry" (R. A. W. Johnstone, ed.), Vol. 4, p. 132. Specialist Periodical Reports, Chemical Society, London.

Desty, D. H. (1965). *Adv. Chromat.* **1**, 218.

Desty, D. H., Haresnape, J. N. and Whyman, B. H. F. (1960). *Anal. Chem.* **32**, 302.

Dijkstra, G. and DeGoey, J. (1958). *In* "Gas Chromatography" (D. H. Desty, ed.), p. 56. Butterworths, London.

DoAmaral, J. (1973). *In* "Serotonin and Behaviour" (J. Barchas and E. Usdin, eds), p. 201. Academic Press, New York and London.

Drozd, J. (1975). *J. Chromat.* **113**, 303.

Ellingboe, J., Almé, B. and Sjövall, J. (1970). *Acta chem. Scand.* **24**, 463.

Ettre, L. S. and Zlatkis, A. (1967). "The Practice of Gas Chromatography." Interscience Publishers, New York.

Eyem, J. (1975). *Chromatographia*, **8**, 456.

Fales, H. M., Nagai, Y., Milne, G. W. A., Brewer, H. B. Jr., Bronzert, T. J. and Pisano, J. J. (1971). *Anal. Biochem.* **43**, 288.

Falkner, F. C., Sweetman, B. J. and Watson, J. T. (1975). *Appl. Spectros. Rev.* **10**, 51.

Falter, H. (1977). *In* "Advanced Methods in Protein Sequence Determination" (S. B. Needleman, ed.), Vol. 25, p. 123. Springer-Verlag, New York.

Field, F. H. (1968). *Adv. mass Spectrom.* **4**, 645.

Fitzpatrick, F. A. (1978). *Anal. Chem.* **50**, 47.

Förster, H.-J., Kelly, J. A., Nau, H. and Biemann, K. (1972). *In* "Chemistry and Biology of Peptides" (J. Meinhoffer, ed), p. 679. Ann Arbor Science Publishers, Michigan.

Fri, C.-G., Wiesel, F.-A. and Sedvall, G. (1974a). *Psychopharmacologia*, **35**, 295.

Fri, C.-G., Wiesel, F.-A. and Sedvall, G. (1974b). *Life Sci.* **14**, 2469.

Frolich, J. C., Sweetman, B. J., Carr, K., Hollifield, J. W. and Oates, J. A. (1975). *Prostaglandins*, **10**, 185.

Gaskell, S. J. and Millington, D. S. (1978a). *Biomed. mass Spectrom.* **5**, 557.

Gaskell, S. J. and Millington, D. S. (1978b). *In* "Quantitive Mass Spectrometry in Life Sciences" (A. P. de Leenheer, R. R. Roncucci and C. Van Peteghem, eds) Vol. II, p. 135. Elsevier, Amsterdam.

Gaskell, S. J. and Pike, A. W. (1978). *In* "Quantitative Mass Spectrometry in Life Sciences" (A. P. de Leenheer, R. R. Roncucci and C. Van Peteghem, eds), Vol. II,

p. 181. Elsevier, Amsterdam.

German, A. L. and Horning, E. C. (1973). *J. chromat. Sci.* **11**, 76.

German, A. L., Pfaffenberger, C. D., Thenot, J.-P., Horning, M. G. and Horning, E. C. (1973). *Anal. Chem.* **45**, 930.

Golay, M. (1958). *In* "Gas Chromatography" (D. H. Desty, ed.), p. 36. Academic Press, New York and London.

Goldyne, M. E. and Hammarström, S. (1978). *Anal. Biochem.* **88**, 675.

Gordon, E. K., Oliver, J., Black, K. and Kopin, I. J. (1974). *Biochem. Med.* **11**, 32.

Gray, W. R., Wojcik, L. H. and Futrell, J. H. (1970). *Biochem. biophys. Res. Commun.* **41**, 1111.

Green, A. R., Koslow, S. H. and Costa, E. (1973). *Brain Res.* **51**, 371.

Gréen, K. (1969). *Chem. Phys. Lipids*, **3**, 254.

Gréen, K. (1972). *Adv. Biosci.* **9**, 91.

Gréen, K. and Granström, E. (1973). *In* "Proceedings of Conference on Prostaglandins in Fertility Control." WHO Research and Training Centre on Human Reproduction, Karolinska Institute, Stockholm, Sweden.

Gréen, K., Granström, E., Samuelsson, B. and Axén, U. (1973). *Anal. Biochem.* **54**, 434.

Gréen, K. and Samuelsson, B. (1967). *In* "Prostaglandin Symposium of the Worcester Foundation of Experimental Biology" (P. W. Ramwell and J. E. Shaw, eds), p. 389. Wiley-Interscience, New York.

Gréen, K. and Steffenrund, S. (1976). *Anal. Biochem.* **76**, 606.

Grob, K. (1965). *Helv. chim. Acta*, **48**, 1362.

Grob, K. (1968). *Helv. chim. Acta*, **51**, 718.

Grob, K. (1975). *Chromatographia*, **8**, 423.

Grob, K. and Grob, G. (1969a). *J. chromat. Sci.* **7**, 584.

Grob, K. and Grob, G. (1969b). *J. chromat. Sci.* **7**, 587.

Grob, K. and Grob, G. (1972). *Chromatographia*, **5**, 3.

Grob, K. and Grob, G. (1976). *J. Chromat.* **125**, 471.

Grob, K. and Grob, K. Jr. (1978). *J. Chromat.* **151**, 311.

Grob, K. Jr. and Grob, K. (1977). *Chromatographia*, **10**, 250.

Grob, K. and Jaeggi, H. (1973). *Anal. Chem.* **45**, 1788.

Groenendijk, H. and Van Kemendade, A. W. C. (1969). *Chromatographia*, **2**, 107.

Grotch, S. (1973). *Anal. Chem.* **45**, 2.

Halasz, I. (1968). *Chromatographia*, **1**, 119.

Hamberg, M. (1972). *Biochem. biophys. Res. Commun.* **49**, 720.

Hamberg, M. (1973). *Anal. Biochem.* **55**, 368.

Hamberg, M. (1974). *Life Sci.* **14**, 247.

Hamberg, M. (1976). *Biochem. biophys. Acta*, **431**, 651.

Hamberg, M. and Samuelsson, B. (1973). *Proc. natn. Acad. Sci. USA*, **70**, 899.

Hamberg, M. and Samuelsson, B. (1974a). *Proc. natn. Acad. Sci. USA*, **71**, 3400.

Hamberg, M. and Samuelsson, B. (1974b). *Proc. natn. Acad. Sci. USA*, **71**, 3824.

Hamberg, M., Svensson, J. and Samuelsson, B. (1975). *Proc. natn. Acad. Sci. USA*, **72**, 2994.

Hamberg, M., Svensson, J., Wakabayashi, T. and Samuelsson, B. (1974). *Proc. natn. Acad. Sci. USA*, **71**, 345.

Hammarström, S., Hamberg, M., Samuelsson, B., Duell, E. A., Stawiski, M. and Voorhees, J. J. (1975). *Proc. natn. Acad. Sci. USA*, **72**, 5130.

Hammer, C. G., Holmstedt, B. and Ryhage, R. (1968). *Anal. Biochem.* **25**, 532.

Hartigan, M. J. and Ettre, L. S. (1976). *J. Chromat.* **119**, 187.

Hastings, C. R., Augl, J. M., Kapila, S. and Aue, W. A. (1973). *J. Chromat.* **87**, 49.

Hatch, F., and Munsun, B. (1977). *Anal Chem.* **49**, 169.

Heki, N., Noto, M., Hosojima, H., Takahashi, S. and Murata, T. (1976). *Folia endocr. jap.* **52**, 149.

Heller, S. R. (1974). *In* "Computer Representation and Manipulation of Chemical Information (W. T. Wipke, S. R. Heller, R. J. Feldmann and E. Hyde, eds), Ch. 8. Wiley-Interscience, New York.

Heller, S. R., Fales, H. M. and Milne, G. W. A. (1973). *Org. mass. Spectrom.* **7**, 107.

Heller, S. R., Fales, H. M., Milne, G. W. A., Feldmann, R. J., Daly, N. R., Maxwell, D. C. and McCormick, A. (1973). Proc. 21st Ann. Conf. Mass Spectrom. Allied Topics, p. 192. San Francisco, California.

Hellström, K., Sjövall, J. and Vihko, R. (1969). *Acta endocr., Copenh.* **60**, 501.

Henneberg, D. (1961). *Anal. Chem.* **183**, 12.

Hertz, H. S., Hites, R. A. and Biemann, K. (1971). *Anal. Chem.* **43**, 681.

Hites, R. A. and Biemann, K. (1968). *Anal. Chem.* **40**, 1217.

Hites, R. A. and Biemann, K. (1970). *Anal. Chem.* **42**, 855.

Horning, E. C., Maddock, K. C., Anthony, K. V. and Vanden Heuvel, W. J. A. (1963). *Anal. Chem.* **35**, 526.

Hudson, G. and Biemann, K. (1976). *Biochem. biophys. Res. Commun.* **71**, 212.

Hunt, D. F. and Crow, F. W. (1978). *Anal. Chem.* **50**, 1781.

Hunt, D. F., Stafford, Jr., G. C., Crow, F. W. and Russell, J. W. (1976). *Anal. Chem.* **48**, 2098.

Ilkova, E. L. and Mistryukov, E. A. (1971). *J. chromat. Sci.* **9**, 569.

Jaffe, B. M., Behrman, H. R. and Parker, C. H. W. (1973). *J. clin. Invest.* **52**, 398.

Jänne, O., Vihko, R., Sjövall, J. and Sjövall, K. (1969). *Clin. chim. Acta*, **23**, 405.

Jeannin, J. F., Bournot, P., Maume, G. and Maume, B. F. (1978). *J. steroid Biochem*, **9**, 615.

Jellum, E., Helland, P., Eldjarn, L., Markwardt, U. and Marhöfer, J. (1975). *J. Chromat.* **112**, 573.

Jenden, D. J. and Cho, A. K. (1973). *Ann. Rev. Pharmacol.* **13**, 371.

Jennings, K. R. (1977). *In* "Mass Spectrometry" (R. A. W. Johnstone, ed.), Vol. 4. Specialist Periodical Reports, Chemical Society, London.

Kaiser, R. (1962). *Z. anal. Chem.* **189**, 1.

Kaiser, R. (1968). *Chromatographia*, **1–2**, 34.

Kaiser, R. and Rieder, R. (1975). *Chromatographia*, **8**, 491.

Karoum, F., Cattabeni, F., Costa, E. and Ruthven, C. R. J. (1972). *Anal. Biochem.* **47**, 550.

Karoum, F., Gillin, J. C., Wyatt, R. J. and Costa, E. (1975). *Biomed. mass Spectrom.* **2**, 183.

Karoum, F., Lefévre, H., Bigelow, L. B. and Costa, E. (1973). *Clin. chim. Acta,* **43**, 127.

Kelly, J. A., Nau, H., Förster, H.-J. and Biemann, K. (1975). *Biomed. mass Spectrom.* **2**, 313.

Kelly, R. W. (1973). *Anal. Chem.* **45**, 2079.

Kelly, R. W. (1974). *Adv. mass Spectrom.* **6**, 193.

Kelly, R. W. (1977). *In* "Quantitative Mass Spectrometry in Life Sciences" (A. P. de Leenheer and R. R. Roncucci, eds), Vol. I, p. 145. Elsevier, Amsterdam.

Kelly, R. W. and Taylor, P. L. (1976). *Anal. Chem.* **48**, 465.

Kennaway, D. J., Frith, R. G., Phillipou, G., Matthews, C. D. and Seamark, R. F. (1977). *Endocrinology*, **101**, 119.

Kiryushkin, A. A., Fales, H. M., Axenrod, T., Gilbert, E. J. and Milne, G. W. A. (1971). *Org. mass Spectrom.* **5**, 19.

Klein, E. R. and Klein, P. D. (1978a). *Biomed. mass Spectrom.* **5**, 91.

Klein, E. R. and Klein, P. D. (1978b). *Biomed. mass Spectrom.* **5**, 321.

Koslow, S. H. (1973). *In* "Frontiers in Catecholamine Research" (E. Usdin and S. Snyder, eds), p. 1085. Pergamon Press, London.

Koslow, S. H. (1974). *Adv. biochem. Psychopharmacol.* **11**, 95.

Koslow, S. H., Cattabeni, F. and Costa, E. (1972). *Science*, **176**, 177.

Koslow, S. H. and Green, A. R. (1973). *Adv. biochem. Psychopharmacol.* **7**, 33.

Koslow, S. H., Racagni, G. and Costa, E. (1974). *Neuropharmacology*, **13**, 1123.

Koslow, S. H. and Schlumpf, M. (1974). *Nature, Lond.* **251**, 530.

Krugers, J. (1968). "Instrumentation in Gas Chromatography." Centrex Publishing Co., Eindhoven.

Laatikainen, T., Peltonen, J. and Nylander, P. (1973). *Steroids*, **21**, 347.

Lawson, A. M., Ramsden, D. B., Raw, R. J. and Hoffenberg, R. (1974). *Biomed. mass Spectrom.* **1**, 374.

Lerner, A. B., Case, J. D. and Heinzelman, R. V. (1959). *J. Am. chem. Soc.* **81**, 6085.

Lerner, A. B., Case, J. D., Takahashi, Y., Lee, T. H. and Mori, W. (1958). *J. Am. chem. Soc.* **80**, 2587.

Lewy, A. J. and Markey, S. P. (1978). *Science*, **20**, 741.

Lhuguenot, J.-C. and Maume, B. F. (1974). *J. chromat. Sci.* **12**, 411.

Lindström, B., Sjöquist, B. and Änggård, E. (1974). *J. lab. Compounds*, **10**, 187.

Littlewood, A. B. (1970). "Gas Chromatography." Academic Press, New York and London.

Maclouf, J., Rigaud, M. Durand, J. and Chebroux, P. (1976). *Prostaglandins*, **11**, 999.

Maganiello, V. and Vaughan, M. (1972). *Proc. natn. Acad. Sci. USA*, **69**, 209.

Malec, E. J. (1971). *J. chromat. Sci.* **9**, 1318.

Malmsten, C., Hamberg, M., Svensson, J. and Samuelsson, B. (1975). *Proc. natn. Acad. Sci. USA*, **72**, 1446.

Marshall, J. L. and Parker, D. A. (1976). *J. Chromat.* **122**, 425.

Martin, A. J. P. and James, A. T. (1952). *Biochem. J.* **50**, 679.

Maume, B. F. and Luyten, J. A. (1973). *J. chromat. Sci.* **11**, 607.

Mayevsky, A., Sjöquist, B., Fri, C.-G., Samuel, D. and Sedvall, G. (1973). *Biochem. biophys. Res. Commun.* **51**, 746.

McDonald, J. A., Callahan, P. X. and Ellis, S. (1972). *In* "Methods in Enzymology" (C. H. W. Hirs and Timashaff, S. N., eds), Vol. 25, p. 272. Academic Press, New York and London.

McKeag, R. G. and Hougen, F. W. (1977). *J. Chromat.* **136**, 308.

Mellon, F. A. (1975). *In* "Mass Spectrometry" (R. A. W. Johnstone, ed.), Vol. 3, p. 117. Specialist Periodical Reports, Chemical Society, London.

Mellon, F. A. (1975). *In* "Mass Spectrometry" (R. A. W. Johnstone, ed.), Vol. 3, p. 59, Specialist Periodical Reports, Chemical Society, London.

Metcalfe, L. D. and Martin, R. J. (1967). *Anal. Chem.* **39**, 1204.

Millard, B. (1977), "Quantitative Mass Spectrometry." Heyden and Son Ltd., London.

Millington, D. S. (1975). *J. steroid Biochem.* **6**, 239.

Millington, D. S., Golder, M. P., Cowley, T., Landon, D., Roberts, H., Butt, W. R. and Griffiths, K. (1976). *Acta endocr., Copenh.* **82**, 561.

Millington, D. S. and Smith, J. A. (1977). *Org. mass Spectrom.* **12**, 264.

Miyazaki, H., Hashimoto, Y., Iwanaga, M. and Kubodera, T. (1974). *J. Chromat.* **99**, 575.

Miyazaki, H., Ishibashi, M., Itoh, M., Morishita, N., Sudo, M. and Nambara, T. (1976). *Biomed. mass Spectrom.* **3**, 55.
Morris, H. R. and Dell, A. (1975). *In* "Instrumentation in Amino Acid Sequence Analysis" (R. N. Perham, ed.), p. 147. Academic Press, New York and London.
Mudgett, M., Bowen, D. V., Field, F. H. and Kindt, T. J. (1975). *Biomed. mass Spectrom.* **5**, 19.
Mudgett, M., Bowen, D. V., Field, F. H. and Kindt, T. J. (1977). *Biomed. mass Spectrom.* **4**, 159.
Munsun, B. (1977). *Anal. Chem.* **49**, 772A.
Murray, S., Baillie, T. A. and Davies, D. S. (1977). *J. Chromat.* **143**, 541.
Muskiet, F. A. J., Fremouw-Ottevangers, D. C., Meulen, J., Wolthers, B. G. and de Vries, J. A. (1978a). *Clin. Chem.* **24**, 122.
Muskiet, F. A. J., Jeuring, H. J., Nagel, G. T., de Bruyn, H. W. A. and Wolthers, B. G. (1978b). *Clin. Chem.* **24**, 1899.
Naegeli, P. R. and Clerc, J. T. (1974). *Anal. Chem.* **46**, 739A.
Narasimhachari, N. (1974). *Biochem. biophys. Res. Commun.* **56**, 36.
Nau, H. (1976a). *J. Chromat.* **121**, 376.
Nau, H. (1976b). *FEBS Lett.* **63**, 154.
Nau, H. (1978). *Adv. mass Spectrom.* **7**, 1518.
Nau, H. and Biemann, K. (1973). *Anal. Lett.* **6**, 1071.
Nau, H. and Biemann, K. (1974). *Anal. Chem.* **46**, 426.
Nau, H. and Biemann, K. (1976a). *Anal. Biochem.* **73**, 154.
Nau, H. and Biemann, K. (1976b). *Anal. Biochem.* **73**, 139.
Nau, H. and Biemann, K. (1976c). *Anal. Biochem.* **73**, 175.
Nau, H., Förster, H.-J., Kelly, J. A. and Biemann, K. (1975). *Biomed. mass Spectrom.* **2**, 326.
Nau, H., Kelly, J. A. and Biemann, K. (1973). *J. Am. chem. Soc.* **95**, 7162.
Neff, N. H., Galli, C. L. and Costa, E. (1977). *Adv. biochem. Psychopharmacol.* **16**, 187.
Nelson, J. C., Weiss, R. M., Lewis, J. E., Wilcox, R. B. and Palmér, F. J. (1974). *J. clin. Invest.* **53**, 416.
Neuner-Jehle, N., Etzweiler, F. and Zarske, G. (1974). *Chromatographia*, **7**, 323.
Nikelly, J. G. and Blumer, M. (1974). *Am. Lab.* **6**, 12.
Novotný, M. and Bartle, K. D. (1970). *Chromatographia*, **3**, 272.
Novotný, M. and Bartle, K. D. (1974a). *J. Chromat.* **93**, 405.
Novotný, M. and Bartle, K. D. (1974b). *Chromatographia*, **7**, 122.
Novotný, M., Blomberg, L. and Bartle, K. D. (1970). *J. Chromat. Sci.* **8**, 390.
Novotný, M. and Grohmann, K. (1973). *J. Chromat.* **84**, 167.
Novotný, M. and Tesařík, K. (1968). *Chromatographia*, **1**, 332.
Novotný, M. and Zlatkis, A. (1971). *Chromat. Rev.* **14**, 1.
Oates, J. A., Seyberth, H. W., Frölich, J. C., Sweetman, B. J. and Watson, J. T. (1978). *In* "Stable Isotopes—Applications in Pharmacology, Toxicology and Clinical Research" (T. A. Baillie, ed.), p. 281. Macmillan, London.
Oates, J. A., Sweetman, B. J., Gréen, K. and Samuelsson, B. (1976). *Anal. Biochem.* **74**, 546.
Onikki, S. and Adlercreutz, H. (1973). *J. steroid Biochem.* **4**, 633.
Ottenstein, D. M. (1968). *J. gas. Chromat.* **6**, 129.
Ovchinnikov, Y. A. and Kiryushkin, A. A. (1972). *FEBS Lett.* **21**, 300.
Peery, C. V., Johnson, G. S. and Pastan, I. (1971). *J. biol. Chem.* **246**, 5785.
Petersen, B. A. and Vouros, P. (1977). *Anal. Chem.* **49**, 1304.
Phillipou, G., Bigham, D. A. and Seamark, R. F. (1975). *Steroids*, **26**, 516.

Pletka, P. and Hickler, R. B. (1974). *Prostaglandins*, **7**, 107.
Priddle, J. D., Rose, K. and Offord, R. E. (1977). *Adv. mass Spectrom. biochem. Med.* **2**, 477.
Prost, M. and Maume, B. F. (1974a). *J. steroid Biochem.* **5**, 133.
Prost, M. and Maume, B. F. (1974b). *In* "Mass Spectrometry in Biochemistry and Medicine" (A. Frigerio and N. Castagnoli, eds), p. 139. Raven Press, New York.
Ramsden, D. B., Raw, P. J. and Hoffenberg, R. (1975). *Proc. R. Soc. Med.* **68**, 69.
Reimendal, R. and Sjövall, J. (1971). *In* "Hormonal Steroids" (V. H. T. James and L. Martini, eds), p. 228. Excerpta Medica Foundation, IC5 209, Amsterdam.
Reimendal, R. and Sjövall, J. (1972). *Anal. Chem.* **44**, 21.
Reimendal, R. and Sjövall, J. (1973). *Anal. Chem.* **45**, 1083.
Reiter, R. J. (1976). *Psychoneuroendocrinology*, **1**, 245.
Reiter, R. J. and Vaughan, M. K. (1977). *Life Sci.* **21**, 159.
Ridley, R. G. (1972). *In* "Biochemical Applications of Mass Spectrometry" (G. Waller, ed.), p. 177. Wiley-Interscience, New York.
Rigaud, M., Chebroux, P., Durand, J., Maclouf, J. and Mandani, C. (1976). *Tetrahedron Lett.* **44**, 3925.
Roeraade, J. (1975). *Chromatographia*, **8**, 511.
Rutten, G. A. F. N. and Luyten, J. A. (1972). *J. Chromat.* **74**, 177.
Ryhage, R. (1964). *Anal. Chem.* **36**, 759.
Ryhage, R. (1965). *Anal. Chem.* **37**, 435.
Ryhage, R. (1973). *Quart. Rev. Biophys.* **6**, 311.
Salmon, J. A. and Flowers. R. J. (1979). *In* "Hormones in Blood" (C. H. Gray and V. H. T. James, eds), Vol. II, p. 237. Academic Press, London and New York.
Samuelsson, B., Granström, E., Gréen, K. and Hamberg, M. (1971). *Ann. N.Y. Acad. Sci.* **180**, 183.
Samuelsson, B. And Gréen, K. (1974). *Biochem. Med.* **11**, 298.
Samuelsson, B., Hamberg, M. and Sweeley, C. C. (1976). *Anal. Biochem.* **38**, 301.
Schomburg, G., Husmann, H. and Weeke, F. (1974). *J. Chromat.* **99**, 63.
Schulte, E. and Acker, L. (1974). *Anal. Chem.* **268**, 260.
Schulten, H.-R. (1978). *Adv. mass Spectrom.* **7A**, 83.
Schulten, H.-R. and Beckley, H. D. (1972). *Org. mass Spectrom.* **6**, 885.
Schultze, P. and Kaiser, K. H. (1971). *Chromatographia*, **4**, 381.
Seamark, R. F., Phillipou, G. and McIntase, J. E. A. (1977). *J. steroid Biochem.* **8**, 885.
Sedvall, G., Bjerkenstedt, L., Swahn, C. G., Wiesel, F. A. and Wode-Helgodt, B. (1977). *Adv. biochem. Psychopharmacol.* **16**, 343.
Sedvall, G., Fyrö, B., Nybäck, H., Wiesel, F. A. and Wode-Helgodt, B. (1974). *J. Psychiat. Res.* **11**, 75.
Senn, M. and McLafferty, F. W. (1966). *Biochem. biophys. Res. Commun.* **23**, 4.
Setchell, K. D. R., Almé, B., Axelson, M. and Sjövall, J. (1976a). *J. steroid Biochem.* **7**, 615.
Setchell, K. D. R., Axelson, M., Sjövall, J. and Gontscharow, N. P. (1976b). *J. steroid Biochem.* **7**, 801.
Setchell, K. D. R., Axelson, M., Sjövall, J., Morgan, R. E. and Kirk, D. N. (1978a). *FEBS Lett.* **88**, 215.
Setchell, K. D. R., Lawson, A. M. and Cummings, A. J. (1978b). *In* "Quantitative Mass Spectrometry in Life Sciences" (A. P. de Leenheer, R. R. Roncucci and C. Van Peteghem, eds), Vol. II, p. 263, Elsevier, Amsterdam.
Setchell, K. D. R., Lawson, A. M., Jones, H. and Cummings, A. J. (1978c). *In* "Recent Advances in Mass Spectrometry and Medicine" (A. Frigerio, ed.) Vol. I, p. 65.

Plenum Publishing Co., New York.

Setchell, K. D. R. and Bonney, R. (1979). *J. steroid Biochem.* (in press).

Setchell, K. D. R., Taylor, N. F., Adlercreutz, H., Axelson, M. and Sjövall, J. (1979). *Res. Steroids*, **8**, 131.

Seyberth, H. W., Segre, G. V., Morgan, J. L., Sweetman, B. J., Potts, J. T. and Oates, J. A. (1975). *New Eng. J. Med.* **293**, 1278.

Seyberth, H. W., Sweetman, B. J., Frölich, J. C. and Oates, J. A. (1976). *Prostaglandins*, **11**, 381.

Siekmann, L. (1974). *J. steroid Biochem.* **5**, 727.

Siekmann, L., Martin, S. and Breuer, H. (1972). *Scand. J. clin. lab. Invest.* **29** (Suppl. 126), 8.8.

Siekmann, L., Martin, S., Siekmann, A. and Breuer, H. (1976a), *Acta. endocr., Copenh.* **82**, 65.

Siekmann, L., Siekmann, A. and Breuer, H. (1978). *Fresenius Z. anal. Chem.* **290**, 122.

Siekmann, L., Siekmann, A., Martin, S. and Breuer, H. (1976b). *In* "Advances in Mass Spectrometry in Biochemistry and Medicine" (A. Frigerio, ed.). Spectrum Publ. Inc., New York.

Simmonds, P. G. and Lovelock, J. E. (1976). *Anal. Chem.* **35**, 1345.

Sjöquist, B. and Änggård, E. (1972). *Anal. Chem.* **44**, 2297.

Sjöquist, B., Lindström, B. and Änggård, E. (1973). *Life Sci.* **13**, 1655.

Sjöquist, B., Lindström, B. and Änggård, E. (1975). *J. Chromat.* **105**, 309.

Sjövall, J. (1975). *J. steroid Biochem.* **6**, 227.

Sjövall, J. and Sjövall, K. (1968). *Steroids*, **12**, 359.

Sjövall, J. and Sjövall, K. (1970). *Annal. clin. Res.* **2**, 1.

Sjövall, J., Sjövall, K. and Vihko, R. (1968). *Steroids*, **11**, 703.

Sjövall, J. and Vihko, R. (1965). *Steroids*, **6**, 597.

Sjövall, J. and Vihko, R. (1966a). *Steroids*, **7**, 447.

Sjövall, J. and Vihko, R. (1966b). *In* "Proceedings of 2nd International Congress on Hormonal Steroids", p. 210. Excerpta Medica International Congress Series 132.

Sjövall, J. and Vihko, R. (1968). *Acta endocr., Copenh.* **57**, 247.

Sjövall, K. (1970a). *Annal. clin. Res.* **2**, 393.

Sjövall, K. (1970b). *Annal. clin. Res.* **2**, 409.

Sjövall, K., Sjövall, J., Maddock, K. and Horning, E. C. (1966). *Anal. Biochem.* **14**, 337.

Smith, A. G., Harland, W. A. and Brooks, C. J, W. (1977). *J. Chromat.* **142**, 533.

Smith, I., Mullen, P. E., Silman, R. E., Snedden, W. and Wilson, B. W. (1976). *Nature, Lond.* **260**, 718.

Supina, W. R., Henley, R. A. and Kruppa, R. F. (1966). *J. Am. Oil chem. Soc.* **43**, 202A.

Swahn, C.-G., Sandgarde, B., Wiesel, F.-A. and Sedvall, G. (1976). *Psychopharmacology*, **48**, 147.

Sweeley, C. C., Elliott, W. H., Fries, I. and Ryhage, R. (1966). *Anal. Chem.* **38**, 1549.

Sweeley, C. C., Young, N. D., Holland, J. F. and Gates, S. C. (1974). *J. Chromat.* **99**, 507.

Sweetman, B. J., Frölich, J. C. and Watson, J. T. (1973). *Prostaglandins*, **3**, 75.

Sweetman, B. J., Watson, J. T., Carr, K., Oates, J. A. and Frölich, J. C. (1973). *Prostaglandins*, **3**, 385.

Takahashi, S., Godse, D. D., Naqvi, A., Warsh, J. J. and Stancer, H. C. (1978). *Clin. chem. Acta,* **84**, 55.

Takahashi, S., Godse, D. D., Warsh, J. J. and Stancer, H. C. (1977). *Clin. chim. Acta,*

81, 183.

Taylor, N. F. and Shackleton, C. H. L. (1979), *J. clin. Endocr. Metab.* **49**

Tesařik, K. and Nečasová, M. (1972). *J. Chromat.* **65**, 39.

Tesařik, K. and Novotný, M. (1968). *In* "Gas Chromatographie" (H. G. Struppe, ed.), p. 575. Akadamie-Verlag GmbH, Berlin.

Thome, F. A. and Young, G. W. (1976). *Anal. Chem.* **48**, 1423.

Thompson, R. (1976). *J. steroid Biochem.* **7**, 845.

Tikkanen, M. J. and Adlercreutz, H. (1970). *Acta chem. Scand.* **24**, 3755.

Van Den Berg, P. M. J. and Cox, T. P. H. (1972). *Chromatographia*, **5**, 301.

Van den Heuvel, W. J. A. and Horning, E. C. (1964). *In* "Biomedical Applications of Gas Chromatography" (H. A. Szymanski, ed.), p. 89. Plenum Press, New York.

Van Hout, P., Szafranek, J., Pfaffenberger, C. D. and Horning, E. C. (1974). *J. Chromat.* **99**, 103.

Venkataraghavan, R., Kwok, K.-S., Pesyna, G. and McLafferty, F. W. (1973). Proc. 21st Ann. Conf. Mass Spectrom. Allied Topics, p. 197.

Verzele, M., Verstappe, M. Sandra, P. Van Luchene, E. and Vuye, A. (1972). *J. chromat. Sci.* **10**, 668.

Vestergaard, P., Sayegh, J. F. and Mowat, J. H. (1975). *Clin. chim. Acta*, **21**, 163.

Voute, P. A. Jr., Wadman, S. K. and van Putten, W. J. (1970). *Clin. Pediatr.* **9**, 206.

Waller, G. R. (1972). "Biochemical Applications of Mass Spectrometry." Wiley-Interscience, New York.

Wang, M.-T., Imai, K., Yoshioka, M. and Tamura, Z. (1975a). *Clin. chim. Acta.* **63**, 13.

Wang, M.-T., Yoshioka, M., Imai, K. and Tamura, Z. (1975b). *Clin. chim. Acta*, **63**, 21.

Ward, S. D. (1971). *In* "Mass Spectrometry" (D. H. Williams, ed.), Vol. 1, p. 253. Specialist Periodical Reports, Chemical Society, London.

Ward, S. D. (1973). *In* "Mass Spectrometry" (D. H. Williams, ed.), Vol. 2, p. 264. Specialist Periodical Reports, Chemical Society, London.

Watson, J. T. (1969). *In* "Ancillary Techniques for Gas Chromatography" (L. S. Ettre and W. H. McFadden, eds), p. 145. Wiley-Interscience, New York.

Watson, J. T. (1971). *In* "Proceedings of Seminar on Use of Stable Isotopes in Clinical Pharmacology" (P. D. Klein and L. J. Roth, eds), p. 239. Conference 711115, National Technical Information Service, Springfield, Virginia.

Watson, J. T. (1972). *In* "Biomedical Applications of Mass Spectrometry" (G. R. Waller, ed.), p. 23. Wiley-Interscience, New York.

Watson, J. T. and Biemann, K. (1964). *Anal. Chem.* **36**, 1135.

Watson, J. T. and Sweetman, B. J. (1974). *Org. mass Spectrom.* **9**, 39.

Weygand, F., Prox, A., Jorgensen, E. C., Axen, R. and Kirchner, P. (1963). *Z. Naturforsch.* **18B**, 93.

Wilson, B. W., Snedden, W., Silman, R. E., Smith, I. and Mullen, P. (1977). *Anal. Biochem.* **81**, 283.

Wilson, B. W., Snedden, W., Tham, K. T. and Willoughby, D. A. (1976). *Agents Actions,* **6**, 176.

Wilson, D. W., John, B. M., Groom, G. V., Pierrepoint, C. G. and Griffiths, K. (1977). *J. endocr.* **74**, 503.

Wilson, J. M. (1977). *In* "Mass Spectrometry" (R. A. W. Johnstone, ed.), Vol. 4, p. 102. Specialist Periodical Reports, Chemical Society, London.

Wood, G. W., Mak, N. and Hobb, A. M. (1976). *Anal. Chem.* **48**, 981.

Zambotti, F., Blau, K., King, G. S., Campbell, S. and Sandler, M. (1975). *Clin. chim. Acta*, **61**, 247.

Zisman, W. A. (1964). *Adv. Chem. Ser.* No. 43, 1.

Zusman, R. M., Caldwell, B. V. and Speroff, L. (1972). *Prostaglandins*, **2**, 41.

Zweig, G. and Sherma, J. (1972). "Handbook of Chromatography." Chemical Rubber Co. Press, Cleveland, Ohio.

IV. Adrenocorticotrophin and Lipotrophin

LESLEY H. REES and P. J. LOWRY

INTRODUCTION

The mammalian pituitary normally contains three zones, pars distalis, pars intermedia and pars nervosa. Several cell types can be recognised in the pars distalis and histochemical and immunohistochemical techniques have distinguished them as the gonadotrophs, thyrotrophs, somatotrophs, lacto-trophs and corticotrophs. Only one cell type is normally found in the pars intermedia, the melanotrophs. Although adrenocorticotrophin (ACTH) and the melanophore-stimulating hormones (MSH's) are structurally related, ACTH is present mainly in the corticotrophs of pars distalis and MSH in the pars intermedia and are secreted as such into the blood from their respective tissues. The normal adult human pituitary does not contain a distinct pars intermedia nor significant quantities of MSH. In the last five years other peptides related to ACTH have been characterised in the human pituitary, these include β- and γ-lipotrophins (β- and γ-LPH), corticotrophin-like intermediate lobe peptide (CLIP) a peptide resembling α-MSH and β-endorphin. The pattern of these peptides in the human pituitary alters during foetal development (Silman, Chard, Lowry, Smith and Young, 1976). Peptides resembling α-MSH and CLIP appear to be present in significant amounts in the pituitary at this time although there is no evidence for the existence of β-MSH (Silman, Chard, Lowry, Smith and Young, 1977). It is somewhat paradoxical that, although there are seven possible biologically active peptides related to ACTH, only the physiology of ACTH is well understood.

A. NOMENCLATURE

The nomenclature of Li (1959) for ACTH and related peptides is employed throughout this chapter. By this system the first ACTH to be isolated from pituitaries of a given species is designated α-ACTH. If a second ACTH were to be found in the pituitaries of the same species it would be designated β-ACTH and so forth. Any polypeptide having an amino acid sequence similar to that of the first isolated ACTH of a given species is also given the name α-ACTH. A superscript is used to indicate the portion of the ACTH molecule which is present in the analogue. If the compound possesses a C-terminal amide this is also indicated in superscript (for example α^{1-17} (NH$_2$)). If the analogue contains portions of the ACTH molecule where species differences occur, the appropriate species is indicated in subscript (for example bovine ACTH = α_b^{1-39} ACTH).

B. CHEMISTRY

One common feature of all these peptides is that they do not contain cysteine and consequently no disulphide bridges. Structurally they can be divided into two groups.

(i) The ACTH-related peptides. ACTH is a peptide consisting of 39 amino acid residues and is the largest characterised peptide of this group. α-MSH has an amino acid sequence that is exactly the same as the NH_2-terminal tridecapeptide of ACTH. In some vertebrates the NH_2-terminal group and COOH-terminal group are blocked by acetylation and amidation respectively. The third peptide in this group is CLIP which has the structure of 18–39 ACTH (Fig. 1). The presence of α-MSH and CLIP in the intermediate lobe led to the postulation that ACTH was synthesised in this lobe serving as the precursor for the two smaller peptides which were formed from it by specific proteolytic cleavages (Scott, Ratcliffe, Rees, Landon, Bennett, Lowry and McMartin, 1973). Yalow and Berson (1971) reported that larger molecular forms of ACTH occur in human pituitaries, and plasma and tumours associated with the ectopic ACTH syndrome (Gewirtz and Yalow, 1974).

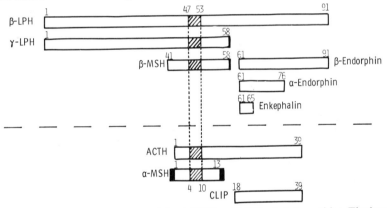

Fig. 1. Schematic representation of the ACTH and LPH related peptides. The hatched area contained within the vertical lines represents the common heptapeptide sequence of amino acids.

They called this material "big ACTH" and demonstrated that a peptide resembling ACTH 1–39 could be generated from it after treatment with trypsin (Yalow and Berson, 1973). Mains and Eipper (1976) have shown larger molecular forms of ACTH in a mouse pituitary tumour cell line using dissociating chromatographic conditions. More recently a study has been made of the molecular forms of ACTH in human plasma using gel filtration under strong acid dissociating conditions. Although the numbers of patient plasmas studied is not large, the presence of significant amounts of "big ACTH" has been demonstrated in patients with the ectopic ACTH syndrome (Ratter, Lowry and Rees, 1979; Ratter, Lowry, Besser and Rees, 1979) and in some patients this is the only form of ACTH immunoreactivity observed. A peptide with the chromatographic properties of 1–39 ACTH predominates in the plasma of patients with pituitary-dependent Cushing's disease, Addison's disease and Nelson's syndrome.

(ii) The lipotrophin-related peptides. The largest peptide of this group is β-lipotrophin, a peptide consisting of some 91 residues. It is structurally related to ACTH by the common sequence of seven amino acids 4–10 in ACTH and 47–53 in β-LPH (Fig. 1). The next largest peptide in this group γ-LPH consists of the first 58 residues of β-LPH and the remaining C-terminal fragment, β-LPH 61–91 (residues 59 and 60 of β-LPH appear to be lost during the proteolytic cleavage) is better known as β-endorphin. The fourth peptide β-MSH is comprised of the 41–58 sequence of β-LPH. The significance of the 22 amino acid residue peptide "human β-MSH" will be discussed later.

In man the plasma levels of ACTH and LPH always parallel each other (Abe, Nicholson, Liddle, Orth and Island, 1969; Jeffcoate, Rees, Lowry and Besser, 1978, 1979; Tanaka, Nicholson and Orth, 1978a; Mullen, Jeffcoate, Linsell, Howard and Rees, 1979) (see below) and are produced in the same cells of the pituitary and appear to be present in the same secretory granules (Phifer, Orth and Spicer, 1974). Preliminary evidence of a large protein containing both ACTH and LPH immunoreactivity has been reported in extracts of human pituitaries (Lowry, Hope and Silman, 1976) in Simian pituitaries (Silman, Holland, Chard, Lowry, Hope, Robinson and Thorburn, 1978) in a mouse pituitary tumour cell line (Mains, Eipper and Ling, 1977) and in a tumour associated with ectopic ACTH secretion (Orth, Guillemin, Ling and Nicholson, 1978). As ACTH and LPH are the putative parent molecules of other peptides this common precursor would be capable of generating at least seven peptides, Eipper, Mains and Guenzi (1976) demonstrated the glycoprotein nature of this high molecular weight precursor and its structure has recently been elucidated by DNA sequencing techniques (Nakanishi, Inoue, Kita, Nakamura, Chang, Cohen and Nurna, 1979).

C. EXTRACTION AND PURIFICATION OF ACTH/LPH

One of the earliest and yet most successful extraction techniques for ACTH was that devised by Lyons in 1937. This employs extraction of fresh pituitary tissue in an acetone and concentrated hydrochloric acid mixture. The water contents of the glands contributes to the aqueous acetone-HCl mixture in which ACTH dissolves. The method has two main advantages in that the high concentration of acetone precipitates much non-specific material and the low pH prevents any enzymic degradation of peptides such as ACTH. Further addition of acetone to the supernatant precipitates ACTH.

The first successful isolation of ACTH was obtained from porcine pituitaries at the Armour laboratories in Chicago (White, 1953) by employing the hot glacial acetic acid extraction and oxycellulose extraction of Astwood, Raben and Payne (1951) followed by exchange chromatography on Amberlite XE 97 (White and Pierce, 1953). This impure preparation was further purified by countercurrent distribution and was claimed to be 90 % homogenous having approximately 120 u/mg by bioassay.

About the same time Bell and his colleagues (Bell, 1954) were also involved in the isolation of porcine ACTH. They used the same procedure as the Armour Group in the initial extraction and the oxycellulose steps. After exhaustive countercurrent distribution (Shepherd, Howard, Bell, Cacciola, Child, Davies, English, Finn, Meisenhelder, Mayer and Van Der Sheer, 1956) several components were isolated, three of which had approximately 100 u/mg by bioassay. Lee and his coworkers described the isolation and purification of human ACTH in several reports (Lee, Lerner and Buettner-Janusch, 1959, 1960, 1961a, b). Again the initial extraction and oxycellulose step of Astwood *et al.* (1951) was followed. Further purification was achieved by ion exchange chromatography on CM and DEAE cellulose. The final product only had 26 u/mg by bioassay and was unstable (Lee *et al.*, 1959). The increasing demand for human growth hormone for therapeutic use led to the investigation of the large scale isolation of human ACTH as a by-product from the isolation of growth hormone. Using CM cellulose ion exchange chromatography and gel filtration on Sephadex, Lerner, Upton and Lande (1968) succeeded in purifying a homogenous fraction with a biological activity of 139 u/mg. Four other fractions of similar high activities with slightly different ion exchange characteristics were also obtained which had amino acid compositions approaching theoretical hACTH. More recently Lowry and Scott (1974) used frozen glands as their starting material and employed the initial extraction method of Lyons (1937). One main peak of biological and immunological activity was found when the crude material was submitted to gel filtration on BioGel P6. However this material separated into two peaks after CM cellulose chromatography. Amino acid analysis of both peaks after acid hydrolysis gave the same theoretical composition for human ACTH. Amino acid analysis after enzymic hydrolysis however suggested that the later eluting peak was true human ACTH and that the second peak was deamidated human ACTH possibly with the β-peptide bond which had been reported to exist in some forms of deamidated ACTH by Riniker, Sieber, Rittel and Zuber (1972). The more basic of the two purified peptides had a biological activity in excess of 200 u/mg in the isolated adrenal cell bioassay (Lowry, McMartin and Peters, 1973).

This would suggest that there is only one ACTH variety in fresh tissue and that all other forms are created during extraction. The different properties on ion exchange chromatography of the the other forms of human ACTH described by Lerner et al. (1968) are difficult to resolve in terms of deamidation as there is only one amide group in human ACTH. An explanation for these other forms is the progressive alkylation of primary amino groups by aldehydes during storage (acetone-dried glands were used in these other studies).

The discovery of β-LPH was an accident. It was isolated during the course of improving the procedure for the isolation of sheep ACTH. Originally (Li, Geshwind, Dixon, Levy and Harris, 1965) absorbed ACTH extracted by the acid-acetone procedure onto oxycellulose before continuing with the final stages of purification (ion exchange, countercurrent distribution). As oxycellulose did not completely remove all the ACTH activity Birk and Li (1964) chose to use ion exchange chromatography on CM cellulose and omitted the oxycellulose step. The yield of ACTH increased considerably and a new peak appeared which was shown to be distinct from other known pituitary hormones in its physico-chemical properties. Its name β-lipotrophin stems simply from the fact that at that time Li and his colleagues were using the isolated rabbit fat pad assay in their search for lipolytic compounds. As it was the second compound isolated which had lipolytic activity (ACTH was the first) it was called β-lipotrophin. If it had first been tested in an MSH assay it would have been called γ-MSH. Another lipolytic hormone was characterised later and was designated γ-LPH (Chrétien and Li, 1967). Subsequently human β- and γ-LPH have been isolated (Cseh, Graf and Goth, 1968; Scott and Lowry, 1974), both groups using acid-acetone extractions of frozen tissue followed by chromatography on cellulose and gel filtration. Bradbury, Smyth and Snell (1976) first reported the isolation of the C-terminal fragment of β-lipotrophin which has subsequently been termed β-endorphin and found to have strong opiate-like activity (Bradbury, Smyth, Snell, Birdsall and Hulme, 1976; Li and Cheung, 1976). Both groups used the acid-acetone extraction of Lyons (1937) followed by the salt fractionation described by Li et al. (1965). The resulting fraction was used as the source of β-endorphin which was isolated in a pure form by ion exchange chromatography and gel filtration.

The structure of the peptide known as $β_h$-MSH comprises 22 amino acids, differing from the β-MSH's of all other species which comprise only 18 amino acids. Their sequences are identical to the 41–58 portion of their corresponding β- and γ-LPH molecules which led Chrétien and Li (1967) to postulate that β-MSH is derived by cleavage from β-LPH by a trypsin-like enzyme, with γ-LPH (N-terminal 58 amino acids of β-LPH) being an intermediate product.

The 22 amino acid peptide sequence of human beta melanocyte stimulating hormone (β_h-MSH) is known to comprise the region 37–58 of β_h- and γ_h-LPH. However, it is now generally accepted that β_h-MSH does not normally occur in human tissues (Bloomfield, Scott, Lowry, Gilkes and Rees, 1974) and that it was artefactually derived from β-LPH as a result of post-mortem autolysis and the mild extraction procedure (5% acetic acid) employed (Scott and Lowry, 1974). Since impure native ACTH presumably contaminated with β-LPH was used to raise antisera to "β-MSH" and since the whole amino acid sequence of β-MSH is contained within β_h-LPH it was quite likely that any resultant antiserum might show cross-reactivity with β_h-and/or γ_hLPH. Indeed, characterisation of the specificity of the antisera employed in early radioimmunoassays for human β-MSH (Abe, Nicholson, Liddle, Island and Orth, 1967) has shown their inability to distinguish between β_h- and γ_h-LPH and β_h-MSH (Gilkes, Bloomfield, Scott, Lowry, Ratcliffe, Landon and Rees, 1975a).

When human pituitaries are collected and extracted under conditions specifically designed to minimise proteolysis no material eluting in the position of the 22 amino acid peptide β_h-MSH is seen but all elutes in the expected position of β_h-LPH (Scott and Lowry, 1974). Similarly, chromatography of plasma from a normal subject after pyrogen administration also confirmed that all the "MSH" immunoreactivity eluted in the position of β-LPH (Gilkes et al., 1975a).

The conclusion that human β-MSH does not exist is further supported by in vitro studies using β_h- and γ_h-LPH and synthetic β_h-MSH in human plasma. β_h-MSH is unstable and its activity disappears rapidly whilst β_h- and γ_h-LPH are more stable and behave like the endogenous material itself (Gilkes et al., 1975a). These data have received subsequent validation by other investigators (Bachelot, Wolfsen and Odell, 1976; Tanaka, Mount and Orth, 1976; Tanaka, Nicholson and Orth, 1977; 1978b).

D. BIOLOGICAL ACTIONS OF ACTH

1. The Adrenal Glands

The effect of hypophysectomy on the adrenal gland is 2 fold, corticosteroidogenesis ceases and the cortex of the gland begins to atrophy. Thus it appears that ACTH stimulates both corticosteroidogenesis and maintains adrenal weight although replacement doses of ACTH will maintain plasma corticosteriods at physiological levels but not adrenal weight. Only pharmacological doses of ACTH are capable of maintaining adrenal weight and plasma taken from patients with Nelson's syndrome or Addison's disease and very high endogenous circulating ACTH levels will also maintain adrenal growth (Segal and Christy, 1968). Preparations of growth hormone have also been shown to act synergistically with ACTH in inducing ornithine decarboxylase (Levine, Nicholson, Liddle and Orth, 1973). Thus it appears that there is a pituitary factor which acts synergistically with, but is distinct from, ACTH.

2. Adipose Tissue

ACTH causes fatty acid release from adipocytes. However, this effect is only observed at pharmacological concentrations and is not considered to be of physiological significance.

E. BIOLOGICAL ACTIONS OF α-MSH AND CLIP

α-MSH is the most potent peptide in darkening the skin of some lower vertebrates. Its biological significance in humans is unknown although a peptide resembling α-MSH is present in the human pituitary only during foetal life. It is also reported to occur in the blood of some, but not all, pregnant women (Clark, Thody, Shuster and Bowers, 1978). After delivery the foetal zone of the human adrenal cortex involutes, while the definitive zone or adult cortex, consisting of a thin layer of cells covering the large foetal zone, hypertrophies. This change may be triggered by a switch in the production of trophic hormones by the foetus from peptides resembling α-MSH and CLIP to ACTH (Silman et al., 1976). It has been reported that α-MSH can stimulate adrenal steroidogenesis in the foetal rabbit (Challis and Torosis, 1977; Glickman, Carson, Naftolin and Challis, 1978) whereas Synacthen does not and in the adult rabbit the converse is true. Studies in the Rhesus monkey in which the changes in morphology of the adrenal gland resemble closely those of man confirm qualitatively similar peptide pattern with the small peptides α-MSH and CLIP in the foetal pituitary and the larger ACTH predominating in the adult (Silman et al., 1978).

The 18–39 ACTH peptide CLIP has been shown to release insulin *in vitro* from isolated pancreatic islets and it is proposed that hypersecretion of CLIP may be the cause of the hyperinsulinaemia observed in genetically obese (*ob/ob*) mouse (Beloff-Chain, Edwardson and Hawthorn, 1976). Porcine ACTH has little or no effect in this system and synthetic α^{1-24} ACTH (Ciba, Synacthen) is devoid of activity. The response to synthetic 17–39 ACTH although significant is variable but this could be due to the generation of the biologically active 18–39 peptide *in situ*. The involvement of CLIP and hypertrophy of the vestigial human pars intermedia in the genesis of the hyperinsulinaemia of human obesity, if any, awaits further clarification. However, control of plasma insulin levels by the pituitary during foetal life, when an active definitive pars intermedia is present could be biologically important, since glucose transport into the blood of the foetus occurs via the placenta rather than via the gut.

F. BIOLOGICAL ACTIONS OF β-LPH AND ENDORPHINS

Although isolated from sheep pituitary glands in 1965 (Li, Barnafi, Chrétien and Chung, 1965) the biological role of β-LPH has remained obscure. The name lipotrophin was chosen by Li (1964) although the evidence for a physiological effect on fat metabolism is slight. The 58 amino acid peptide, γ-LPH, was isolated by Chrétien and Li (1967) and subsequently both were isolated from human pituitary tissue (Cseh, Gráf and Goth, 1968; Scott and Lowry, 1974). Although the true function of β-LPH awaits definition, it is possible that it acts as a precursor for β-endorphin (amino acids 61–91 of β-LPH), a substance which binds strongly to opiate receptors in brain and elsewhere (Bradbury, Smyth, Snell, Birdsall and Hulme, 1976; Ling, Burgus and Guillemin, 1976; Lazarus, Ling and Guillemin, 1976).

The concept of an endogenous analgesic was given a considerable boost when Hughes, Smith, Kosterlitz, Fothergill, Morgan and Morris (1975) reported the identification of two small peptides extracted from porcine brain tissue with strong opiate-like analgesic and receptor-binding activity. These substances are pentapeptides and differ from one another by a single amino acid (methionine enkephalin and leucine enkephalin; Met-enkephalin and Leu-enkephalin). Soon after their discovery the amino acid sequence of methionine enkephalin was noted to be identical with amino acids 61–65 of β-LPH. Subsequently, β-endorphin was shown to be at least 30 times more potent than enkephalin in its binding to opiate receptors and in experimental animals is a more powerful analgesic.

It is interesting to speculate that chronic opiate abuse in man might be expected to cause a sustained suppression of endogenous analgesic and that sudden opiate withdrawal would lead to unoccupied receptors and the clinical features of opiate withdrawal. Thus, it is possible that the biological basis for the efficacy of electro-acupuncture in relieving the symptoms of heroin withdrawal (Wen and Cheung, 1973; Wen and Teo, 1975) might be due to stimulation of release of an endogenous opiate.

After hypophysectomy, opiate agonist activity resembling β-endorphin, can still be found in brain tissue (Cheung and Goldstein, 1976) and both β-LPH and ACTH have been found in the brains of several species independent of the presence of pituitary tissue, suggesting a dissociated distribution for these two peptides (Krieger, Liotta, Suda, Palkovits and Brownstein, 1977). Furthermore recent demonstration of β-endorphin in cerebrospinal fluid from hypopituitary patients, without either LPH or ACTH in their blood (Jeffcoate, Rees, McLoughlin, Ratter, Hope, Lowry and Besser, 1978), would also support synthesis by the brain itself. Thus, the two long held premises that ACTH and β-LPH are synthesised only in pituitary tissue, and that they are always synthesised together, may require revision.

The physiological roles of brain β-LPH and β-endorphin may differ from their pituitary counterparts. It may be that they should be viewed more as neurotransmitters and modulators of behaviour than as hormones. In this regard, peptide fragments of ACTH are known to alter behaviour in some mammalian species (De Wied, 1976) and some of the effects of β-endorphin are similar to those of morphine in that they can cause both prolactin and growth hormone release in rats via a hypothalamic action (Cocci, Santagostino, Gil-Ad and Müller, 1977). Because of technical difficulties in the radioimmunoassay of β-endorphin it remains unclear as to whether this peptide is found in the human peripheral circulation. Data obtained in rats suggests that the blood levels observed would be insufficient for significant opiate agonist activity (Guillemin, Vargo, Rossier, Minick, Ling, Rivier, Vale and Bloom, 1977).

G. MEASUREMENT OF ACTH

At the outset it should be clearly understood that the measurement of circulating ACTH levels involves the use of assays that are considerably more complicated, expensive and less precise than the fluorimetric, competitive protein binding and radioimmunoassays for plasma cortisol. Since under steady state conditions a cortisol measurement can be regarded as a bioassay for ACTH this measurement should always be performed in preference to an ACTH assay. However, exceptions to the above do occur when this relationship does not hold true. Thus, when the adrenal cortex is under maximal stimulation, a further increase in ACTH levels (> 300 pg/ml) will not cause a further rise in plasma cortisol. Liddle, Island and Meador (1962), demonstrating that the rate-limiting step in the hypothalamic–pituitary–adrenal axis is the adrenal cortex. Dissociation between ACTH and cortisol levels occurs:

(i) in a patient with the ectopic ACTH syndrome or after administration of pyrogen, when ACTH levels may be very high and the adrenal cortex is maximally stimulated;

(ii) in a patient who has Cushing's syndrome due to an autonomous adrenal source of cortisol (adenoma/carcinoma) in whom ACTH levels will be suppressed although cortisol levels will be high,

(iii) in the presence of adrenocortical failure due to either Addison's disease or an inherited enzyme defect (congenital adrenal hyperplasia, CAH) when ACTH levels will be high and cortisol levels low.

In all circumstances other than these a cortisol level serves as a bioassay for ACTH and for technical reasons should be performed in preference.

All currently available assays for ACTH employ either biological or immunological techniques. Since the steroidogenic (biological) activity resides within the N-terminal region of the molecule and antisera raised against ACTH by immunisation with intact $\alpha_h{}^{1-39}$ACTH usually results in C-terminally directed antibodies (Imura, Sparks, Grodsky and Forsham, 1965; Imura, Sparks, Tosaka, Hane, Grodsky and Forsham, 1967) a dissociation between results obtained by immunoassay and bioassay may occur.

Table 1

Current ACTH assays.

Method	Index of precision (λ)	Sensitivity (mu)	References
Adrenal ascorbic acid content in hypophysectomised rats	0·176	0·20	Sayers et al. (1948)
Corticosterone levels in the adrenal vein of hypophysectomised rats	0·298	0·005	Lipscomb and Nelson (1962)
In vitro steroidogenesis in isolated adrenal cells	0·01–0·06	0·0001	Sayers and Giordano (1973)
Cytochemical bioassay	0·09	2·5 fg (0·00025 μu)	Chayen et al. (1972)
Radioreceptor assay		0·0001	Lefkowitz et al. (1970)
Radioimmunoassay		0·0001	Berson and Yalow (1968); Landon and Greenwood (1968)

Usually, immunoassay values tend to be higher than bioassay values, an observation which could be due to the presence either of partially degraded ACTH which has lost biological activity but retained immunological activity (Besser, Orth, Nicholson, Byyny, Abe and Woodham, 1971; May-suyama, Ruhmann-Wennhold and Nelson, 1971) or to the presence of higher molecular weight precursors such as big ACTH with reduced biological activity (Gewirtz and Yalow, 1974; Ratter, Hogan, Lowry, Edwards and Rees, 1977).

Since the last edition of this book several new assays for ACTH have been developed some of which are sufficiently sensitive to measure ACTH in unextracted plasma samples (Table 1).

1. ACTH Standards

The First International Standard (IS) of ACTH was established by WHO in 1950; it had been prepared from the most highly purified preparation then available and was assigned a unitage of 1 u/mg. This standard was superseded by the 2nd IS in 1956 (assigned a potency of 1·14 u/mg) and by the current 3rd IS (Bangham, Mussett and Stack-Dunne, 1962).

The 3rd IS of ACTH differed from the earlier two standards in that it was prepared from ACTH further purified on oxycellulose, resulting in material with a potency (in terms of 2nd IS) of approximately 30 u/mg by i.v. bioassay, and of approximately 100 u/mg by s.c. bioassay. The unitage of the IS was then assigned on the basis of its potency by s.c. assays (5·0 u/ampoule). The difference between the i.v.:s.c. potency ratio of the oxycellulose purified material and that (1:1) observed with the 1st and 2nd IS, led to a discontinuity of the i.v. unitage because of the need to maintain continuity of unitage for preparations for therapeutic use, nearly all of which are administered subcutaneously.

The s.c.:i.v. potency ratio of batches of corticotrophins of various species has been variable and unpredictable and the cause has not yet been satisfactorily explained.

Measurement of corticotrophin has meanwhile been stabilised by the availability of an international working standard (which has also been the basis for the USP standards) of the same material as the (3rd) International Standard. Some research workers have caused some confusion by using this working standard for assays in which the dose is given intravenously with an unofficial unitage of 1·5 u/ampoule instead of the 5·0 u designated by WHO.

It has also become clear that the 3rd IS, which is of porcine origin, is not suitable in all assay systems for the immunoassay of ACTH. Work is in progress to establish an IRP of human ACTH for immunoassay.

2. ACTH Bioassays

Readers are referred to several comprehensive reviews of ACTH measurement by bioassay (Vernikos-Danellis, 1965; Sayers, 1967). The rapidity of progress in this field is well illustrated by the fact that, of the assays described then, only a modified Lipscomb-Nelson assay is now ever used clinically. Many of the earlier bioassays were technically complex, insensitive and imprecise which meant that it was not really until the advent of radioimmunoassay and concurrently with it improved bioassay techniques, that any substantial information regarding ACTH levels in body fluids in health and disease became available.

The very early bioassays depending on adrenal maintenance or repair in intact or hypophysectomised animals are only of historic interest. The introduction of the adrenal ascorbate depletion assay described by Sayers *et al.* (1948) represented a major advance and enabled the very first determinations of circulating ACTH to be made in patients with elevated levels due to adrenocortical failure (Sydnor, Sayers, Brown and Tyler, 1953).

(a) Bioassays employing hypophysectomised animals

In all these assay systems endogenous hormone is removed either by hypophysectomy before assay or by pharmacological suppression by the use of exogenous corticosteroids. Thus, Nelson and Hume (1955) described an assay using measurement of corticosteroids in the adrenal venous effluent of hypophysectomised dogs. For obvious reasons this constituted a very expensive system as well as being insensitive and hypophysectomised dogs were soon replaced by hypophysectomised rats (Lipscomb and Nelson, 1962). Most of our understanding of the physiology and pathophysiology of ACTH secretion has been established using this assay (Lipscomb and Nelson, 1962; Williams, Island, Oldfield and Liddle, 1961; Liddle and Williams, 1962; Ney, Shimizu, Nicholson, Island and Liddle, 1963).

Two hours after hypophysectomy, male Sprague-Dawley rats are injected intravenously with either saline, standard ACTH or the sample to be assayed. Blood is collected via a cannula inserted into the left-adrenal vein.

In each assay, three rats receive saline (to provide base line data), three the standard ACTH at each of two dose levels, and the others samples (plasma or tissue extracts). Corticosterone in adrenal venous plasma is measured by a fluorimetric technique (Mattingly 1962), and the end-point determined as the amount of steroid liberated per minute. The mean potency and 95% confidence limits for each sample are then calculated.

Although the use of this assay allowed Liddle *et al.* (1962) to undertake classical studies on the physiological mechanisms controlling ACTH

F

secretion and also to assess the value of ACTH measurements to the clinician, the large volumes of blood required as well as technical difficulties precluded its widespread clinical use. However, subsequent modifications (Nicholson and Van Loon, 1973) have resulted in an assay with improved sensitivity.

Two other *in vivo* bioassays are worthy of comment. Thus, removal of the need to cannulate the adrenal vein was introduced (Vernikos-Danellis, Anderson and Trigg, 1966). In this assay endogenous ACTH secretion is inhibited by exogenous corticosteroids or hypophysectomy, unilateral adrenalectomy is performed and after administration of the standard ACTH or test sample the other adrenal is removed. The difference in corticosterone content of the two adrenal glands is the assay end-point. Espiner, Beaven and Hart (1963) described a more sensitive although less practical procedure in which a bilaterally adrenalectomised Merino ewe was used in which one adrenal was transplanted into the neck. The ability to directly inject the test sample into the blood supply of the transplanted adrenal results in greatly improved sensitivity.

(b) In vitro bioassays

ACTH bioassays based on the use of adrenal tissue in non-proliferative organ culture have inherent advantages when compared with the bioassays described above. Thus, the presence of endogenous ACTH does not pose a problem and the sample for assay is brought into direct contact with its target organ and is also protected both from circulating proteolytic enzymes as well as from sites of *in vivo* degradation such as kidney and liver. Saffran and Schally (1955) were the first to employ this type of assay in which adrenal segments were incubated in Krebs–Ringer bicarbonate glucose solution. Fluorogenic corticosteroid output into the medium was measured. However the use of isolated adrenocortical cells rather than whole adrenals or adrenal segments or slices has resulted in greatly improved sensitivity (Table 1).

(1) Isolated adrenal cell bioassay. Rat adrenal tissue is dispersed by a combination of tryptic digestion and mechanical agitation, and the cells are either suspended in Krebs–Ringer bicarbonate solution containing bovine serum albumin and a high concentration of calcium ions (Swallow and Sayers, 1969; Sayers, Swallow and Giordano, 1971) or perfused suspended in a column of Biogel beads (Lowry, McMartin and Peters, 1973; Lowry and McMartin, 1974). Corticosterone output in the perfusate is measured by a fluorimetric technique. Although such assays can detect as little as 10 pg ACTH, plasma interferes in the system. This problem has been studied by Sayers and Giordano (1973) who observed that, whilst small volumes of serum (5–20 µl) did not

inhibit steroidogenesis, addition of larger volumes had a marked inhibitory effect so that this assay system cannot be used for measurement of ACTH in unextracted plasma although prior extraction of ACTH onto Quso glass and subsequent assay is a feasible approach.

(2) *The cytochemical assay.* This bioassay is the most sensitive described for any hormone and was developed by Chayen, Loveridge and Daly (1971, 1972). The general principle, that is the precise measurement of biochemical changes induced by hormones in their specific target organs using quantitative cyto-chemistry (Chayen and Bitensky, 1968) has been applied to the measurement of other peptide hormones (LH, TSH, TRH, gastrin and PTH; Chayen, Daly, Loveridge and Bitensky, 1976; Rees and Ratter, 1978) and because of the great sensitivity obtained is available for the measurement of hormones which circulate in low molar concentrations (such as ACTH, PTH, TSH, etc.). The general schemes for the measurement of any hormone by cyto-chemical bioassay is to remove target organs and cut into segments, maintain each segment separately *in vitro*, treat with standard or plasma, chill and section, react for cytochemical response and measure by microdensitometry (from Chayen *et al.*, 1976). Another advantage of the great sensitivity of the technique is that basal circulating ACTH levels can be measured after the sample has been diluted 100 times.

In the initial development of this assay four segments of guinea pig adrenals were employed for the production of a standard curve and the remaining two for dilutions of plasma (1:100 and 1:1000). Obviously, the assay throughput was greatly limited by the size of these adrenal glands and thus by the availability of adequate numbers of segments. However, increased throughput has been achieved by modification of the segment assay to a section assay, in which the hormone reaction takes place on a microscope-slide sections of adrenal tissue rather than on whole segments (Alaghband-Zadeh, Daly, Bitensky and Chayen, 1974).

The cytochemical ACTH bioassay depends upon the ability of the ACTH to deplete the adrenals of ascorbate (Sayers, Sayers and Woodbury, 1948). Although the significance of this reaction in relationship to steroidogenesis is obscure, there is good evidence that the amount of cortisol produced by different adrenal segments exposed to various ACTH concentrations is directly related to loss of ascorbate from the adrenal tissue (Chayen *et al.*, 1976). The response of the adrenals to ACTH is measured using the Prussian blue reaction which measures total reducing potency, most of which is due to ascorbate. The reaction that occurs is as follows:

ferricyanide + reducing moiety → ferrocyanide + oxidised moiety

ferrocyanide + ferric ions → ferric ferrocyanide (Prussian blue)

Since Prussian blue is insoluble, precipitation occurs within the adrenal cells according to how much ascorbate they originally contained. The absorption spectrum of Prussian blue in the cells of the guinea pig zona reticularis has been determined. The effect is measured in cells of the zona reticularis because the maximal response to ACTH occurs here, whereas the zona fasciculata is either non-responsive or demonstrates a reversed effect. Thus, the zona reticularis cells exposed to high concentrations of ACTH are depleted of ascorbate, and contain less Prussian blue compared to those exposed to lower ACTH concentrations. The concentration of Prussian blue (expressed as integrated extinction × 100) and ACTH are inversely related and provide the typical ACTH bioassay standard curve.

The index of precision varies between 0·02–0·1 (Holdaway, Bloomfield, Ratcliffe, Hinson, Rees and Rees, 1974) comparing well with most other hormone bioassays. Similarly, fiducial limits vary between 87–115% and 98–102% (Daly, Loveridge, Bitensky and Chayen, 1972). The detectable concentration of standard ACTH over blank value is approximately 5 fg/ml and the lowest plasma ACTH level ever measured by this technique is 34 fg/ml (Rees, Ratcliffe, Besser, Kramer, Landon and Chayen, 1973).

ACTH levels measured in the cytochemical bioassay rise and fall in accordance with established ACTH physiology. Thus, after the acute administration of cortisol to a normal volunteer, ACTH levels fell from 50 pg/ml to 34 fg/ml at the end of 4 hr, allowing for the first time the calculation of the half-time for disappearance of endogenous ACTH from a basal level (10·4 min; Rees, Ratcliffe, Besser, Kramer, Landon and Chayen, 1973). In a similar study disappearance of endogenous injected synthetic α^{1-24} ACTH gave similar half-times (Daly, Fleischer, Chambers, Bitensky and Chayen, 1974).

Overall agreement between values obtained in the cytochemical assay and in other assays is excellent (Rees, Ratcliffe, Besser, Kramer, Landon and Chayen, 1973). However, immunological/biological dissociations have been observed both during dynamic physiological testing and in patients with pathologically raised ACTH levels (Daly, Fleischer, Chambers, Bitensky and Chayen, 1974). Even with the section assay the sample throughput is limited making it unsuitable for routine clinical use. However the very small sample volumes required (µl plasma) means that measurements in heel-prick samples from babies is feasible, and could possibly be of value in the early detection of congenital adrenal hyperplasia (CAH) (Holdaway, Rees and Landon, 1973). Obviously this microbiological approach is ideal for use in small animal research work, for example measuring ACTH in blood samples obtained by cannulating a rat tail vein.

(c) Radioimmunoassays

The first radioimmunoassay for ACTH was reported by Felber (1963) and subsequently an assay capable of measurement of ACTH in plasma samples was reported by Yalow, Glick, Roth and Berson (1964). The outstanding problem of all radioimmunoassays for ACTH has been the difficulty in developing antisera of the affinity necessary to measure the low circulating levels of ACTH. Thus, although the reported estimates of the normal basal ACTH levels in man differ between laboratories, nonetheless the consensus view is that levels are below 80 pg/ml at 09.00 hr and below 10 pg/ml at midnight.

(1) Antisera production. ACTH is a poor immunogen, antisera production only being successful when ACTH is conjugated to a larger carrier protein, such as heterologous serum albumin, thyroglobulin etc. before immunisation. Orth (1974) has described his method for raising anti-ACTH antisera in detail. In this method, synthetic α^{1-24} ACTH is conjugated to bovine serum albumin using the carbodiimide reaction (McGuire, McGill, Leeman and Goodfriend, 1965), dialysed and the conjugate emulsified with Freund's adjuvant. Rabbits or sheep are used for immunisation with a single i.v. injection of conjugated ACTH with adjuvant (250 µg) being given first followed by multiple site intradermal injection (Vaitukaitis, Robbins, Nieschlag and Ross, 1971) of 1 mg of antigen in adjuvant given in 20 or more sites in volumes of 0·1–0·2 ml/site. This technique is obviously preferable to the older methods in which unpleasant painful footpad injections were employed which usually became infected. Booster injections of conjugate are given after a two week interval and the animals bled after another two or three weeks. Although with this protocol, antisera of high sensitivity and titre are reproducibly obtained (Orth, 1974), nonetheless in most hands only a small percentage of antisera will be sufficiently sensitive to measure ACTH in plasma even after prior extraction and reports of antisera capable of measuring basal ACTH levels in unextracted plasma are few (Berson and Yalow, 1968; Orth, 1974).

Thus, extraction and concentration of ACTH in plasma may be required, which of necessity results in added complexity and hence to the introduction of extra sources of error. Nonetheless major advantages of this approach include removal of non-specific interference by plasma components and the avoidance of tracer damage by proteolytic enzymes in plasma. Several relatively simple extraction procedures are available including absorption onto either talc (Rosselin, Assan, Yalow and Berson, 1966), silicic acid or leached silica (Vycor) glass (Stouffer and Lipscomb, 1963; Donald, 1967; Ratcliffe and Edwards, 1971; Rees, Cook, Kendall, Allen, Kramer, Ratcliffe and Knight, 1971). It must be born in mind however, that all extraction procedures for ACTH have been validated for either α^{1-39} ACTH or α^{1-24} ACTH. In the light of current knowledge of the heterogeneous nature of circulating immunoreactive ACTH the proportion of these other uncharacterised ACTH-related peptides extracted by such procedures remains unknown.

(2) *Characterisation of antisera.* Since the structure of the α_h^{1-39} ACTH is defined and a wide variety of synthetic analogues are available it is possible to define the antigenic determinant of a particular antiserum with confidence by the use of the type of cross-reactivity studies which are well described (Landon, Girard and Greenwood, 1968; Orth, 1974). Although most anti-ACTH antisera do not show cross-reactivity with the β-LPH-related peptides, occasionally a core antiserum may be produced which shows cross-reactivity with both ACTH and LPH. Although ACTH and LPH are secreted together in all physiological and pathological situations the use of such an antiserum in clinical practice remains to be evaluated.

(3) *Preparation of ACTH tracer.* ACTH tracer of high specific activity is easily prepared by the use of the classical chloramine T method. However, solid-phase lactoperoxidase is preferable (Karonen, Mörsky, Siren and Seuderling, 1975) since it causes less iodination damage thus improving the shelf-life and overall quality of the tracer. Purification procedures have usually exploited the absorption properties of ACTH using cellulose (Yalow, Glick, Roth and Berson, 1964) or silicates (Rosselin et al., 1966; Rees et al., 1971) as absorbant. Pure iodinated ACTH will absorb, whereas damaged ACTH or unreacted iodide will not, or the small amounts that do can be removed by washing. Pure tracer is removed by elution with either plasma, acetone–acetic acid or acetone–water mixtures. However, the recent description by Bennett, Hudson, McMartin and Purdon (1977) of the use of octadecyl silyl silica (ODS silica) resin which separates on the basis of hydrophobicity rather than ionic charge allows not only separation of mono from diiodinated ACTH but from non-iodinated ACTH so allowing addition of a very small amount of purified undamaged tracer in the assay tube. The use of Iodogen (1,3,4,6-tetrachloro-3α,6α-diphenylglycouril) as alternative iodination procedure is under present evaluation (Salacinski, Hope, McClean, Clement-Jones, Sykes, Price and Lowry, 1979). Theoretically this has the property of an ideal electron acceptor and preliminary data suggest that virtual complete incorporation of radioiodine into peptide can occur without damage, thus overriding the requirement for tracer purification. Apart from this obvious major advantage the technique is very simple: 20 µl of 1 mg/ml solution of Iodogen in methylene chloride is allowed to dry in the bottom of a small polypropylene tube. 0·5 nmole of protein or peptide in 10 µl of 0·1 M PO_4 plus 1 mCi of ^{125}I are added and the tube is tapped gently at

1 min intervals. After 10 min the solution is aspirated.

(4) *Clinical use of ACTH assays.* With the introduction of radioimmuno-assay for ACTH the use of ACTH measurement has assumed a small although important role in clinical practice (Besser and Landon, 1968: Rees, 1976). Some clinical applications of basal plasma ACTH measurements are:

(i) to obtain information not provided by other means (in differentiating between the causes of Cushing's syndrome, in monitoring progress following the treatment of Cushing's disease, in monitoring the treatment of ectopic ACTH secreting tumours):

(ii) to obtain information more easily than can be elicited by alternative means (in differentiating between primary and secondary adrenocortical insufficiency, in monitoring steroid replacement therapy for congenital adrenal hyperplasia).

Collection of the blood samples must be undertaken with care to minimise both loss of ACTH due to adsorption onto glass surfaces as well as to prevent proteolytic destruction of ACTH in blood (Besser, Orth, Nicholson, Byyny, Abe and Woodham, 1971). This is particularly important if a bioassay for ACTH is employed since bioactivity declines more rapidly than immuno-reactivity. Thus, ideally samples should be collected into cooled plastic lithium heparin tubes, centrifuged at 4° and the plasma decanted into a plastic (polystyrene) tube and snap frozen in dry ice and stored at −20° until assayed. The presence of any haemolysis leads to rapid ACTH destruction and may result in spuriously low levels.

Initial attempts to stabilise ACTH immunoreactivity in blood and plasma appeared promising with the use of the proteolytic enzyme inhibitor N-ethyl-maleimide (NEM; Hogan, Rees, Lowry, Ratter and Snitcher, 1976) in that stabilisation for up to 72 hr was achieved by the immediate addition of 10^{-3}M NEM to the blood. However, most of these studies employed the use of purified human ACTH (α_h^{1-39} ACTH) added to blood. Subsequent studies using blood taken from patients with disorders of the pituitary–adrenal axis and raised ACTH levels showed major discrepancies, in that the addition of NEM to some samples resulted in successful stabilisation whereas degradation was observed with others. Others (Jubiz and Nolan, 1978) have also suggested that the use of NEM is effective. Our inability to reproducibly stabilise endogenous ACTH may reflect the heterogeneity of circulating molecular forms of ACTH mentioned earlier in this chapter occurring in different pathological conditions.

In normal adults, immunoreactive ACTH levels at 09.00 hr lie between 10-80 pg/ml and fall to undetectable levels (< 10 pg/ml) at 24.00 hr. Obviously normal ranges for ACTH values will depend upon the specificity of the antisera employed and may therefore vary from laboratory to laboratory. In patients with ACTH-dependent Cushing's syndrome, ACTH is detected in the circulation whereas when an autonomous adrenal tumour (adenoma or carcinoma) is the cause, levels are undetectable (< 10 pg/ml) (Fig. 2). Thus,

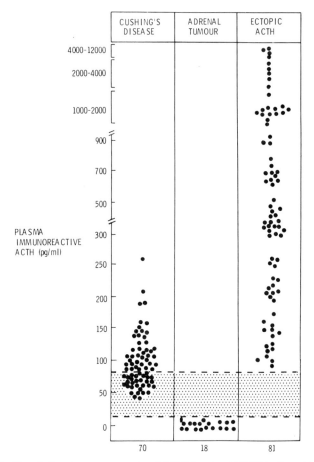

Fig. 2. Circulating immunoreactive ACTH levels at 09.00 hr in patients with proven Cushing's syndrome. Stippled area represents the normal range of plasma ACTH at 09.00 hr.

this single measurement is of itself clinically invaluable in establishing the aetiology of Cushing's syndrome and no patient with this condition should receive definitive treatment without at least one plasma ACTH determination. Nonetheless, there is certainly one exception to the above clear definition, which occurs in patients with pituitary-dependent Cushing's disease and nodular hyperplasia of the adrenal glands, in whom ACTH measurements may be intermittently detectable and then undetectable, presumably due to the relative autonomy of adrenal cortisol production.

A basal 09.00 hr ACTH measurement is also useful in the differentiation between primary and secondary adrenocortical failure, although because of the complexity and expense of ACTH measurements, this is required only as a backup to conventional tests of steroid reserve. Thus, in Addison's disease and congenital adrenal hyperplasia (CAH), ACTH levels are raised (although a diurnal variation will exist) whereas in secondary hypoadrenalism ACTH levels lie either within the normal range or below the limits of detection of the assay. Although a wide variety of dynamic test procedures are employed in the investigation of hypothalamic–pituitary–adrenal function a detailed discussion of the advantages and disadvantages of any particular approach will not be given here since this subject has been extensively reviewed elsewhere (James and Landon, 1968; Edwards and Besser, 1974; Rees, 1977a,b). Only those tests of relevance will be discussed in relationship to particular pathological disorders later in this chapter.

(5) *Measurement of LPH/endorphin.* Several radioimmunoassays for β_h-MSH have been described (Abe, Nicholson, Liddle, Island and Orth, 1967; Donald and Toth, 1973; Donnadieu and Sevaux, 1973; Thody and Plummer, 1973; Gilkes, Bloomfield, Scott, Lowry, Ratcliffe, Landon and Rees, 1975a). Most of the antisera employed in these studies show full cross-reaction with β-LPH and γ-LPH on a molar basis (Rees, 1977a). Interestingly the antiserum used by Donald and Toth (1973) only shows partial cross-reaction with β-LPH (3%) whilst showing equimolar cross-reactivity with β-MSH and γ-LPH. Such differences in antisera specificity probably accounts for the report of discrepancy between ACTH and β-MSH levels during insulin hypoglycaemia in man (Donald and Toth, 1973). More recently, a radioimmunoassay has been described in which the antiserum employed measures β_h- and γ_h-LPH but shows no cross-reaction with β_h-MSH (Jeffcoate, Rees, Lowry and Besser, 1978a). Presumably, the antiserum employed is directed towards the N-terminal 1–36 amino acid sequence of β_h-LPH. As with ACTH, extraction of plasma is required before assay to achieve adequate sensitivity to measure basal circulating LPH levels. Levels reported at 09.00 hr in normal subjects lie between 20–200 pg/ml falling to < 20–80 pg/ml at 23.00 hr.

Like ACTH, LPH secretion is episodic (Tanaka, Nicholson and Orth, 1978a) and secretion of ACTH/LPH is tightly coupled (Gilkes, Rees and Besser, 1977; Rees, Bloomfield, Gilkes, Jeffcoate and Besser, 1977; Tanaka, Nicholson and Orth, 1978a; Mullen et al., 1979) (Fig. 3). Studies on the half-time for disappearance of ACTH and MSH/β-LPH in patients with pathologically elevated levels of both peptides (Nelson's syndrome, Addison's disease) show dissociation between the two (Gilkes, 1975; Rees, Gilkes and Jeffcoate, 1977; Tanaka, Nicholson and Orth, 1978a) Thus, mean half-times for disappearance for immunoreactive ACTH of 40 min and MSH/LPH of 95 min in seven patients with Nelson's syndrome was observed by Rees *et al.* (1977). In patients with Addison's disease mean half-times for disappearance for ACTH of 34 min (range 30–37 min) and MSH/LPH of 59 min (range 45–72) are reported by Gilkes (1975) and times of 40 min for ACTH (range 20–51 min

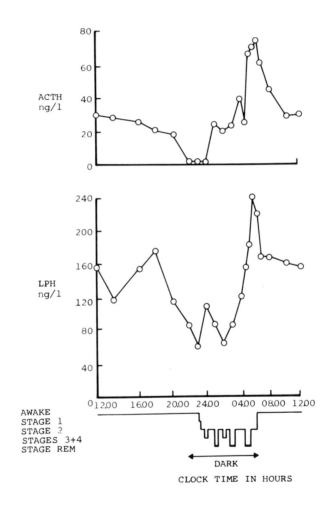

Fig. 3. Levels of immunoreactive lipotrophin and immunoreactive ACTH measured in the same plasma samples over 24 hr in a 31-yr-old male volunteer. The patterns over 24 hr show a close correlation (product moment correlation 0·81). (By permission of the eds, *Clin. Endocr.*)

and 83 min for MSH/LPH (range 44–133 min demonstrating considerable agreement (Tanaka, Nicholson and Orth, 1978a). Infusion studies by Liotta *et al.* (1978b) confirmed the longer half-time for disappearance of β-LPH than of ACTH.

Because of the excellent correlation observed between immunoreactive ACTH and plasma cortisol levels in normal individual subjects (Tanaka, Nicholson and Orth, 1978a; $r = 0.62$–0.75, n = 3) and since ACTH/MSH/LPH levels correlate well in patients with diseases of the pituitary–adrenal axis (Rees, Bloomfield, Gilkes, Jeffcoate and Besser, 1977; $r = 0.88$, n = 43) and in individual subjects (Tanaka, Nicholson and Orth, 1978a; $r = 0.66$–0.75, n = 3) an excellent correlation between plasma cortisol and MSH/LPH levels is also observed; making the measurement of LPH an alternative to ACTH in clinical practice.

Since the β-endorphin sequence of amino acids is contained within the β-LPH molecule it would be expected that most antisera used in radio-immunoassay might detect the β-endorphin sequence whether present as a separate entity or as part of the larger molecule. This problem bedevils the whole field of β-endorphin research in which radioimmunoassays are employed. An attempt to overcome this problem has been made by the use of two radioimmunoassays for β-LPH, one which measures the N-terminal LPH sequence (vide supra) which does not contain the β-endorphin sequence and another, C-terminally directed antiserum (Jeffcoate *et al.*, 1978). Using this system the presence of greater amounts of material reacting with the C-terminal antiserum would suggest the presence of β-endorphin. The use of such antisera in combination with gel chromatography means that more specific identification of β-endorphin in blood becomes a possibility (Guillemin *et al.*, 1977).

Although the correlation between ACTH and LPH ($r = 0.88$) reported by Gilkes *et al.* (1975a) in patients with diseases of the pituitary–adrenal axis appeared excellent, nevertheless closer examination of the data suggested that in normal subjects and patients with excess secretion of pituitary ACTH/LPH, ACTH levels were equal to or higher than MSH/LPH levels whereas in patients with ectopic ACTH secretion the reverse occurred (Gilkes, Rees and Besser, 1977). These studies were carried out using an antiserum (67 patients) which measures β_h-LPH, γ_h-LPH and β_h-MSH equally on a molar basis (Gilkes *et al.*, 1975a).

Subsequent data obtained using an antiserum measuring β_h-LPH and γ_h-LPH but not β_h-MSH (Jeffcoate, Rees, Lowry and Besser, 1978b) so far do not show such a clear distinction although inadequate data as yet are available for statistical analysis (Jeffcoate, Tomlin, McLoughlin, Rees and Besser, 1979). Any explanation for such findings and their discrepancies remains totally speculative at this time.

H PHYSIOLOGY OF ACTH SECRETION

1. Circadian Rhythmicity

The establishment of a circadian rhythm of ACTH and hence of cortisol secretion in humans occurs around the age of 3 and persists throughout life. ACTH and cortisol levels rise to a maximum between 06.00 and 09.00 hr with light playing a major role in the peak of ACTH observed immediately after rising, and fall progressively throughout the day. However studies of both ACTH and cortisol levels taken during frequent blood sampling show that both cortisol (Krieger, Allen, Rizzo and Krieger, 1971) and ACTH levels oscillate throughout the day with secretory peaks increasing in height occurring between 02.00 and 08.00 hr (J. R. Daly, personal communication; Rees, 1977a). Such fluctuations of cortisol secretion do not appear to be due to either altered metabolic clearance of cortisol or any change in the responsiveness of the adrenal to ACTH (McDonald, Weise and Patrick, 1956).

Although the factor postulated to control ACTH secretion, corticotrophin releasing factor (CRF), was the first hypothalamic regulatory factor to be demonstrated (Guillemin and Rosenberg, 1955; Saffran and Schally, 1955) it has still not been positively identified. The reasons for this include lack of specificity and sensitivity of bioassay systems used, the loss and instability of CRF activity during multiple fractionation procedures and the identification of several different factors with CRF activity. Additionally, the neurohypophyseal peptide arginine vasopressin (AVP) has been proposed as a CRF although the generally accepted view is that this is distinct from CRF (Schally and Bowers, 1964; Burgus and Guillemin, 1970). There is little doubt, however, that vasopressin does release ACTH in a dose-dependent manner from isolated pituitary cells (Portanova and Sayers, 1973; Gillies and Lowry, 1978) and can do so at concentrations of AVP which have been found in portal blood. Recent immunological studies have shown that nearly all CRF activity can be removed from crude rat hypothalmic extracts by binding to specific AVP antisera. The dose response curve of synthetic AVP however is less steep than that of the crude extract (Gillies, Van Wimersma Greidanus and Lowry, 1979). However, the major peak of this crude extract after gel filtration runs in exactly the expected position of synthetic AVP and gives the typical shallow dose response curve produced by AVP in this bioassay. Thus it is indistinguishable immunologically, biologically and chromatographically from AVP (Gillies and Lowry, 1979). It has been proposed that the main CRF activity found in rat hypothalami is vasopressin plus a synergistic factor raising the attractive hypothesis that ACTH release and thus its concentration in blood is controlled by a peptide whose potency can be increased by the presence of a factor which alone has no significant effect on ACTH secretion. This factor could also be involved in the release of other hormones e.g. growth hormone and prolactin which are known to be secreted simultaneously with ACTH in response to certain stresses. This type of control has adaptive advantages, especially for a hormone like ACTH which is under feedback control by circulating corticosteroids, since it would provide the facility to respond to acute stress even in the presence of high circulating steroid levels. This type of control appears to be lost in Cushing's disease where there is usually no response to insulin-induced hypoglycaemia (James, Landon, Wynn and Greenwood, 1968; Krieger and Luria, 1977). However, such patients exhibit significantly greater increments in plasma ACTH concentration in response to exogenous administration of vasopressin than do normal subjects. Using immunohistochemistry hypothalamic vasopressin concentration in rats can be seen to alter in response to the circulating levels of corticosterone (Zimmerman, 1976), adrenalectomy leading to an increase and cortisol administration a decrease. Thus, one can postulate that it is the synergistic factor that causes the increase in response to insulin hypoglycaemia and that in Cushing's disease this factor is already maximally released. The high circulating levels of glucocorticoids in such patients would suppress release of hypothalamic vasopressin so that exogenously administered vasopressin would exert a greater effect in the presence of excessive concentrations of the putative synergistic factor.

2. Feedback Control

Although the reciprocal relationship between circulating cortisol and ACTH constitutes a major homeostatic mechanism, much controversy exists regarding the major site of feedback (for a detailed review see Kendall, 1971). Corticosteroid receptors have been demonstrated both in the hypothalamus and pituitary although for obvious reasons most data relate not to man but to experimental animals. For example, binding of ^{3}H-corticosterone to cell nuclei and soluble macromolecules in both rat anterior pituitary and hypothalamic tissues has been demonstrated and in both *in vivo* and *in vitro* bioassay systems, CRF release from rat hypothalami can be suppressed by dexamethasone, corticosterone and cortisol. Similarly, increase in rat median eminence CRF-activity can be suppressed by prior administration of corticosterone (Jones, Hillhouse and Burden, 1976).

Two components of cortisol/ACTH feedback have been postulated, one occurring immediately after the steroid administration (fast feedback) and the other occurring more slowly and related to the actual dose of steroid administered (slow feedback) (Dallman and Yates, 1969; Jones, Hillhouse and Burden, 1976). Fast feedback has been clearly demonstrated in man with cessation of ACTH secretion occurring within 2 min of an i.v. bolus of cortisol (Rees, Ratcliffe, Kramer, Besser, Landon and Chayen, 1973). More detailed data concerning the finer control of corticosteroid feedback in man are sparse although the effects of continued exogenous corticosteroid administration have been studied (Landon, Snitcher and Rees, 1976). Prolonged administration of a variety of natural and synthetic cortico- steroids usually results in adrenal atrophy subsequent upon suppression of ACTH secretion; overall this is related to the duration of treatment and steroid dosage administered. Thus, a small dose of prednisolone (2·5 mg daily) will cause little, if any, suppression, whereas larger doses (20 mg daily) result in rapid adrenal atrophy. Undoubtedly the time of day of steroid administration has a profound influence on the resultant severity of ACTH suppression and subsequently of adrenal atrophy. Thus, a dose of exogenous steroid given in the evening (18.00 hr) will suppress the early morning ACTH rise. To circumvent this problem clinically intermittent steroid administration (say 2–3 day intervals) is therefore desirable.

When steroid treatment is discontinued, ACTH and hence cortisol levels may remain suppressed for weeks or months and subsequent failure to respond to insulin-induced hypoglycaemia with an adequate rise in ACTH/ cortisol has been observed for 1–2 yr. However, this should be regarded as an unusual event since a study by Plumpton, Besser and Cole (1969) on 20 patients who received exogenous steroids for 3–30 months previously, showed that cortisol levels during insulin-induced hypoglycaemia and surgical stress were no different from a control group of patients who had never received steroids. Thus, complete recovery of the hypothalamic–pituitary–adrenal axis must have occurred. In this respect it is of interest that ACTH levels rise during the recovery phase confirming that atrophy of the adrenal glands takes longer to resolve than any suppression of ACTH secretion.

Conversely, lowering of circulating corticosteroid levels either due to primary adrenocortical failure (Addison's disease), due to an intra-adrenal enzyme defect (CAH) or due to the exogenous administration of drugs which interfere with cortisol biosynthesis in the adrenal cortex (e.g. metyrapone) all results in elevations of circulating ACTH levels.

3. Stress Control

A variety of different stressors will result in rapid ACTH release. In such circumstances both circadian rhythmicity and feedback control are overridden and break-through ACTH secretion, and hence cortisol secretion, will occur. Thus, early observations demonstrated clearly that ACTH release during operative stress occurs, even during the simultaneous infusion of high doses of both dexamethasone (5 mg/hr) and cortisol (50 mg/hr). For example, the induction of hypoglycaemia by the administration of exogenous insulin in the face of a continuous infusion of dexamethasone (1 mg/hr) resulted in a marked rise in plasma cortisol levels. A similar effect was observed following pyrogen administration (James, Landon and Fraser, 1968).

I. CONTROL OF LPH/ENDORPHIN SECRETION

Originally it had been thought that it was plasma β-MSH which mirrored ACTH blood levels in nearly every physiological and pathophysiological situation with only one or two reports suggesting divergence of secretion (Donald and Toth, 1973). With the observation that β-MSH did not exist in human pituitaries (Lowry and Scott, 1974) but that β-MSH immuno-reactivity was due to a larger molecule β-LPH, Bloomfield, Scott, Lowry, Gilkes and Rees (1974) suggested that plasma β-MSH immunoreactivity in humans was due to LPH. It was subsequently shown that the β-MSH antiserum used by Donald and Toth (1973) did not, in fact, fully cross-react with β_h-LPH (Gilkes et al., 1975a). As discussed earlier, this antisera does, however, fully cross-react with γ-LPH so it would appear that in the situation studied (insulin hypoglycaemia) the peptide released is predominantly β-LPH and not its fragments. The only other situation in which ACTH/LPH levels appear dissociated is in patients with chronic renal failure on maintenance haemodialysis (Gilkes, Eady, Rees, Munro and Moorhead, 1975b) and the β-MSH levels could be correlated, both with the number of years that patients had been on dialysis and also with the degree of skin pigmentation. Jeffcoate et al. (1978) have confirmed these elevated levels with a different anti-LPH antiserum.

The C-terminal 61-91 fragment β-LPH β-endorphin (Fig. 1) has been shown to have potent in vitro and in vivo opiate activity (Bradbury, Smyth, Snell, Birdsall and Hulme, 1976; Li and Cheung, 1976; Ling, Burgus and Guillemin, 1976) whilst β-LPH has little or no opiate activity. Thus, it is important when considering levels of lipotrophin to know in which molecular forms these peptides exist. Circulating levels may not simply mirror the molecular forms found in the pituitary gland: γ-LPH has been purified from extracts of human pituitaries although insignificant amounts of β-endorphin only were obtained (Hope and Lowry, unpublished observations). Although there appears to be considerable circumstantial evidence that ACTH and LPH/endorphin are under the same hypothalamic control in man, little experimental data exist to substantiate this hypothesis.

The isolated rat anterior pituitary cell column provides an ideal system for the simultaneous study of the control of ACTH and LPH/endorphin peptides (Estivariz, Gillies and Lowry, 1979). Using a radioimmunoassay which cross-reacts with both rat β-LPH and β-endorphin and an ACTH radioimmunoassay it has been shown that ACTH and β-LPH/endorphin release responds to crude stalk median eminence (SME) extracts and synthetic vasopressin (AVP) in exactly the same fashion. Preincubations of SME extracts with a specific anti-AVP antiserum quenched the β-LPH/endorphin releasing activity of these extracts in a parallel manner to that observed for ACTH. Gel chromatography of the material released by the pituitary cell column after stimulation with either SME or AVP gave the same pattern of peptides. Most of the immunoreactive β-endorphin eluted in the expected position of β-LPH. There was however a significant peak of β-endorphin. ACTH eluted in the expected position of 1–39 ACTH. As the pituitary cell column eluate was collected under ideal conditions (it was acidified to pH 1·5 within seconds of secretion) it appears that the normal secretion of endorphin-like material is mainly in the form of β-LPH with small but significant amounts of β-endorphin, and that the release of these peptides from the pars distalis is under exactly the same hypothalamic control. The significance of such a pattern of peptides is not yet clear especially in relationship to the presence of an inactive precursor which has the facility to generate peripherally an active opiate. This possibility would, of course, offer an increased flexibility for the generation of the opiate active peptides, only under stress conditions, where there might be an associated release of peptidases capable of cleaving β-endorphin from β-LPH. These peptidases need not be of pituitary origin but could be released in the periphery (for example at the site of injury).

J. TESTS OF THE HYPOTHALAMO–PITUITARY–ADRENAL AXIS

Corticotrophin is one link in a highly integrated control system of the hypothalamo–pituitary–adrenal axis, the end products of which are the glucocorticoid hormones, in the human mainly cortisol. Before direct assays of corticotrophin and corticotrophin releasing factor (Vol. I, Ch. I) became available, corticotrophin activity had to be measured indirectly from the effect of various manipulations of the axis of plasma cortisol or the daily excretion of cortisol or its metabolites. In general, the levels of plasma cortisol and excretion of cortisol and its metabolites relate to the cortisol secretion rate. ACTH levels are usually raised in pituitary dependent Cushing's disease and the ectopic ACTH syndrome and are undetectable in patients with Cushing's syndrome and an adrenal adenoma or carcinoma.

1. Dynamic Tests

Many dynamic tests have been developed to assess the functional integrity and reserve capacity of all, or some of, the components of the HPA axis. Indeed their multiplicity is such that individual investigators may differ in their choice of test for use in a given clinical situation. Thus it must be stressed that this section reflects the authors' personal views.

The tests used include suppression of cortisol production by dexamethasone or metyrapone, and stimulation of cortisol production by ACTH or its synthetic analogues, or insulin hypoglycaemia. In our view, the limited information obtainable by the vasopressin and pyrogen stimulation tests is not sufficient to justify the severe side effects that may be experienced by some patients.

2. Steroid Suppression Tests

These tests depend on the oral administration of the synthetic glucocorticoid dexamethasone and the measurement of plasma cortisol and urinary free and 17-oxogenic steroids and are used in the diagnosis of Cushing's syndrome. Dexamethasone is employed since it has the advantage of high potency and is not detected by the methods used for the measurements of corticosteroids in blood or urine. Thus, the effect of the glucocorticoid on endogenous corticosteroid secretion can be studied. A variety of regimes for giving dexamethasone have been described (Table 2). The most valuable is that described by Liddle *et al.* (1960) in which a dose of 0·5 mg given 6 hourly for 48 hr was observed to suppress urinary Porter-Silber chromogens to below 8·5 μmol/day in normal subjects. Patients with Cushing's syndrome due to adrenocortical tumours did not suppress on this dose although with higher doses (2 mg

Table 2

Dexamethasone suppression tests

Diagnosis of Cushing's syndrome
    (i) 0·5 mg oral dexamethasone 6 hourly (09.00, 15.00, 21.00 and 03.00 hr) for 48 hr. Urinary 17-oxogenic steroids should fall below 14 μmol/day and plasma fluorogenic cortisol levels to less than 200 nmol/l
    (ii) 1·0–2·0 mg oral dexamethasone at midnight and plasma fluorogenic cortisol measured at 09·00 hr should be less than 200 nmol/l
Differential diagnosis of Cushing's syndrome
    (i) 2·0 mg oral dexamethasone 6 hourly for 48 hr. Plasma cortisol and urinary 17-oxogenic steroids should fall by at least 50% in the majority of patients with Cushing's disease

---

6 hourly for 48 hr) patients with Cushing's disease suppress by at least 50% whereas patients with Cushing's syndrome due to ectopic ACTH secretion or an adrenal tumour do not. However, it is important to note that exceptions are well recorded with some patients with Cushing's disease failing to suppress (Cope, 1966) and also patients with adrenocortical tumours and the ectopic ACTH syndrome showing supression (Kendall and Sloop, 1968). Occasionally paradoxical responses are observed with a rise in urinary 17-oxogenic steroids occurring (Cope, 1956; James, Landon and Wynn, 1965). Thus, the value of this test is in establishing the diagnosis of Cushing's syndrome rather than its aetiology. Occasionally patients with Cushing's disease show intermittent suppression of plasma and urinary corticosteroids and patients with severe mental depression may show resistance to suppression (Butler and Besser, 1968). Since this group may have other stigmata of Cushing's syndrome (for example weight gain) they may provide diagnostic difficulties. The overnight, or single dose dexamethasone suppression test is a useful screening test and has recently been reassessed (Shimizu and Yashida, 1977). However it must be emphasised that it is only a screening test and lack of full suppression of plasma cortisol does not confirm Cushing's syndrome, since false positives are found.

3. Insulin Stimulation Test

Intravenous administration of insulin results in a rapid decrease in blood glucose levels which, in normal subjects, causes a marked rise in plasma ACTH and cortisol levels once the glucose has fallen to below 2·2 mmol/l (Landon, Wynn and James, 1963; Greenwood, Landon and Stamp, 1966). This test has the major advantage that it assesses the integrity of the entire HPA axis and its responsiveness to stress, while hypoglycaemia is a potent stimulus to both growth hormone and prolactin secretion. Indeed an absent or impaired growth hormone response is one of the earliest indications of hypothalamic or pituitary malfunction.

The subject should be fasted and an amount of insulin chosen to induce satisfactory hypoglycaemia without causing severe side-effects. This is best achieved by giving the insulin as a single intravenous injection at a dosage based on body weight and related to the tentative clinical diagnosis. The usual dose is 0·15 u/kg. This should be decreased to 0·1 u/kg in patients suspected to be suffering from conditions associated with increased insulin sensitivity (for example patients with hypothalamic, pituitary or adrenal hypofunction or malnourished subjects). Obese patients or patients who have Cushing's syndrome or acromegaly may require 0·2 or 0·3 u/kg. Blood samples are taken immediately before and at 30 min intervals for 2 hr after the injections, for glucose and cortisol determinations. The maximum plasma cortisol level reached should exceed 580 nmol/l with an increment above the basal value of at least 100%.

In Cushing's syndrome, whatever the aetiology there is no rise (James, Landon, Wynn and Greenwood, 1968). Although patients with mental depression may also require larger insulin doses to achieve hypoglycaemia normal responses are seen in this group (Besser and Edwards, 1972). The insulin stimulation test is the most reliable test for the diagnosis of Cushing's syndrome but gives no information regarding aetiology.

The test is safe providing it is not performed on patients with epilepsy or ischaemic heart disease, a doctor is present, intravenous glucose is kept available and a carbohydrate-containing meal is given at its conclusion.

4. Vasopressin and Pyrogen Stimulation Tests

In our view, the limited information that can be obtained by these two tests is not sufficient to justify the severe side-effects that may be experienced by the patient.

5. Metyrapone Test

Metyrapone (2-methyl-l,2-bis(3-pyridyl)-l-propanone inhibits (among other enzyme systems), the 11β-hydroxylase involved in the final step of cortisol synthesis (Liddle, Estep, Kendall, Williams and Townes, 1959). The resultant fall in circulating cortisol stimulates ACTH secretion via the negative feedback mechanism which, in turn, stimulates steroid biosynthesis and the release of 11-deoxycortisol (the main precursor of cortisol) into the circulation. The test is based on the fact that 11-deoxycortisol, unlike cortisol, does not suppress ACTH secretion while its metabolites are determined by the commonly employed urinary 17-oxogenic steroid assay.

Urinary 17-oxogenic steroid levels are determined for complete 24 hr collections on four consecutive days. The first two serve as control periods and on day 3 the subject is given 750 mg of Metyrapone by mouth at 4-hourly intervals for six doses. An increment above basal excretion of at least 36µmol/ 24 hr on day 3 or day 4 provides the essential criterion of normality. It is important to confirm a fall in plasma cortisol and fluorimetric cortisol measurements are made at 0, 1, 2, 3, 4 and 24 hr. This test is of value in helping to determine the aetiology in patients with proven Cushing's syndrome. Thus, a greatly enhanced response is observed in those with pituitary-dependent Cushing's disease, urinary levels rising to greater than twice basal levels on the day of or the day after the administration of metyrapone reflecting the hyperplastic adrenal cortex. No response occurs in patients with adrenocortical tumours. Patients with ectopic ACTH secretion usually show no rise although exceptions are well recorded. Some patients report epigastric discomfort whilst taking metyrapone so each dose should be taken with food. Since the patient is rendered adrenocortically insufficient during this test it should only be performed with the patient in bed under close supervision.

6. ACTH Stimulation Tests

These tests are of value in the investigation both of hyper- and hypofunction and assess the reserve capacity of the adrenal cortex directly. Until recently they involved the administration of ACTH (usually of porcine origin) and the determination of the urinary steroid responses. The preparations available occasionally evoked allergic reactions while the collection of the total 24 hr urine saves is notoriously difficult. Thus most tests today employ Synacthen (since it is a pure substance and dosage can be calculated accurately by weight) and are based on the plasma cortisol response.

(a) Synacthen screening test

The procedure can be performed on out-patients and involves only the collection of a blood sample followed by a single intravenous (or intramuscular) injection of 250 µg Synacthen and the taking of a second blood sample exactly 30 min later. In normal subjects the 30 min level is at least 550 nmol/l with an increment above the basal value of at least 200 nmol/l. This simple procedure is normally used ohly for screening purposes and an abnormal result requires confirmation by a more prolonged Synacthen stimulation test.

(b) Two or five hour Synacthen test

Blood samples are taken before and at hourly intervals for either 2 or 5 hr following a single intramuscular injection of 1 mg Synacthen depot (a long acting form of Synacthen in which the peptide is absorbed onto a zinc phosphate complex). In normal subjects plasma cortisol levels more than double in the first hour and then rise more slowly during the remainder of the test.

(c) Three-day Synacthen test

This is used only to differentiate between primary and secondary adrenocortical insufficiency. A 30 min Synacthen test is performed at 09.00 hr on the first day. The subject then receives, once daily, an intramuscular injection of Synacthen depot (1 mg) and a second short Synacthen test is performed at 09.00 hr on day 4. No response is found in patients with primary andrenocortical insufficiency whereas those with the secondary form show a marked improvement in their second test (James and Landon, 1968).

K. CUSHING'S SYNDROME

The commonest cause of Cushing's syndrome is iatrogenic i.e. due to the exogenous administration of corticosteroids or ACTH to patients with disease such as rheumatoid arthritis and asthma. This will not be discussed further.

Although Cushing's syndrome is a rare disorder, nonetheless the investigation, management and treatment still represents a major challenge for both the clinical endocrinologist and chemical pathologist. It seems fair to state that every patient with Cushing's syndrome is unique and that the biochemistry and clinical features of any two patients never seem identical. The investigation of each patient is directed towards ascertaining the underlying aetiology. The two ACTH-dependent causes are pituitary-dependent bilateral adrenal hyperplasia (Cushing's disease) and the ectopic ACTH syndrome and ACTH-independent causes, adrenal adenoma and carcinoma.

When making the diagnosis and determining the aetiology of Cushing's syndrome all the clinical features and the results of a series of basal measurements and of dynamic test procedures must be considered together. Suggested protocol for the investigation of a patient with a provisional diagnosis of Cushing's syndrome is as follows:

(i) making the diagnosis: (clinical assessment, circadian rhythm of plasma cortisol, measurement of urinary steroid secretion (especially free cortisol), overnight or low dose (0·5 mg 6 hourly for 48 hr) dexamethasone suppression test;

(ii) making the differential diagnosis: (clinical assessment, ACTH measurement, high dose dexamethasone suppression test, and metyrapone test).

Plasma cortisol levels are usually raised or lie within the normal range but with loss of diurnal rhythm. Characteristically both plasma and urinary cortisol levels fail to suppress on dexamethasone (0·5 mg 6 hourly for 48 hr) and marked suppression is good evidence against the diagnosis. Patients with active Cushing's syndrome lose their ability to respond to stress so that no response is observed during the production of insulin-induced hypoglycaemia with a rise in circulating ACTH and hence cortisol secretion. In this instance, measurement of plasma ACTH is not required since cortisol measurements alone will suffice.

Two diagnostic pitfalls should be mentioned: firstly, patients with primary psychiatric disease, especially endogenous depression, have both raised plasma and urinary cortisol levels, loss of diurnal rhythm of plasma cortisol and show resistance to suppression by dexamethasone (Butler and Besser, 1968) although responsiveness to insulin hypoglycaemia is maintained. Patients who excessively abuse alcohol also develop many of the physical and biochemical characteristics of Cushing's syndrome, sometimes with very high circulating corticosteroid levels and again with loss of diurnal rhythm. This disorder has been called alcoholic pseudo-Cushing's syndrome (Smals, Kloppenborg, Njo, Knoben and Ruland, 1976; Rees, Besser, Jeffcoate, Goldie and Marks, 1977) and its increasing recognition has led to the inclusion of a blood ethanol measurement in our protocol for the investigation of a suspected case of Cushing's syndrome.

1. Cushing's Disease; Nelson's Syndrome

The underlying aetiology of pituitary-dependent Cushing's disease remains unknown. It is probable that it represents a group of disorders some caused by primary hypothalamic and some by primary pituitary disease which may help to explain the diverse nature of the different forms of treatment which have been advocated. Radiological evidence for the presence of a pituitary tumour is rarely seen, and in a recent review radiological abnormalities were not observed in 66 of 86 patients with Cushing's disease (MacErlean and Doyle, 1976). However, pathological and histological evidence of microadenoma formation is reported in 64–86% of such patients (Cushing, 1932; Doniach, 1977; Tyrrell, Brooks, Fitzgerald, Cofoid, Forsham and Wilson, 1978).

In patients with Cushing's disease ACTH levels are suppressible with higher doses of exogenous corticosteroids and most patients will show a 50% reduction of basal urinary 17-oxogenic (17-OGS) steroids following dexamethasone 2 mg 6 hourly for 48 hr. In contrast a patient with an underlying adrenal adenoma or carcinoma or with the ectopic ACTH syndrome usually fails to suppress on 8 mg dexamethasone/day although well-documented exceptions exist. A further demonstration that feedback remains intact in patients with Cushing's disease is provided by the observation that urinary 17-OGS show an excessive increase after the administration of metyrapone which causes a rise in the circulating ACTH level which stimulates large, hyperactive adrenal glands causing excessive secretion of cortisol precursors. ACTH is always detected in the circulation of patients with Cushing's disease and either lie within the normal range (30–80 pg/ml) or are elevated. However, it is unusual to see ACTH levels above 300 pg/ml although considerable fluctuations are the rule, and serial sampling for ACTH measurements with blood taken through an indwelling cannula (every 15 min for 4 hr) will reveal the extent of this periodicity. In most patients with Cushing's disease a good correlation of immunoreactive ACTH with bioactive ACTH is observed (Ratter, Hogan, Lowry, Edwards and Rees, 1977).

Different clinicians will recommend particular treatments for patients with Cushing's disease. Thus, bilateral adrenalectomy, yttrium 90 (^{90}Y) pituitary implantation, external pituitary irradiation with or without medical adrenalectomy, transphenoidal adenomectomy or hypophysectomy, cyproheptadine and bromocriptine all have their protagonists. The very diversity of treatments speaks to the unsatisfactory nature of any one particular approach as well as to a fundamental lack of understanding of the underlying cause of the excessive ACTH secretion. In some patients cure can be demonstrated by resolution of the clinical and biochemical features of Cushing's syndrome and return of circadian rhythmicity of ACTH secretion.

Nelson's syndrome is characterised by radiological evidence of the presence of a pituitary tumour and skin pigmentation in a patient after bilateral adrenalectomy for Cushing's disease (Nelson, Sprunt and Morris, 1966). Although estimates vary on the number of patients who will develop such a complication it should be avoided (see below) at all costs since some tumours may be aggressive and invasive and difficult to treat effectively. Circulating immunoreactive ACTH levels are high (usually > 500 pg/ml) and dissociation between immunoreactive and bioactive ACTH is observed although the reasons for this are unclear since in a dissociating chromatographic system the majority of circulating ACTH appears to resemble α_h^{1-39} ACTH (Ratter et al., 1977, 1979). ACTH levels will respond to insulin-induced hypoglycaemia with a further rise and are readily suppressible with exogenous corticosteroids, although on normal replacement regimes (30 mg cortisol daily and 0·1 mg fludrocortisone alternate days or daily) escape occurs so that ACTH levels remain high for most of the day. If pituitary irradiation is given immediately after adrenalectomy, Nelson's syndrome does not occur (Orth and Liddle, 1971).

2. Ectopic ACTH Syndrome

The secretion of ACTH by non-endocrine tumours (the ectopic ACTH syndrome; Liddle, Nicholson, Island, Orth, Abe and Lowder, 1969) is probably a more common cause of Cushing's syndrome than previously recognised (Rees and Ratcliffe, 1974; Rees, 1975, 1977c; Rees, Bloomfield, Gilkes, Jeffcoate and Besser, 1977). Although ectopic ACTH appears biochemically and biologically to be similar to pituitary ACTH (Liddle et al., 1969; Lowry, Rees, Tomlin, Gillies and Landon, 1976) the full amino acid sequence of ectopic ACTH is not known, and it seems clear that both the larger molecular weight precursor forms of ACTH/LPH as well as ACTH and LPH-related fragments may also be synthesised and sometimes secreted. In this regard it seems possible that the production of such substances could account for some of the unusual clinical and biochemical features observed in patients with ectopic ACTH secretion although this remains speculative. For example, the almost invariable presence of hypokalaemia in such patients has always been explained as a manifestation of the greater severity of the hypercortisolaemia or to the excessive secretion of deoxycorticosterone (Scham-belan, Slaton and Biglieri, 1971).

Bloomfield (1975) studied a large number of tumours associated with ectopic ACTH production using a combination of gel chromatography with a variety of radioimmunoassays for ACTH and LPH and related fragments and have demonstrated that many tumours contain substantial amounts of CLIP and α-MSH-related peptides resembling those previously described (Orth, Nicholson, Mitchell, Island and Liddle, 1973). However, whether any or all of these peptides are secreted into the blood is still unknown. As discussed earlier Yalow and Berson (1971) first described the presence of big ACTH in both blood and tumour tissues from patients with ectopic ACTH secretion. More recent studies (Himsworth, Bloomfield, Coombes, Ellison, Gilkes, Lowry, Setchell, Slavin and Rees, 1977; Ratter, Lowry and Rees, 1979) suggest that some of these precursors do circulate.

When the ectopic ACTH syndrome is associated with an oat cell carcinoma of the lung. ACTH levels are usually very high and the rapid progression of severe Cushing's syndrome results in the early demise of the patient. In contrast, an increasing awareness of the possibility of an underlying occult neoplasm (often benign) as a cause of Cushing's syndrome has resulted in attempts at anatomical localisation by the use of catheterisation studies with selective venous sampling for ACTH and LPH measurements (Schteingart,

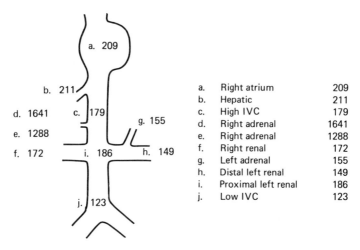

a.	Right atrium	209
b.	Hepatic	211
c.	High IVC	179
d.	Right adrenal	1641
e.	Right adrenal	1288
f.	Right renal	172
g.	Left adrenal	155
h.	Distal left renal	149
i.	Proximal left renal	186
j.	Low IVC	123

Fig. 4. Selective venous catheterisation of patient WH with the ectopic ACTH syndrome. Immunoreactive ACTH measurements in pg/ml at the places indicated. High spots were recorded when the catheter was in the right adrenal vein. Subsequently a benign right adrenal phaeochromocytoma was removed which did not secrete catecholamines. (By permission of the ed., *Adv. Med.*)

Conn, Orth, Harrison, Fox and Bookstein, 1972; Rees, Bloomfield, Gilkes, Jeffcoate and Besser, 1977; Rees, Tomlin, Ratter, Jeffcoate and Nichol, 1978). (Fig. 4). Thus, thymic carcinoid tumours, adrenal phaeochromocytomas and pancreatic islet cell tumours have all been localised and successfully resected by the use of this technique.

An alternative limited form of catheter study has been advocated (Corrigan, Schaaf, Whaley, Czerwinski and Earll, 1977) in which very high internal jugular vein sampling with simultaneous removal of a peripheral vein sample for ACTH measurements is undertaken. High ACTH levels in the internal jugular samples should be suggestive of a pituitary source of ACTH (Cushing's disease) whereas the converse would suggest an ectopic origin. However, caution must be exercised since the ectopic elaboration of materials by the tumour which might stimulate pituitary ACTH release (cortico-trophin-releasing factor(s) could cause diagnostic confusion (Upton and Amatruda, 1971; Suda, Demura, Demura, Wakabayshi, Ogadiri and Shizume, 1977). A similar phenomenon has recently been reported in patients with raised calcitonin levels and non-endocrine neoplasia, in which the origin of the calcitonin appears to be the thyroid gland and not the tumour itself (Silva, personal communication).

Measurement of circulating ACTH by radioimmunoassay is of value in following the response to treatment in patients with ectopic ACTH secretion. In particular the presence of a small amount of detectable ACTH not sup-pressible by dexamethasone is indicative of tumour recurrence and may be present in the absence of overt Cushing's syndrome (Rees, Bloomfield, Gilkes, Jeffcoate and Besser, 1977). Such measurement should allow the earlier detection and hence initiation of a more effective earlier treatment.

The low incidence of overt ectopic ACTH secretion in patients with oat cell carcinoma of the lung contrasts with the biochemical observations that 51% of 43 patients with proven oat cell carcinoma of the lung have raised midnight plasma cortisol levels are not suppressed at 09.00 hr after oral administration of 2 mg dexamethasone given at 11.00 hr the previous night (Gilby, Rees and Bondy, 1976). Supportive data for a higher incidence of occult ectopic ACTH secretion in patients with oat cell carcinoma of the lung has been observed in a study of patients with a variety of histological types of lung tumours, with the patients with oat cell carcinomas or bronchial carci-noids having plasma cortisol levels in excess of 280 nmol/l at midnight (Bloom-field, Holdaway, Corrin, Ratcliffe, Rees, Ellison and Rees, 1977). Gewirtz and Yalow (1974) have also shown raised plasma ACTH levels in the afternoon in 53% of patients with bronchial cancer (tumour types unspecified), and others have reported significantly higher basal plasma and urinary 17OGS in patients with non-malignant lung disease.

Thus, the true incidence of ectopic ACTH secretion is unknown and estimates will depend upon whether clinical or biochemical criteria are employed. The factors operating to obscure the true incidence are multiple. For example, in the early stages of the disease the operation of normal feedback mechanisms will tend to maintain plasma cortisol levels within the normal range and the secretion of relatively biologically inactive ACTH precursors or fragments will remain unrecognised. A study of the occurrence of different molecular forms of ACTH and related peptides in the blood of patients with lung cancer may possibly provide the clue towards detection of the elusive biological marker for lung cancer.

3. Adrenal Tumours

The diagnosis of autonomous cortisol secretion from an adrenal adenoma or carcinoma is usually made during the routine investigations of a patient with Cushing's syndrome. In this instance an ACTH determination is of immense value since an undetectable level by radioimmunoassay (< 10 pg/ml) in the presence of proven Cushing's syndrome is virtually diagnostic. When ACTH levels are measured in such patients using the highly sensitive cytochemical bioassay discussed earlier (Chayen et al., 1972; Holdaway, Rees and Landon. 1973) levels of around 80 fg/ml are recorded. The finding of an undetectable ACTH level by radioimmunoassay (vide supra) is indispensable for any clinician investigating a patient with Cushing's syndrome, since immediate attention can be directed towards lateral localisation of the tumour. However, it is advisable to have at least two ACTH measurements since the adrenals of some patients (approximately 10%) with pituitary dependent Cushing's disease undergo adenomatous change, and relative autonomy of such adenomata may suppress ACTH to low or intermittently undetectable levels. Conventional clinical assessment and the use of intravenous pyelography, adrenal isotope scanning, computerised axial tomography (EMI scanning) and adrenal venous sampling for cortisol and other corticosteroids are all employed for tumour lateralisation. Approximately 10% of tumours are bilateral and the size of the tumour is the best guide to its malignancy (Neville and Symington, 1967).

L. ADRENOCORTICAL FAILURE

Primary failure of the adrenal cortex is most commonly caused by destruction of the adrenal glands, due either to an autoimmune process, tuberculosis or more rarely destruction by metastatic carcinoma. Primary adrenal failure may also be due to inborn errors of the adrenal enzyme involved in cortisol biosynthesis (CAH) or due more rarely to childhood diseases such as Addison–Schilder's disease. Secondary adrenocortical failure results from hypothalamic or pituitary failure causing impaired ACTH secretion or can be a direct result of ACTH suppression caused by exogenous administration of glucocorticosteroids.

It is essential to make this differentiation between primary and secondary adrenocortical failure for two reasons. Firstly patients with primary adrenocortical failure (Addison's disease) usually have impaired secretion of all the adrenal steroids, including aldosterone, so that it is essential to give a mineralocorticoid (such as 9α-fluorocortisol) as well as a corticosteroid for replacement purposes. In contrast, circulating aldosterone levels are not significantly decreased in patients with secondary adrenocortical insufficiency because production of this steroid is controlled predominantly by the renin–angiotensin system (and not ACTH). Secondly, unlike patients with primary adrenocortical insufficiency, those with the secondary form may be deficient in other hormones and may require replacement hormones such as thyroxine.

Clinical evaluation and basal urinary and plasma steroid measurements as well as assessment of their response to exogenously administered ACTH usually result in a rapid diagnosis. A protocol for the investigation of any patient with suspected adrenocortical insufficiency is shown in Table 3. In difficult circumstances a single ACTH measurement will distinguish primary from secondary adrenocortical failure since levels are high if the disease is primary and low or undetectable in the secondary group (Besser, Cullen, Irvine, Ratcliffe and Landon, 1971; Rees, 1977a). However, ACTH measurements are complex and expensive and are usually unnecessary since the long and short Synacthen tests alone should suffice. In this regard, ACTH levels have been raised in two patients with possibly compensated primary adrenocortical failure, when both basal and stimulated plasma corticosteroids lay within normal limits (Edwards, 1977).

Determination of ACTH levels in blood may be of value in patients with Addison's disease or CAH in assessing the response to a given replacement dose of glucocorticoid. The best biochemical assessment of any patient on cortisol replacement (usual maintenance dose 30 mg daily) involves the serial determination of plasma cortisol levels throughout the day to obtain a cortisol profile with measurements of immunoreactive ACTH, particularly before the morning dose of cortisol. This latter dose should be given before the patient gets out of bed since rising results in the biggest surge of ACTH. Such information concerning cortisol/ACTH levels throughout the day in any individual patient with Addison's disease or CAH will allow finer adjustments of cortisol replacement to be made and usually results in adequate control and abolition of undesirable surges of ACTH. Undoubtedly, failure to maintain adequate circulating cortisol levels throughout the day is most often observed in patients treated with cortisone acetate when both inadequate

Table 3

Suggested protocol for the investigation of patients with suspected adrenocortical insufficiency.

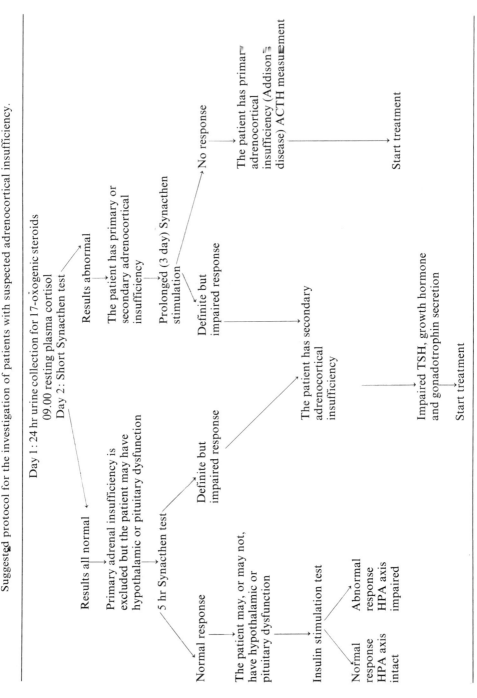

Day 1 : 24 hr urine collection for 17-oxogenic steroids
09.00 resting plasma cortisol
Day 2: Short Synacthen test

Results all normal

Primary adrenal insufficiency is
excluded but the patient may have
hypothalamic or pituitary dysfunction

5 hr Synacthen test

Normal response

The patient may, or may not,
have hypothalamic or
pituitary dysfunction

Insulin stimulation test

Normal
response
HPA axis
intact

Abnormal
response
HPA axis
impaired

Definite but
impaired response

The patient has secondary
adrenocortical
insufficiency

Impaired TSH, growth hormone
and gonadotrophin secretion

Start treatment

Results abnormal

The patient has primary or
secondary adrenocortical
insufficiency

Prolonged (3 day) Synacthen
stimulation

Definite but
impaired response

No response

The patient has primary
adrenocortical
insufficiency (Addison's
disease) ACTH measurement

Start treatment

absorption and/or hepatic conversion to cortisol may result in inadequate circulating cortisol levels. This may cause chronic ill-health, skin pigmention and more rarely enlargment of the pituitary gland with development of radiological evidence of a pituitary tumour/hyperplasia with both high circulating ACTH and prolactin (Himsworth, Slavin and Rees, 1978); the latter being reversible by adequate replacement therapy with cortisol alone.

Occasionally however, it proves very difficult to abolish undesirable surges of ACTH secretion and the use of reversed circadian administration of a glucocorticoid should be tried (for example prednisolone before rising 2·5 mg and 5 mg at 06.00 hr or occasionally dexamethasone is required. The use of the latter has sometimes been required for treating children with CAH when a fine balance between controlling the sometimes severe clinical and biochemical problems resulting from inadequate ACTH suppression (virilisation, saltwasting, etc.) must be weighed against overtreatment which may suppress not only ACTH but also growth hormone secretion and result in stunting of growth. However, there is also good evidence that dexamethasone may have an accumulative effect, providing further problems for the paediatrician. It is therefore helpful to the clinician caring for any child with CAH to have access to frequent ACTH determinations although in practice, because of the complexity of most ACTH radioimmunoassays, it proves difficult to provide as much data as might seem desirable.

1. Congenital Adrenal Hyperplasia

Reports on the incidence of CAH vary greatly throughout the world and suggest that it may be much higher than previously recognised (Mauthe, Laspe and Knorr, 1977). CAH in male infants may go undiagnosed since virilisation at birth will not be observed and the infant may appear to be completely normal. It has recently been suggested that undiagnosed CAH, especially where adrenal enzyme defects may be only partial, could be a cause of unexplained death in early infancy, especially in male infants. Attempts at screening for CAH, especially in at risk infants born to families with a history of CAH could be based either on the measurement of 17-α-hydroxyprogesterone in cord blood (Hughes, Williams and Birch, 1977) in dried blood obtained from heel-prick samples (Pang, Hotchkiss, Drash, Levine and New, 1977), in saliva (Walker and Fahmy, 1978) or alternatively the measurement of ACTH by cytochemical bioassay in heel-prick samples (Holdaway et al., 1973). Experience with screening for congenital hypothyroidism by measurement of TSH in dried blood spots has already been successfully instituted in many countries. TSH is quite stable in whole blood adsorbed to filter paper and the possibility exists that ACTH is similar in this respect cannot be discounted.

2. The Steroid-treated Patient

Treatment with natural or synthetic corticosteroids, such as cortisol, prednisolone, triamcinolone or betamethasone, is by far the most common cause
of secondary adrenocortical insufficiency and, as such, merits its own section.
Suppression of the HPA axis, with resultant adrenal atrophy, is an almost
invariable consequence of their administration (whether given orally,
parenterally or topically), the degree being related to steroid dose and length
of treatment. A variable time elapses after cessation of such therapy before
the functional integrity of the HPA axis is restored and the adrenal atrophy
is corrected.

The most common clinical situations in which assessment of pituitary–
adrenal function may be required is if such patients require surgery; encounter
some other stressful situation; present with signs and symptoms suggestive of
an acute adrenal crisis; or if the physician wishes to determine that adequate
function has been restored after termination of treatment. The most valuable
procedures for these purposes are the determination of basal circulating
cortisol levels and their responses to Synacthen (to assess the function of the
adrenal) and to insulin-induced hypoglycaemia (to assess stress responsiveness) (Plumpton and Besser, 1969).

(a) Pituitary–adrenal function during and following steroid withdrawal

Physicians need not anticipate problems on discontinuing corticosteroid
therapy since the occurrence of severe signs and symptoms is extremely rare,
with most reported cases being insufficiently documented to discount other
disorders which produce a similar clinical picture. Thus tests are seldom
necessary, especially if steroids are withdrawn slowly both to avoid an acute
exacerbation of the disorder for which they were given and to allow sufficient
time for recovery of the HPA axis. Under no circumstances should ACTH be
added to the treatment regime at this time since, while it will rapidly reverse
the adrenal atrophy, it further impairs hypothalamic and/or pituitary
function.

(b) The steroid-treated patient requiring surgery

A second problem is the steroid treated subject who requires surgery or who
is subjected to other stressful situations such as infection or a fracture. There
is now adequate information available to set out certain guidelines. Within
three months of stopping corticosteroids, HPA function is usually fully
recovered and there is no need to perform any investigations. In patients
receiving corticosteroids or those who are within three months of their dis-

continuation, it is wise to determine the plasma cortisol response to insulin-induced hypoglycaemia. If normal, surgery can be undertaken without steroid cover. If impaired, a satisfactory regime is to give 100 mg of cortisol by intramuscular injection at the same time as the premedication. This is the only cover required for simple procedures such as endoscopy, while further 100 mg injections 6 hourly for 24 hr are sufficient for minor surgery and their continuation for 72 hr will cover major operations such as gastrectomy or hip replacement.

M. PATHOPHYSIOLOGY OF β-LPH/ENDORPHIN SECRETION

Circulating levels of LPH mirror ACTH levels in patients with Cushing's disease, Nelson's syndrome, the ectopic ACTH syndrome and Addison's disease, and are undetectable in patients with hypopituitarism and Cushing's syndrome due to autonomous adrenal cortisol production (Abe *et al.*, 1967; 1969; Gilkes *et al.*, 1975a; Tanaka, Nicholson and Orth, 1977; Jeffcoate *et al.*, 1978; Tanaka *et al.*, 1978; Mullen *et al.*, 1979). However, the overlap between levels of ACTH observed in patients with pituitary-dependent Cushing's disease and the normal ACTH range is not observed, LPH levels always being elevated possibly allowing clearer differentiation between normals and those with Cushing's disease (Jeffcoate, Tomlin, McLoughlin, Rees and Besser, 1979).

For the technical reasons discussed, virtually no data exist regarding the presence of β-endorphin in human blood although using two antisera directed at different parts of the LPH molecule (an N-terminal antiserum measuring β_h- and γ-LPH and a C-terminal antiserum measuring β_h-LPH and β_h-endorphin) Jeffcoate, Rees, McLoughlin, Ratter, Hope, Lowry and Besser (1978) failed to find evidence for β-endorphin in blood although immunoassay and chromatographic evidence for β_h-endorphin in human CSF was obtained even in patients with panhypopituitarism and undetectable circulating ACTH and LPH in blood. In a similar study, Liotta, Suda and Krieger (1978) failed to identify immunoreactive β-endorphin in human pituitary tissue or blood obtained from normal subjects during insulin hypoglycaemia and following Metyrapone administration.

However, until careful chromatographic characterisation of LPH-like peptides in blood has been accomplished, both positive and negative data based solely on the use of radioimmunoassay must be viewed with great caution.

REFERENCES

Abe, K., Nicholson, W. E., Liddle, G. W., Island, D. P. and Orth, D. N. (1967). *J. clin. Invest.* **46**, 1609.

Abe, K., Nicholson, W. E., Liddle, G. W., Orth, D. N. and Island, D. P. (1969). *J. clin. Invest.* **48**, 1580.

Alaghband-Zadeh, J., Daly, J. R., Bitensky, L. and Chayen, J. (1974). *Clin. Endocr.* **3**, 319.

Astwood, G. B., Raben, M. S., Payne, R. W. and Grady, A. B. (1951). *J. Am. chem. Soc.* **73**, 2969.

Bachelot, I. G., Wolfsen, A. R. and Odell, W. D. (1976). Abst. 58th Ann. Meet. Am. Endocr. Soc., p. 120.

Bangham, D. R., Mussett, M. V. and Stack-Dunne, M. P. (1962). *Bull. W. H. Org.* **27**, 395.

Bell, P. H. (1954). *J. Am. chem. Soc.* **76**, 5565

Beloff-Chain, A., Edwardson, J. A. and Hawthorn, J. (1976). *J. Endocr.* **73**, 288.

Bennet, H. P. J., Hudson, A. M., McMartin, C. and Purdon, G. E. (1977). *Biochem. J.* **168**, 9.

Berson, S. A. and Yalow, R. S. (1968). *J. clin. Invest.* **47**, 2725.

Besser, G. M. and Landon, J. (1968). *Br. med. J.* **iv**, 552.

Besser, G. M. and Edwards, C. R. W. (1972). *Clin. Endocr. Metab.* **1**, 451.

Besser, G. M., Cullen, D. R., Irvine, W. J., Ratcliffe, J. G. and Landon, J. (1971). *Br. med. J.* **i**, 374.

Besser, G. M., Orth, D. N., Nicholson, W. E., Byyny, R. L., Abe, K. and Woodham, J. P. (1971). *J. clin. Endocr. Metab.* **32**, 595.

Birk, Y. and Li, C. H. (1964). *J. biol. Chem.* **239**, 1048.

Bloomfield, G. A. (1975). Ph.D. thesis, London University.

Bloomfield, G. A., Scott, A. P., Lowry, P. J., Gilkes, J. J. H. and Rees, L. H. (1974). *Nature, Lond.* **252**, 492.

Bloomfield, G. A., Holdaway, I. M., Corrin, B., Ratcliffe, J. G., Rees, G. M., Ellison, M. and Rees, L. H. (1977). *Clin. Endocr.* **6**, 95.

Bradbury, A. F., Smyth, D. G. and Snell, C. R. (1976). *Biochem. biophys. Res. Commun.* **69**, 950.

Bradbury, A. F., Smyth, D. G., Snell, C. R., Birdsall, N. J. M. and Hulme, E. C. (1976). *Nature, Lond.* **252**, 492.

Br. med. J. (1978). Leading Article, **2**, 155.

Burgus, R. and Guillemin, R. (1970). *Ann. Rev. Biochem.* **39**, 499.

Butler, P. W. P. and Besser, G. M. (1968). *Lancet*, **i**, 1234.

Challis, J. R. G. and Torosis, J. D. (1977). *Nature, Lond.* **269**, 818.

Chayen, J. and Bitensky, L. (1968). *In* "The Biological Basis of Medicine" (E. E. Bittar and N. Bittar, eds), pp. 337, Academic Press, London and New York.

Chayen, J., Loveridge, N. and Daly, J. R. (1971). *Clin. Sci.* **41**, 2P.

Chayen, J., Loveridge, N. and Daly, J. R. (1972). *Clin. Endocr.* **1**, 219.

Chayen, J., Daly, J. R., Loveridge, N. and Bitensky, L. (1976). *Rec. Prog. Horm. Res.* **32**, 33.

Cheung, A. L. and Goldstein, A. (1976). *Life Sci.* **19**, 1005.

Chrétien, M. and Li, C. H. (1967). *Can. J. Biochem.* **45**, 1163.

Clark, D., Thody, A. J., Shuster, S. and Bowers, H. (1978). *Nature, Lond.* **273**, 163.

Cocci, D., Santagostino, A., Gil-Ad, I., Ferri, S. and Müller, E. E. (1977). *Life Sci.*

20, 2041.

Cope, C. L. (1956). *Br. med. J.* **ii**, 193.

Cope, C. L. (1966). *Bri. med. J.* **ii**, 847.

Corrigan, D. F., Schaaf, M., Whaley, R. A., Czerwinski, C. L. and Earll, J. M. (1977). *New Engl. J. Med.* **296**, 861.

Cseh, G., Graf, L. and Goth, E. (1968). *FEBS Lett.* **2**, 42.

Cushing, H. (1932. *Bull. Johns Hopkins Hosp.* **50**, 127.

Dallman, M. F. and Yates, F. E. (1969). *Ann. N. Y. Acad. Sci.* **156**, 696.

Daly, J. R., Loveridge, N., Bitensky, L. and Chayen, J. (1972). *Ann. clin. Biochem.* **9**, 81.

Daly, J. R., Fleisher, M. R., Chambers, D. J. Bitensky, L. and Chayen, J. (1974). *Clin. Endocr.* **3**, 335.

De Wied, D. (1976). Proc. 5th Int. Cong. Endocr., Vol. 7, pp. 18–24, Excerpta Medica, Amsterdam.

Doe, R. P., Vennes, J. A. and Flink, F. S. (1960). *J. clin. Endocr. Metab.* **20**, 253.

Donald, R. A. (1967). *J. Endocr.* **39**, 451.

Donald, R. A. and Toth, A. (1973). *J. clin. Endocr. Metab.* **36**, 925.

Doniach, I. (1977). *Clin. Endocr. Metab.* **6**, 21.

Donnadieu, M. and Sevaux, D. (1973). *Biomedicine,* **19**, 272.

Edwards, C. R. W. (1977). Personal communication.

Edwards, C. R. and Besser, G. M. (1974). *Clin. Endoc. Metab.* **3**, 475.

Eipper, B. A., Mains, R. E. and Guenzi, D. (1976). *J. biol. Chem.* **251**, 4115.

Ekman, H., Hokansson, B., McCaulty, J. D., Lehmann, J. and Sjorgren, B. (1961). *J. clin. Endocr. Metab.* **21**, 684.

Espiner, E. A., Beaven, D. W. and Hart, D. S. (1963). *J. Endocr.* **27**, 267.

Estivariz, F. E., Gillies, G. and Lowry, P. J. (1979). *J. Endocr.* **80**, 4p.

Felber, J. P. (1963). *Experientia,* **19**, 227.

Gewirtz, G. and Yalow, R. S. (1974). *J. clin. Invest.* **53**, 1022.

Gilby, E. D., Rees, L. H. and Bondy, P. J. (1976). Excerpta Med. Int. Cong. Ser. No. 375, pp. 132–138. Excerpta Medica, Amsterdam.

Gilkes, J. J. H. (1975). M.D. thesis, University of London.

Gilkes, J. J. H., Bloomfield, G. A., Scott, A. P., Lowry, P. J., Ratcliffe, J. G., Landon, J. and Rees, L. H. (1975a). *J. clin. Endocr. Metab.* **40**, 450.

Gilkes, J. J. H., Eady, R. A. J., Rees, L. H., Munro, D. ·D. and Moorhead, J. F. (1975b). *Br. med. J.* **i**, 656.

Gilkes, J. J. H., Rees, L. H. and Besser, G. M. (1977). *Br. med. J.* **i**, 996.

Gillies, G. E. and Lowry, P. J. (1978). *Endocrinology,* **103**, 521.

Gillies, G. E., Van Wimersma Greidanus, Tj. B. and Lowry, P. J. (1979). *Endocrinology,* **103**, 528.

Gillies, G. E. and Lowry, P. J. (1979). *Nature, Lond.* **278**, 463.

Glickman, J. A., Carson, G. D., Naftolin, F. and Challis, J. G. R. (1978). Abst. 60th Ann. Meet. Endocr. Soc., p. 347.

Greenwood, F. C., Landon, J. and Stamp, T. C. B. (1966). *J. clin. Invest.* **45**, 429.

Guillemin, R. and Rosenberg, B. (1955). *Endocrinology,* **57**, 599.

Guillemin, R., Vargo, T., Rossier, J., Minick, S., Ling, N., Rivier, C., Vale, W. and Bloom, F. (1977). *Science,* **197**, 1367.

Himsworth, R. L., Bloomfield, G. A., Coombes, R. C., Ellison, M., Gilkes, J. J. H., Lowry, P. J., Setchell, K. D. R., Slavin, G. and Rees, L. H. (1977). *Clin. Endocr.* **7**, 45.

Himsworth, R. L., Slavin, G. and Rees, L. H. (1978). *Clin. Endocr.* **9**, 131.

Hogan, P., Rees, L. H., Lowry, P. J., Ratter, S. and Snitcher, E. J. (1976). *J. Endocr.*

G

71, 63p.

Holdaway, I. M., Rees, L. H. and Landon, J. (1973). *Lancet*, **ii**, 1170.

Holdaway, I. M., Bloomfield, G. A., Ratcliffe, J. G., Hinson, K. W. F., Rees, G. M. and Rees, L. H. (1974). *In* "Endocrinology 1973" (S. Taylor, ed.), p. 309. Heinemann, London.

Hughes, J., Smith, T. W., Kosterlitz, H. W., Fothergill, L. A., Morgan, B. A. and Morris, H. R. (1975). *Nature, Lond.* **258**, 577.

Hughes, I. A., Williams, D. H. and Birch, A. D. (1977). *Lancet*, **i**, 487.

Imura, H., Sparks, L. L., Grodsky, G. M. and Forsham, P. H. (1965). *J. clin. Endocr. Metab.* **25**, 1361.

Imura, H., Sparks, L. L., Tosaka, M., Hane, S., Grodsky, G. M. and Forsham, P. H. (1967). *J. clin. Endocr. Metab.* **27**, 15.

James, V. H. T. and Landon, J. (1968). *In* "Recent Advances in Endocrinology" (V. H. T. James, ed.), p. 50. Churchill Livingstone, Edinburgh.

James, V. H. T., Landon, J. and Wynn, V. (1965). *J. Endocr.* **33**, 515.

James, V. H. T., Landon, J. and Fraser, R. (1968). *Mem. Soc. Endocr.* **17**, 141.

James, V. H. T., Landon, J., Wynn, V. and Greenwood, F. C. (1968). *J. Endocr.* **40**, 15.

Jeffcoate, W. J., Rees, L. H., Lowry, P. J. and Besser, G. M. (1978a). *J. Endocr. Metab.* **47**, 160.

Jeffcoate, W. J., Rees, L. H., Lowry, P. J. and Besser, G. M. (1978b). *J. Endocr.* **77**, 27P.

Jeffcoate, W. J., Rees, L. H., McLoughlin, L., Ratter, S. J., Hope, J., Lowry, P. J. and Besser, G. M. (1978). *Lancet*, **ii**, 119.

Jeffcoate, W. J., Tomlin, S. J., McLoughlin, L., Rees, L. H. and Besser, G. M. (1979). *J. Endocr.* **80**, 6p.

Jones, M. T., Hillhouse, E. and Burden, J. (1976). *In* "Frontiers in Neuroendocrinology" (L. Martini and W. F. Ganong, eds), Vol. 4, pp. 196–254. Raven Press, New York.

Jubiz, W. and Nolan, G. (1978). *Clin. Chem.* **24**, 826.

Karonen, S. L., Mörsky, P., Siren, M. and Seuderling, U. (1975). *Anal. Biochem.* **67**, 1.

Kendall, J. W. (1971). *In* "Frontiers in Neuroendocrinology" (W. F. Ganong, ed.), pp. 177–207. Oxford University Press, Oxford.

Kendall, J. W. and Sloop Jr., P. R. (1968). *New Eng. J. Med.* **279**, 532.

Krieger, D. T. and Luria, M. (1977). *J. clin. Endocr. Metab.* **44**, 361.

Krieger, D. T., Allen, W., Rizzo, F. and Krieger, H. P. (1971). *J. clin. Endocr.* **32**, 266.

Krieger, D. T., Liotta, A., Suda, T., Palkovits, M. and Brownstein, M. J. (1977). *Biochem. biophys. Res. Commun.* **76**, 930.

Landon, J. and Greenwood, F. C. (1968). *Lancet*, **i**, 273.

Landon, J., Wynn, V. and James, V. H. T. (1963). *J. Endocr.* **27**, 183.

Landon, J., Snitcher, E. and Rees, L. H. (1976). *Br. J. Dermat.* **94**, 61.

Lazarus, L. H., Ling, N. and Guillemin, R. (1976). *Proc. nat. Acad. Sci. USA*, **73**, 2156.

Lee, T. H., Lerner, A. B. and Buettner-Janusch, V. (1959). *J. Am. chem. Soc.* **81**, 6084.

Lee, T. H., Lerner, A. B. and Buettner-Janusch, V. (1960). *Ciba Found. Coll.* **13**, 251.

Lee, T. H., Lerner, A. B. and Buettner-Janusch, V. (1961a). *J. biol. Chem.* **236**, 2970.

Lee, T. H., Lerner, A. B. and Buettner-Janusch, V. (1961b). *J. Biol. Chem.* **236**, 1390.

Lefkowitz, R. J., Roth, J. and Pastan, I. (1970). *Science*, **170**, 633.

Lerner, A. B., Upton, G. V. and Lande, S. (1968). *In* "Pharmacology of Hormonal Polypeptides and Proteins" (N. Back, L. Martini and R. Paoletti, eds), pp. 203–212. Plenum Press, London.

Levine, J. H., Nicholson, W. E., Liddle, G. W. and Orth, D. N. (1973). *Endocrinology*,

92, 1089.

Li, C. H. (1959). *Science*, **129**, 969.

Li, C. H. (1964). *Nature, Lond.* **201**, 924.

Li, C. H. and Cheung, D. (1976). *Nature, Lond.* **260**, 622.

Li, C. H., Geschwind, I. I., Dixon, J. S., Levy, A. L. and Harris, J. I. (1965). *J. Biol. Chem.* **213**, 171.

Li, C. H., Barnafi, L., Chrétien, M. and Chung, D. (1965). *Nature, Lond.* **208**, 1093.

Liddle, G. W. (1960). *J. clin. Endocr. Metab.* **20**, 1539.

Liddle, G. W. and Williams Jr., W. C. (1962). *In* "The Human Adrenal Cortex" (A. R. Currie, T. Symington and J. K. Grant, eds), pp. 461. Churchill Livingstone, Edinburgh.

Liddle, G. W., Estep, A. L., Kendall, J. W., Williams, W. C. and Townes, A. W. (1959). *J. clin. Endocr. Metab.* **19**, 875.

Liddle, G. W., Island, D. P. and Meador, C. K. (1962). *Rec. Prog. Horm. Res.* **18**, 125.

Liddle, G. W., Nicholson, W. E., Island, D. P., Orth, D. N., Abe, K. and Lowder, S. C. (1969). *Rec. Prog. Horm. Res.* **25**, 283.

Ling, N., Burgus, R. and Guillemin, R. (1976). *Proc. nat. Acad. Sci. USA*, **73**, 3942.

Liotta, A. S., Suda, T. and Krieger, D. T. (1978a). *Proc. nat. Acad. USA*, **75**, 2950.

Liotta, A. S., Li, C. H., Schussler, G. C. and Krieger, D. T. (1978b). *Life Sci.* **23**, 2323.

Lipscomb, H. S. and Nelson, D. H. (1962). *Endocrinology*, **71**, 13.

Lowry, P. J. and McMartin, C. (1974). *Biochem. J.* **142**, 287.

Lowry, P. J. and Scott, A. P. (1974). *Biochem. J.* **139**, 593.

Lowry, P. J., Mc Martin, C. and Peters, J. (1973). *J. Endocr.* **59**, 43.

Lowry, P. J., Hope, J. and Silman, R. E. (1976). Excerpta Med. Cong. Ser. No. 402, Proc. 5th Int. Cong. Endocr., Vol I (V. H. T. James, ed.). Excerpta Medica, Amsterdam.

Lowry, P. J., Rees, L. H., Tomlin, S., Gillies, G. and Landon, J. (1976). *J. clin. Endocr. Metab.* **43**, 831.

Lyons, W. R. (1937). *Proc. Soc. exp. Biol. Med.* **35**, 645.

McDonald, R. K., Weise, V. K. and Patrick, R. W. (1956). *Proc. Soc. exp. Biol. Med.* **93**, 348.

MacErlean, D. P. and Doyle, F. H. (1976). *Br. J. Radio*, **49**, 820.

McGuire, J., McGill, R., Leeman, S. and Goodfriend, T. (1965). *J. Clin. Invest.* **44**, 1672.

Mains, R. E. and Eipper, B. A. (1976). *J. biol. Chem.* **251**, 4115.

Mains, R. E., Eipper, B. A. and Ling, M. (1977). *Proc. nat. Acad. Sci. USA*, **74**, 3014.

Matsuyama, H., Ruhmann-Wennhold, A. and Nelson, D. H. (1971). *Endocrinology*, **88**, 692.

Mattingly, D. (1962). *J. Clin. Pathol.* **15**, 374.

Mattingly, D. and Tyler, C. (1976). *Br. med. J.* **2**, 668.

Mauthe, I., Laspe, H. and Knorr, D. (1977). *Klin. Padiat. Diag.* **189**, 172.

Mullen, P.E., Jeffcoate, W. J., Linsell, C., Howard, R. and Rees, L. H. (1979). *Clin. Endocr.* (in press).

Nakanishi, S., Inoue, A., Kita, T., Nakamura, M., Chang, A. C. Y., Cohen, S. and Numa, S. (1979). *Nature, Lond.* **278**, 423.

Nelson, D. H. and Hume, D. M. (1955). *Endocrinology*, **57**, 184.

Nelson, D. H., Sprunt, J. G. and Morris, R. B. (1966). *J. clin. Endocr. Metab.* **26**, 722.

Neville, A. M. and Symington, T. (1967). *J. Pathol. Endocr.* **93**, 19.

Ney, R. L., Shimizu, N., Nicholson, W., Island, D. and Liddle, G. W. (1963). *J. clin. Invest.* **42**, 1669.

Nicholson, W. E. and Van Loon, G. R. (1973). *J. lab. Clin. Med.* **81**, 803.

Orth, D. N. (1974). *In* "Methods of Hormone Radioimmunoassay" (B. M. Jaffe and H. R. Behrman, eds), pp. 125–159. Academic Press, London and New York.

Orth, D. N. and Liddle, G. W. (1971), *New Engl. J. Med.* **285**, 243.

Orth, D. N., Nicholson, W. E., Mitchell, W. M., Island, D. P. and Liddle, G. W. (1973). *J. clin. Invest.* **52**, 1756.

Orth, D. N., Guillemin, R., Ling, N. and Nicholson, W. E. (1978). *J. clin. Endocr. Metab.* **46**, 849.

Pang, S., Hotchkiss, J., Drash, A. L., Levine, L. S. and New, M. I. (1977). *J. clin. Endocr. Metab.* **45**, 1003.

Phifer, R. F., Orth, D. N. and Spicer, S. S. (1974). *J. clin. Endocr. Metab.* **39**, 684.

Plumpton, F. S. and Besser, G. M. (1969). *Br. J. Surg.* **3**, 215.

Plumpton, F. S., Besser, G. M. and Cole, P. V. (1969). *Anaesthesia*, **24**, 3.

Portanova, R. and Sayers, F. (1973). *Proc. Soc. exp. Biol. Med.* **143**, 661.

Ratcliffe, J. G. and Edwards, C. R. W. (1971). *In* "Radioimmunoassay Methods" (W. M. Hunter and K. R. Kirkham, eds), pp. 502–512. Churchill Livingstone, Edinburgh.

Ratter, S. J., Hogan, P., Lowry, P. J., Edwards, C. R. W. and Rees, L. H. (1977). *J. Endocr.* **75**, 30.

Ratter, S. J., Lowry, P. J. and Rees, L. H. (1979). *J. Endocr.* (in press).

Ratter, S. J., Lowry, P. J., Besser, G. M. and Rees, L. H. (1979). *J. Endocr.* (in press).

Rees, L. H. (1975). *J. Endocr.* **67**, 143.

Rees, L. H. (1976). *Curr. clin. Chem.* **3**, 384.

Rees, L. H. (1977a). *In* "Clinical Neuroendocrinology" (L. Martini and G. M. Besser, eds), pp. 401–441. Academic Press, London and New York.

Rees, L. H. (1977b). *Clin. Endocr. Metab.* **6**, 137.

Rees, L. H. (1977c). *In* "Advanced Medicine" (G. M. Besser, ed.), pp 78–98. Pitman Medical, London.

Rees, L. H. and Ratcliffe, J. G. (1974). *Clin. Endocr.* **3**, 263.

Rees, L. H. and Ratter, S. J. (1978). *Br. J. hosp. Med.* March, 229.

Rees, L. H., Cook, D., Kendall, J. W., Allen, C., Kramer, R. M., Ratcliffe, J. G. and Knight, R. A. (1971). *Endocrinology*, **89**, 259.

Rees, L. H., Ratcliffe, J. G., Besser, G. M., Kramer, R., Landon, J. and Chayen, J. (1973). *Nature New Biol.* **241**, 84.

Rees, L. H., Besser, G. M., Joffcoate, W. J., Goldie, D. J. and Marks, V. (1977). *Lancet*, **i**, 726.

Rees, L. H., Bloomfield, G. A., Gilkes, J. J. H., Jeffcoate, W. J. and Besser, G. M. (1977). *Ann. N. Y. Acad. Sci.* **297**, 603.

Rees, L. H., Gilkes, J. J. H. and Jeffcoate, W. J. (1977). *In* "Frontiers of Hormone Research" (Tj. B. van Wimersama Greidanus, ed.) Vol. 4, p. 21. S. Karger, Basel.

Rees, L. H., Tomlin, S. J., Ratter, S. J., Jeffcoate, W. J. and Nichol, W. (1978). Abst. 60th Ann. Meet. Endocr. Soc. p. 197.

Riniker, B., Sieber, P., Rittel, W. and Zuber, H. (1972). *Nature New Biol.* **235**, 114.

Rosselin, G., Assan, R., Yalow, R. S. and Berson, S. A. (1966). *Nature, Lond.* **212**, 355.

Saffran, M. and Schally, A. V. (1955). *Can. J. Biochem. Physiol.* **33**, 408.

Saffran, M. and Schally, A. V. (1955). *Endocrinology*, **56**, 523.

Salacinski, P., Hope, J., McClean, C., Clement-Jones, V., Sykes, J., Price, J. and Lowry, P. J. (1979). *J. Endocr.* (in press).

Sayers, G. (1967). *In* "Hormones in Blood" (C. H. Gray and A. L. Bacharach, eds), p. 169. Academic Press, London and New York.

Sayers, G. and Giordano, N. D. (1973). In "Methods in Investigative and Diagnostic Endocrinology" (S. A. Berson and R. S. Yalow, eds), pp. 359–366, North Holland Publishing Co., Amsterdam.

Sayers, G., Swallow, R. L. and Giordano, N. D. (1971). Endocrinology, 88, 1063.

Sayers, M. A., Sayers, G. W. and Woodbury, P. L. (1948). Endocrinology, 42, 379.

Schally, A. V. and Bowers, C. Y. (1964). Metabolism, 13, 1190.

Schambelan, M., Slaton, P. E. and Biglieri, E. G. (1971). Am. J. Med. 51, 299.

Schteingart, D. E., Conn, J. W., Orth, D. N., Harrison, T. S., Fox, F. E. and Bookstein, J. J. (1972). J. clin. Endocr. Metab. 34, 676.

Scott, A. P. and Lowry, P. J. (1974). Biochem. J. 139, 593.

Scott, A. P., Ratcliffe, J. G., Rees, L. H., Landon, J., Bennett, H. P. J., Lowry, P. J. and McMartin, C. (1973). Nature New Biol. 224, 65.

Segal, B. M. and Christy, N. P. (1968). J. clin. Endocr. Metab. 28, 1465.

Shepherd, R. G., Howard, K. S., Bell, P. H., Cacciola, A. R., Child, R. G., Davies, M. C., English, J. P., Finn, B. M., Meisenhelder, J. H., Moyer, A. W. and Van der Sheer, J. (1956). J. Am. chem. Soc. 78, 5051.

Shimizu, N. and Yashida, H. (1977). Endocr. Jap. 23, 479.

Silman, R. E., Chard, T., Lowry, P. J., Smith, I. and Young, I. M. (1976). Nature, Lond. 260, 716.

Silman, R. E., Chard, T., Lowry, P. J., Smith, I. and Young, I. M. (1977). In "Frontiers of Hormone Research. Melanocyte Stimulating Hormone: Control, Chemistry and Effects" (Tj. B. van Wimersma Greidanus, ed.), pp. 179–187. S. Karger, Basel.

Silman, R. E., Holland, D., Chard, T., Lowry, P. J., Hope, J., Robinson, J. S. and Thorburn, G. D. (1978). Nature, Lond. 276, 526.

Smals, A. G., Kloppenborg, P. W., Njo, K. T., Knoben, J. M. and Ruland, C. M. (1976). Br. med. J. 2, 1298.

Stouffer, J. E. and Lipscomb, H. S. (1963). Endocrinology, 72, 91.

Suda, T., Demura, H., Demura, R., Wakabayashi, K. N., Odagiri, E. and Shizume, K. (1977). J. clin. Endocr. Metab. 44, 440.

Swallow, R. L. and Sayers, G. (1969). Proc. Soc. exp. Biol. Med. 131, 1.

Sydnor, K. L., Sayers, G., Brown, H. and Tyler, F. H. (1953). J. clin. Endocr. Metab. 13, 891.

Tanaka, K., Mount, C. D. and Orth, D. N. (1976). Abst. 58th Ann. Meet. Am. Endocr. Soc., p. 121.

Tanaka, K., Nicholson, W. E. and Orth, D. N. (1977). Front. Horm. Res. 4, 208.

Tanaka, K., Nicholson, W. E. and Orth, D. N. (1978a). J. clin. Endocr. Metab. 46, 883.

Tanaka, K., Nicholson, W. E. and Orth, D. N. (1978b). J. clin. Invest. 62, 94.

Thody, A. J. and Plummer, N. A. (1973). J. Endocr. 58, 263.

Tyrell, J. B., Brooks, R. M., Fitzgerald, P. A., Cofoid, P. B., Forsham, P. H. and Wilson, C. B. (1978), New Engl. J. Med. 298, 753.

Upton, G. V. and Amatruda, T. T. (1971), New Engl. J. Med. 285, 419.

Vaitukaitis, J. L., Robbins, J. B., Nieschlag, E. and Ross, G. T. (1971). J. clin. Endocr. Metab. 33, 988.

Vernikos-Danellis, J. (1965). Vit. Horm. 23, 97.

Vernikos-Danellis, J., Anderson, E. and Trigg, L. (1966). Endocrinology, 79, 624.

Visser, M. and Swaab, D. F. (1977). In "Frontiers of Hormone Research" (Tj. B. van Wimersma Greidanus, ed.), pp. 42–45, S. Karger, Basel.

Walker, R. F. and Fahmy, D. R. (1978). J. Endocr. 79, 64P.

Wen, H. L. and Cheung, S. Y. C. (1973). Asian J. Med. 9, 138.

Wen, H. L. and Teo, S. W. (1975). *Mod. Med. Asia*, **11**, 23.

White, W. F. (1953). *J. Am. Chem. Soc.* **75**, 503.

White, W. F. and Pierce, W. L. (1953). *J. Am. chem. Soc.* **75**, 245.

Williams, W. C., Island, D., Oldfield, R. A. A. and Liddle, G. W. (1961). *J. clin. Endocr. Metab.* **21**, 426.

Yalow, R. S. and Berson, S. A. (1971). *Biochem. Biophys. Res. Commun.* **44**, 439.

Yalow, R. S. and Berson, S. A. (1973). *J. clin. Endocr. Metab.* **36**, 415.

Yalow, R. S., Glick, S. M., Roth, J. and Berson, S. A. (1964). *J. clin. Endocr. Metab.* **24**, 1219.

Zimmerman, E. A. (1976). *In* "Frontiers of Neuroendocrinology" (L. Martini and W. F. Ganong, ed.), Vol. 4. Raven Press, New York.

V. Corticosteroids

DIANA RIAD-FAHMY,

G. READ and I. A. HUGHES

INTRODUCTION

Steroid hormones synthesised and secreted by the adrenal cortex are essential for life, and are intimately concerned in a wide range of metabolic processes. They include the glucocorticosteroids like cortisol and cortisone which influence carbohydrate and protein metabolism (Thompson and Lippman, 1974). Aldosterone, the mineralocorticosteroid controlling electrolyte balance is considered in Ch. X. Sensitive assays for determining the major adrenal steroids have been developed and are now in widespread use for studying the mechanisms controlling adrenal secretory activity. Many of these assays are simple high-throughput procedures of clinical value in the diagnosis and treatment of adrenal dysfunction. The results of these assays can sometimes be difficult to interpret without an understanding of the factors controlling the activity of the hypothalamo–pituitary–adrenal system. A knowledge of the enzyme systems involved in adrenocorticosteroid biosynthesis and their location within adrenal cells is also helpful when attempting to extrapolate from results of *in vitro* experimentation to the *in vivo* situation in both man and mammals. Inhibitors of these enzyme systems have been synthesised and found to be clinically useful in the diagnosis and treatment of adrenal dysfunction. The following sections will therefore be concerned with the more fundamental aspects of adrenal steroid biochemistry; methods for determining circulating steroid concentrations and the clinical significance of the results obtained are discussed later in this chapter.

A. NOMENCLATURE OF ADRENAL STEROIDS

Although more than 40 steroids have been isolated from adrenal tissue (Briggs and Brotherton, 1970a; Wettstein, 1959) not all are secreted by the adrenal gland. Some are now known to be intermediates formed during biosynthesis, and others are metabolic degradation products. Some may even be artifacts formed after removal of the gland from the body. It is generally accepted (Pincus, 1958) that only steroids present in adrenal venous blood in higher concentrations than in the peripheral circulation, are true adrenal secretory products. The nomenclature of these adrenal steroids is based on the IUPAC convention (1970) and is rationalised by considering all steroids to derive from basic saturated parent hydrocarbons (Klyne, 1957). Pregnane is the parent hydrocarbon of the C_{21}-steroids such as cortisol, whereas the C_{19}-steroids are considered as derivatives of androstane. The formula of cortisol, with the agreed identification of the ring system and numbering of the carbon atoms is shown in Fig. 1. Cortisol differs from pregnane in having a double bond at C-4 and is therefore de-

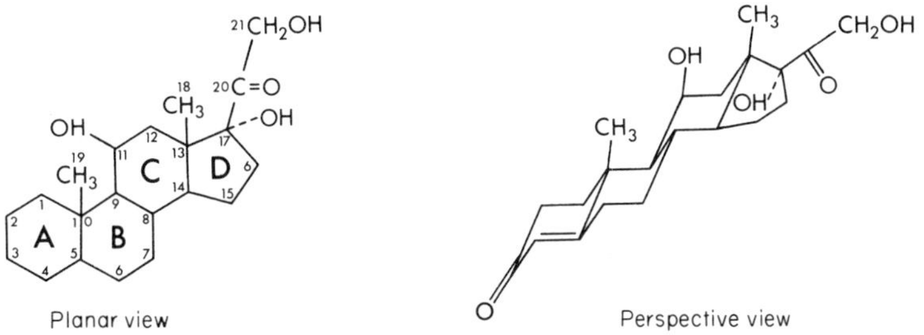

Fig. 1. Cortisol ($11\beta,17\alpha,21$-trihydroxypregn-4-ene-3,20-dione).

scribed as a pregnene derivative with various attached substituent groups; it is given the systematic name of $11\beta,17\alpha,21$-trihydroxypregn-4-ene-3,20-dione. The angular methyl groups attached to carbon atoms 10 and 13 are shown as projecting above the plane of the molecule. The orientation of the substituent hydroxyl groups is given relative to these methyl groups. The spatial arrangement of substituents when they project in the same direction as the angular methyl groups is described as *cis* or β-orientated and on the flat representation of the steroid molecule are drawn as a solid line (C—OH). If, however, the substituent groups project below the plane of the molecule they are *trans* or α-orientated and the bond is drawn as a dashed line (C———OH). The nomenclature therefore allows adequate identification of the various corticosteroids secreted by the adrenal gland.

It was Borth (1956) who proposed that the term corticosteroid should apply to those C_{21} steroids, containing three or more oxygen atoms, which are found in the adrenal gland, blood or urine. The structures of the more important corticosteroids secreted by the adrenal gland, together with their systematic and trivial names are illustrated in Fig. 2. These biologically active compounds are all Δ^4-3-ketones, since they have a keto group ($>C=O$) at C-3 and a double bond originating at C-4. All corticosteroids have a side chain at C-17 which may be that of an α-ketol or a dihydroxy acetone grouping.

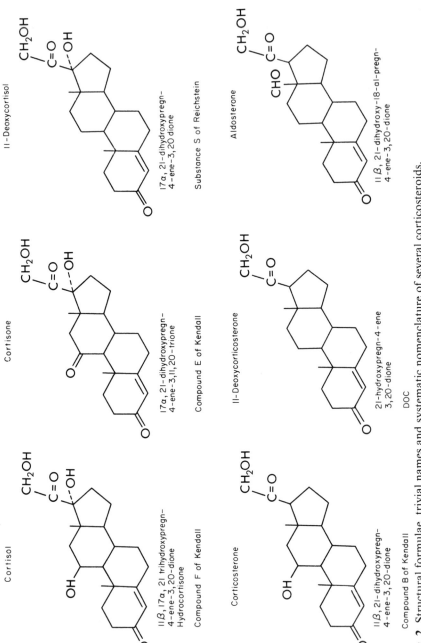

Fig. 2. Structural formulae, trivial names and systematic nomenclature of several corticosteroids.

$$\text{CH}_2\text{OH}$$
$$\text{CH}_3 \quad \text{C} = \text{O}$$
$$D$$

α-Ketol
side-chain

$$\text{CH}_2\text{OH}$$
$$\text{CH}_3 \quad \text{C} = \text{O}$$
$$\text{--OH}$$
$$D$$

Dihydroxyacetone
side-chain

Aldosterone, the most important mineralocorticosteroid, secreted by cells of the zona glomerulosa of the adrenal cortex differs from the majority of corticosteroids in having an aldehyde group at C-18. The glucocorticosteroids including cortisol and cortisone have a methyl group at C-18. Synthesis and secretion of these steroids by the zona reticularis and zona fasciculata of the adrenal cortex is largely controlled by adrenocorticotrophin (ACTH).

B. THE ADRENAL GLAND

1. Structure and Function

The lipid-rich adrenal cortex in man, illustrated in Fig. 3, is divided into three concentric zones, the zona glomerulosa, zona fasciculata and zona reticularis

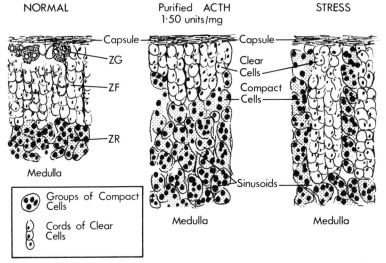

Fig. 3. Artists representation of the human adrenal gland. The changes in cell type following ACTH administration and stress are shown on the right: ZG = zona glomerulosa, ZF = zona fasciculata, ZR = zona reticularis. (After Griffiths *et al.*, 1963.)

(Arnold, 1866). The zona fasciculata constitutes most of the cortex, being composed of long regular columns of cells, rich in lipid, but containing few mitochondria and little endoplasmic reticulum. The reticular cells are arranged in alveoli separated by thin-walled prominent sinuses. The cells are lipid poor but have abundant mitochondria and endoplasmic reticulum (Symington, 1969; Malamed, 1975). A similar lipid-rich cortex is seen in the monkey, rat and rabbit; in other mammals such as the cow, sheep and hamster, the adrenal cortex contains little lipid and the zona fasciculata and zona reticularis are less well defined (Symington, 1960). The zona glomerulosa, prominent in the glands of sheep and rat, is often ill-defined in the human adrenal cortex. It may be confined to scattered islets of cells immediately next to the capsule so that sections of the human adrenal often show the zona fasciculata directly under the capsule (Symington, 1962).

Other zones have been described in various animals (Cater and Lever, 1954; Chester Jones, 1957; Howard and Migeon, 1962) and the foetal zone has also been extensively studied in previable and still-born infants and children dying in the neonatal period (Bloch et al., 1956; Ross, 1962). Just prior to birth, the foetal zone is the most prominent region in the cortex, being composed of cells closely resembling those of the zona reticularis of the adult cortex (Luse, 1967). The width of the foetal zone accounts for the disproportionately large size of the foetal adrenal gland at this period of life. After birth, however, it undergoes rapid involution and during the neonatal period the adult zone increases in size and differentiates into the classical zones (Lanman, 1953).

Early attempts to correlate structure of the adrenal gland with function were largely based on histological and histochemical studies. The cell migration theory introduced by Gottschau (1883) suggested that cells formed in the subcapsular region migrate to the zona fasciculata, elaborate their secretions and die in the zona reticularis, cells of the senescent zone being removed by the extensive vascular channels in this region of the cortex. Failure to demonstrate centripetal cell migration (Calma and Foster, 1943) together with the finding of active enzyme systems in reticular cells (Yoffey, 1955) threw doubt on this theory.

Stimulus for development of the zonation theory (Swann, 1940; Chester Jones, 1957) came with the demonstration that electrolyte imbalance results from adrenalectomy but not from hypophysectomy. The theory proposed that the zona glomerulosa, relatively independent of pituitary control, was the site of mineralocorticosteroid formation, and the glucocorticosteroids were formed by the fascicular tissue, while adrenal androgen production was restricted very largely to the zona reticularis. The demonstration of the 11β-hydroxylase activity throughout adrenal tissue led Symington and coworkers to suggest that the zona fasciculata and zona reticularis acts as a single unit, the main function being the formation of C_{21}-steroids and to a lesser extent androgens and possibly oestrogens (Grant and Griffiths, 1962; Griffiths et al., 1963). Reticular and fascicular cells were found to produce cortisol equally well but only fascicular cells responded to ACTH stimulation. The cholesterol-rich zona fasciculata may therefore be a storage zone for steroid hormone precursors to be utilised in times of stress or following ACTH stimulation (Griffiths and Glick, 1966). Morphological changes (Fig. 3) occurring after ACTH stimulation or in stressed glands obtained post-mortem support this concept (Symington et al., 1955; Symington, 1962). The change in cell type from fascicular to reticular as lipid reserves are depleted is first observed at the interface between the zona fasciculata and zona reticularis. The apparent widening of the zona reticularis is paralleled by an increased secretion of cortisol in adrenal venous blood (Grant, 1968).

2. Control of Adrenal Secretory Activity

Cortisol biosynthesis in adrenal tissue is controlled primarily by adreno-corticotrophic hormone (ACTH) which may sometimes be called corticotrophin or adrenocorticotrophin (Atcheson and Tyler, 1975; Rees and Landon, 1976). This 39 amino acid polypeptide, synthesised and stored in the anterior pituitary gland, is secreted in response to a corticotrophin releasing factor originating in the hypothalamus and transported via a portal system to the pituitary gland. In the short term, ACTH increases blood flow to the gland (Symington, 1969) and increases steroidogenesis and secretion of most adrenal steroid hormones (Hechter, 1949; Dixon et al., 1967). More prolonged exposure to ACTH depletes reserves of cholesterol in the zona fasciculata (Symington, 1969) and finally causes marked adrenal hypertrophy (Studzinski et al., 1963). In the absence of ACTH, the adrenal gland becomes atrophic and cortisol secretion is very much reduced (James and Landon, 1968).

(a) Mode of action of ACTH

Adrenal tissue responds promptly to ACTH stimulation, increased steroid levels being observed in venous blood within 5 min of administration (Haynes, 1975). Since side chain cleavage of cholesterol to form pregnenolone is generally accepted as the rate limiting reaction in adrenal steroid bio-synthesis (Stone and Hechter, 1954), theories on the mode of action of ACTH centre on factors limiting this reaction. The second messenger, cyclic 3′,5′-AMP, is thought to mediate ACTH action, for when the protein hormone is bound to specific receptors on the surface of adrenal cells, adenyl cyclase is stimulated thereby increasing the conversion of ATP to the cyclic nucleotide. The short term effect of ACTH, mediated by the action of AMP on phosphorylase or glucose-6-phosphate dehydrogenase, allows shunting of intermediary metabolites into the pentose phosphate pathway. Metabolism of intermediates via this pathway provides increased NADPH, an essential cofactor for the side chain cleaving enzyme system.

Haynes and Berthet (1957), and McKern (1966) therefore suggest that ACTH increases steroidogenesis by making additonal NADPH available to the side-chain splitting enzyme system. Koritz and Hall (1964), however, believe that the role of 3'5'-AMP is to increase permeability of the mitochondrial membrane: pregnenolone may therefore pass more readily into the cytoplasm and its inhibitory effect on side chain cleavage is thereby reduced. Studies by Ferguson (1963) and Garren et al. (1965) with known inhibitors of protein synthesis including puromycin and cycloheximide indicated that these abolish the stimulatory effect of ACTH. Thus part of the initial action of ACTH on steroid biosynthesis would seem to be controlled by mechanisms involving protein synthesis and recent studies have been directed to the effect of ACTH on RNA synthesis and nuclear transcription. In an excellent review, Haynes (1975) suggested that theories on the mode of action of ACTH were better designated as hypotheses and that no single hypothesis was completely satisfactory.

(b) Mechanisms controlling adrenal steroid secretion

Excellent reviews (Mess and Martini, 1968; Sayers and Portanova, 1975) of the mechanisms controlling adrenal secretory activity, illustrated diagrammatically in Fig. 4, indicate that both the hypothalamo–pituitary axis and neuronal impulses from the central nervous system (CNS) are involved. The long loop feedback system depends on the inhibitory action of circulating steroids at the hypothalamic level. Short loop feedback systems would also seem to be involved, since ACTH influences release of hypothalamic corticotrophin releasing factor (CRF), and cortisol itself also directly reduces the synthesis and secretion of ACTH by the pituitary gland. Furthermore, CRF activity does not appear to be restricted to the hypothalamus, since crude extracts of cerebral cortex and liver influence ACTH release in a similar manner (Egdahl, 1960), the activity of these extracts being modified by adrenal steroids (Brodish, 1973). External stimuli, for example trauma, hypoglycaemia, infection, cause a dramatic rise in circulating cortisol levels, an effect thought to be mediated by neuronal impulses from the CNS acting on the hypothalamus. Even in the absence of undue environmental disturbance, spontaneous secretory episodes occur (Hellman et al., 1970) although the purpose served by the episodic secretion remains obscure. It certainly does not appear to be directed towards maintaining steady state

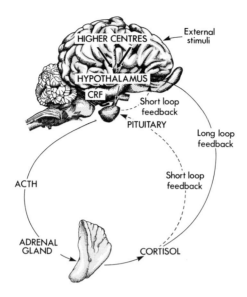

Fig. 4. Feedback systems controlling adrenal secretory activity.

cortisol levels, since a well defined temporal pattern of episodic secretion over a 24 hr period has been demonstrated (Fig. 5). This so called circadian rhythm in adrenal secretory activity falls into four well defined phases (Table 1), and results in widely fluctuating cortisol levels. A 6 hr period of minimal secretory activity, associated with the start of the sleep period, results in low circulating cortisol concentrations. Maximal activity occurs just prior to waking and cortisol levels at this time are high (Weitzman *et al.*, 1971; Gutai *et al.*, 1977).

Rhythmic variation in plasma cortisol levels appears to depend on changes in the duration and frequency of adrenal secretory episodes rather than on differences in the rate of secretion (Weitzman *et al.*, 1971). Acute alterations in waking times have no influence on the rhythm and it is unlikely to be an inborn rhythm since it may be altered to one of 12, 19 or 32 hr provided sufficient time is allowed for this new pattern to be established (Orth *et al.*, 1967). In this connection, however, it is interesting to note that isolated hamster adrenal cells in culture maintain rhythmic secretion of corticosterone for several days in the absence of ACTH (Shiotsuka *et al.*, 1974).

(c) Control of foetal adrenal growth and activity

Recent evidence (Jost, 1975) suggests that the foetal hypothalamo–pituitary system controls the later stages of foetal adrenal development and activity.

Table 1

Cortisol secretory activity analysed by descriptive phases (from Weitzman et al., 1971).

Phase	Title	Start to end of phase (hr) (0 hr is time of sleep onset)	Duration (hr)	Min of secretory activity/hr	Average total cortisol secreted phase (mg); (1 mg = 2·76 μmol)
I	Minimal secretory activity	−4 to 2	6	2	0·28
II	Preliminary nocturnal episode	3 to 5	3	16	1·70
III	Main secretory	6 to 9	4	31	6·30
IV	Intermittent waking activity	10 to −5	11	15	7·20

In the first 20 weeks of gestation foetal weight is similar in normal and anencephalic pregnancy (Benirschke, 1956). As illustrated in Fig. 6, however, adrenal weight continues to increase throughout the latter stages of gestation in the normal foetus but remains static in anencephalics. Since some anterior pituitary tissue is present in almost all human anencephalics (Angevine, 1938; Lanman, 1953) it is possible that release of hypothalamic CRF may limit endocrine activity in certain cases. Although at one time, human chorionic gonadotrophin (IICG) was thought to influence foetal adrenal development (Lanman, 1962), this is no longer generally accepted, since HCG levels are within the normal range in anencephalic pregnancy and in

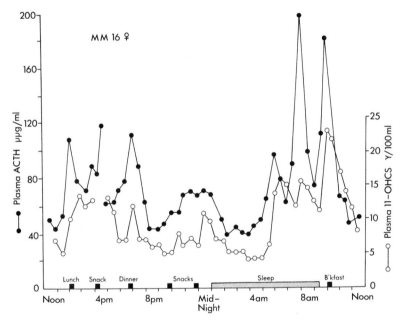

Fig. 5. Circadian periodicity of plasma 11-hydroxycorticosteroid (11-OHCS) and plasma adrenocorticotrophic hormone (ACTH) levels over a 24-hr period, as determined by half-hourly sampling. Meal times and sleep as indicated. Symbols in upper left corners of graphs refer to initials, age, and sex of subject (from Krieger *et al.*, 1971).

the latter stages of gestation HCG levels decrease whereas foetal adrenal weight increases (Frandsen and Stakeman, 1964; Jost, 1975).

Foetal hypothalamo–pituitary–adrenal activity is controlled by feedback systems that appear relatively autonomous since physiologically effective amounts of maternal ACTH do not readily cross the placental barrier (Lanman, 1962). Transport of corticosteroids across the placenta is, however, unrestricted, since mothers with Cushing's syndrome (Kreines and de Vaux,

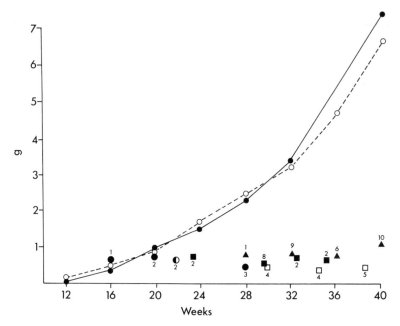

Fig. 6. Weight of adrenals in normal and anencephalic American and Japanese human foetuses. Solid line = normal American foetuses, dotted line = normal Japanese foetuses, other symbols = anencephalic foetuses (from Jost, 1975).

1971), or undergoing high dose glucocorticosteroid therapy (Simmer *et al.*, 1966), give birth to infants having atrophic adrenal glands. In these patients, the high circulating levels of maternal corticosteroids are thought to suppress the secretion of foetal ACTH (Oakey, 1970).

Studies in sheep and other ruminants by Liggins (1969) and Liggins *et al.* (1973) indicate that activity of the foetal pituitary–adrenal system may well be involved in controlling the onset of parturition; corticosteroid levels increase dramatically in the foetal circulation and premature delivery can be induced by injecting ACTH or glucocorticosteroids into the foetus. The role of cortisol in the initiation of parturition in human pregnancy remains obscure despite intensive study (Turnbull *et al.*, 1977; Chard *et al.*, 1977). It is, however, noteworthy that anencephalic pregnancies are usually prolonged (Comerford, 1965) as are those in mothers with Addison's disease (Osler, 1962).

3. Assessment of Adrenal Function

It is now generally accepted that tests of adrenal function should include those designed to investigate basal levels of adrenal activity together with dynamic procedures indicating the ability of the hypothalamo–pituitary–adrenal system to respond to stress. The commonly used tests of adrenal function, outlined in Fig. 7 are only briefly considered in this section since detailed information is readily available (James and Landon, 1976; Briggs and Brotherton, 1970b; Gold, 1977).

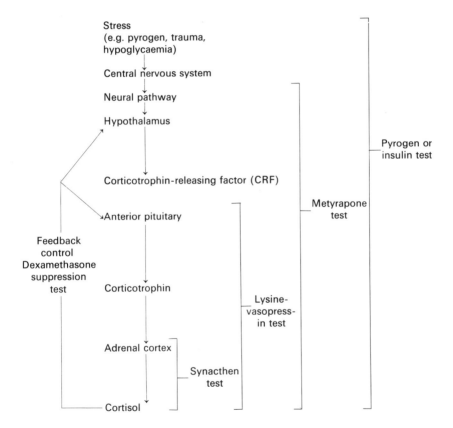

Fig. 7. Clinical tests for adrenal–pituitary–hypothalamic function (from Briggs and Brotherton, 1970b).

(a) ACTH (Synacthen) stimulation

Synacthen, a synthetic analogue (containing the biologically active N-terminal 1–24 amino acid sequence of naturally occurring ACTH) is widely used for short term (30–60 min) screening procedures and long term (3 day) stimulation tests. The simple procedure is useful since a normal rise in plasma cortisol excludes primary adrenocorticosteroid insufficiency. An abnormal result requires confirmation by more prolonged stimulation.

(b) Lysine vasopressin test

This test is not popular since it can have unpleasant side effects. It is also of doubtful clinical value because although vasopressin administration is associated with a marked rise in adrenal secretory activity the exact mode and site of action of vasopressin on the hypothalamo–pituitary–adrenal axis remains obscure.

(c) Dexamethasone suppression test

Potent synthetic steroids can be used for investigating the feedback regulation of pituitary ACTH secretion and dexamethasone is generally the steroid of choice since it causes no significant interference in the majority of plasma and urinary assay techniques. A widely used screening procedure to exclude Cushing's syndrome is the overnight test using 1 mg dexamethasone; a suppressed early morning plasma cortisol level indicates normal adrenal function. In another short term test using a single dose (2 mg; 5·1 μmol) of dexamethasone, patients with hypercortisolism, irrespective of its aetiology, fail to show normal suppression. A larger dose (8 mg; 20·3 μmol) of dexamethasone is helpful in establishing a differential diagnosis since patients having an ectopic source of ACTH, or with adrenal neoplasia, do not achieve the low levels observed in cases where excessive ACTH is of pituitary origin.

(d) Metyrapone (Metopirone) test

Metyrapone administration, by inhibiting the activity of 11β-hydroxylase, the enzyme system involved in the final stage of cortisol biosynthesis, decreases circulating cortisol levels. In normal circumstances, the metyrapone-induced fall in the plasma cortisol concentration causes increased secretion of ACTH, which in turn stimulates the adrenal secretion of relatively inactive 11-deoxycorticosteroids. This response is usually monitored by measuring the excretion in the urine of the metabolites of these steroids, which are excreted as 17-oxogenic steroids (see also p. 221). Provided care is taken to ensure that adequate circulating levels of metyrapone are achieved, an impaired response suggests hypothalamic, pituitary or adrenal hypofunction. A reduced response is also observed with Cushing's syndrome caused by an autonomous adrenocortical tumour or by the production of ectopic ACTH in amounts causing maximal adrenal stimulation. In patients with hypercortisolism due to a primary excess of ACTH secreted by the pituitary, the response to metyrapone is generally normal or may even be excessive.

(e) Insulin "stress" test

Intravenous administration of insulin reduces circulating glucose levels to less than 50% of basal values, within 30 min. This hypoglycaemia-induced stress, normally associated with a marked rise in plasma ACTH and circulating cortisol concentrations, provides a test for assessing the integrity of the complete hypothalamo–pituitary–adrenal axis. An inadequate response in this test is observed in patients having hypo-function of the hypothalamus, the pituitary or the adrenal gland, and in all cases of hyper-cortisolism with the possible exception of some ectopic ACTH producing syndromes.

(f) Pyrogen tests

The intravenous administration of certain highly purified non-antigenic bacterial endotoxins stimulates adrenal steroid secretion. Since their exact site of action remains somewhat uncertain, however, and unpleasant side effects frequently occur, this test is rarely used.

4. Synthetic Inhibitors of Adrenal Steroidogenesis

Adrenal steroid biosynthesis may be reduced by inhibitors acting directly on enzyme systems or indirectly by suppressing hypothalamo–pituitary activity. This section is restricted to a brief account of synthetic compounds, which act directly on adrenal enzyme systems. Some of these inhibitors are com-paratively specific and act mainly on one enzyme system. Inhibition of a single enzyme system such as that effecting hydroxylation at C-11 frequently blocks the formation of all 11β-hydroxysteroids including cortisol, corti-costerone and aldosterone. Synthetic inhibitors acting on enzyme systems involved in the initial stages of steroidogenesis may cause reduced bio-synthesis of all hormones including those of the adrenal gland as well as those originating in testicular and ovarian tissue. Synthetic inhibitors have proved to be of value in both the diagnosis and treatment of adrenal dys-function (Temple and Liddle, 1970; Samuels and Nelson, 1975).

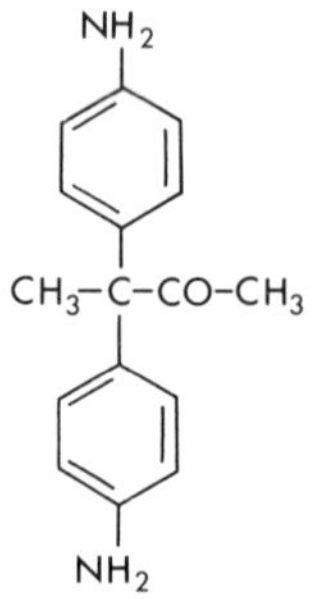

Amphenone B
3,3-bis (*p*-aminophenyl) 2-
butanone dihydrochloride

Although amphenone was one of the earliest inhibitors investigated (Hertz *et al.*, 1955) its mode of action remains obscure. In animals, amphenone caused cholesterol to accumulate in adrenal tissue and reduced the secretion of cortisol and aldosterone (Hoet and Molineaux, 1960). Interest in this compound waned when clinical trials indicated extensive toxic side effects (Hertz *et al.*, 1956).

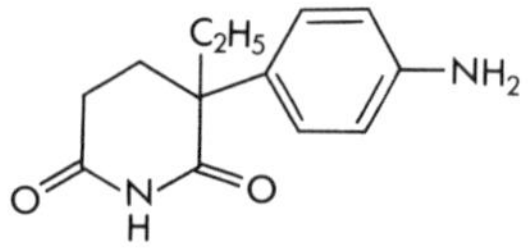

Aminoglutethimide
"Elipten" (CIBA)
α-Ethyl-α-*p*-aminophenylglutarimide

Aminoglutethimide inhibits the conversion of cholesterol to 20α-hydroxy-cholesterol (Kahnt and Neher, 1966) and reduces the activity of the cholesterol side chain-splitting enzyme system (Cash *et al.*, 1967). Cholesterol therefore accumulates in the adrenal cortex and since steroid formation at an undifferentiated step in the biosynthetic pathway is inhibited, production of all adrenal steroids including cortisol, corticosterone and aldosterone is reduced (Dexter *et al.*, 1967; Camacho *et al.*, 1967). Aminoglutethimide has therefore been used to reduce circulating steroid concentrations in patients having hypercortisolism (Fishman *et al.*, 1967) and hyperaldosteronism (Cash *et al.*, 1967). Aminoglutethimide co-administered with dexamethasone has been used to achieve medical adrenalectomy in patients with breast cancer and early studies report encouraging responses (Newsome *et al.*, 1977; Santen *et al.*, 1977).

Triparanol
1-[4-(Diethylaminoethoxy) phenyl] -1,1-
(p-ptolyl) -2-(p-chlorophenyl)ethanol

Clofibrate
Atromid-S
Ethyl α-p-chlorophenyl-α-methylpropionate
Ethyl chlorophenoxyisobutyrate

Studies of Holloszy and Eisenstein (1961) suggest that triparanol decreases cholesterol biosynthesis by inhibiting the enzyme system involved with the reduction of the double bond in the side chain of desmosterol. Although this inhibitor effectively reduced the secretion of adrenal steroids (Melby *et al.*, 1961), extensive side effects led to its withdrawal from clinical use. Clofibrate is considered a more useful inhibitor which also blocks the earlier stages of cholesterol biosynthesis (Briggs and Brotherton, 1970c).

o,p'DDD
1,1- Dichloro-2-(O-chlorophenyl)-2-
(p-chlorophenyl)-ethane

o,p'-DDD appears to be a highly selective cytotoxic agent inducing degenerative changes in adrenal mitochondria leading, eventually, to the destruction of the fascicular and reticular cells, yet leaving the zona glomerulosa largely intact (Nelson and Woodard, 1949; Nichols, 1961). Degenerative changes in the zona fasciculata and zona reticularis are paralleled by reduced cortisol synthesis following ACTH stimulation (Nichols, 1961; Gaunt *et al.*, 1965). Clinical experience with o,p'-DDD reviewed by Hutter and Kayhoe (1966) indicated the value of this adrenocorticolytic agent in treating adrenal neoplasia.

Cyanoketone

Cyanoketone appears to be a comparatively specific agent, blocking only 3β-hydroxysteroid dehydrogenase activity in adrenal tissue of both man and mammals (Goldman, 1968). Acting most probably as a stoichiometric inhibitor it decreases the conversion of pregnenolone to progesterone and therefore inhibits the synthesis of adrenocorticosteroids. Synthesis of Δ^5-3β-hydroxysteroids is unimpaired. Since cyanoketone has been reported to increase androgen production (Bongiovani et al., 1967), its use in women and children may be restricted.

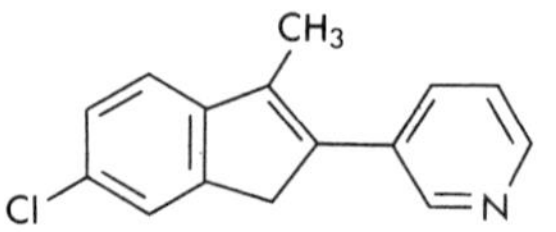

Su-8000 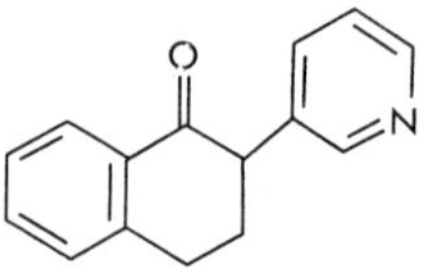   Su-9055

Chart et al. (1962) investigated inhibitors of the 17α-hydroxylase enzyme system and found that in canine adrenal tissue, SU 9055 inhibited the secretion of cortisol and its 11-deoxysteroid precursor, which was paralleled by a compensatory rise in corticosterone and 11-deoxycorticosterone secretion. Later studies (Bledsoe et al., 1964; Raman et al., 1966) indicate that these inhibitors also reduced the conversion of corticosterone to aldosterone. Side effects, including abdominal distress and diarrhoea, preclude the use of SU 9055 in man (Bledsoe et al., 1964).

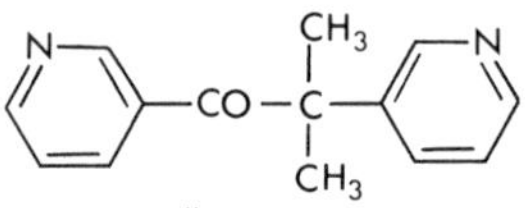

"Metyrapone" (CIBA)
Metopirone
2-Methyl-1,2-bis-(3-pyridyl)-1-propanone

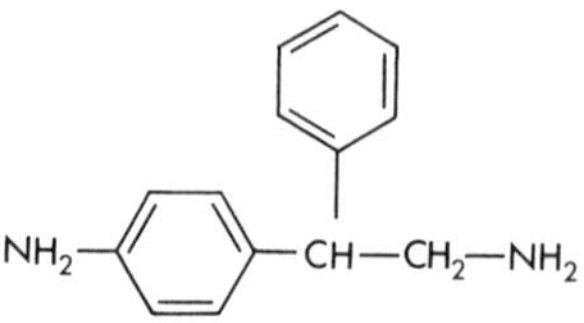

SKF 12185

Metyrapone, a derivative of amphenone, and SKF 12185 inhibit the adrenal secretion of cortisol, corticosterone and aldosterone in both man and mammals (Liddle et al., 1958; Chart et al., 1958). SKF 12185 although more potent, has received comparatively little attention since it only became available after the clinical usefulness of metyrapone was well established. At low doses, metyrapone appears to be a specific competitive inhibitor of 11β-hydroxylase activity (Dominguez and Samuels, 1963) possibly due to interaction of metyrapone with cytochrome P-450, a protein involved in the electron transport system essential for hydroxylation (Sweat et al., 1969; Williamson and O'Donnell, 1969).

Metyrapone has been widely used for the diagnostic evaluation of pituitary–adrenal reserve and for distinguishing patients having hyper-cortisolism due to pituitary or adrenal dysfunction (Liddle and Island, 1962). Metyrapone has also been used in the treatment of patients with autonomous adrenal neoplasms and successful management of patients with the ectopic ACTH syndrome has been reported (Temple and Liddle, 1970).

5. Synthetic Compounds Acting on Feedback Systems to Inhibit Adrenal Secretion

(a) Steroid analogues

Naturally occurring physiologically active adrenal steroids can be syn-thesised in quantity (Fieser and Fieser, 1959; Hems, 1962; Briggs and Brotherton, 1970d). These compounds, however, are known to have unwanted side effects including gastric irritation, activation of latent ulcers and latent infection; they also have the additional defect of increased sodium retention. Many cortisol analogues having additional double bonds, halogen atoms, methyl and hydroxyl groups have been prepared and tested.

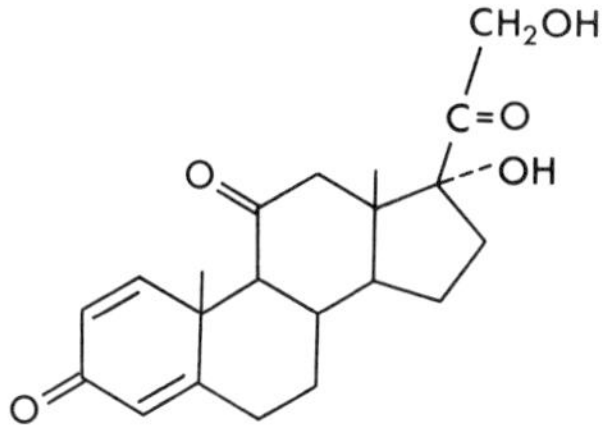

Prednisone

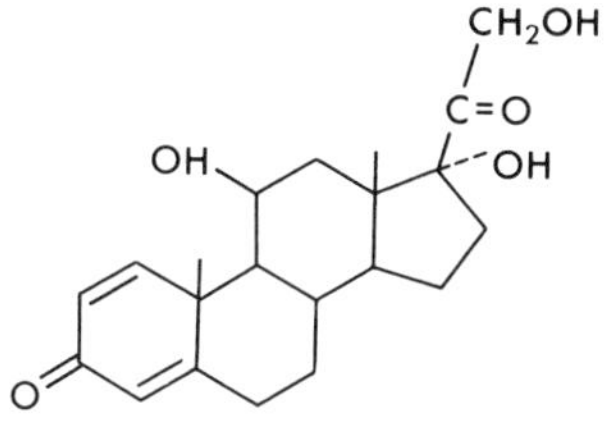

Prednisolone

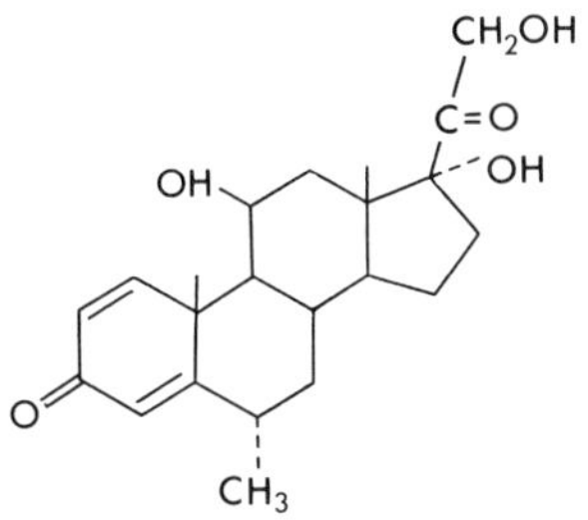

Methyl prednisolone

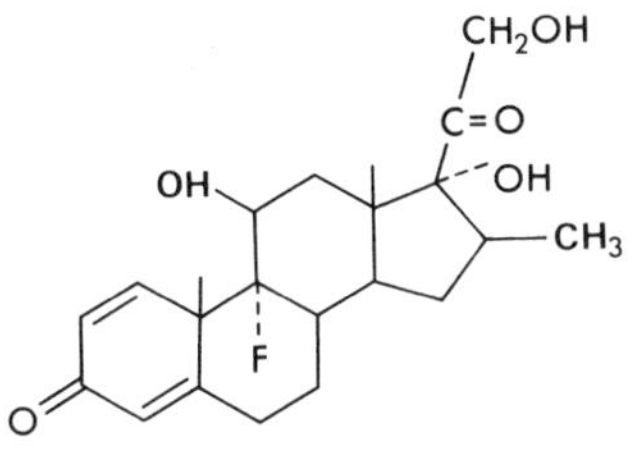

β- Methasone

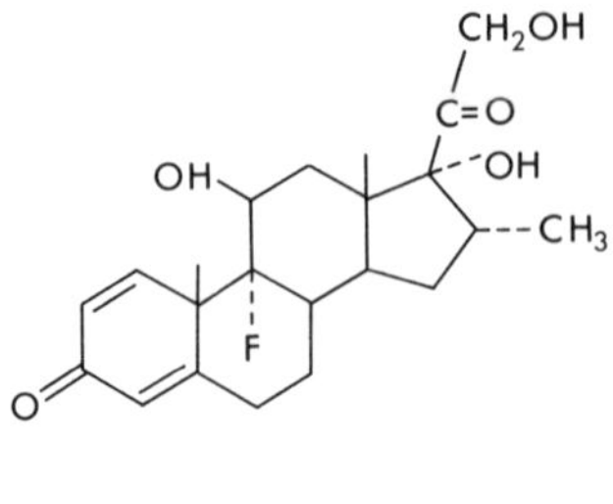

Dexamethasone

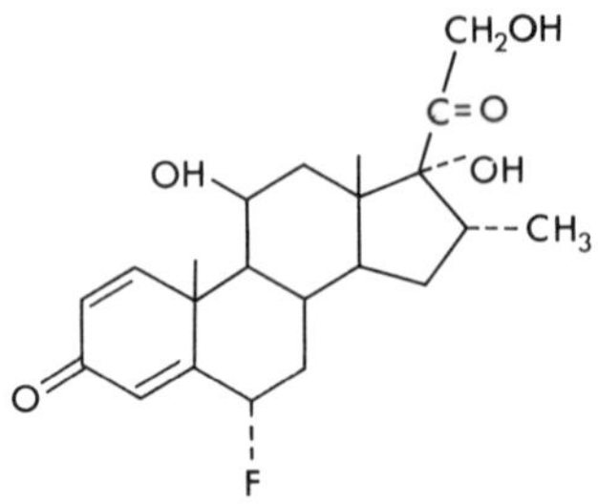

p-Methasone

Two double bonds in ring A, as in prednisone and prednisolone, represent the optimum in unsaturation, activity being reduced by altering the position and number of double bonds. These compounds synthesised by Hershberg and coworkers (Herzog *et al.*, 1955; Nobile *et al.*, 1955) were the first analogues to have greater physiological activity, and to cause less sodium retention than cortisol.

Experience has shown that a suitable balance of effects can be achieved by appropriate dual substitution since fluorination increases anti-inflammatory activity whereas methylation or hydroxylation reduces sodium retention. In many cases where more than one favourable modification has been made to the cortisol molecule the biological effects are additive (Hems, 1962).

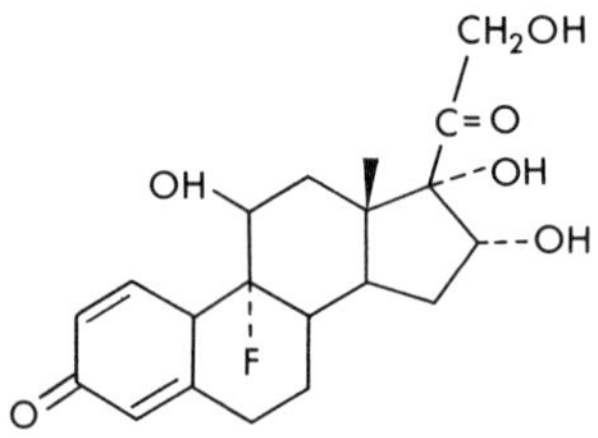

Triamcinolone

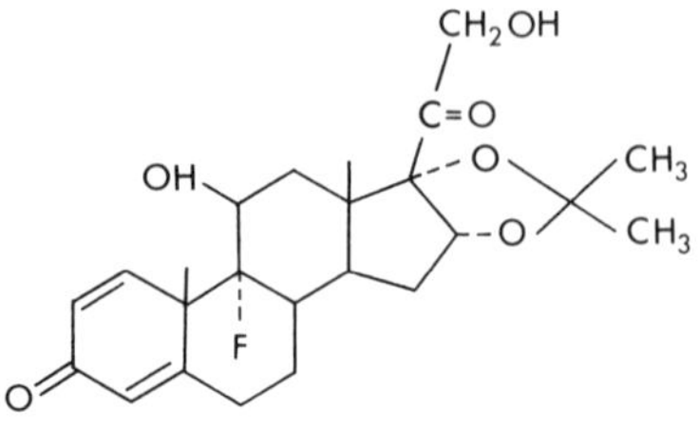

Triamcinolone acetonide

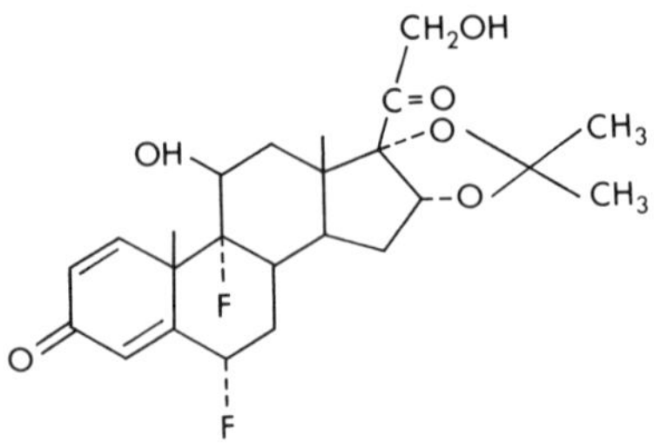

Fluocinolone acetonide

Most cortisol analogues having the 11β-hydroxy group possess systemic and topical activity; however, combination of the 16α, 17α hydroxyl groups of triamcinolone with acetone, forming the acetonide, greatly increase topical activity. Fluocinolone acetonide is recommended for topical use only (Phillips, 1976).

(b) Monoamine oxidase inhibitors

Experimental evidence of Krieger (1972, 1973), on the neurotransmitter regulation of ACTH release, suggested that hypercortisolism due to excessive pituitary ACTH secretion may originate from defective CNS regulation. It is therefore not surprising to find that some monoamine oxidase inhibitors used in the treatment of depression (nialamide, etryptamine, tranylcypromine) may inhibit adrenal secretory activity (Briggs and Brotherton, 1970b). A cyproheptadine-induced remission in Cushing's disease has also been reported (Krieger *et al.*, 1975).

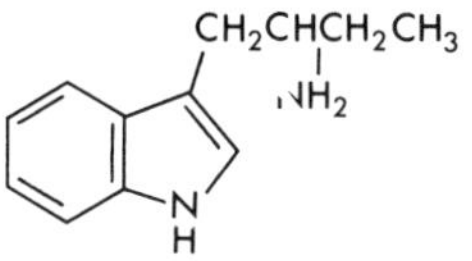

"Monase" etryptamine α-ethyltryptamine

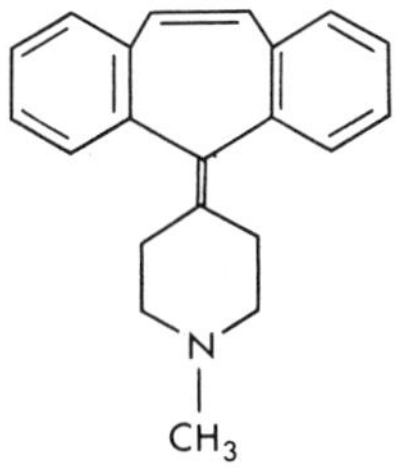

Cyproheptadine

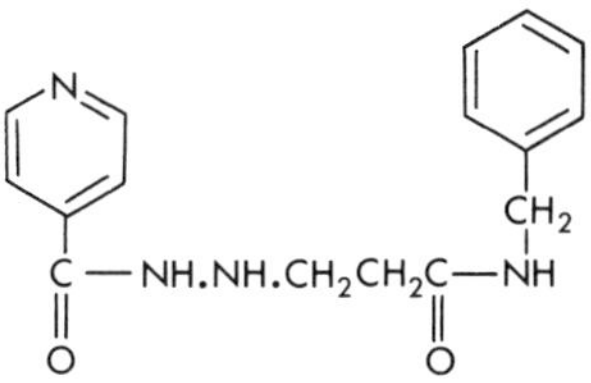

Nialamide "niamid"

$$\text{CH—CH—NH}_2$$
$$\text{CH}_2$$

"Parnate" tranylcypromine

C. CORTISOL BINDING GLOBULIN

Adrenal steroids, like other biologically active compounds, circulate in plasma either free or protein bound, the two forms being in equilibrium. Although most adrenal steroids are loosely bound to albumin, cortisol and cortisone are also specifically bound to the protein generally referred to as cortisol binding globulin (CBG) or transcortin (Daughaday, 1956; Bush, 1957; Sandberg and Slaunwhite, 1958). Accumulating evidence, reviewed by Westphal (1970), suggests that biological activity is a function of the non-protein bound steroid concentration and not of the total circulating concentration. Slaunwhite et al. (1962) have provided good direct evidence that CBG-bound cortisol is biologically inactive. It was shown that partially purified CBG, when administered intravenously to adrenalectomised animals, blocked the cortisol-induced increase in liver glycogen and decreased the reduction of cortisol by liver microsomal preparations when added to the incubation medium.

Human CBG has been isolated, purified and shown to be a glycoprotein having a molecular weight of approximately 50,000 with one binding site per molecule (Seal and Doe, 1962; Slaunwhite et al., 1966). As indicated in Table 2, binding affinity is very largely dependent on the spatial configuration of the substituents in the steroid nucleus. Integrity of the Δ^4-3-oxo group and the presence of the C-20 oxo group are essential for high avidity binding; the 11β, 17α and 21-hydroxyl groups also contribute to the strength of the binding. Involvement of the 11β-hydroxyl group in the hemi-acetal structure of aldosterone could well relate to the decreased binding of this steroid compared with corticosterone (Daughaday, 1967). Modification of ring A in synthetic steroids causes little change in binding, but introduction of 16α-substituents, or fluoro-groups at C-6 and C-9 markedly reduces binding affinity (De Moor et al., 1963).

The concentration of CBG in human plasma has been determined by a variety of methods, recently reviewed by Westphal (1975) and previously by Daughaday (1967). The results obtained are in good agreement and indicate a normal CBG concentration of approximately 35 mg/l in both male and female plasma. Foetal CBG concentrations are low (De Moore et al., 1962), as are those in new born infants (Sandberg et al., 1966). Doe

Table 2

fluence of various steroids *in vitro* on the transcortin binding of cortisol (De Moor *et al.*, 1963).

eroid examined	Cortisol 'displaced' %
iamcinolone: 9α-fluoro-11β,16α,17α,21-tetrahydroxypregna-1,4-dicne-3,20-dione	2
estrone	3
trahydrocortisone	3
trahydrocortisol	4
trahydro-DOC	4
tamethasone: 9α-fluoro-16β-methyl-11β,17α,21-trihydroxypregna-1,4-diene-3,20-dione	5
dosterone	6
Pregnenolone	8
egnane-3α,17α,20α-triol	9
trahydro S	10
xamethasone: 9α-fluoro-16α-methyl-11β,17α,21-trihydroxypregna-1,4-diene-3,20-dione	10
ednisone: 17α,21-dihydroxypregna-1,4-diene-3,11,20-trione	11
soxycorticosterone	11
stradiol	11
hydroepiandrosterone	16
ogesterone	23
stosterone	25
hydroandrosterone	27
egnanediol	29
drosterone	31
Deoxycortisol	36
Desoxycortisol	38
ednisolone: 11β,17α,21-trihydroxypregna-1,4-diene-3,20-dione	41
x-OH-Progesterone	46

et al., (1965) have reported low plasma concentrations of CBG affecting three generations of the same family, with correspondingly low plasma 17α-hydroxycorticosteroid levels. Low CBG concentrations have also been reported in cases of severe liver cirrhosis, dysproteinaemias, which may or may not be associated with hypoalbuminaemia, and in multiple myeloma. Although low concentrations of this protein have been associated with Cushing's syndrome, it is far more usual to find CBG levels within the normal range in both Cushing's syndrome and Addison's disease (Dixon *et al.*, 1967).

The binding capacity of CBG is limited and under normal circumstances approximates to 20 μg cortisol/100 ml (552 nmol/l) plasma. When cortisol concentrations are elevated and exceed the binding capacity of CBG, disproportionately high levels of free cortisol are found in plasma, Fig. 8. At

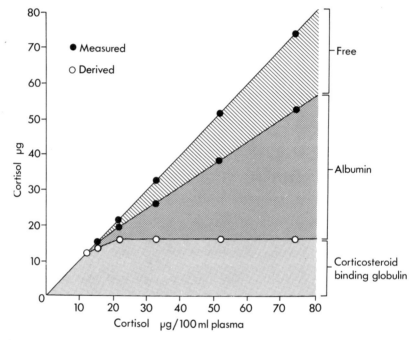

Fig. 8. The distribution of unbound, albumin-bound and CBG bound cortisol in serum at 4° (1 μg/100 ml = 27·6 nmol/1, 1 μg = 2·76 nmol) (from Daughaday and Mariz, 1961).

low steroid concentrations, a proportion of the circulating cortisol remains unbound, the amount varying slightly with concentration but usually approximating to 10% of the total (Daughaday, 1967; Lavelle, 1974). The binding of cortisol by CBG may well influence the equilibrium concentration of cortisol across capillary membranes (Florini and Buyske, 1961; Daughaday, 1967) and possibly accounts for the decreased metabolism of cortisol when CBG concentrations are high (Migeon *et al.*, 1957; Cohen *et al.*, 1958).

The low steroid concentrations in extracellular fluids may also relate to their low CBG content (Daughaday, 1959; Cope, 1964a).

Oestrogens, both naturally occurring and synthetic, induce increased synthesis of CBG (Mills *et al.*, 1960; Booth *et al.*, 1961; Doe *et al.*, 1964). In pregnancy, therefore, levels of CBG start to rise at approximately three months gestation and reach mean values of 70 mg/l during the last trimester. Following delivery, binding protein concentrations fall to non-pregnant levels within 14 days. Patients with cancer of the prostate on diethylstilboestrol therapy (5 mg/day; 18·6 μmol/day) also have markedly elevated CBG levels (92 mg/l) seven days after starting treatment. Women taking oestrogen-containing preparations for contraceptive purposes were similarly found to have elevated binding protein concentrations (Durber and Daly, 1976). A concomitant rise in plasma cortisol occurs during pregnancy, following diethylstilboestrol treatment and in women taking oestrogens; clinical manifestations of cortisol excess are rarely observed in these subjects since the oestrogen-induced rise in cortisol is associated with the biologically inactive protein bound fraction. Elevated cortisol concentrations are also found in Cushing's syndrome due to adrenal hyperplasia, adrenal adenoma and "oat-cell" carcinoma of the lung. However, in these patients CBG levels are within the normal range (Doe *et al.*, 1964). There is therefore a disproportionate rise in the free steroid fraction and symptoms characteristic of hypercortisolism are usually observed.

Investigation of the renal excretion of [^{14}C]cortisol (Peterson *et al.*, 1955) indicated that little ($<1\%$) of the intravenously administered dose was excreted unchanged in the urine, the major proportion ($>90\%$) of the administered dose being recovered as free and conjugated metabolites of cortisol. Later studies (Beisel *et al.*, 1964) showed that the cortisol levels in urine accurately reflected the non-protein-bound cortisol concentration in plasma. The clearance rate of plasma cortisol was about 20 ml/min in the early morning, when cortisol levels were high but decreased during the day with the corresponding fall in circulating cortisol concentrations. Figure 9 illustrates the removal of unbound cortisol from the plasma on glomerular filtration and the subsequent passive reabsorption by the tubule of a large proportion of the filtered cortisol. The term urinary free cortisol is frequently used to emphasise that it is the steroid and not its metabolites that is being determined in the urine. There is evidence to suggest that urinary free cortisol is clinically useful as an index of the non-protein-bound cortisol circulating in plasma (Burke and Beardwell, 1973). However, since urinary estimations are complicated by "complete collection" difficulties it is possible that determination of cortisol levels in saliva, which also reflect the biologically active fraction in plasma will prove to be a practical alternative as is suggested later in this chapter.

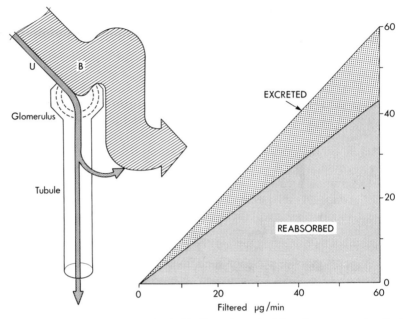

Fig. 9. The urinary loss of cortisol. Binding of cortisol by plasma proteins limits glomerular filtration to the unbound fraction. The larger portion of this is reabsorbed from the tubule, with excreted and reabsorbed cortisol varying proportionately with the filtered load as shown to the right (from Beisel *et al.*, 1964).

D. STEROID BIOSYNTHESIS IN THE ADRENAL CORTEX

It is now generally accepted that adrenal steroids are synthesised almost exclusively from cholesterol (see Fig. 10; Werbin *et al.*, 1959; Werbin and Chaikoff, 1961; Krum *et al.*, 1964). The sole precursor role assigned to cholesterol may, however, be a question of availability rather than absolute

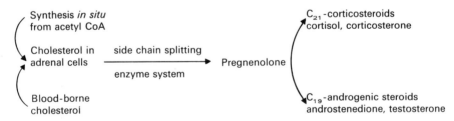

Fig. 10. Diagrammatic overview of adrenal hormone biosynthesis.

specificity of the enzyme systems involved, since adrenal tissue readily converts desmosterol to pregnenolone (Steinberg et al., 1961; Goodman et al., 1962). Furthermore, since the concentration of cholesteryl esters, rather than free cholesterol is reduced on ACTH stimulation it would seem that the ester form, stored in the zona fasciculata of the adrenal cortex may be utilised in times of stress for adrenal steroidogenesis (Grant, 1968).

Cholesterol, present in the adrenal cortex, may arise by direct uptake of the sterol circulating in blood or by synthesis within adrenal cells from C-2 fragments (acetylCoA) formed directly within the tissue during intermediate metabolism (Hechter et al., 1953; Caspi et al., 1962). Since the relative importance of these sources of adrenal cholesterol in man and other mammals has been previously discussed (Vinson and Whitehouse, 1970) and details of the biosynthesis of cholesterol from acetate has also been presented in other reviews (Samuels and Uchikawa, 1967; Griffiths and Cameron, 1975), detailed consideration of these aspects of adrenocorticosteroid synthesis in this chapter is unnecessary. It is, however, noteworthy to briefly record that cholesterol, a C_{27}-sterol, is built up from isoprene units, C_5 fragments which join to form squalene, a linear C_{30}-compound that cyclises with molecular rearrangement to form lanosterol. Zymosterol and desmosterol are further intermediates formed during the conversion of lanosterol to cholesterol.

1. Conversion of Cholesterol to Pregnenolone

$[4\text{-}^{14}C]$- and $[26\text{-}^{14}C]$-labelled cholesterol were used to show the conversion of cholesterol to $(4\text{-}^{14}C]$ pregnenolone and a labelled C_6-fragment, isocaproic acid after incubation with adrenal tissue (see Fig. 11; Lynn et al., 1954; Saba et al., 1954; Constantopoulos and Tchen, 1961). Formation of the C_6-fragment indicates that activation of the bond between C-20 and C-22 is essential for side chain splitting and since the lyase requires both NADPH and molecular O_2 (Solomon et al., 1956; Halkerston et al., 1961), some of the enzyme systems involved must be mixed function oxidases/hydroxylases (Mason, 1957). Various hydroxy- and oxo-derivatives of cholesterol have been incubated with adrenal preparations to assess their role as possible precursors of pregnenolone (Dorfman and Unger, 1965; Burstein and Gut, 1971). Of the four possible monohydroxy compounds, the 20α- and the 22R-hydroxyderivatives were readily converted to prenolone, whereas the isomeric 20β- and 22S-compounds were not. Since the dihydroxy compound, 20, 22R-dihydroxycholesterol was also metabolised (Shimizu et al., 1961; Constantopoulos et al., 1962) the preferred reaction sequence may be that shown in Fig. 12.

H

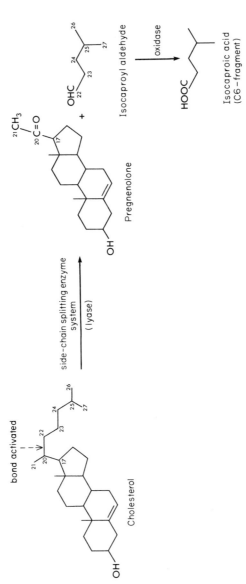

Fig. 11. Conversion of cholesterol to pregnenolone.

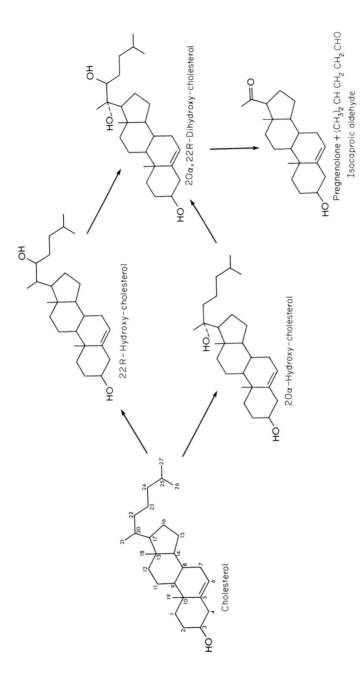

22R-Hydroxy-cholesterol

20α,22R-Dihydroxy-cholesterol

20α-Hydroxy-cholesterol

Cholesterol

Pregnenolone + (CH₃)₂ CH CH₂ CH₂ CH₂ CHO
Isocaproic aldehyde

Fig. 12. Possible intermediates in the conversion of cholesterol to pregnenolone.

Hall and Koritz (1964) were, however, unable to confirm the formation of these intermediates. They found no radioactivity associated with 20α-hydroxycholesterol on incubating adrenal tissue with [³H] cholesterol and an excess of the unlabelled 20α-hydroxysteroid. This discrepancy could arise if exogenous 20α-hydroxycholesterol did not equilibrate with the labelled material formed on hydroxylation of [³H]cholesterol. More recent evidence (Luttrel et al., 1972) suggests that the intermediates formed during preg-nenolone formation involve reactive transient intermediate complexes which may be represented as radical or ionic species. Hydroxylated compounds may therefore not be obligatory intermediates but simply by-products of the true intermediates. Evidence that hydroxylation of cholesterol at C-17 may also precede side-chain cleavage (Shimizu, 1965; Burstein et al., 1968) indicates a possibility for the direct formation of 17α-hydroxypregnenolone from cholesterol without the intermediate formation of pregnenolone. The relative importance of this pathway remains to be determined (Vinson and Whitehouse, 1970).

2. Conversion of Pregnenolone to Corticosteroids

Pregnenolone is now generally accepted to be the precursor of all mammalian steroid hormones. It may be converted to corticosteroids by two possible pathways (Fig. 13) depending on whether oxidation of the Δ^5-3β-hydroxy group of pregnenolone occurs before or after hydroxylation at C-17. The classical, or Δ^4-pathway, for cortisol biosynthesis in human adrenal tissue is based on perfusion studies of ox adrenal glands (Hechter and Pincus, 1954; Hechter, 1958). Pregnenolone, when metabolised by way of the Δ^4-pathway, is first oxidised to progesterone and following a series of hydroxylation reactions occurring in the sequence 17α, 21, 11β finally leads to synthesis of cortisol. The introduction of a 21-hydroxyl group would appear to preclude subsequent hydroxylation at C-17. The 11β-hydroxylation of 11-deoxycorticosterone (DOC) gives rise to corticosterone. Hydroxylation of the angular methyl group at C-18 leads to formation of 18-hydroxy DOC and 18-hydroxycorticosterone. The relative importance of these steroids as aldosterone precursors has been the subject of much debate (Wettstein et al., 1955; Ayres et al., 1958; Stachenko and Giroud, 1962; Pasqualini, 1964; Sharma, 1970).

It would appear that when pregnenolone is metabolised by the classical pathway progesterone is an obligatory intermediate from which all other C_{21}-steroids are synthesised (Samuels and Uchikawa, 1967). Later studies (Lipsett and Hokfelt, 1961; Weliky and Engel, 1962) which indicated ready conversion of 17α-hydroxypregnenolone to cortisol, suggested the possibility of an alternative pathway for cortisol biosynthesis. It has now been estab-

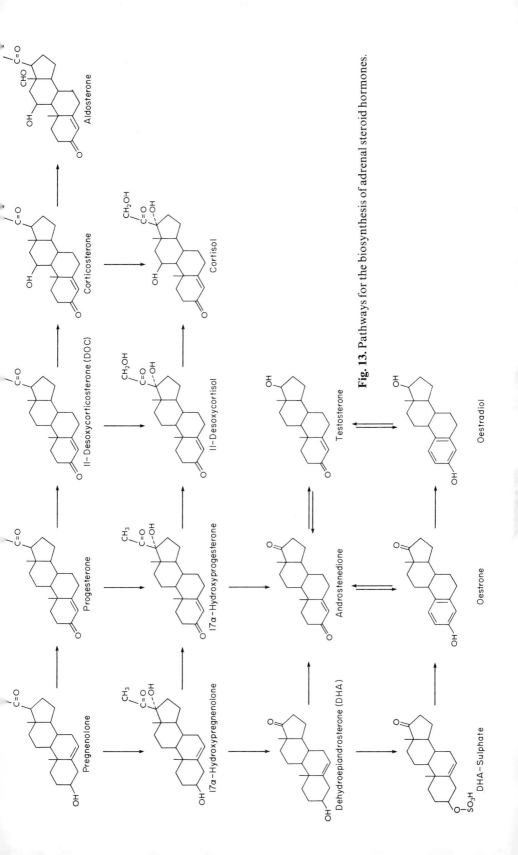

Fig. 13. Pathways for the biosynthesis of adrenal steroid hormones.

lished (Mulrow *et al.*, 1962; Cameron *et al.*, 1968; Griffiths and Cameron, 1970) that this alternative Δ^5-pathway, in which pregnenolone is first converted to 17α-hydroxypregnenolone and subsequently oxidised to 17α-hydroxyprogesterone, could well be the main route for cortisol biosynthesis in human adrenal tissue. Other mammals have adrenal enzyme systems which are essentially similar to those in man; the ratio of cortisol to corticosterone secreted is, however, species-specific. In some mammals (rabbit, mouse and rat) corticosterone predominates whereas in others cortisol is the major secretory product (Chester Jones, 1976).

3. Conversion of Pregnenolone to Adrenal Androgens and Oestrogens

Human adrenal tissue when incubated with radiolabelled pregnenolone and progesterone, synthesises androgenic C_{19}-steroids including dehydro-epiandrosterone (DHA), androstenedione and testosterone (Gaul *et al.*, 1962; Kase and Kowal, 1962; Ward and Grant, 1963; Axelrod and Gold-zieher, 1968). In an excellent report of adrenal androgen biosynthesis, Griffiths and Cameron (1970) note the importance of cell type when interpreting results from incubations of normal, hyperplastic and neoplastic adrenal tissue preparations. The major adrenal androgen is DHA, largely secreted as the sulphate (Baulieu, 1962; Vande Wiele *et al.*, 1962; Gurpide *et al.*, 1963); similar amounts of androstenedione and testosterone are also secreted (Baird *et al.*, 1969). Direct evidence for adrenal oestrogen secretion has been presented (Baird *et al.*, 1969; Millington *et al.*, 1976) and *in vitro* incubation of adrenal tissue with androgens (Baggett *et al.*, 1959; Cameron *et al.*, 1969) showed small but significant oestrogen biosynthesis.

4. Enzyme Systems

As indicated earlier the enzyme systems involved in the biosynthesis of adrenal steroids include the hydroxylases and the side-chain splitting enzymes, the lyases, both of which require NADPH and molecular O_2; the 3β-hydroxysteroid dehydrogenases, requiring $NADP^+$ or NAD^+ and the isomerases, for which no coenzyme has been identified.

(a) Δ^5-3β-Hydroxysteroid dehydrogenase/isomerase enzyme system

This enzyme system effecting oxidative changes in ring A is confined almost exclusively ($>90\%$) to microsomal preparations of adrenal tissue (Beyer and Samuels, 1956; Inano *et al.*, 1969). Although Ward and Engel (1964) have shown reversibility of the 3β-hydroxysteroid-dehydrogenase/isomerase enzyme system in sheep adrenal microsomal preparations, the system is generally considered irreversible under normal physiological conditions (Samuels and Nelson, 1975). Dehydrogenation, converting the 3-hydroxy to the 3-oxo group is thought to precede the enzyme-catalysed isomeric shift of the double bond from C-5 to C-4 since Δ^4-3-hydroxyallylic alcohols are not intermediates in the reaction (Ward and Engel, 1966). The dehydrogenase preferentially utilises NAD^+ as the hydrogen acceptor; $NADP^+$ may be used but rates are markedly reduced (Koritz, 1964). Although the question of substrate specificity of the 3β-hydroxysteroid-dehydrogenases remains unanswered, the studies of Ewald et al. (1964, 1965) suggest the probability of three distinct isomerases in bovine adrenal tissue. Specificity in these enzyme systems may therefore reside in the isomerase rather than the dehydrogenase.

(b) Hydroxylating enzyme systems

Adrenal hydroxylating enzyme systems are all mixed function oxidases, located in both the mitochondria and the microsomes. They are not, as was first supposed, single proteins. Omura et al. (1966) have shown that at least three proteins are involved in mitochondrial hydroxylations. These have now been identified as a specific flavoprotein, a non-haeme iron protein (adrenodoxin) and a haemeprotein (cytochrome P-450). The pathway for electron transport and activation of molecular O_2 in mitochondrial hydroxylations reviewed by Samuels and Nelson (1975) is illustrated in Fig. 14.

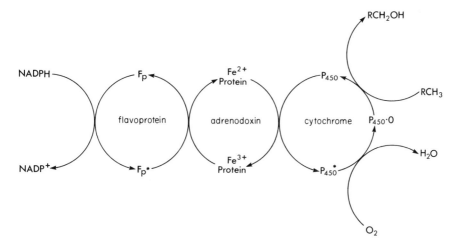

Fig. 14. Pathway for electron transport and activation of molecular O_2 in mitochondrial hydroxylations.

Microsomal hydroxylases differ from those in the mitochondria in that adrenodoxin is absent and the specific flavoprotein reduces cytochrome C directly. It is generally thought, but not yet proved, that specificity is conferred by the terminal oxidase of the hydroxylation sequence, i.e. the protein directly responsible for introducing the hydroxyl radical into the steroid molecule.

5. Distribution of Steroidogenic Enzyme Systems within Adrenal Cells

The well defined spatial distribution of steroidogenic enzyme systems in adrenal cells has been reviewed by Malamed (1975); the location of the enzyme systems involved in the classical pathway for adrenal steroid hormone biosynthesis is illustrated in Fig. 15.

The hydroxylases and lyases involved in the side-chain splitting of cholesterol and the 11β-hydroxylase are associated with the inner mitochondrial membrane. The 17α- and 21-hydroxylases and the 3β-hydroxysteroid dehydrogenase/isomerase enzyme systems are associated with the smooth endoplasmic reticulum. This spatial arrangement necessitates the shuttling of intermediates between mitochondria and endoplasmic reticulum. Thus pregnenolone must pass from the mitochondria for conversion to progesterone and 17α-hydroxypregnenolone, which must then return to the mitochondria for introduction of the 11β-hydroxyl group. The details of this shuttle remain obscure. Matsumoto and Samuels (1969) have shown that although the cytosol contains no specific binding protein for pregnenolone, strong binding to the endoplasmic reticulum occurs and at equilibrium high concentrations of pregnenolone relative to the cytosol are achieved.

E. STEROID BIOSYNTHESIS IN THE FOETAL ADRENAL GLAND

In the human foetal adrenal cortex all the enzyme systems required for cortisol and androgen biosynthesis are present as early as 12 weeks gestation (Bloch and Benirschke, 1959; Villee et al., 1959; Villee et al., 1961). The foetal adrenal cortex, however, differs from the adult cortex in that activity of the 3β-hydroxysteroid dehydrogenase enzyme system is low whereas that of the 16α-hydroxylase and sulphatase enzymes is comparatively high (Villee et al., 1961; Simmer et al., 1964). The foetus therefore produces mainly pregnenolone, DHA and 16α-hydroxymetabolites in preference to progesterone, cortisol, corticosterone and aldosterone. Foetal sulphatase activity converts the potent steroid hormones, oestradiol and oestrone, synthesised in the

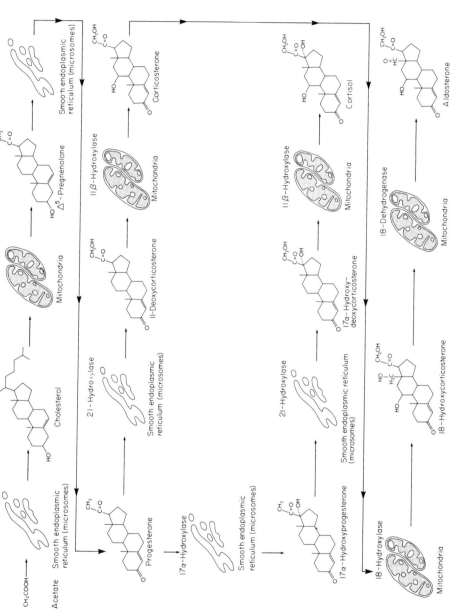

Fig. 15. Simplified scheme of steroidogenesis and its intracellular pathways. Corticosterone and cortisol are end products in the zona fasciculata and reticularis. Corticosterone produced in zona glomerulosa is converted to aldosterone. (from Malamed, 1975).

placenta and present in high concentrations in umbilical venous blood, to relatively inert sulphate esters (Schwers *et al.*, 1965). Sulphation may therefore be an effective mechanism for preventing excessive oestrogenic action in the foetus. Clinically useful tests of foetal well-being rely very largely on the increased biosynthetic capacity of foetal adrenal tissue with advancing gestation. The steady rise in secretion of foetal C_{19}-steroids, particularly DHA and 16α-hydroxyDHA provides increased amounts of precursors for placental oestrogen formation. Assay of maternal oestrogens in either plasma or urine therefore reflects functional integrity of the foetoplacental unit, foetal jeopardy being associated with low oestrogen levels (Oakey, 1974).

F. METABOLISM OF CORTISOL

Radiolabelled cortisol when injected into the general circulation disappears rapidly having a half-life of from 70–100 min (Edwards and Landon, 1976). Hellman *et al.* (1971) suggest that the reversible uptake of cortisol by peripheral tissues may involve cyclic oxidation and reduction of the 11β-hydroxyl group. Some unchanged cortisol appears in the urine (Lindholm, 1973) but by far the largest proportion of the daily cortisol output is irreversibly removed by the liver (Briggs and Brotherton, 1970e). The complex metabolic interconversions effected by hepatic tissue lead to formation of the biologically inactive, water soluble, cortisol metabolites found in urine. The more important intermediates formed during the course of cortisol metabolism are illustrated in Fig. 16. Activity of the hepatic 11β-hydroxy oxido-reductase enzyme system converts cortisol to cortisone. Metabolism of these steroids therefore follows a common pathway (Rosenfeld, 1967). Reduction of the oxo-group at C-3 and the Δ^{4-5}-double bond forms compounds of the 3β-hydroxypregnane series in which the 3α, 5β isomers predominate. These two reduced metabolites of cortisol are generally known as tetrahydrocortisol and allotetrahydrocortisol; a similar nomenclature is followed for cortisone. Further reduction of these tetrahydro compounds at C-20 yields the isomeric 20α- and 20β-compounds known as the cortols and cortolones depending on the oxygen function present at C-11. Cortisol and cortisone may also be reduced at C-20, the corresponding trihydroxy alcohols being formed. Loss of the side chain at C-17 occurs to a limited extent resulting in the formation of 11-oxygenated-17-oxosteroids. Although hydroxylation can occur in both the A and B rings of the steroid nucleus, only 6β-hydroxycortisol is formed to any appreciable extent.

Cortisol, cortisone, their 20-dihydrometabolites, together with 6β-hydroxycortisol, are all excreted as free steroids (Bulaschenko *et al.*, 1960; Cope, 1964b). Levels are generally low, the reported values for 6β-hydroxy-

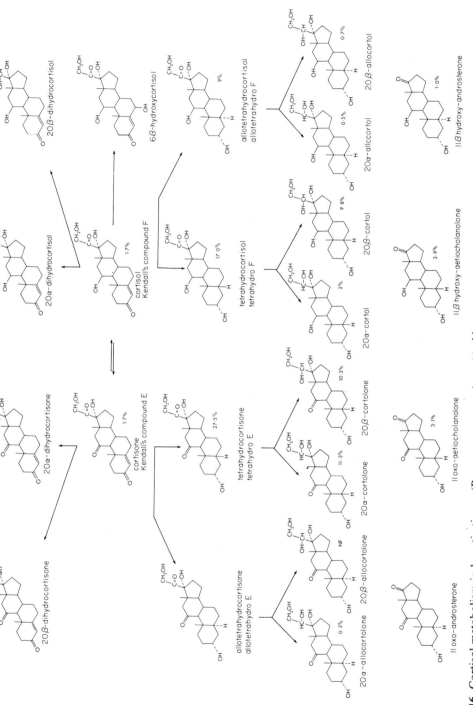

Fig. 16. Cortisol metabolism in hepatic tissue. (Percentage conversion of [4-^{14}C]-cortisol to various metabolites; from Fukushima *et al.*, 1960.)

cortisol, the principal free steroid normally present in male and female urine, usually being less than 500 µg/24 hr (1·3 µmol/24 hr) (Katz *et al.*, 1962). Urinary levels of 6β hydroxycortisol may have some diagnostic significance since values are increased following administration of ACTH and oestrogens; elevated levels have also been associated with Cushing's syndrome (Pal, 1978). In marked contrast ring A-reduced metabolites are excreted mainly as conjugates (Romanoff *et al.*, 1961). By far the largest proportion are conjugated with glucuronic acid, though some may be excreted as sulphates. Conjugates at C-3 predominate, but limited conjugation with the C-21 hydroxyl group may also occur. Classic studies (Fukushima *et al.*, 1960) in which [4-^{14}C] cortisol was injected intravenously into a group of normal men indicated that most (> 80%) of the injected dose appeared in the urine within 24 hr. Of the radioactivity recovered, 64% was associated with the neutral fraction following β-glucuronidase hydrolysis. The distribution of radioactivity in the spectrum of metabolites isolated is illustrated in Fig. 16.

G. METHODS FOR THE DETERMINATION OF CORTICOSTEROID CONCENTRATIONS

Typical results obtained for the following corticosteroids are summarised in Table 3.

1. "Corticosteroids"

The earliest procedures for determining the adrenocorticosteroids, based on chemical reactions with colorimetric end-points, were highly insensitive. These methods were therefore applied to urine, which was readily available to the analyst in much greater volume. Since the major proportion of the cortisol secreted by the adrenal gland is excreted in the urine as cortisol metabolites, the determination of the amount of these compounds in a 24-hr urine sample provided an assessment of the daily secretion rate of cortisol. The chemical procedures used were not specific, but determined metabolites of other adrenal steroid hormones in addition to those of cortisol; the class of compound determined depending on the assay procedure used, as indicated in Fig. 17.

In the United States the method of Porter-Silber (1950) was widely used for the assay of urinary cortisol metabolites. The group of metabolites determined were known as the urinary 17-hydroxycorticosteroids. In this method conjugates were hydrolysed enzymatically and the free steroids were determined following reaction with a concentrated sulphuric acid/phenyl-hydrazine reagent. Since this reagent reacted only with the dihydroxyacetone

Table 3

Corticosteroid levels in normal subjects (1 μg/100 ml = 27·5 nmol/l).

Corticosteroid	Method	Time	Range	No. of subjects	References
Plasma					
11-Hydroxycorticoid	Fluorimetry	09.00–10.00	6·5–26·3 μg/100 ml M = 14·2 μg/100 ml	52	Mattingly (1962)
Cortisol	Double isotope derivative	Random	3·1–20·2 μg/100 ml M = 9·8	17	Fraser and James (1968)
	CPB	09.00 09.00	15·2 ± 5·1 μg/100 ml 17·6 ± 4·3 μg/100 ml	12♂ 12♀	Murphy et al. (1963) Murphy et al. (1963)
	CPB	a.m.	11·7 ± 3·7 μg/100 ml	20	Iturzaeta et al. (1970)
	RIA	08.00	10·6–25 μg/100 ml M = 17·7	1?	Dash et al. (1975)
	RIA	08.00	8–18 μg/100 ml	22	Kao et al. (1975)
	RIA	08.00	5·5–20 μg/100 ml M = 12·6	30	Rolleri et al. (1976)
	RIA	09.00	4·4–35 μg/100 ml	19	Seth and Brown (1978)
11-Deoxycortisol	CPB		0·8 ± 0·8 μg/100 ml		Spark (1971)
	CPB		0·18 ± 0·01		Newsome et al. (1972)
Following single o/night Metyrapone 30 mg/kg	RIA	08.00	8–22·3 μg/100 ml M = 13·7	54 sick controls	Mahajan et al. (1972)
Following 6 × 750 mg Metyrapone	CPB	—	16·8 ± 4·4 μg/100 ml	32	Spark (1971)

Table 3—*continued*

Corticosteroid	Method	Time	Range	No. of subjects	References
Following single o/night Metyrapone 2–3 g	RIA	08.00	7–25 µg/100 ml	12	Kao (1975)
Corticosterone	CPB	08.00	400 ± 30 ng/100 ml		Newsome et al. (1972)
	RIA	08.00	396 ± 228 ng/100 ml 655 ± 271 ng/100 ml	15♂ 15♀	Nabors et al. (1974) Nabors et al. (1974)
11-Deoxycorticosterone	RIA	Random	1–12 ng/100 ml M = 5	10	Arnold and James (1971)
	Double isotope derivative	Random	4–18 ng/100 ml M = 7	24	Arnold and James (1971)
18-Hydroxycorticosterone	RIA	Random	6–16 ng/100 ml 13–42 ng/100 ml	6-recumbent 17-standing	Martin et al. (1975)
	glc		3–25 ng/100 ml	18	Wilson et al. (1976)
18-OH-DOC	glc	?	20–160 ng/100 ml	7	Mason and Fraser (1975)
	RIA	a.m.	3·3–16 ng/100 ml M = 8·5	18	Chandler et al. (1976)
	RIA	08.00	10·1 ± 6·5 ng/100 ml	20-supine	Sulon and Sparano (1978)
			9·4 ± 4·2 ng/100 ml	20-movement	Sulon and Sparano (1978)
17α-Hydroxyprogesterone	CPB	Age 15 hr–3 day Age 3–15 day	1·1–2·1 µg/100 ml <1·0 µg/100 ml	3 46	Atherden et al. (1974) Atherden et al. (1974)
	RIA	Age 0·5 yr–16 yr	<0·2 µg/100 ml	500	Hughes and Winter (1976)

Urine					
17-Oxogenic steroid (17-OGS)	Colorimetric	—	8–18 mg/24 hr 6–16 mg/24 hr	♂ ♀	Edwards and Landon (1976)
11-Hydroxycorticosteroids	Fluorimetry	—	229 ± 66 µg/24 hr 174 ± 53 µg/24 hr	♂ ♀	Mattingly et al. (1964)
Free cortisol	CPB	—	56 ± 33 µg/24 hr 41 ± 30 µg/24 hr	♂ ♀	Murphy (1968)
	RIA	—	43 ± 15 µg/24 hr	8	Ruder et al. (1972)
6β-OH-Cortisol	RIA	—	286 ± 54 µg/24 hr 233 ± 80 µg/24 hr	10♂ 8♀	Park (1978) Park (1978)
Saliva					
Cortisol	RIA	09.00	$9 \cdot 7 \pm 4 \cdot 04$ nmol/l	41	Walker et al. (1978b)
17α-OH-Progesterone	RIA	09.00	90–1500 pmol/l		Walker et al. (1979)

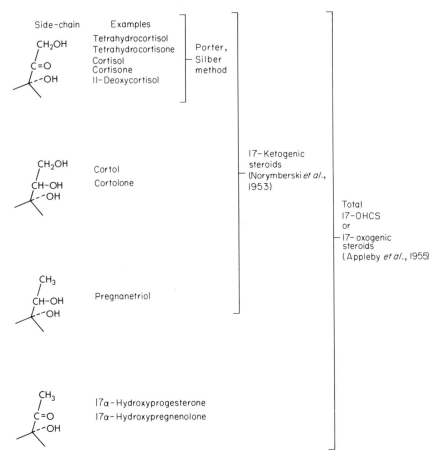

Fig. 17. Specificity of various corticosteroid colorimetric assay procedures.

side-chain, this method determined only cortisol, 11-deoxycortisol, cortisone and their reduced tetrahydrometabolites. In the United Kingdom the procedure of Norymberski *et al.* (1953) was in general use. This method relied on sodium bismuthate oxidation, a reaction which not only cleaved the ketols and diols of the C_{21}-steroid side chain forming 17-oxosteroids, but also removed the glucuronide moiety of the steroid conjugates, thereby obviating the need for hydrolysis. The 17-oxosteroids formed were reacted with the Zimmermann reagent to give a coloured product; a correction factor excluded interference from the 17-oxosteroids originally present in the urine. An improved assay was introduced by Appleby *et al.* (1955) in which sodium borohydride was used to reduce the endogenous 17-oxosteroids, thereby obviating the need for a correction factor; this reagent also reduced those steroids with a C-20 oxo-group to the corresponding hydroxyl compounds. Subsequent treatment with periodate led to the formation of 17-oxosteroids which were then determined, as before, with the Zimmermann reagent. The group of urinary steroids measured by the Appleby modification, which included compounds having the 21-deoxyketol side-chain in the determination, were originally referred to as total 17-hydroxycorticosteroids. This, however, caused confusion with the results obtained by the Porter-Silber method and following a recommendation by a Medical Research Council working party (Gray et al., 1969), the metabolites determined by the Appleby procedure became generally known as the 17-oxogenic steroids.

Some attempts were made to increase the specificity of the urinary procedures. The most successful have featured fractionation of the 17-oxosteroids, formed following sodium borohydride/periodate or bismuthate degradation, by gas–liquid chromatography, into those with and those without an 11-hydroxyl group. The ratio, known as the 11-oxygenation index, has proved to be of value in the diagnosis of congenital adrenal hyperplasia (Clayton et al., 1971). The application of gas chromatography with capillary columns has made it possible to determine a number of steroid metabolites in a single urine specimen and thus to construct a urinary steroid "profile" (Fantl and Gray, 1977). This technique has the advantage of revealing simultaneously the excretion pattern of a number of steroid metabolites.

Several of the earlier methods for determining plasma cortisol concentration were also based on the Porter-Silber colour reaction. Again, such methods generally lacked sensitivity, required considerable technical expertise, and their use was therefore restricted to specialised laboratories. Greater devolution of such assays became possible when procedures for cortisol determination were introduced which were based on the principle of acid-induced fluorescence. In an early paper Sweat (1954) reported a fluorimetric procedure for determining individual plasma corticosteroids following separation by column chromatography on silica. This complex, time-consuming methodology was simplified by the efforts of many workers but the procedure most widely adopted was that developed by Mattingly (1962). This consisted essentially of extracting plasma with carefully purified methylene chloride, reacting this extract with a sulphuric acid/ethanol reagent and determining the fluorescence developed at exactly 13 min after mixing. This method, capable of determining 18–24 samples a day, has unquestionably been of great clinical value for assessing cortisol levels in plasma. The assay, however, lacks specificity. Corticosterone, for example, was shown to produce a fluorescence, relative to cortisol, of approximately 250%, but this was less likely to be of significance than interference by various drugs, of which spironolactone was the most notorious. Equally important was the production of a non-specific plasma fluorescence and James *et al.* (1967) have shown, by comparison of results obtained by a fluorimetric procedure with those obtained by a reference double isotopic derivative technique, that only 59% of the total fluorescence produced was due to cortisol. The semi-automated procedure of Townsend and James (1968), which has a throughput of 23 samples/hr, provided significantly better agreement between the isotopic and fluorimetric procedures with a mean of 83% of the fluorescence being due to cortisol. The fluorimetric assays in routine use produced results which correlated well with changes in plasma cortisol, but did not measure cortisol alone. Results from these assays were therefore referred to as plasma 11-hydroxy-corticoids (11-OHCS). Certain practical details of the fluorescence procedure are discussed in a report by a Medical Research Council working party (James *et al.*, 1971).

2. Cortisol

(a) Protein binding assays

Assays based on the principle of competitive protein binding (Diczfalusy, 1970) were first introduced by Murphy and her coworkers. The original reported method for determining cortisol (Murphy *et al.*, 1963) was, however, insensitive and time-consuming, since low specific activity [^{14}C]cortisol was used as the radioactive label, and equilibrium dialysis was used to separate free and bound steroid. The assay was markedly simplified when gel filtration replaced dialysis (Murphy and Pattee, 1964) but the assay only became attractive for routine plasma corticosteroid measurement when tritiated steroids of high specific activity were introduced and the unbound fraction was separated by adsorption (Murphy, 1967). In this form the assay has excellent sensitivity and allows precise determination of cortisol concentrations using only 50 μl of plasma. Plasma from subjects undergoing oestrogen treatment or in the third trimester of pregnancy contains markedly increased transcortin concentrations and is therefore suitable for use in the binding assay. Removal of endogenous corticosteroid by gel filtration at elevated temperatures increases the number of available binding sites and is claimed to increase assay precision (Baranczuk *et al.*, 1973). Transcortins from various animals show varying binding affinity for the different cortico-steroids; the specificity in competitive protein binding (CPB) assays has been improved in some instances by varying the source of the transcortin. Although Murphy (1967) recommended human CBG, with Fuller's earth as the absorbent, for maximum specificity for cortisol, Ficher *et al.* (1973) later showed that horse serum provides better specificity and sensitivity.

In certain instances the specificity of the conventional CPB assay is inadequate. Plasma cortisol concentrations determined by the CPB procedure in newborn infants, cord blood and in patients with the adrenogenital syndrome were significantly different from those determined by a double isotope derivative assay (Iturzaeta et al., 1970). Additional specificity may be obtained by incorporating a purification step before the CPB procedure. Selective extraction (Murphy, 1967), paper chromatography (Iturzaeta et al., 1970), reverse phase thin layer chromatography (Turner et al., 1973) or column chromatography on LH-20 (Murphy and d'Aux, 1972) have been used, but these procedures all add considerably to the time taken to perform the assay and decrease its value as a routine method.

The use of a $[^{75}Se]$ gamma-emitting label in a CPB procedure has recently been recommended (Baum et al., 1974) since radioactivity in the tubes can be counted directly avoiding the time-consuming addition of expensive scintillant. These workers destroyed the binding to endogenous proteins by heat denaturation, thus releasing cortisol and obviating the need for extraction. They further simplified the assay by using Sephadex for separating free and bound steroid. The reagents for this procedure have been made available commercially ("Cortipac", Radiochemical Centre, Amersham) and results obtained using the CPB assay kit and a fluorimetric procedure have been compared (Gore and Lester, 1975; Crowley et al., 1975).

(b) Radioimmunoassay

The general principles of radioimmunoassay have been well summarised in several reviews (Skelley et al., 1973; Abraham, 1974; Cameron et al., 1975) and will therefore not be considered in detail in this section. It is, however, noteworthy that the specificity of all radioimmunoassays (RIA) is critically dependent on the quality of the antibody. Antibodies can not be produced by immunising an animal against the steroid itself, since steroids have too low a molecular weight to be antigenic. A suitable derivative of the steroid is therefore conjugated to a large antigenic carrier molecule, such as bovine serum albumin, and it is this conjugate which is used for immunisation (Fig. 18). Conjugation is achieved by introducing a bifunctional bridging group into the steroid molecule. The position on the steroid through which it is coupled to the carrier molecule is a critical factor in determining the specificity of the antiserum. In general, antisera are comparatively "blind" to changes in the hapten molecule close to the site of conjugation, and have good discrimination against changes distal to the site of conjugation. Thus, if the steroid is coupled via one of its functional groups, this group will not be able to act as a strong antigenic determinant, and antisera generated by such an antigen will be "blind" to changes near the conjugation site.

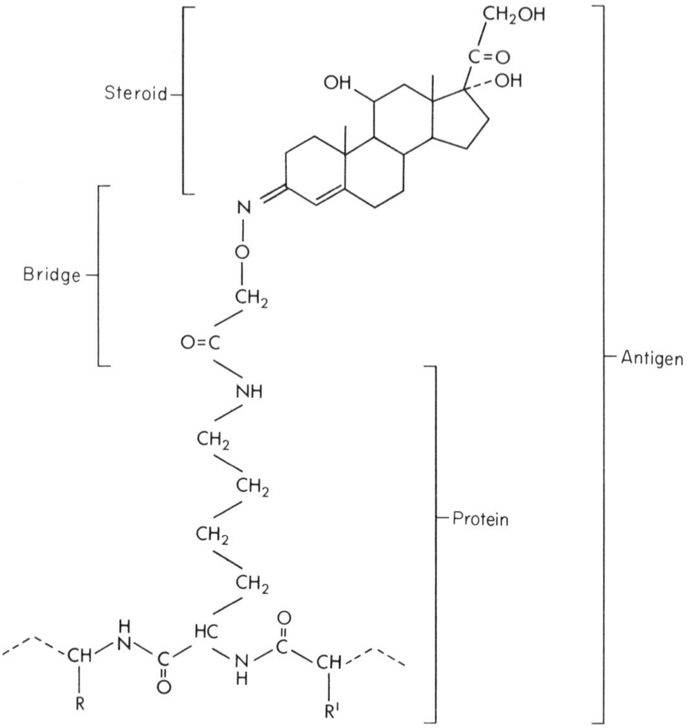

Fig. 18. Structure of the cortisol immunogen cortisol-3-(*O*-carboxymethyl)-oxime/ bovine serum albumin conjugate.

The first radioimmunoassays for cortisol employed the hapten, cortisol-21-hemisuccinate. This compound is comparatively easy to synthesise (Campuzano *et al.*, 1973) but would not be expected to give assays of high specificity with respect to the C-17, C-20 and C-21 positions, since these are close to the site of conjugation. In particular, significant cross-reactions with progesterone and 17α-hydroxyprogesterone would be anticipated.

Although some of the published procedures appear to have adequate specificity, the data in Table 4 show that it is obviously difficult to reproducibly generate specific antisera using the cortisol 21-hemisuccinate hapten. An antiserum raised to a hapten coupled through the A ring would seem likely to show considerably better discrimination against endogenous corticosteroids such as corticosterone. Cortisol-3-(*O*-carboxymethyl)-oxime may be prepared by the procedure of Arnold and James (1971) or that of Janoski *et al.* (1974). Antisera raised to conjugates of this hapten show

Table 4

Cross reactivity of various antisera raised against cortisol-21-hemisuccinate haptens.

Cortisol	100	100	100	100	100
11-Deoxycortisol	—	9	10	100	100
Corticosterone	48	8	1·4	—	30
Cortisone	35	12	—	40	—
17α-Hydroxyprogesterone	—	2·5	—	56	—
Progesterone	—	1	5·5	28	7
Testosterone	7·5	0·3	—	13	6
References	Nieschlag et al. (1974)	Abraham et al. (1972)	Vecsei et al. (1972)	Ruder et al. (1972)	Farmer and Pierce (1974)

considerable specificity and may be produced reproducibly. Data drawn from several independent laboratories are shown in Table 5.

Table 5

Cross reactions of competing steroids with anticortisol-3-BSA sera.

Cortisol	100	100	100
11-Deoxycortisol	7·1	3·8	14
Corticosterone	4·0	12·5	1·7
Cortisone	0·7	6·6	0·29
17α-Hydroxyprogesterone	0·01	0·06	0·04
Progesterone	0·01	0·001	0·18
Testosterone	0·01	0·001	0·01
	Fahmy et al. (1975a)	Dash et al. (1975)	Hasler et al. (1976)

These assays employed an ethanol (Fahmy et al., 1975a) or methylene chloride (Dash et al., 1975) extraction step, and a commercially available [^{3}H]cortisol radioligand. Preassay purification by LH-20 column chromatography was shown not to significantly alter the results obtained.

Further developments in cortisol plasma assays have been directed towards improving robustness, simplicity, cost effectiveness and sample turnover rather than specificity. Introduction of a gamma-emitting radioligand, obviating the use of the expensive scintillation cocktail and disposable counting vials, substantially reduces running costs. The introduction of a [^{75}Se]radioligand (2-methylselenoprednisolone acetate) with cortisol-3 antisera seriously reduces the specificity of the assay (Fahmy et al., 1975b). However, the use of an [^{125}I]radioligand has led to an assay with reduced running costs and an increased potential for automation. Homologous radioligands are available for assays utilising both cortisol-21 (Brombacher et al., 1975) and cortisol-3 (Read et al., 1977) antisera.

Assay simplification has been achieved by using a solid-phase system, to separate the free and bound steroid fractions. This system is extremely tolerant of variation in time and temperature, allowing good results to be achieved by inexperienced technicians. Also antisera, when coupled to a solid phase support, have excellent stability to a reduction in pH. The differential in stability between coupled antisera and endogenous cortisol binding proteins has been exploited to achieve a direct assay for plasma cortisol using both [^{3}H] (Rolleri et al., 1976) and [^{125}I] (Seth and Brown, 1978) radioligands. Other methods used to achieve direct assays for plasma cortisol include heat denaturation (Foster and Dunn, 1974), addition of alcohol (Gomez-Sanchez et al., 1977) and use of proteolytic enzymes (Hasler et al., 1976). All these procedures are directed against the endogenous binding proteins. The use of a direct assay combining a solid phase antiserum and an [^{125}I]radioligand is probably the method of choice for determining plasma cortisol at present (Hindawi et al., 1979; Riad-Fahmy et al., 1979). Laboratories having large numbers of samples to process and adequate staff and facilities, are likely to prepare their own reagents whilst smaller centres will find it economic to arrange supplies from a larger laboratory.

(c) Future developments

Further developments are likely in the field of immunoassays utilising non-radioactive tracers. Enzymeimmunoassays (EIA) have major intrinsic advantages, including removal of any possible radiation hazard, the relative stability of the label, and lower capital costs. A major factor in the cost of beta and gamma-scintillation counters is the sample-changing mechanism. Colourimetric read-out in enzyme assays is essentially instantaneous, and thus manual sampling is practical, and automated sample-change unnecessary. The cheapness and robustness of the capital equipment required is a major factor in the growth of enzymeimmunoassays, especially in Third World countries. The whole topic of enzymeimmunoassay has been recently reviewed (Pal, 1978b; Schuurs and van Weemen, 1977; Wisdom, 1976).

Although the cortisol enzymeimmunoassays reported thus far have lacked sensitivity, it is possible to establish EIAs meeting all usual assay validation criteria, including a sensitivity equal to that of the equivalent

RIA (Joyce *et al.*, 1978). Reported enzymeimmunoassays for cortisol have used antisera raised to cortisol 21-hemisuccinate with cortisol 21-hemisuccinate/β-galactasidase (Comoglio and Celada, 1976), cortisol 21-hemisuccinate/alkaline phosphatase (Ogihara *et al.*, 1977), or cortisol 21-amine/alkaline phosphatase (Kobayashi *et al.*, 1978) conjugates. As previously noted, earlier methods based on the use of cortisol-21 antisera have shown limited specificity. The development of specific EIAs, however, using appropriate cortisol haptens linked to an enzyme via the A ring, could well make enzymeimmunoassay for the determination of cortisol the method of choice for many laboratories.

Another area likely to see important developments is that of fluorimmunoassay. A major factor impeding automation and simplification of immunoassays is the necessity to separate free and bound label before measuring the response parameter. It is feasible, using fluorescence labels, to eliminate the separation stage by, for example, spin polarisation fluorescence (Watson *et al.*, 1976) or by the radiationless energy transfer technique using labelled antibody and labelled ligand (Ullman *et al.*, 1976). Application of fluorescence immunoassays to cortisol is to be anticipated in the near future.

The general problems and applications of non-isotopic immunoassays is considered in some detail in Ch. I.

(d) Cortisol reference procedures

A growing awareness of the importance of quality control of hormone assays has led to a need for the provision of pools of plasma with an accurately known hormone concentration. Whilst known amounts of pure steroid may be added to plasma of low steroid content this is an inadequate measure since such samples will fail to discriminate between various assay procedures of different specificity. The requirements of a reference procedure are essentially different from those of a routine clinical assay procedure. Simplicity and rapid sample turnover may be neglected if the assay is improved with respect to accuracy, precision and specificity.

The double isotope derivative technique of James *et al.* (1967) has been mentioned previously. Another reference assay is that of gas chromatography with electron capture detection (Mason and Fraser, 1975). However, in this procedure cortisol is oxidised prior to derivatisation, yielding the androstenedione heptafluorobutyrate derivative. Since other corticosteroids such as cortisone and 21-deoxycortisol will yield the same derivative, the specificity of the procedure is heavily dependent on the efficiency of the first paper chromatography step.

Gas chromatography–mass spectrometry is currently accepted as the reference procedure of choice for steroids (Bjorkhem *et al.*, 1974; Breuer and

Siekmann, 1975; Brooks and Gaskell, 1979). Use of high resolution ion monitoring confers an additional selectivity on a technique which has high intrinsic accuracy and a reference procedure, using high resolution mass spectrometry with gas chromatography, has been established in the Tenovus Institute laboratories, for the measurement of plasma cortisol. A simplified assay scheme is shown in Fig. 19.

Deuterated. cortisol is added as a recovery standard to each plasma. Cortisol is extracted with methylene chloride and then derivatised to give the methyloxime. Cortisol ethyloxime is then added as a reference standard and the trimethylsilyl derivatives formed. Selected ion detection at 605.3626, 608.3814 and 619.3782 atomic mass units of the derivatives of cortisol, deuterated cortisol, and the ethyloxime standard then allowed the determination of the cortisol content of the plasma.

While this reference procedure is relatively slow, requiring considerable technical skill, and extremely expensive equipment, these factors are not of overriding importance since only small numbers of samples are required to validate an assay or to establish reference materials for national or even international quality control schemes. A reference procedure must give high specificity and accuracy, and the excellent agreement of data produced by Dr S. Gaskell in the Tenovus Institute using the procedure outlined above, with results produced by four other European laboratories using independent GC–MS procedures, suggest that the high resolution GC–MS method fulfils these requirements. The comparison of data forms part of a programme for the production of reference materials which has been established under the auspices of the European Economic Community Bureau of Reference (Hjelm, 1978).

3. 6β-Hydroxycortisol

This polar steroid is the major unconjugated cortisol metabolite in urine and is excreted in increased amounts during late pregnancy and by neonates (Pal, 1978). Although limited hydroxylation at C-6 apparently occurs in adrenal tissue, hepatic hydroxylating enzyme systems would seem to be largely responsible for this biotransformation. Since similar enzyme systems metabolise many drugs, it has been suggested (Park, 1978) that changes in the urinary output of 6β-hydroxycortisol may provide an index of hepatic drug metabolising enzymes. Use of the urinary levels of 6β-hydroxycortisol for this purpose presupposes a simple, precise and specific assay procedure and until recently such a method has not been available. However, this steroid can now be determined by a fluorimetric method following chromatography (Pal, 1979), or by a direct radioimmunoassay (Park, 1978). The latter uses an antiserum raised against an antigen in which 6β-hydroxycortisol

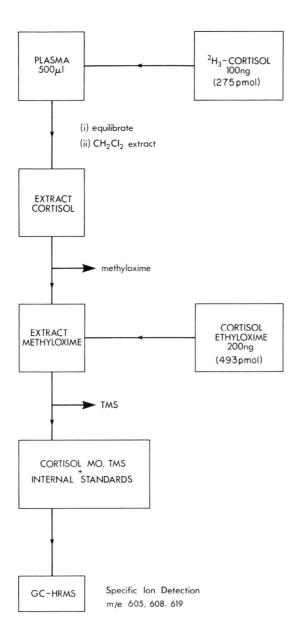

Fig. 19. Flow chart of the reference assay procedure for determination of plasma cortisol concentrations by GC-hr MS.

was linked to bovine serum albumin through the 3-position (Park *et al.*, 1976). The antiserum shows good discrimination against cortisol metabolites formed by reduction of the A ring. Preassay purification, using either thin layer or paper chromatography, did not significantly alter the concentrations determined.

4. 11-Deoxycortisol (Reichstein's Compound S)

Interest in the determination of this steroid has largely reflected its use in the evaluation of pituitary–adrenal reserve by the metyrapone (Metopirone) test. Metyrapone blocks conversion of 11-deoxycortisol to cortisol: the fall in circulating cortisol levels stimulates ACTH release which feeds back to stimulate adrenal steroidogenesis. Since 11-hydroxylation remains pharmacologically blocked the net result is an increase in synthesis and secretion of 11-deoxycortisol. A normal response to metyrapone was formerly assessed by determination of urinary oxogenic steroids or by an equivalent nonspecific colourimetric procedure. Subjects with an intact pituitary–adrenal axis will show a significant rise in urinary corticosteroid metabolites. Assessment of an adequate response using urinary analyses requires from two to five, complete 24-hr urine collections, a time-consuming, expensive procedure. The use of competitive protein binding assays to measure 11-deoxycortisol in plasma was therefore advantageous (Strott *et al.*, 1969) but it is important to ensure that the dose of metyrapone administered will effectively block 11-hydroxylation. This is achieved by determining cortisol in addition to 11-deoxycortisol, using specific assays for each hormone. Both steroids may be measured by competitive protein binding assays following differential extraction using carbon tetrachloride then dichloromethane (Spark, 1971) or after separation on an LH-20 Sephadex column (Newsome *et al.*, 1972).

Both steroids have also been measured by a radioimmunoassay procedure using commercially available reagents, also after LH-20 chromatography (Brown *et al.*, 1976). An elegant procedure has been described by Kao *et al.* (1975) where direct radioimmunoassays are used to determine cortisol and 11-deoxycortisol using antibodies having negligible cross-reactions with the other steroid. Whilst this appears to be a very useful technique, its general applicability must be questioned since most cortisol antisera previously described have demonstrated significant cross-reaction with 11-deoxycortisol.

5. Corticosterone

A radioimmunoassay procedure for determining corticosterone has been reported, using an antiserum raised to a corticosterone-21-hemisuccinate conjugate (Gross *et al.*, 1972). The specificity of the antiserum is not high but the simple RIA of mouse plasma samples was claimed to give results in good agreement with those obtained in an assay incorporating a chromatographic procedure. While it appears unlikely that corticosterone in human plasma could be measured accurately by the simple assay, since cortisol has a 17% cross reaction with the antiserum used, it can be measured by a competitive protein-binding assay procedure after LH-20 chromatography (Newsome *et al.*, 1972), or by radioimmunoassay after paper chromatography (Nabors *et al.*, 1974). A gas liquid chromatography procedure with electron capture detection is also available as a reference procedure for this steroid (Mason and Fraser, 1975).

6. 11-Deoxycorticosterone (DOC)

Two excellent reference procedures are available for assay of this steroid in plasma. The original double isotope derivative procedure (Arnold and James, 1971) allowed the measurement of the concentration range in normal subjects. In brief [^{14}C]DOC was added to plasma (20–25 ml), which was then extracted with methylene chloride. Following acetylation with [^{3}H] acetic anhydride, the [^{3}H]DOC-acetate was purified by two-dimensional thin-layer chromatography, diluted with carrier, then repurified by paper chromatography. The product was reduced enzymatically and the derivative purified by two further paper chromatography steps before determination of the [^{14}C]/[^{3}H] ratio. The procedure lacks sensitivity (4 ng/ml; 12.1 nmol/l) and therefore relatively large volumes of plasma are required.

The second reference procedure is that of Wilson and Fraser (1971), which employs gas-liquid chromatography (GLC). Deoxycorticosterone is extracted from plasma and acetylated, the product being purified by thin-layer chromatography. After hydrolysis, the steroid is rechromatographed, then derivatised to yield the heptafluorobutyrate (HFB). Progesterone HFB is used as the internal standard for the GLC step which uses an electron capture detector. This is an excellent reference procedure requiring rather less plasma than the double isotope derivative method, but is too time-consuming for a routine clinical assay and the method makes high demands on the technical ability of the analyst.

The low sensitivity and intense labour requirements of the reference procedures are largely overcome in the radioimmunoassay described by Arnold and James (1971). The specificity of the antiserum, raised to a 11-deoxycorticosterone 3-(*O*-carboxymethyl)oxime/bovine serum albumin conjugate, was disappointing; complete cross reaction being demonstrated with progesterone and major interference from corticosterone. A paper chromatography step was therefore incorporated in the assay procedure and excellent agreement with both the reference methods was demonstrated.

7. 18-Hydroxy-11-deoxycorticosterone

The role of 18-hydroxy-11-deoxycorticosterone (18-OH-DOC) in human hypertension is still unclear but lack of a simple and specific assay capable of measuring circulating plasma levels of this steroid has undoubtedly hindered the elucidation of its physiological function.

Circulating levels were first measured directly by Mason and Fraser (1975), using gas chromatography and electron capture detection. The steroid was extracted from plasma using dichloromethane, purified by paper chromatography, oxidised to the gamma-lactone, repurified by a second paper chromatography step and then derivatised to yield the heptafluoro-butyrate, before GLC quantitation using an aldactone internal standard. The method is obviously technically demanding and requires 5 ml of plasma.

Assay of this steroid was simplified by the introduction of a radio-immunoassay procedure by Chandler et al. (1976) who raised an antiserum to an 18-OH-DOC-3-(O-carboxymethyl)oxime/bovine serum albumin con-jugate. Specificity of the antiserum appeared to be satisfactory except for the significant cross-reaction (60%) with 18-hydroxycorticosterone. This inter-ference was completely eliminated by routinely incorporating a single paper chromatography preassay purification step, since an additional paper chromatography step in a different solvent system did not significantly lower the concentrations determined. Similar conclusions were reached by Dale et al. (1976). Using an antiserum raised to a similar conjugate, the cross-reaction of 18-hydroxycorticosterone was only 7% but a thin-layer chromatography step was routinely performed before radioimmunoassay. Again Sulon and Sparano (1978) report a RIA using an antiserum raised to a similar conjugate but the cross reaction of 18-hydroxycorticosterone is only 0·9%. The authors therefore advocate a non-chromatographic radio-immunoassay and support the specificity of their procedure by the excellent agreement demonstrated in concentrations determined by the direct RIA and by a GLC procedure based on that of Mason and Fraser (1975). However, the normal range (20–160 ng/100 ml; 0·6–4·6 nmol/l) is significantly higher than that reported by Sulon and Sparano (1978) (10·1 ± 6·5 ng/100 ml (291 ± 188 pmol/l) in the supine subject, 9·4 ± 4·2 ng/100 ml (271 ± 121 pmol/l) after movement). After prolonged dexamethasone treatment, Mason and Fraser (1975) reported levels of 37 ± 18 ng/100 ml (1068 ± 519 pmol/l) whereas Sulon and Sparano (1978) quote levels of 2·3 ± 0·8 ng/100 ml (66 ± 23 pmol/l). The agreement among Sulon and Sparano (1978), Dale et al. (1976) and Chandler et al. (1976) as to the normal level (approximately 9 ng/100 ml; 260 pmol/l) would appear to cast enough doubt on the data of Mason and Fraser (1975) to rule out use of the GLC method as a reference procedure. It is possible that the differences in reported normal ranges are not methodological but due to differences in sampling due to salt load, stress, time of day, and posture, and to variation caused by episodic secretion. Variation in these factors may also significantly alter the plasma concentrations of steroids which will cross-react with the antiserum. Until more data are available it would appear advisable to use the highest specificity antisera available and to continue to incorporate a chromatography step if accurate results are to be reported.

8. 18-Hydroxycorticosterone

This steroid is the putative precursor of aldosterone although evidence that it is indeed a true intermediate is equivocal. The endocrinology of the steroid has been reviewed recently (Fraser and Lantos, 1978). As with 18-OH-DOC circulating levels of the steroid have been determined by GLC using electron capture detection and by radioimmunoassay. In the procedure using GLC (Wilson et al., 1976), the steroid was oxidised to the 11-oxo-gamma lactone and then purified by paper chromatography before derivatisation to the 3-enyl heptafluorobutyrate. The RIA similarly uses the formation of the gamma lactone to reduce problems of ring isomerisation (Martin et al., 1975). Antisera were raised to the 3-(O-carboxymethyl)-oxime derivative of the gamma lactone and are highly specific, apart from a 100% cross-reaction with the gamma lactone of 18-hydroxy-DOC. The label used in the radioimmunoassay was prepared using the mitochondrial fraction from Aylesbury duck adrenal glands to convert [³H]corticosterone to [³H]18-hydroxy-corticosterone. A paper chromatography purification was included routinely to eliminate interference from 18-OH-DOC. The normal ranges quoted for the GLC procedure (6–16 ng/100 ml (166–441 pmol/l) in recumbent subjects, 13–42 ng/100 ml (359–1159 pmol/l) in the standing position) and the RIA (3–25 ng/100 ml; 83–690 pmol/l) appear to be in excellent agreement, given the problems in assessing comparability of sampling. The technically simple radioimmunoassay would appear to be the assay of choice at this time.

9. 17α-Hydroxyprogesterone

Estimations of 17α-hydroxyprogesterone are principally of use in the diagnosis and management of congenital adrenal hyperplasia (CAH). Urinary analyses for these purposes, based on the determination of pregnanetriol (Shackleton et al., 1972), or the 11-oxygenation index (Clayton et al., 1971), can give misleading results in the neonatal period and the collection of urine in neonates often presents difficulties. In contrast, measurement of 17α-hydroxyprogesterone in plasma has diagnostic significance in CAH during the first days of life (Youssefnejadian and David, 1975). An assay for the accurate measurement of 17α-hydroxyprogesterone in plasma was first described by Strott and Lipsett (1968). Alkalinised plasma was ether extracted and the extracted steroid was purified by thin-layer chromatography both before and after an acetylation procedure. The 17α-hydroxyprogesterone concentration in the final eluate was determined by a competitive protein binding assay. The assay has good specificity, but lacks sensitivity, 3 ml of plasma being required, and is obviously slow and technically demanding. A modification of this method by Stone et al. (1971), using Celite column chromatography was claimed to have the advantages of simultaneously assaying progesterone and 17α-hydroxyprogesterone, lower assay blanks, and a greater sample throughput. The method was simplified further by replacing the chromatographic step by a simple partition between water and carbon tetrachloride (Pham-Huu-Trung et al., 1973) or by the use of a relatively non-polar solvent for extraction such as 2% ethanol in petroleum spirit (Barnes and Atherden, 1972). These simplified procedures lack specificity for 17α-hydroxyprogesterone; progesterone in particular will interfere. This limited specificity will not prevent accurate diagnosis of CAH but could possibly affect its use in monitoring treatment, especially in the pubertal female.

The first radioimmunoassays introduced for determination of 17α-hydroxyprogesterone contributed little to specificity. Early antisera were raised to an 11-deoxycortisol-21-hemisuccinate hapten (Abraham et al., 1971) and the specificity of these antisera was such that preassay purification was essential. Purification may be effected by thin layer (Wickings, 1975) or column chromatography (Jänne et al., 1975) procedures. Specificity of an antiserum raised to a 6-(O-carboxymethyl)-oxime derivative of 17α-hydroxyprogesterone appears to be superior (Hughes and Winter, 1976), but LH-20 column chromatography purification was advocated. Satisfactory cross reactions were reported by Pang et al. (1977) for an assay using a hapten conjugated at C-7 but the nature of the hapten, and the necessity or otherwise of preassay chromatography, are poorly described. Cross reactions of an antiserum raised to 17α-hydroxyprogesterone-3-(O-carboxymethyl)-oxime have been described (Youssefnejadian et al., 1972) but an LH-20 column chromatography step was considered necessary to remove progesterone. However, chromatography has been shown not to be necessary to obtain accurate concentrations of plasma 17α-hydroxyprogesterone in children when using an antiserum provided by Dr Loriaux's group at the National Institutes of Health Bethesda (Walker et al., 1979) and similar results have been obtained recently using an antiserum raised in our laboratories to a

17α-hydroxyprogesterone-3-(*O*-carboxymethyl)-oxime conjugate.

Radioimmunoassays appear likely to steadily displace competitive protein binding procedures in the determination of 17α-hydroxyprogesterone since the specificity of the antisera becoming available will facilitate assay simplification, and the increased sensitivity will be of value in monitoring the low levels seen in adequately treated patients and in identifying heterozygote carriers with a partial 21-hydroxylase deficiency (Lee and Gareis, 1975).

10. Urinary Free Cortisol

It is well known that isolated plasma samples taken from patients with clinically proven Cushing's disease may have cortisol concentrations that fall in the normal range. In such cases determination of the 24-hr urinary free cortisol output is a more reliable index of adrenocortisol hyperfunction. A procedure was described by Murphy (1968) in which cortisol was extracted from urine using methylene chloride and determined in a simple competitive protein binding assay using CBG. Although the assay is claimed to be highly specific for cortisol little evidence is presented: the suppression of urinary free cortisol by dexamethasone to low concentrations is a necessary, but by no means sufficient, criterion of specificity. The use of competitive protein binding determination of urinary free cortisol in the diagnosis of Cushing's syndrome has been reviewed (Burke and Beardwell, 1973). A radioimmunoassay procedure was introduced by Ruder *et al.* (1972), using antisera generated to cortisol 21-hemisuccinate antigens. The antisera had comparatively poor specificity, and a thin-layer chromatography purification was essential if accurate urine concentrations were to be determined. However, the assay was more sensitive and had a greatly improved dynamic range compared with the CPB procedure. Data from another group using a similar antiserum (Chattaraj *et al.*, 1976) demonstrated significantly lower apparent cortisol concentrations when LH-20 chromatography was replaced by a thin-layer chromatographic purification procedure. It is possible that use of the more specific cortisol antisera currently available, raised to cortisol-3-(*O*-carboxymethyl)oxime antigens, will significantly reduce the discrepancy between assays performed with and without preassay chromatographic purification.

It has been suggested (Mattingly and Tyler, 1976) that since circadian rhythm is abnormal in Cushing's syndrome an overnight urine collection, rather than a complete 24-hr collection, is adequate to identify subjects producing excess cortisol: urinary 11-hydroxycorticosteroid concentrations, measured fluorometrically, were shown to be significantly higher in women with Cushing's syndrome than in normal, hirsute or obese controls. It appears probable that overnight collections could be applied to the urinary free cortisol determination with equal success. Obviously concomitant kidney disease, with altered renal handling, may give highly misleading results in any determination using urinary concentrations.

11. Salivary Cortisol

The importance of stimulation and suppression tests in the accurate assessment of adrenal status is now well accepted but repeated venepuncture is unpopular with both physicians and patients. The measurement of cortisol concentrations in either mixed saliva or in parotid fluid provides an attractive alternative. Collection of saliva is stress-free and therefore well suited to tests requiring multiple sampling. Because the cortisol concentration in saliva reflects the free or non-protein-bound fraction in plasma, normal salivary cortisol concentrations are seen in conditions where there is an abnormality in the level of plasma cortisol binding protein, such as in women taking contraceptive steroid preparations. Normal urinary free cortisol levels are also found, but determination of salivary cortisol may replace determination of urinary free cortisol since the newer procedure eliminates the difficulties of ensuring a complete 24-hr urine collection whilst providing similar clinical data.

A sensitive direct RIA has been established for the measurement of salivary cortisol concentrations (Walker, et al., 1978). Responses to dexamethasone suppression and Synacthen stimulation have been determined in normal subjects, low levels established in patients with adrenal insufficiency, and high concentrations with abolished diurnal rhythm in patients with Cushing's syndrome. The salivary steroid levels accurately reflected concomitant changes in plasma concentrations, in particular a clear circadian rhythm was demonstrated. Since saliva is readily collected, and salivary cortisol can be measured accurately by a simple, direct RIA this procedure appears likely to achieve wide usage, particularly in screening procedures.

12. Salivary 17α-Hydroxyprogesterone

Determination of the concentration of 17α-hydroxyprogesterone in plasma is of established value in the initial diagnosis of congenital adrenal hyperplasia and has also been advocated for monitoring the adequacy of treatment (Lippe et al., 1974; Bacon et al., 1977). However, repeated venepuncture in children is stressful and requires the patient to attend a clinic. Development of a sensitive RIA (Walker et al., 1979) has facilitated determination of a provisional "normal range" for the 17α-hydroxyprogesterone concentration in saliva. Concentrations in saliva from patients with proven CAH were up to 38 fold higher than those in normal subjects, and showed a good correlation with concentrations in matched plasma samples. Since saliva can be collected easily by a stress-free procedure, use of salivary 17-hydroxy-progesterone assays will permit more detailed monitoring of therapy in patients with CAH. This will facilitate optimum corticosteroid therapy, providing each child with the opportunity to achieve its growth potential.

H. PATHOLOGICAL VARIATIONS IN CORTICOSTEROID PRODUCTION

Clinically, the most important corticosteroids produced by the adrenal cortex are cortisol and aldosterone. Diseases of the adrenal cortex are associated in the main with increased or decreased production of these two hormones. These topics are considered here, and also in Ch. IV. Abnormal aldosterone production is discussed in Ch. X.

1. Increased Cortisol Production

Cushing's syndrome refers to the constellation of symptoms and signs which occur as a result of increased circulating concentrations of cortisol from whatever cause. Cushing, in 1932, described 12 cases of a disorder which he suggested were due to pituitary basophilism. The eponym, Cushing's disease, should therefore only apply to cases of hypercortisolism of pituitary or hypothalamic origin, whereas other cases of hypercortisolism of endogenous or exogenous origin are examples of Cushing's syndrome. The availability of assays for measurement of plasma ACTH concentrations has provided a useful aetiological classification for Cushing's syndrome or hypercortisolism.

ACTH dependent:

(i) bilateral adrenocortical hyperplasia (Cushing's disease) secondary to increased pituitary ACTH secretion,

(ii) ectopic ACTH syndrome resulting in hypercortisolism secondary to increased ACTH secretion of non-pituitary origin,

(iii) iatrogenic hypercortisolism secondary to treatment with ACTH or its synthetic analogues.

Non-ACTH dependent:

(i) tumours of the adrenal cortex, either adenomas or carcinomas,

(ii) iatrogenic hypercortisolism secondary to treatment with excessive amounts of cortisol or its synthetic analogues.

I

The clinical features of hypercortisolism include truncal obesity, plethoric moon face, striae formation, ecchymoses, hypertension and glucose intolerance. Females, in addition, may be hirsute and amenorrhoeic. The cardinal feature of Cushing's syndrome in children is growth failure. There are numerous laboratory tests available for confirming the diagnosis of hypercortisolism. It is essential to document increased concentrations of circulating cortisol. Some centres still rely on measurement of urinary metabolites of cortisol and a 24-hr urinary 17-oxogenic steroid determination when expressed as a function of creatinine excretion can be a reliable indicator of the presence or absence of hypercortisolism (Streeton et al., 1969). Values in excess of 6·5 mg/g creatinine are suggestive of hypercortisolism. The measurement of 24-hr urinary free cortisol has been shown to be of value in the diagnosis of hypercortisolism (Burke and Beardwell, 1973). Normal values range from 0–95 µg/day (0–262 nmol/day) in adults. Urinary free cortisol is normal in obesity, which can occasionally be confused with Cushing's syndrome.

Measurement of urinary corticosteroid excretion is now being replaced by determination of plasma cortisol concentrations for the investigation of hypercortisolism. The various methods available to determine plasma cortisol concentrations have been detailed previously. Random measurements of plasma cortisol or corticosteroids are seldom useful in confirming a clinical diagnosis of hypercortisolism. It is necessary to demonstrate, if possible, a loss of the normal diurnal rhythm in plasma concentrations of corticosteroids. This is illustrated in Fig. 20. Two patients with Cushing's disease and one patient with Cushing's syndrome due to an adrenal adenoma

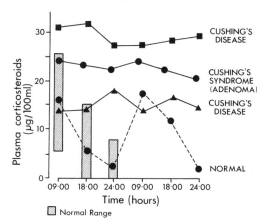

Fig. 20. Diurnal rhythm of plasma corticosteroids in normal subjects, Cushing's disease and adrenal adenoma (1 µg/100 ml ≃ 28 nmol/l) (from Besser and Edwards, 1972).

demonstrate an absence of a diurnal pattern in plasma corticosteroid concentrations, in contrast to a normal subject who shows the usual fall in plasma corticosteroid concentrations during the late afternoon and evening, and a subsequent rise during the early hours of the morning. As a general rule, the midnight plasma corticosteroid level should be about 50% of its early morning value (normally 7–22 µg/dl (195–610 nmol/l) as measured by the competitive protein binding method). Some of the highest plasma corticosteroid concentrations are found in patients with Cushing's syndrome due to the ectopic ACTH syndrome (Nugent and Mayes, 1966). It is important to establish whether an elevated plasma corticosteroid level can be suppressed by exogenous corticosteroids. A useful screening test for Cushing's syndrome is the measurement of plasma cortisol at 08.00 hr following the administration of 1 mg (2·5 µmol) dexamethasone by mouth the previous night (Nichols et al., 1965). Most normal subjects and those with simple obesity suppress to plasma cortisol levels < 6 µg/dl (< 166 nmol/l) (Pavlatos et al., 1965). Recently, this test, although extremely useful as an out-patient investigation, has been shown not to be completely reliable since it has failed to detect one of an unknown number of patients with Cushing's syndrome, probably due to an unusually slow turnover of the dexamethasone (Meikle et al., 1975). The dexamethasone suppression test devised by Liddle (1960) has been used extensively as a diagnostic test in Cushing's syndrome. Classically, normal subjects and obese patients suppress plasma and urinary corticosteroid levels following low dose dexamethasone therapy (0·5 mg (1·3 µmol) every 6 hr for 2 days). Urinary 17-oxogenic steroid levels should fall to less than 4 mg/24 hr or less than 1–2 mg/g creatinine. A higher dose of dexamethasone (2 mg (5·1 µmol) every 6 hr for 2 days) is employed if no suppression has occurred in order to distinguish adrenal hyperplasia as a result of pituitary hyperfunction from Cushing's syndrome due to a non-pituitary cause. In the former case, suppression of plasma or urinary corticosteroid levels usually occurs with the high dose of dexamethasone, whereas no suppression occurs with an adrenal tumour or the ectopic ACTH syndrome. Unfortunately, the dexamethasone suppression test is not entirely reliable and there are reports of patients with bilateral adrenocortical hyperplasia failing to suppress on the high dose of dexamethasone (Cope, 1972) and cases of adrenal carcinoma which do suppress with dexamethasone administration (Rayfield et al., 1971). Rarely, a patient with Cushing's syndrome may exhibit a paradoxical response to dexamethasone by demonstrating a marked increase in plasma and urinary corticosteroid levels (French et al., 1969). Treatment should not be based, therefore, on the results of this test alone. The metyrapone test can sometimes be useful in distinguishing bilateral adrenal hyperplasia from Cushing's syndrome secondary to an adrenal tumour (Tyler and West, 1972). In the former, there is an exaggerated response in plasma 11-deoxycortisol and urinary 17-OHCS levels when compared to levels in normal subjects. When given to patients with adrenal tumours, metyrapone fails to elicit a rise in plasma 11-deoxycortisol levels and its urinary metabolites, due to the chronically suppressed hypothalamic–pituitary axis failing to release ACTH. However, it is possible to have a normal response with adrenal tumours (Crystal et al., 1970) and a positive response in the ectopic ACTH syndrome. The response to exogenous ACTH stimulation is not reliable in distinguishing the various types of Cushing's syndrome. Probably the most useful test now available to discriminate between bilateral adrenal hyperplasia (Cushing's disease) and adrenal tumour is measurement of plasma ACTH concentrations. The basal levels of plasma ACTH in patients with bilateral adrenal hyperplasia, adrenal tumour and the ectopic ACTH syndrome are shown in Fig. 21. In Cushing's disease, morning plasma ACTH concentrations can be normal (up to 80 ng/l) or elevated up to 250 ng/l. In contrast, plasma ACTH levels in cases due to adrenal tumour are invariably suppressed below the lower limit of sensitivity of the immunoassay. The highest ACTH levels are usually seen in Cushing's syndrome caused by ectopic ACTH production. The sources of ACTH in this syndrome include tumours of the lung and bronchi, thymus, pancreas, liver, ovary, breast and thyroid. Despite the markedly elevated plasma corticosteroid levels often seen in the ectopic ACTH syndrome, the clinical features of Cushing's syndrome are usually absent. Instead, the patients with this syndrome exhibit signs of marked weight loss and cachexia as a result of the underlying malignancy. They are often pigmented and have marked muscle wasting and weakness, oedema and a hypokalaemic alkalosis. The last feature is probably associated with the higher plasma cortisol concentrations found in this syndrome, but some of these patients do produce large quantities of the mineralocorticosteroids, corticosterone and 11-deoxycorticosterone (Schambelan et al., 1971).

The cortisol secretion rate is usually elevated in patients with hypercortisolism. The normal cortisol secretion rate ranges from 6·3–28·6 mg/day (17·4–78·9 µmol/day) (Cope and Pearson, 1965) and when expressed in relation to body surface area, it is independent of age. Thus the normal cortisol secretion rate in children and adults is 11·8 ± 2·5 (S.E.M.) mg/M^2/day (31·7 ± 6·9 (S.E.M.) µmol/M^2/day) (Kenny et al., 1966). Cope and Pearson (1965) found a mean cortisol secretion rate of 64 mg/day (176 µmol/day) (range 36–138 (99–381 µmol)) in 26 cases of bilateral adrenal hyperplasia. The highest secretion rates occur in cases with adrenal tumour and in the ectopic ACTH syndrome. Since measurement of the cortisol secretion rate requires the administration of isotopically labelled cortisol and chromatographic purification of urinary cortiscosteroids, the technique is seldom used in clinical practice.

There is an abundance of tests available for the investigation of suspected Cushing's syndrome. The currently most frequently used tests include the following:

(i)   basal 24-hr urinary free cortisol,
(ii) plasma cortisol determination at midnight and 08.00 hr,
(iii) overnight dexamethasone suppression test,
(iv) low and high dose dexamethasone suppression test of Liddle,
(v)   Metyrapone test,
(vi) insulin hypoglycaemia (see p. 193),
(vii) plasma ACTH determinations.

Recently, with the use of sensitive and specific radioimmunoassays, it has been possible to determine cortisol concentrations in saliva (Walker *et al.*, 1978). The ease of saliva collection by non-stressful techniques is a distinct advantage in the assessment of adrenocortical function. Preliminary studies (Figs 22 and 23) indicate that saliva cortisol concentrations closely reflect concentrations of cortisol in plasma. Thus two patients with Cushing's

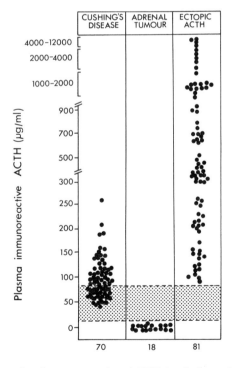

Fig 21. Plasma morning immunoreactive ACTH levels in patients with Cushing's disease, adrenal tumour and the ectopic ACTH syndrome. The shaded area is the normal range at 09.00 hr (from Rees and Landon, 1976).

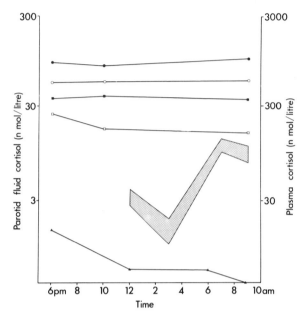

Fig. 22. Diurnal variation of parotid fluid cortisol concentration in four normal subjects, (shaded area), diurnal variation in plasma (filled symbols) and parotid fluid (open symbols) cortisol in two patients with Cushing's syndrome (subjects 1 and 2), and cortisol suppression in parotid fluid by dexamethasone ($\blacktriangle$) (1 nmol/l = 36·25 ng/dl).

disease showed an absence of diurnal rhythm in saliva cortisol levels, one patient with primary adrenal insufficiency failed to demonstrate an increase in saliva cortisol concentrations following ACTH stimulation and a normal subject had suppressed saliva cortisol levels after dexamethasone administration. Since cortisol in saliva is non-protein bound, the use of a saliva as a biological fluid to study adrenocortical function has the added advantage that it reflects the free or biologically active cortisol concentration.

Pituitary dependent bilateral adrenal hyperplasia (Cushing's disease) accounts for 80% of the cases of Cushing's syndrome, excluding the ectopic ACTH syndrome and Cushing's syndrome resulting from exogenously administered glucocorticoid and ACTH preparations. However, iatrogenic causes of Cushing's syndrome as a result of treatment are the most common. Systemic glucocorticoid therapy is used for a wide variety of clinical conditions. When administered in pharmacologic amounts, they suppress the release of CRF and ACTH and result in functional adrenal insufficiency. Their suppressive effect is related to dosages, duration of therapy and mode of administration. The clinical signs are indistinguishable from those produced by an excess of endogenous cortisol. The most potent glucocorticoid when compared with cortisol on a weight basis, and commonly used in clinical practice is dexamethasone. It is at least 30 times as potent as cortisol in terms of glucocorticoid potency. In an attempt to prevent adrenal insufficiency pharmacologic doses of corticosteroids can be administered on alternate days with some degree of success (MacGregor et al., 1969). The withdrawal of steroid therapy and the assessment of hypothalamic–pituitary–adrenal reserve is discussed later.

Non-pathological changes in plasma cortisol concentrations can occur due to alterations in the concentration of corticosteroid binding globulin (CBG). Since nearly 80% of plasma cortisol is bound to CBG, total plasma cortisol levels will vary with changes in CBG concentrations. Thus with oestrogen administration (Sandberg et al., 1964) and during pregnancy (Rosenthal et al., 1969) quite marked increased levels of CBG occur. Consequently, the concentration of plasma cortisol rises several-fold during pregnancy or oestrogen administration and is not the result of increased cortisol secretion by the adrenal cortex (Migeon et al., 1968). Concentrations of CBG can be affected by various drugs (Nelson, 1969), protein-losing states and hepatic dysfunction. Inherited variations in CBG concentrations occur with either decreases (Doe et al., 1965) or increases (Lohrenz et al., 1968) in the levels of this binding protein. Since the unbound or free cortisol is unaltered in these situations, no clinical abnormalities are associated with the changes in CBG concentration.

2. Decreased Cortisol Production

The adrenal cortex synthesises three classes of steroid hormones—glucocorticosteroids (cortisol), mineralocorticosteroids and androgens. This section deals mainly with disorders resulting in decreased cortisol production. Adrenal insufficiency may be primary (Addison's disease) in which production of all three classes of steroids is deficient or secondary to reduced trophic hormone stimulation by ACTH, when the disorder is usually confined to subnormal cortisol production. Congenital adrenal hyperplasia is functionally a disorder of adrenal insufficiency and is discussed in this section.

(a) Primary adrenal insufficiency (Addison's disease)

Before clinical signs of adrenal insufficiency appear, more than 90% of the adrenal glands must be destroyed. Idiopathic atrophy (probably auto-immune) and tuberculous destruction of the adrenal glands account for more than 90% of cases. Other causes include histoplasmosis, amyloidosis and metastatic carcinoma involving the adrenals. The major clinical features of primary adrenal insufficiency are weakness, weight loss, increased skin pigmentation, hypotension, gastro-intestinal symptoms and menstrual disorders in females. The diagnosis is established by demonstrating a sub-normal response of the adrenal cortex to ACTH stimulation. Basal plasma cortisol concentrations are usually less than 3 µg/dl (83 nmol/l), but it is essential to examine the plasma cortisol response to administration of ACTH. In a short-term ACTH test, plasma cortisol is measured 30 and 60 min after an i.v. or i.m. injection of 250 µg synthetic β^{1-24} corticotrophin (Synacthen). In general, plasma cortisol concentrations range from 18–40 µg/dl (497–1104 nmol/l) at 30 min and 25–50 µg/dl (690–1380 nmol/l) at 60 min in normal subjects (Grieg et al., 1969). At least a 2 fold increase over base-line plasma cortisol levels should be obtained. A suboptimal response does not necessarily indicate adrenal insufficiency and a more pro-longed ACTH stimulation should be performed either using a 4–6 hr i.v. infusion of ACTH (Landon et al., 1964) or a long-acting preparation of ACTH such as tetracosactrin depot (Besser et al., 1967). Some patients with secondary adrenal insufficiency will only respond following prolonged ACTH stimulation. Plasma concentrations of ACTH are markedly elevated in primary adrenal insufficiency (up to 1200 ng/l) whereas they are usually undetectable in adrenal insufficiency secondary to hypopituitarism and to excessive systemic steroid therapy (Besser et al., 1971).

There have been several reports of cases in whom clinical symptoms and signs of adrenal insufficiency occur in association with elevated ACTH levels and decreased cortisol production. There is no response to exogenous ACTH stimulation, but in contrast to true Addison's disease, salt-wasting is not a feature and patients are able to retain sodium in the face of a low salt diet (Migeon et al., 1968; Thistlethwaite et al., 1975). There is a familial pattern to these cases and it has been suggested that the primary defect is at the adrenal ACTH receptor or post-receptor site (Spark and Etzkorm, 1977).

Congenital adrenal hypoplasia is an inherited disorder which presents clinically in early life as salt-losing adrenal insufficiency (Pakravan et al., 1974). The absence of increased plasma concentrations of adrenal steroid precursors distinguishes it from the more common salt-losing congenital adrenal hyperplasia affecting a male infant. The pattern of inheritance can either be autosomal recessive (Karenyi, 1961) or X-linked recessive (Weiss and Mellinger, 1970); both exhibit distinct types of histology. Management of this disorder is similar to Addison's disease, requiring replacement therapy with glucocorticosteroids and mineralocorticosteroids.

Isolated defects in the terminal pathway of aldosterone biosynthesis with unimpaired cortisol biosynthesis have also been described, i.e. a defect in 18-hydroxylation of corticosterone (Visser and Cost, 1964) and a defect in the dehydrogenation of 18-hydroxycorticosterone (Ulick *et al.*, 1964). More recent studies of further cases have documented decreased aldosterone production and increased plasma renin activity (Hamilton *et al.*, 1976; Milla *et al.*, 1977). The predominant clinical features are salt-wasted infants who fail to thrive. The exact defect is important to recognise since therapy requires replacement with mineralocorticoids only and not glucocorticosteroids.

(b) *Secondary adrenal insufficiency*

Secondary adrenal insufficiency can be a consequence of panhypopituitarism or more rarely can result from an isolated ACTH deficiency (Aynsley-Green *et al.*, 1978). The most important test in this situation is an assessment of hypothalamic–pituitary–adrenal function. This is best accomplished by measuring the plasma cortisol response to insulin-induced hypoglycaemia as a standard test of pituitary ACTH reserve (Greenwood *et al.*, 1966). It can also be combined with other hormone stimulation tests for a full profile of pituitary function (Mortimer *et al.*, 1973). Peak plasma cortisol levels exceeding 20 μg/dl (552 nmol/l) following hypoglycaemia indicate adequate pituitary ACTH secretion. The metyrapone test, by its inhibition of the 11 β-hydroxylase enzyme, has also been used to assess pituitary–adrenal function (Keenan *et al.*, 1973). Specific assays for measuring the expected rise in plasma 11-deoxycortisol and fall in plasma cortisol concentrations should be available for this test; otherwise the response can be documented using measurement of 24-hr urinary 17-oxogenic steroid excretion. The results are often misleading and the test can be dangerous in hypopituitarism. Its use has largely been superseded by the insulin-induced hypoglycaemia test. There is also no place now for the use of vasopressin stimulation as a test of pituitary ACTH secretion (Gwinup, 1965). The test produces unpleasant side effects and can be dangerous. Similarly, pyrogen tests should no longer be used.

The commonest cause of secondary adrenal insufficiency is prolonged therapy with pharmacological doses of glucocorticosteroids. Suppression is greater at the hypothalamic–pituitary level than at the level of the adrenal gland. Normal function may not return for up to one year after steroid therapy has been stopped (James, 1970). Suppression and atrophy of the contralateral adrenal gland also occurs with a unilateral autonomous cortisol-secreting adrenal adenoma or carcinoma. Graber *et al.* (1965) performed serial measurements of plasma cortisol and ACTH in patients before and after removal of adrenal tumours (Fig. 24). Before surgery, plasma cortisol levels were elevated and ACTH levels were suppressed. Plasma cortisol levels fell after surgery, but ACTH levels remained suppressed. Over the next few months, plasma ACTH levels returned to normal and then became elevated. Plasma cortisol levels, however, remained subnormal, indicating that adrenal recovery lags behind pituitary recovery. About nine months after removal of the source of excess cortisol, plasma cortisol and ACTH levels returned to normal and there was a normal response to the metyrapone test. It is important to realise that any patient who has received suppressive doses of steroids for more than a week should have therapy withdrawn gradually over a period of weeks. Such patients if stressed (infection, anaesthetics, etc.) can develop acute adrenal insufficiency for up to a year after steroid therapy has been withdrawn.

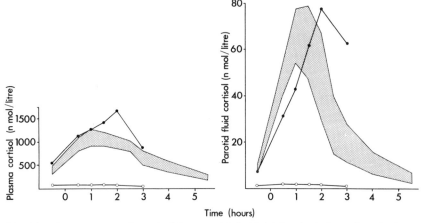

Fig. 23. The response of cortisol in parotid fluid (right shaded area) and plasma (left shaded area) to stimulation with 250 µg of Synacthen (i.m.) in normal subjects, subjects taking an oestrogen contraceptive preparation (filled circles), and a subject with secondary adrenal atrophy (open circles).

Isolated deficiencies of anterior pituitary hormones have been described (Odell, 1966). Thus isolated ACTH deficiency, although uncommon, is well documented. Patients exhibit typical features of adrenal insufficiency, but lack the characteristic pigmentation of Addison's disease. In children, the condition is associated with hypoglycaemia which appears to be due to a combination of impaired alanine metabolism and a decreased rate of gluconeogenesis (Anysley-Green et al., 1978).

3. Congenital Adrenal Hyperplasia

Congenital adrenal hyperplasia (CAH) or the adrenogenital syndrome is an inherited disorder of cortisol biosynthesis. The mode of inheritance is autosomal recessive. The normal pathways of adrenal steroid biosynthesis have been discussed earlier in this chapter and are illustrated in Fig. 11. Five specific enzyme deficiencies can result in varying forms of CAH (Zurbrugg,

1975). More than 90% of cases are due to a deficiency of C-21 hydroxylase, but there are well documented clinical and biochemical reports of cases resulting from deficiencies of the enzymes, C-20–22 desmolase (Prader and Siebermann, 1957), 3β-hydroxysteroid dehydrogenase (Bongiovanni, 1962), 17α-hydroxylase (Biglieri et al., 1966; New, 1970) and 11β-hydroxylase (Eberlein and Bongiovanni, 1956). Some of these enzymes are also necessary for testosterone biosynthesis and hence failure of masculinisation may occur in male infants.

Deficiency of the 21-hydroxylase enzyme results in failure to convert 17α-hydroxyprogesterone (17 OHP) to 11-deoxycortisol and finally to cortisol. The decreased cortisol production in turn, leads to increased pituitary ACTH secretion due to a failure in negative feedback control. This results in hyperplastic adrenal glands, excessive production of steroid precursors and increased synthesis of androgens. The latter causes the clinical signs of virilisation seen in CAH. About 50% of cases with 21-hydroxylase deficiency are salt-losers owing to an additional defect in the synthesis of mineralocorticosteroids. The enzymatic block causes an increased production of 17 OHP and the liver metabolises 17 OHP to pregnanetriol which can be measured either in plasma or urine and used as a diagnostic test (Bongiovanni, 1953; Bongiovanni et al., 1964). In the early newborn period, measurement of urinary 17-oxosteroids and prenanetriol can be a misleading test for the diagnosis of CAH. In normal infants, urinary 17-oxosteroid excretion may be as high as 2·5 mg/day, but only 1–2 mg/day in an affected infant. Urinary pregnanetriol excretion may be normal in an infant with CAH during the first week of life (Shackleton et al., 1972). Problems with interpreting results of urinary steroid determinations in the newborn period and the difficulties with obtaining accurate urine collections has led to the use of direct measurement of plasma concentrations of steroid precursors in CAH. Thus, measurement of plasmas 17 OHP concentrations is now well established as a diagnostic test in CAH due to 21-hydroxylase deficiency (Strott et al., 1969; Youssefnejadian and David, 1975; Hughes and Winter, 1976). The concentrations of plasma 17 OHP during the first few days of life in normal infants and those with untreated CAH are shown in Fig. 25. Immediately after birth, plasma concentrations of 17 OHP exceed 50 nmol/l (1·65 μg/dl) in newborn infants but fall rapidly over the next 24 hr following removal of the placental supply of this steroid. By 36 hr of age, mean levels of plasma 17 OHP are 6 nmol/l (0·20 μg/dl). In untreated infants with CAH, plasma 17 OHP concentrations exceed 100 nmol/l (3·30 μg/dl) in early life and remain elevated prior to glucocorticoid replacement therapy. In an infant with suspected CAH, a blood sample collected at 24 hr of age for determination of plasma 17 OHP concentration should readily distinguish CAH from normals.

As expected, plasma 17 OHP concentrations decrease following gluco-corticoid replacement therapy, but normal levels may not be achieved until there has been more than one week of treatment (Hughes and Winter, 1976). It is possible to utilise measurements of plasma 17 OHP concentrations to monitor the efficacy of glucocortoid replacement therapy in CAH patients, in a similar fashion to the use of plasma glucose levels in patients with diabetes mellitus. However, because of the intrinsic diurnal rhythm in plasma concentrations of this steroid, due care must be given to such factors as the time of sampling and its relationship to the previous glucocorticoid dose when interpreting the results (Hughes and Winter, 1977). Recently, a radio-immunoassay for 17 OHP in saliva has been developed which, because of the ease of frequent saliva collections, may be extremely useful in the longer term management of these patients (Walker et al., 1979).

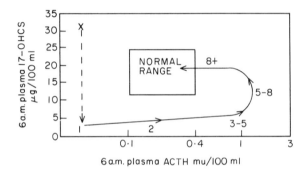

Fig. 24. Relationship between plasma corticosteroid and plasma ACTH levels during recovery (in months) from prolonged pituitary–adrenal suppression (after Graber et al., 1965).

Several steroid hormones apart from 17 OHP are elevated in untreated or poorly controlled CAH. Thus, marked elevations in the plasma concentrations of progesterone, 17α OH-pregnenolone, androstenedione, 21-deoxy-cortisol, testosterone and dehydroepiandrosterone have been documented in this condition (Lippe et al., 1974; McKenna et al., 1976; Hughes and Winter, 1978; Franks, 1974; Korth-Schutz et al., 1978). Plasma concentrations of testosterone are increased mainly through peripheral conversion of androstenedione to testosterone (Horton and Frasier, 1967). Consequently, there is a significant correlation between plasma concentrations of 17 OHP and testosterone in prepubertal and adolescent female patients (Hughes and Winter, 1978). Plasma testosterone concentrations do not usually exceed normal values until plasma concentrations of 17 OHP exceed 30 nmol/l (0·99 μg/dl). Thus simultaneous determinations of plasma concentrations of 17 OHP and testosterone can be useful as an index of therapeutic control in CAH patients. There is no correlation between plasma concentrations of

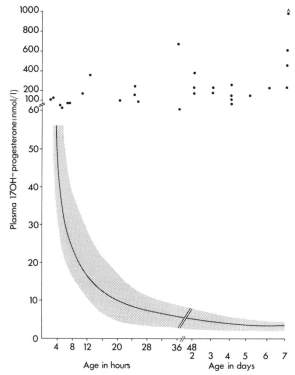

Fig 25. Plasma concentrations of 17α-hydroxyprogesterone in normal and untreated CAH infants during the first week of life. The line and shaded area represents the mean and range of values in normal infants, 1 nmol/l = 33·05 ng/dl. (from Hughes *et al.*, 1979).

17 OHP and testosterone in adolescent males due to the increased testicular testosterone secretion which occurs during puberty and in adult life.

4. Corticosteroids in Non-endocrine Disease

This subject is discussed extensively in the previous edition (Dixon *et al.*, 1967) with particular reference to obesity, diabetes mellitus, thyroid, liver and renal diseases.

The clinical distinction between simple obesity and Cushing's syndrome can sometimes be difficult. Urinary 17-OHCS excretion is elevated in patients with obesity (Schteingart *et al.*, 1963), but urinary free cortisol (Streeten *et al.*, 1969) and plasma cortisol levels (Schteingart and Conn, 1965) are essentially normal. The cortisol production rate is frequently increased in obesity even when expressed per unit surface area. Thus Migeon *et al.* (1963) found a mean cortisol production rate of $15\cdot0 \pm 5\cdot6$ mg/M^2/day ($41\cdot4 \pm 15\cdot4$ μmol/M^2/day) in a group of obese subjects to be significantly higher than the mean production rate of $11\cdot3 \pm 1\cdot6$ mg/M^2/day ($31\cdot2 \pm$

4·4 µmol/M²/day) determined in a group of normal subjects. The plasma half-life of cortisol is shortened in obesity (Schteingart and Conn, 1965) and therefore the cortisol production rate must be increased in order to maintain normal plasma levels of cortisol. Conversely, the urinary excretion of cortisol metabolites is decreased in starvation and malnutrition (Bliss and Migeon, 1957). Protein restriction reduces cortisol turnover and metabolite excretion (Schteingart and Conn, 1965). Starvation in the obese subject leads to elevated plasma cortisol concentrations and a partial loss in the normal diurnal rhythm (Galvao-Teles et al., 1976).

Thyroid diseases may affect adrenocortical function, although obvious symptoms and signs of adrenal dysfunction do not usually occur. In hyperthyroidism, the adrenal cortex is hyperplastic and the metabolic turnover of corticosteroids is increased (Peterson, 1958), while the reverse occurs in hypothroidism. In both forms of thyroid disease, plasma cortisol concentrations are normal (Brien, 1976). The effects of thyroid hormone on steroid hormone metabolism have recently been reviewed by Gordon and Southren (1977). Adrenal corticosteroids have a depressing effect on thyroid function. Dexamethasone suppresses baseline thyrotropin (TSH) levels and a rebound increase in TSH levels occurs when the medication is withdrawn (Nicoloff et al., 1970). There is a blunted TSH response to TRH (thyrotrophin releasing hormone) in patients on high doses of glucocorticosteroids and in patients with Cushing's syndrome (Otsuki et al., 1973). In addition, pharmacological doses of glucocorticosteroids leads to a reduction in basal circulating serum triiodothyronine levels without significantly affecting serum thyroxine levels (Sowers et al., 1977). This suggests that glucocorticosteroids may interfere with the peripheral conversion of thyroxine to triiodothyronine.

The liver plays a central part in the metabolism of corticosteroids. Consequently, it is not surprising that in liver disease there is an impaired removal of cortisol from plasma. The main defect in liver cell failure is in reduction of the A ring and not in conjugation (Brown and Englert, 1961). The urinary output of corticosteroids is therefore reduced in liver disease. A steady state is maintained by decreasing cortisol production such that plasma cortisol levels are usually normal in liver disease (Peterson, 1960).

The effect of alcohol on pituitary–adrenal function has recently been studied in detail. Excessive alcohol ingestion can simulate the clinical signs of Cushing's syndrome. Rees et al. (1977) reported four patients in whom there were definite clinical and biochemical features of Cushing's syndrome associated with alcohol abuse. Plasma cortisol concentrations were elevated and there was a loss of diurnal rhythm. Some patients also showed elevated plasma ACTH levels with absent diurnal rhythm. Impaired hepatic function following excess alcohol ingestion might be expected to result in a lower metabolic clearance rate for cortisol. However, it is unlikely that this is the cause of the adrenocortical dysfunction in these patients. The liver damage is often minimal and acute ingestion of excess alcohol can stimulate adrenocortical activity in normal subjects. It is more likely that the clinical and biochemical features of alcohol-induced pseudo-Cushing's syndrome are associated with increased stimulation of pituitary ACTH secretion. With abstinence from alcohol, the clinical and biochemical abnormalities usually resolve spontaneously. Recently, there has been a case report of a breast-fed infant who developed pseudo-Cushing's syndrome as a result of excessive maternal ingestion of alcohol (Binkiewicz *et al.*, 1978).

Patients with severe depression may show elevated plasma cortisol levels, loss of the normal diurnal rhythm and failure to suppress plasma cortisol levels with dexamethasone administration (Butler and Besser, 1968). These biochemical disturbances usually resolve following successful treatment of the underlying depressive illness. It is difficult to determine how much of the increased cortisol production in depressed patients is secondary to nonspecific stress factors. Specific clinical characteristics which appear to correlate most closely with increased cortisol production include active suicidal impulses and severe anxiety. Apathetic depressed patients, in general, do not have marked cortisol hypersecretion. It has been hypothesised that there is a functional depletion of brain noradrenaline in depressed patients which may result in increased ACTH and cortisol secretion (Van Loon, 1973).

REFERENCES

Abraham, G. E. (1974). *Acta endocr., Copenh.* **75** (Suppl. 183).
Abraham, G. E., Hopper, K., Tulchinsky, D., Swerdloff, R. S. and Odell, W. D. (1971). *Anal. Lett.* **4**, 325.
Abraham, G. E., Buster, J. E. and Teller, R. C. (1972). *Anal. Lett.* **5**, 757.
Angevine, D. M. (1938). *Arch. Pathol.* **26**, 507.
Appleby, J. I., Gibson, G., Norymberski, J. K. and Stubbs, R. D. (1955). *Biochem. J.* **60**, 453.
Arnold, J. (1866). *Virchows Arch. path. Anat. Physiol.* **35**, 64.
Arnold, M. L. and James, V. H. T. (1971). *Steroids*, **18**, 789.
Atcheson, J. B. and Tyler, F. H. (1975). *In* "Handbook of Physiology Sect. 7: Endocrinology, Vol. VI. Adrenal Gland" (R. D. Greep and E. B. Astwood, eds), pp. 127–134. American Physiological Society, Washington.
Atherden, S. M., Edmunds, A. T. and Grant D. B. (1974). *Arch. dis. Childh.* **49**, 192.
Axelrod, L. R. and Goldzieher, J. W. (1968). *Biochem. biophys. Acta*, **152**, 391.
Aynsley-Green, A., Moncrieff, M. W., Ratter, S., Benedict, C. R., Storrs, C. N. and Wilkinson, R. H. (1978). *Arch. dis. Childh.* **53**, 499.
Ayres, P. J., Perlman, W. H., Tait, J. F. and Tait, S. A. S. (1958). *Biochem. J.* **70**, 230.
Bacon, G. E., Spencer, M. L. and Kelch, R. P. (1977). *Clin. Endocr.* **6**, 113.
Baggett, B., Engel, L. L., Balderas, L., Lanman, G., Savard, K. and Dorfman, R. I. (1959). *Endocrinology*, **64**, 600.
Baird, D. T., Uno, A. and Melby, J. G. (1969). *J. Endocr.* **45**, 135.

Baulieu, E.-E. (1962). *J. clin. Endocr. Metab.* **22**, 501.
Baranczuk, R., Muldoon, T. G. and Mahesh, V. B. (1973). *Steroids*, **22**, 273–284.
Barnes, N. D. and Atherden, S. M. (1972). *Arch. dis. Childh.* **47**, 62.
Baum, C. K., Tudor, R. and Landon, J. (1974). *Clin. chim. Acta*, **55**, 147.
Beisel, W. R., DiRaimondo, V. C. and Forsham, P. H. (1964). *Ann. int. Med.* **60**, 641.
Benirschke, K. (1956). *Obstet. Gynec. N.Y.* **8**, 412.
Besser, G. M., Butler, P. W. P. and Plumpton, F. S. (1967). *Br. med. J.* **ii**, 391.
Besser, G. M., Cullen, D. R., Irvine, W. J., Ratcliffe, J. G. and Landon, J. (1971). *Br. med. J.* **i**, 374.
Besser, G. M. and Edwards, C. R. W. (1972). *Clin. Endocr. Metab.* **1**, 451.
Beyer, K. F. and Samuels, L. T. (1956). *J. biol. Chem.* **219**, 69.
Biglieri, E. G., Hervon, M. A. and Brust, N. (1966). *J. clin. Invest.* **45**, 1946.
Binkiewicz, A., Robinson, M. J. and Senior, B. (1978). *J. Pediatr.* **93**, 965.
Björkhem, I., Blömstrand, R., Lantto, O., Löf, A. and Svensson, L. (1974). *Clin. chim. Acta*, **56**, 241.
Bledsoe, T., Island, D. P., Riondel, A. M. and Liddle, G. W. (1964). *J. clin. Endocr. Metab.* **24**, 740.
Bliss, E. L. and Migeon, C. J. (1957). *J. clin. Endocr. Metab.* **17**, 760.
Bloch, E. and Benirschke, K. (1959). *J. biol. Chem.* **234**, 1085.
Bloch, E., Benirschke, K. and Rosemberg, E. (1956). *Endocrinology*, **58**, 626.
Bongiovanni, A. M. (1953). *Bull. Johns Hopkins Hosp.* **92**, 244.
Bongiovanni, A. M. (1962). *J. clin. Invest.* **41**, 2086.
Bongiovanni, A. M., Eberlein, W. R., Goldman, A. S. and New, M., (1967). *Rec. Prog. Horm. Res.* **23**, 375.
Bongiovanni, A. M., Root, A. W. and Eberlein, W. R. (1964). *J. clin. Endocr. Metab.* **24**, 1312.
Booth, M., Dixon, P. F., Gray, C. H., Greenaway, J. M. and Holness, N. J. (1961). *J. Endocr.* **23**, 25.
Borth, R. (1956). *Acta endocr., Copenh.* **22**, 125.
Breuer, H. and Siekmann, L. (1975). *J. steroid Biochem.* **6**, 685.
Brien, T. G. (1976). *Clin. Endocr.* **5**, 97.
Briggs, M. H. and Brotherton, J. (1970a). "Steroid Biochemistry and Pharmacology", pp. 1–22. Academic Press, London and New York.
Briggs, M. H. and Brotherton, J. (1970b). "Steroid Biochemistry and Pharmacology", pp. 192–264. Academic Press, London and New York.
Briggs, M. H. and Brotherton, J. (1970c). "Steroid Biochemistry and Pharmacology", pp. 171–191. Academic Press, London and New York.
Briggs, M. H. and Brotherton, J. (1970d). "Steroid Biochemistry and Pharmacology", pp. 301–327. Academic Press, London and New York.
Briggs, M. H. and Brotherton, J. (1970e). "Steroid Biochemistry and Pharmacology", pp. 52–83. Academic Press, London and New York.
Brodish, A. (1973). *In* "Brain–Pituitary–Adrenal Interrelationships" (A. Brodish and E. S. Redgate, eds), pp. 128–151. Karger, Basel.
Brombacher, P. J., Gijzen, A. H. J., Janssens, H. H. P. and Soons, M. P. J. (1975). *Clin. chim. Acta*, **58**, 173.
Brooks, C. J. W. and Gaskell, S. J. (1979). Hormones. *In* "Biochemical Applications of Mass Spectrometry" (G. Waller, ed.), Suppl. Vol. 1. Wiley Interscience, New York.
Brown, H. and Englert, E., Jr. (1961). *Arch. int. Med.* **107**. 773.
Brown, J. R., Cavanaugh, A. H. and Farnsworth, W. E. (1976). *Steroids*, **28**, 487.

Bulaschenko, H., Richardson, E. M. and Dohan, F. C. (1960). *Arch. biochem. biophys.* **87**, 81.

Burke, C. W. and Beardwell, C. G. (1973). *Q. J. Med. New Ser.* **XLII**, 175.

Burstein, S., Kimball, H. L., Chaudhuri, N. K. and Gut, M. (1968). *J. biol. Chem.* **243**, 4417.

Burstein, S. and Gut, M. (1971). *Rec. Prog. horm. Res.* **27**, 303.

Bush, I. E. (1957). *Rec. Prog. horm. Res.* **11**, 263.

Butler, P. W. P. and Besser, G. M. (1968). *Lancet*, **i**, 1234.

Calma, I. and Foster, C. L. (1943). *Nature, Lond.* **152**, 536.

Camacho, A. M., Cash, R., Brough, A. J. and Wilroy, R. S. (1967). *J. Am. med. Assoc.* **202**, 114.

Cameron, E. H. D., Hillier, S. G. and Griffiths, K. (eds) (1975). "Steroidimmunoassay", Proc. 5th Tenovus Workshop. Alpha Omega Alpha, Cardiff.

Cameron, E. H. D., Jones, T., Jones, D., Anderson, A. B. M. and Griffiths, K. (1969). *J. Endocr.* **45**, 215.

Cameron, E. H. D., Beynon, M. A. and Griffiths, K. (1968). *J. Endocr.* **41**, 319.

Campuzano, H. C., Wilkerson, J. E., Raven, P. B., Schabram, T. and Horvath, S. M. (1973). *Biochem. Med.* **7**, 350.

Cash, R., Brough, A. J., Cohen, M. N. P. and Satoh, P. S. (1967), *J. clin. Endocr. Metab.* **27**, 1239.

Caspi, E. R., Dorfman, R. I., Khan, B. T., Rosenfeld, G. and Schmid, W. (1962). *J. biol. Chem.* **237**, 2085.

Cater, D. B. and Lever, J. D. (1954). *J. Anat.* **88**, 437.

Chandler, D. W., Tuck, M. and Mayes, D. M. (1976). *Steroids,* **27**, 235.

Chard, T., Silman, R. E. and Rees, L. H. (1977). *Ciba Found. Symp.* **47**, 359.

Chart, J. J., Allen, M. J., Bencze, W. T. and Gaunt, R., (1958). *Experientia,* **14**, 151.

Chart, J. J., Sheppard, H., Mowles, T. and Howie, N. (1962). *Endocrinology,* **71**, 479.

Chattoraj, S. C., Turner, A. K., Pinkus, J. L. and Charles, D. (1976). *Am. J. Obstet. Gynec.* **124**, 848.

Chester Jones, I. (1976). *Proc. Soc. Endocr.* **71**, 3P.

Chester Jones, I. (1957). "The Adrenal Cortex." University Press, Cambridge.

Clayton, B. E., Edwards, R. W. H. and Makin, H. L. J. (1971). *J. Endocr.* **50**, 251.

Cohen, M., Stiefel, M., Reddy, W. J. and Laidlaw, J. C. (1958). *J. clin. Endocr. Metab.* **18**, 1076.

Comerford, J. B. (1965). *Lancet*, **i**, 679.

Comoglio, S. and Celada, F. (1976). *J. immunol. Meth.* **10**, 161.

Constantopoulos, G., Satoh, P. S. and Tchen, T. T. (1962). *Biochem. biophys. Res. Commun.* **8**, 50.

Constantopoulos, G. and Tchen, T. T. (1961). *J. biol. Chem.* **236**, 65.

Cope, C. L. (1964a). "Adrenal Steroids and Disease", pp. 60–72. Pitman, London.

Cope, C. L. (1964b). "Adrenal Steroids and Disease", pp. 85–112. Pitman, London.

Cope, C. L. (1972). "Adrenal Steroids and Disease", 2nd Edition. Pitman Medical, London.

Cope, C. L. and Pearson, J. (1965). *J. clin. Path.* **18**, 82.

Crowley, M. F., Garbien, K. J. T. and Tuttlebee, J. W. (1975). *Ann. clin. Biochem.* **12**, 66.

Crystal, R. G., Rose, L. I., Jagger, P. I. and Lauler, D. P. (1970). *J. clin. Endocr. Metab.* **31**, 199.

Dale, S. L., Komanicky, P., Pratt, J. H. and Melby, J. (1976). *J. clin. Endocr. Metab.* **43**, 803.

Dash, R. J., England, B. G., Midgely, A. R. and Niswender, G. D. (1975). *Steroids*, **26**, 647.

Daughaday, W. H. (1956). *J. lab. Clin. Med.* **48**, 799.

Daughaday, W. H. (1959). *Physiol. Rev.* **39**, 885.

Daughaday, W. H. (1967). *In* "The Adrenal Cortex" (A. B. Eisenstein, ed.), pp. 385–403, Little, Brown and Co., Boston.

Daughaday, W. H. and Mariz, I. K. (1961). *Metabolism*, **10**, 936.

Dexter, R. N., Fishman, L. M., Ney, R. L. and Liddle, G. W. (1967). *J. clin. Endocr. Metab.* **27**, 473.

Diczfalusy, E. (1970). "Steroid Assay by Protein Binding", Trans. 2nd Karolinska Symp. (E. Diczfalusy, ed.). Also published as *Acta endocr., Copenh.* (Suppl. 147).

Dixon, P. F., Booth, M. and Butler, J. (1967). The corticosteroids. *In* "Hormones in Blood" (C. H. Gray and A. L. Bacharach, eds), Vol. 2, pp. 306–389. Academic Press, London and New York.

Doe, R. P.,Fernandez, R. and Seal, U. S. (1964). *J. clin. Endocr. Metab.* **24**, 1029.

Doe, R. P., Lohrenz, F. N. and Seal, U. S. (1965). *Metabolism*, **14**, 940.

Dominguez, O. V. and Samuels, L. T. (1963). *Endocrinology*, **73**, 304.

Dorfman, R. I. and Ungar, F. (1965). "Metabolism of Steroid Hormones." Academic Press, New York and London.

Durber, S. M. and Daly, J. R. (1976). *Clin. chim. Acta*, **68**, 43.

Durber, S. M., Lawson, J. and Daly, J. R. (1976). *Br. J. Obstet. Gynaec.* **83**, 814.

Eberlein, W. R. and Bongiovanni, A. M. (1956). *J. biol. Chem.* **223**, 85.

Edwards, C. R. W. and Landon, J. (1976). *In* "Hormone Assays and Their Clinical Application" (J. A. Loraine and E. T. Bell, eds), 4th edition, pp. 519–579. Churchill Livingstone, Edinburgh.

Egdahl, R. H. (1960). *Endocrinology*, **66**, 200.

Ewald, W., Werbin, H. and Chaikoft, I. L. (1964). *Steroids*, **4**, 759.

Ewald, W., Werbin, H. and Chaikoft, I. L. (1965). *Biochem. biophys. Acta*, **111**, 306.

Fahmy, D. R., Read, G. F. and Hillier, S. G. (1975). *Steroids*, **26**, 267.

Fahmy, D., Read, G. and Hillier, S. G. (1975b). *Proc. Soc. Endocr.* **65**, 45P.

Fantl, V. and Gray, C. H. (1977). *Clin. chim. Acta*. **79**, 237.

Farmer, R. W. and Pierce, C. E. (1974). *Clin. Chem.* **20**, 411.

Ferguson, J. J. (1963). *J. biol. Chem.* **238**, 2754.

Ficher, M., Curtis, G. C., Ganjam, V. K., Joshlin, L. and Perry, S. (1973). *Clin. Chem.* **19**, 511.

Fieser, L. F. and Fieser, M. A. (1959). "Steroids." Chapman and Hall, London.

Fishman, L. M., Liddle, G. W., Island, D. P., Fleischer, N. and Kuchel, O. (1967). *J. clin. Endocr. Metab.* **27**, 481.

Florini, J. R. and Buyske, P. A. (1961). *J. biol. Chem.* **236**, 247.

Foster, L. B. and Dunn, R. T. (1974). *Clin. Chem.* **20**, 365.

Frandsen, V. A. and Stakeman, G. (1964). *Acta endocr., Copenh.* **47**, 265.

Franks, R. C. (1974). *J. clin. Endocr. Metab.* **39**, 1099.

Fraser, R. and James, V. H. T. (1968). *J. Endocr.* **40**, 59.

Fraser, R. and Lantos, C. P. (1978). *J. steroid Biochem.* **9**, 273.

French, F. S., Macfie, J. A., Baggett, B., Williams, T. F. and Van Wyk, J. J. (1969). *Am. J. Med.* **47**, 619.

Fukushima, D. K., Bradlow, L. H., Hellman, L., Zumoff, B. and Gallagher, T. F. (1960). *J. biol. Chem.* **235**, 2246.

Galvao-Teles, A., Graves, L., Burke, C. W., Fotherby, K. and Fraser, T. R. (1976). *Acta endocr., Copenh.* **81**, 321.

Garren, L. D., Ney, R. L. and Davies, W. W. (1965). *Proc. natn. Acad. Sci. USA*, **53**, 1443.

Gaul, G., Lemus, A. E., Kline, I. T., Gut, M. and Dorfman, R. I. (1962). *J. clin. Endocr. Metab.* **22**, 1193.

Gaunt, R., Chart, J. J. and Renzi, A. A. (1965). *Rev. Physiol.* **56**, 114.

Gold, E. M. (1977). *Postgrad. Med.* **62**, 105.

Goldman, A. S. (1968). *J. clin. Endocr. Metab.* **28**, 1539.

Gomez-Sanchez, C., Milewich, L. and Holland, O. B. (1977). *J. lab. Clin. Med.* **89**, 902.

Goodman, D. S., Avigan, J. and Wilson, H. (1962). *J. clin. Invest.* **41**, 2135.

Gordon, G. G. and Southren, A. L. (1977). *Bull. N.Y. Acad. Sci.* **53**, 241.

Gore, M. and Lester, E. (1975). *Ann. clin. Biochem.* **12**, 160.

Gottschau, M. (1883). *Arch. Anat. Physiol. (Anatom Abt)*, 412.

Graber, A. L., Ney, R. L., Nicholson, W. E., Island, D. P. and Liddle, G. W. (1965). *J. clin. Endocr. Metab.* **25**, 11.

Grant, J. K. and Griffiths, K. (1962). *In* "The Human Adrenal Cortex" (A. R. Currie, T. Symington and J. K. Grant, eds), pp. 26–29. E. and S. Livingstone, Edinburgh.

Grant, J. K. (1968). *J. Endocr.* **41**, 111.

Gray, C. H., Baron, D. N., Brooks, R. V. and James, V. H. T. (1969). *Lancet,* i, 124.

Greenwood, F. C., Landon, J. and Stamp, T. C. B. (1966). *J. clin. Invest.* **45**, 429.

Grieg, W. R., Boyle, J. A., Maxwell, J. D., Lindsey, R. M. and Browning, M. C. K. (1969). *Postgrad. med. J.* **45**, 307.

Griffiths, K. and Cameron, E. H. D. (1970). *In* "Advances in Steroid Biochemistry and Pharmacology" (M. H. Briggs, ed.), Vol. 2, pp. 223–265. Academic Press, London and New York.

Griffiths, K. and Cameron, E. H. D. (1975). *In* "The Cell in Medical Science. Vol. 3. Cellular Specialisation" (F. Beck and J. B. Lloyd, eds), pp. 155–191. Academic Press, London and New York.

Griffiths, K. and Glick, D. (1966). *J. Endocr.* **35**, 1.

Griffiths, K., Grant, J. K. and Symington, T. (1963). *J. clin. Endocr. Metab.* **23**, 776.

Gross, H. A., Ruder, H. J., Brown, K. S. and Lipsett, M. B. (1972). *Steroids,* **20**, 681.

Gurpide, E., Macdonald, P. C., Vande Wiele, R. L. and Lieberman, S. (1963). *J. clin. Endocr. Metab.* **23**, 346.

Gutai, J. P., Meyer III, W. J., Kowarski, A. and Migeon, C. J. (1977). *J. clin. Endocr. Metab.* **44**, 116.

Gwinup, G. (1965). *Lancet,* ii, 572.

Halkerston, I. D. K., Eichhorn, J. and Hechter, O. (1961). *J. biol. Chem.* **236**, 374.

Hall, P. F. and Koritz, S. B. (1964). *Biochim. biophys. Acta,* **93**, 441.

Hasler, M. J., Painter, K. and Niswender, G. D. (1976). *Clin. Chem.* **22**, 1850.

Hamilton, W., McCandless, A. E., Ireland, J. T. and Gray, C. E. (1976). *Arch. dis. Childh.* **51**, 576.

Haynes, R. C. J. (1975). *In* "Handbook of Physiology, Sec. 7, Endocrinology, Vol. VI. Adrenal Gland" (R. O. Greep and E. B. Astwood, eds), pp. 69–76. American Physiological Society, Washington.

Haynes, R. C. J. and Berthet, L. (1957). *J. biol. Chem.* **225**, 115.

Hechter, O. (1949). *Fed. Proc.* **8**, 70.

Hechter, O. (1958). *In* "Cholesterol: Chemistry, Biochemistry and Pathology" (R. P. Cook, ed.), p. 547. Academic Press, New York and London.

Hechter, O. and Pincus, G. (1954). *Physiol. Res.* **34**, 459.

Hechter, O., Soloman, M. M., Zaffaroni, A. and Pincus, G. (1953). *Arch. biochem.*

Biophys. **46**, 201.

Hellman, L., Nakada, F., Zumoff, B., Fukushima, D., Bradlow, L. and Gallagher, T. F. (1971). *J. clin. Endocr. Metab.* **33**, 52.

Hellman, L., Nakada, F., Curti, J., Weitzman, E. D., Kream, S., Roffwarg, H., Ellman, S., Fukushima, D. K. and Gallagher, T. F. (1970). *J. clin. Endocr. Metab.* **30**, 411.

Hems, B. A. (1962). *Br. med. Bull.* **18**, 93.

Hertz, R., Allen, M. J., Schricher, F. G., Doyse, F. G. and Hallman, L. F. (1955). *Rec. Prog. horm. Res.* **11**, 119.

Hertz, R., Pittman, J. A. and Graff, M. M. (1956). *J. clin. Endocr. Metab.* **16**, 705.

Herzog, H. L., Nobile, A., Tolksdorf, S., Charney, W., Hershberg, E. B. and Perlman, P. L. (1955). *Science*, **121**, 176.

Hindawi, R., Dyas, J., Read, G. F., Gaskell, S. and Riad-Fahmy, D. (1979). *Proc. Soc. Endocr.* **81**, 130p.

Hjelm, M. (1978). *In* "Quantitative Mass Spectrometry in Life Sciences" (A. P. de Leenheer, R. Roncucci and C. van Peteghem, eds) Vol. II. Elsevier, Amsterdam.

Hoet Jr., J. J. and Molineaux, L. (1960). *Acta endocr., Copenh.* **33**, 375.

Holloszy, J. and Eisenstein, A. B. (1961). *Proc. Soc. exp. Biol. Med.* **107**, 347.

Horton, R. and Frasier, S. D. (1967). *J. clin. Invest.* **46**, 1003.

Howard, E. and Migeon, C. J. (1962). *Handb . Exp. Pharmacol.* **14**, 570.

Hughes, I. A., Fahmy, D. R. and Griffiths, K. (1979). *Arch. dis. Childh.* **54**, 347.

Hughes, I. A. and Winter, J. S. D. (1976). *J. Pediat.* **88**, 766.

Hughes, I. A. and Winter, J. S. D. (1977). *In* "Congenital Adrenal Hyperplasia" (P. A. Lee, L. P. Plotnick, A. A. Kowarski and C. J. Migeon, eds), pp. 141–156. University Park Press, London.

Hughes. I. A. and Winter, J. S. D. (1978). *J. clin. Endocr. Metab.* **46**, 98.

Hutter, A. M. Jr., and Kayhoe, D. E. (1966). *Am. J. Med.* **41**, 581.

Inano, H., Machino, A. and Tamaoki, B. (1969). *Steroids*, **13**, 357.

Iturzaeta, N. F., Hillman, D. A. and Colle, E. (1970). *J. clin. Endocr. Metab.* **30**, 185.

IUPAC (1970). IUPAC-IUB 1967 Revised Tentative Rules for Steroid Nomenclature. *J. steroid Biochem.* **1**, 143.

Jackson, C. M. (1909). *Am. J. Anat.* **9**, 119.

James, V. H. T. (1970). *Pharm. Clin.* **2**, 182.

James, V. H. T. and Landon, J. (1968). *In* "Recent Advances in Endocrinology" (V. H. T. James, ed.), pp. 50–94. J. and A. Churchill, London.

James, V. H. T. and Landon, J. (1976). "Hypothalamic–Pituitary–Adrenal Function Tests." Ciba, London.

James, V. H. T., Mattingly, D. and Daly, J. R. (1971). *Br. med. J.* **ii**, 310.

James, V. H. T., Townsend, J. and Fraser, R. (1967). *Proc. Soc. Endocr.* **37**, xxviii.

Jänne, O., Perheentupa, J., Viinikka, L. and Vihko, R. (1975). *Clin. Endocr.* **4**, 39.

Janoski, A. H., Schulman, F. C. and Wright, G. E. (1974). *Steroids*, **23**, 49.

Jost, A. (1975). *In* "Handbook of Physiology, Sect. 7: Endocrinology, Vol. VI. Adrenal Gland" (R. O. Greep and E. B. Astwood, eds), pp. 107–115. American Physiological Society, Washington.

Joyce, B. G., Wilson, D. W., Read, G. F. and Riad-Fahmy, D. (1978). *Clin. Chem.* **24**, 2099.

Kahnt, F. W. and Neher, R. (1966). *Helv. chim. Acta*, **49**, 725.

Kao, M., Voina, S., Nichols, A. and Horton, R. (1975). *Clin. Chem.* **21**, 1644.

Karenyi, N. (1961). *Arch. Pathol.* **71**, 336.

Kase, K. and Kowal, J. (1962). *J. clin. Endocr. Metab.* **22**, 925.

Katz, F. H., Lipman, M. M., Franz, A. G. and Jailer, J. W. (1962). *J. clin. Endocr. Metab.* **22**, 71.

Keenan, B. S., Beitius, D., Lee, P. A., Kowerski, A., Blizzard, R. M., and Migeon, C. J. (1973). *J. clin. Endocr. Metab.* **37**, 540.

Kenny, F. M., Preeyasombat, C. and Migeon, C. J. (1966). *Pediatrics*, **37**, 34.

Klyne, W. (1957). "The Chemistry of the Steroids." Methuen, London.

Kobayashi, Y., Ogihara, T., Amitani, K., Watanabe, F., Kiguchi, T., Ninomiya, I. and Kumahara, Y. (1978). *Steroids*, **32**, 137.

Kondo, S. (1959). *Bull. exp. Biol.* **9**, 51.

Koritz, S. B. (1964). *Biochemistry*, **3**, 1098.

Koritz, S. B. and Hall, P. F. (1964). *Biochemistry*, **3**, 1298.

Korth-Schutz, S., Virdis, R., Saenger, P., Chow, D. M., Levine, L. S. and New, M. I. (1978). *J. clin. Endocr. Metab.* **46**, 452.

Kreines, K. and de Vaux, W. D. (1971). *Pediatrics*, **47**, 516.

Krieger, D. T. (1972). *Mt Sinai J. Med.*, N.Y. **39**, 416.

Krieger, D. T. (1973). *Mt Sinai J. Med.*, N.Y. **40**, 302.

Krieger, D. T., Allen, W., Rizzo, F. and Krieger, H. P. (1971). *J. clin. Endocr. Metab.* **32**, 266.

Krieger, D. T., Amorosa, L. and Linick, F. (1975). *New Engl. J. Med.* **293**, 893.

Krum, A. A., Morris, M. D. and Bennett, L. L. (1964). *Endocrinology*, **74**, 543.

Landon, J., James, V. H. T., Cryer, R. J., Wynn, V. and Frankland, A. W. (1964). *J. clin. Endocr. Metab.* **24**, 1206.

Lanman, J. T. (1953). *Medicine (Balt.)* **32**, 389.

Lanman, J. T. (1962). *In* "Human Adrenal Cortex" (A. R. Currie, T. Symington and J. K. Grant. eds), pp. 547–558. Livingstone, Edinburgh.

Lavelle, M. J. (1974). *In* "Biochemistry of Women: Methods for Clinical Investigation" (A. S. Curry and J. V. Hewitt, eds), pp. 129–150. CRC Press, Cleveland.

Lee, P. A. and Gareis, F. J. (1975). *J. clin. Endocr. Metab.* **41**, 415.

Levell, M. J., Mitchell, F. L., Paine, C. G. and Jordan, A. (1957). *J. clin. Path.* **10**, 72.

Liddle, G. W. (1960). *J. clin. Endocr. Metab.* **20**, 1539.

Liddle, G. W. and Island, D. P. (1962). *In* "The Human Adrenal Cortex" (A. R. Currie, T. Symington and J. K. Grant, eds), pp. 217–223. Livingstone, Edinburgh.

Liddle, G. W., Lowe, E. M. and Harris, A. P. (1958). *J. clin. Endocr. Metab.* **18**, 906.

Liggins, C. G. (1969). *In* "Foetal Autonomy: A Ciba Foundation Symposium" (G. E. W. Wolstenholme and M. O'Connor, eds), pp. 218–224. J. and A. Churchill, London.

Liggins, C. G., Fairclough, R. J., Grieves, S. A., Kendall, J. Z. and Knox, B. S. (1973). *Rec. Prog. horm. Res.* **29**, 111.

Lindholm, J. (1973). *Scand. J. clin. Lab. Invest.* **31**, 115.

Lippe, B. M., LaFranchi, S. H., Lavin, N., Parlow, A., Coyotupa, J. and Kaplan, S. A. (1974). *J. Pediat.* **85**, 782.

Lipsett, M. B. and Hokfelt, B. (1961). *Experientia*, **15**, 449.

Lohrenz, F., Doe, R. P. and Seal, U. S. (1968). *J. clin. Endocr. Metab.* **28**, 1073.

Luse, S. (1967). *In* "The Adrenal Cortex" (A. B. Eisenstein, ed.), pp. 1–61. Little, Brown and Co. Boston.

Luttrell, B., Hochberg, R. B., Dixon, W. R., McDonald, P. D. and Lieberman, S. (1972). *J. biol. Chem.* **247**, 1462–1472.

Lynn, W. S. Jr., Staple, E. and Gurin, S. (1954). *J. Am. chem. Soc.* **76**, 4048.

MacGregor, R. R., Sheagren, J. N., Lipsett, M. B. and Wolff, S. M. (1969). *New Engl. J. Med.* **280**, 1427.

Mahajan, D. K., Wahlen, J. D., Tyler, F. H. and West, C. D. (1972). *Steroids*, **20**, 609.
Malamed, B. (1975). *In* "Handbook of Physiology, Sect. 7: Endocrinology, Vol. VI. Adrenal Gland" (R. O. Creep and E. B. Astwood, eds), pp. 25–39. American Physiological Society, Washington.
Martin, V. I., Edwards, C. R. W., Biglieri, E. G., Vinson, G. P. and Bartter, F. C. (1975). *Steroids*, **26**, 591.
Mason, H. S. (1957). *Adv. Enzymol.* **19**, 79.
Mason, P. A. and Fraser, A. (1975). *J. Endocr.* **64**, 277.
Matsumoto, K. and Samuels, L. T. (1969). *Endocrinology*, **85**, 402.
Mattingly, D. (1962). *J. clin. Path.* **15**, 374.
Mattingly, D., Dennis, P. M., Pearson, J. and Cope, C. L. (1964). *Lancet*, **ii**, 1046.
Mattingly, D. and Tyler, C. (1976). *Br. med. J.* **ii**, 668.
McKenna, T. J., Jennings, A. S., Liddle, G. W. and Burr, I. M. (1976). *J. clin. Endocr. Metab.* **42**, 918.
McKern, K. W. (1966). *Biochim. biophys. Acta*, **121**, 207
Meikle, A. W., Lagerquist, L. G. and Tyler, F. H. (1975). *J. Lab. clin. Med.* **86**, 472.
Melby, J. C., St. Cyr, M. and Dale, S. L. (1961). *New Engl. J. Med.* **264**, 583.
Mess, B. and Martini, L. (1968). *In* "Recent Advances in Endocrinology" (V. H. T. James, ed.), pp. 1–49. J. and A. Churchill, London.
Migeon, C. J., Bertrand, J. and Wall, P. E. (1957). *J. clin. Invest.* **36**, 1350.
Migeon, C. J., Green, O. C. and Eckert, J. P. (1963). *Metabolism*, **12**, 718.
Migeon, C. J., Kenny, F. M. and Taylor, F. H. (1968). *J. clin. Endocr.* **28**, 661.
Milla, P. J., Trompeter, R., Dillon, M. J., Robins, D. and Shackleton, C. (1977). *Arch. dis. Childh.* **52**, 580.
Millington, D. S., Golder, M. P., Cowley, T., London, D., Roberts, H., Butt, W. R. and Griffiths, K. (1976). *Acta endocr., Copenh.* **82**, 561.
Mills, I. H. (1962). *Br. med. Bull.* **18**, 127.
Mills, I. H., Schedl, H. P., Chen, P. S. and Barther, F. C. (1960). *J. clin. Endocr. Metab.* **20**, 515.
De Moor, P., Heirwegh, K., Heremans, J. and Declerck-Raskin, M. (1962). *J. clin. Invest.* **41**, 816.
De Moor, P., Deckx, R. and Steeno, O. (1963). *J. Endocr.* **27**, 355.
Mortimer, C. H., Besser, G. M., McNeilly, A. S., Tunbridge, W. M. E., Gomez-Pan, A. and Hall, R. (1973). *Clin Endocr.* **2**, 317.
Mulrow, P. J., Cohn, G. L. and Kuljian, A. (1962). *J. clin. Invest.* **40**, 1584.
Murphy, B. E. P. (1967). *J. clin. Endocr. Metab.* **27**, 973.
Murphy, B. E. P. (1968). *J. clin. Endocr. Metab.* **28**, 343.
Murphy, B. E. P. and Diez d'Aux, R. C. (1972). *J. clin. Endocr. Metab.* **35**, 678.
Murphy, B. E. P., Engelberg, W. and Pattee, C. J. (1963). *J. clin. Endocr. Metab.* **23**, 293.
Murphy, B. E. P. and Pattee, C. J. (1964). *J. clin. Endocr. Metab.* **24**, 919.
Nabors, C. J., West, C. D., Mahajan, D. K. and Tyler, F. H. (1974). *Steroids*, **23**, 363.
Nelson, D. H. (1969). *Postgrad. Med.* **46**, 135.
Nelson, A. A. and Woodard, G. (1949). *Arch. Pathol.* **48**, 387.
New, M. I. (1970). *J. clin. Invest.* **49**, 1930.
Newsome, H. H., Brown, P. W., Terz, S. S. and Lawrence, W. (1977). *Cancer*, **39**, 542.
Newsome, H. H., Clements, A. S. and Borum, E. H. (1972). *J. clin. Endocr. Metab.* **34**, 473.
Nichols, J. (1961). *In* "The Adrenal Cortex" (H. D. Moon, ed.), pp. 315. Paul B. Hoeben Inc., New York.
Nichols, T., Nugent, C. A. and Tyler, F. H. (1965). *J. clin. Endocr. Metab.* **25**, 343.

Nicoloff, J. T., Fisher, D. A. and Appleman, M. D., Jr. (1970). *J. clin. Invest.* **49**, 1922.

Nieschlag, E., Usadel, K. H., Kley, H. K., Schwedes, U., Schöffling, K. and Krüskemper, H. L. (1974). *Acta endocr., Copenh.* **76**, 556.

Nobile, A., Charney, W., Perlman, P. L., Herzog, H. L., Payne, C. C., Tully, M. E., Jeunik, M. A. and Hershberg, E. B. (1955). *J. Am. chem .Soc.* **77**, 4184.

Norymberski. J. K., Stubbs, R. D. and West, H. F. (1953). *Lancet*, **i**, 1276.

Nugent, C. A. and Mayes, D. M. (1966). *J. clin. Endocr. Metab.* **26**, 1116.

Oakey, R. E. (1970). *Vit. Horm.* **28**, 1.

Oakey, R. E. (1974). *In* "Biochemistry of Women: Methods for Clinical Investigation" (A. S. Curry and J. V. Hewitt, eds), pp. 19–44. CRC Press, Cleveland.

Odell, W. D. (1966). *J. Am. med. Assoc.* **197**, 1006.

Ogihara, T., Miyai, K., Nishi, K., Ishibashi, K. and Kumahara, Y. (1977). *J. clin. Endocr. Metab.* **44**, 91.

Omura, T., Sanders, E., Esterbrook, R. W., Cooper, D. Y., and Rosenthal, O. (1966). *Anal. biochem. Biophys.* **117**, 660.

Orth, D. N., Island, D. P. and Liddle, G. W. (1967). *J. clin. Endocr. Metab.* **27**, 549.

Osler, M. (1962). *Acta endocr., Copenh.* **41**, 67.

Otsuki, M., Dakoda, M. and Baba, S. (1973). *J. clin Endocr. Metab.* **36**, 95.

Pakravan, P., Kenny, F. M., Depp, R. and Allen, A. C. (1974). *J. Pediatr.* **84**, 74.

Pal, S. B. (1978). *Metabolism*, **27**, 1003.

Pal, S. B. (Ed.) (1978b), "Enzyme Labelled Immunoassay.of Hormones and Drugs." Walter de Gruyter, Berlin and New York.

Pal, S. B. (1979). Pers. comm.

Pang, S., Hotchkiss, J., Drash, A. L., Levine, L. S. and New, M. I. (1977). *J. clin. Endocr. Metab.* **45**, 1003.

Park, B. K. (1978). *J. steroid Biochem.* **9**, 963.

Park, B. K., Rowe, P. H., Osbourne, M. and Dean, P. D. G. (1976). *FEBS Lett.* **68**, 237.

Pasqualini, J. R. (1964). *Nature, Lond.* **201**, 501.

Pavlatos, F. C., Smilo, R. P. and Forsham, P. H. (1965). *J. Am. med.Assoc.* **193**, 720.

Peterson, R. E. (1958). *J. clin. Invest.* **37**, 736.

Peterson, R. E. (1960). *J. clin. Invest.* **39**, 320.

Peterson, R. E., Wyngaarden, J. B., Guerra, S. I. Brodie, B. B. and Bunim, J. J. (1955). *J. clin. Invest.* **34**, 1779.

Pham-Huu-Trung, M. T., Gourmelen, M. and Girard, F. (1973). *Acta endocr., Copenh.* **74**, 316.

Phillips, G. M. (1976). *In* "Mechanisms of Topical Corticosteroid Activity" (L. Wilson and R. Marks, eds), pp. 1–18. Churchill Livingstone, Edinburgh.

Pincus, G. (1959). *In* "Proc. 4th Int. Cong. Biochem. Vienna, 1958", Vol. 4, pp. 1–11. Pergamon Press, Oxford.

Porter, C. C. and Silber, R. H. (1950). *J. biol. Chem.* **185**, 201.

Prader, A. and Siebermann, R. E. (1957). *Helv. paed. Acta*, **12**, 569.

Raman, P. B., Sharma, D. C. and Dorfman, R. I. (1966). *Biochemistry*, **5**, 1795.

Rayfield, E. J., Rose, L. I., Cain, J. P., Dluhy, R. G. and Williams, G. H. (1971). *New Engl. J. Med.* **284**, 591.

Read, G. F., Fahmy, D. R. and Walker, R. F. (1977). *Ann. clin. Biochem.* **14**, 343.

Rees, L. H., Besser, G. M., Jeffcoate, W. J., Goldie, D. J. and Marks, V. (1977). *Lancet*, **i**, 726.

Rees, L. H. and Landon, J. (1976). *In* "Hormone Assays and their Clinical Application" (J. A. Loraine and E. T. Bell, eds), 4th edition, pp. 193–220. Churchill Livingstone, Edinburgh.

Riad-Fahmy, D., Read, G. F., Gaskell, S. J., Dyas, J. and Hindawi. R. (1979). *Clin. Chem.* **25**, 655.

Rolleri, E., Zannino, M.; Orlandini, S. and Malvano, A. (1976). *Clin. chim. Acta,* **66**, 319.

Romanoff, L. P., Morris, C. W., Welch, P., Rodriguez, R. M. and Pincus, G. (1961). *J. clin. Endocr. Metab.* **21**, 1413.

Rosenfeld, R. S., Fukushima, D. K. and Gallagher, T. F. (1967). *In* "The Adrenal Cortex" (A. B. Eisenstein, ed.), pp. 103–131. Little, Brown and Co., Boston.

Rosenthal, H. E., Slaunwhite, W. R. J. and Sandberg, A. A. (1969). *J. clin. Endocr.* **29**, 352.

Ross, M. H. (1962). *In* "The Human Adrenal Cortex" (A. R. Currie, T. Symington and J. K. Grant, eds), pp. 558–569. E. and S. Livingstone, Edinburgh.

Ruder, H. J., Guy, R. L. and Lipsett, M. B. (1972). *J. clin. Endocr. Metab.* **35**, 219.

Saba, N., Hechter, O. and Stone, D. (1954). *J. Am. chem. Soc.* **76**, 3862.

Samuels, L. T. and Nelson, D. H. (1975). *In* "Handbook of Physiology, Sect. 7: Endocrinology, Vol. VI. Adrenal Gland" (R. O. Greep and E. B. Astwood, eds), pp. 55–68. American Physiological Society, Washington.

Samuels, L. T. and Uchikawa, T. (1967). *In* "The Adrenal Cortex" (A. B. Eisenstein, ed.), pp. 61–102. Little, Brown and Co., Boston.

Sandberg, A. A., Rosenthal, H., Schneider, S. L. and Slaunwhite, W. R. Jr., (1966). *In* "Steroid Dynamics" (G. Pincus, T. Nakao and J. F. Tait, eds), pp. 1–61. Academic Press, New York and London.

Sandberg, A. A. and Slaunwhite Jr., W. R. (1958). *J. clin. Invest.* **37**, 928.

Sandberg, A. A., Woodruff, M., Rosenthal, H., Nienhouse, S. L. and Slaunwhite Jr., W. R. (1964). *J. clin. Invest.* **43**, 461.

Santen, R. J., Samojlik, E., Lipton, A., Harvey, H., Ruby, E. B., Wells, S. A. and Kendall, J. (1977). *Cancer,* **39**, 2948.

Sayers, G. and Portanova, R. (1975). *In* "Handbook of Physiology, Sect. 7: Endocrinology, Vol. VI. Adrenal Gland" (R. O. Greep and E. B. Astwood, eds). American Physiological Society, Washington.

Schambelan, M., Slaton Jr., P. E. and Biglieri, E. G. (1971). *Am. J. Med.* **51**, 299.

Schteingart, D. E. and Conn, J. W. (1965). *Ann. N.Y. Acad. Sci.* **131**, 388.

Schteingart, D. E., Gregerman, R. I. and Conn, J. W. (1963). *Metabolism,* **12**, 484.

Schuurs, A. H. W. M. and van Weemen, B. K. (1977). *Clin. chim. Acta,* **81**, 1.

Schwers, J., Erikson, G. and Diczfalusy, E. (1965). *Acta endocr., Copenh,* **49**, 65.

Seal, U. S. and Doe, R. P. (1962). *J. biol. Chem.* **237**, 3136.

Seth, J. and Brown, L. M. (1978). *Clin. chim. Acta,* **86**, 109.

Shackleton, C. H., Mitchell, F. L. and Farquar, J. W. (1972). *Pediatrics,* **49**, 198.

Sharma, D. C. (1970). *Acta endocr., Copenh.* **63**, 299.

Shimizu, K. (1965). *J. biol. Chem.* **240**, 1941.

Shimizu, K., Gut, M. and Dorfman, R. I. (1961). *J. biol. Chem.* **237**, 699.

Shiotsuka, R., Jovonovich, J. and Jovonovich, J. (1974). *Chronobiologia,* 1 (Suppl. 1), 109.

Simmer, H. H., Easterling Jr., W. E., Pion, R. J. and Dignam, W. J. (1964). *Steroids,* **4**, 125.

Simmer, H. H., Dignam, W. J., Easterling, W. E., Frankland, M. V. and Naftolin, F. (1966). *Steroids,* **8**, 179.

Skelley, D. S., Brown, L. P. and Besch, P. K. (1973). *Clin. Chem.* **19**, 146.

Slaunwhite Jr., W. R., Lockie, G. N., Black, N. and Sandberg, A. A. (1962). *Science,* **135**, 1062.

Slaunwhite Jr., W. R., Schneider, S., Wissler, F. C. and Sandberg, A. A. (1966).

Biochemistry, **5**, 3527.

Solomon, S., Levitan, P. and Lieberman, S. (1956). *Rev. Can. Biol.* **15**, 282.

Sowers, J. R., Carlson, H. E., Brantbas, N. and Hershman, J. M. (1977). *J. clin. Endocr. Metab.* **44**, 237.

Spark, R. F. (1971). *Ann. int. Med.* **75**, 717.

Spark, R. F. and Etzkorn, J. R. (1977). *New Engl. J. Med.* **297**, 917.

Stachenko, J. and Giroud, C. J. P. (1962). *In* "The Human Adrenal Cortex" (A. R. Currie, T. Symington and J. K. Grant, eds), pp. 30–43. Livingstone, Edinburgh.

Steinberg, D., Avigan, J. and Feigelson, E. B. (1961). *J. clin. Invest.* **40**, 884.

Stone, D. and Hechter, O. (1954). *Arch. biochem. Biophys.* **51**, 457.

Stone, S., Kharma, K. M., Nakamura, R. M., Mishell, D. R. and Thorneycroft, I. H. (1971). *Steroids*, **18**, 161.

Streeten, D. H. P., Stevenson, C. T., Dalakos, T. G., Nicholas, J. J., Dennick, L. G. and Fellerman, H. (1969). *J. clin. Endocr. Metab.* **29**, 1191.

Strott, C. A. and Lipsett, M. B. (1968). *J. clin. Endocr. Metab.* **28**, 1426.

Strott, C. A., West, C. D., Nakagawa, K., Kondo, T. and Tyler, F. H. (1969). *J. clin. Endocr. Metab.* **29**, 6.

Strott, C. A., Yoshima, T. and Lipsett, M. B. (1969). *J. clin. Invest.* **48**, 930.

Studzinski, G. P., Hay, D. C. F. and Symington, T. (1963). *J. clin. Endocr. Metab.* **23**, 248.

Sulon, J. and Sparano, F. (1978). *J. Steroid Biochem.* **9**, 253.

Swann, H. G. (1940). *Physiol. Rev.* **20**, 493.

Sweat, M. L. (1954). *Anal. Chem.* **26**, 773.

Sweat, M. L., Young, R. B. and Bryson, M. J. (1969). *Arch. biochem. Biophys.* **130**, 60.

Symington, T. (1960). *Biochem. Soc. Symp.* **18**, 40.

Symington, T. (1962). *Br. med. Bull.* **18**, 117.

Symington, T. (1969). "Functional Pathology of the Human Adrenal Gland", pp. 13–21. E. and S. Livingstone, Edinburgh.

Symington, T., Currie, A. R., Curran, R. C. and Davidson, J. N. (1955). *In* "Ciba Foundation Colloquia in Endocrinology, Vol. 8: The Human Adrenal Cortex" (G. E. W. Wolstenholme and M. P. Cameron, eds), pp. 70–87. J. and A. Churchill, London.

Temple, T. E., Dexter, R. N., Liddle, G. W. and Jones, D. J. (1969). *Clin. Res.* **17**, 24.

Temple, T. E. and Liddle, G. W. (1970). *Ann. Rev. Pharmacol.* **10**, 199.

Thistlethwaite, D., Darling, J. A. B., Fraser, R., Mason, P. A., Rees, L. H. and Harkness, R. A. (1975). *Arch. dis. Childh.* **50**, 291.

Thompson, E. B. and Lippman, M. E. (1974). *Metabolism*, **23**, 159.

Townsend, J. and James, V. H. T. (1968). *Steroids*, **11**, 497.

Turnbull, A. C., Anderson, A. B. M., Flint, A. P. F., Jeremy, J. Y., Keirse, M. J. N. C. and Mitchell. M. D. (1977). *Ciba Found. Symp.* **47**, 427.

Turner, A. K., Carroll, C. J., Pinkus, J. L., Charles, D. and Chattoraj, S. C. (1973). *Clin. Chem.* **19**, 731.

Tyler, F. H. and West, C. D. (1972). *Am. J. Med.* **53**, 664.

Ulick, S., Gautier, E., Vetter, K. K., Markello, J. R., Yaffe, S. and Lowe, C. U. (1964). *J. clin. Endocr.* **24**, 669.

Ullmann, E. F., Schwarzberg, M. and Rubenstein, K. E. (1976). *J. biol. Chem.* **251**, 4172.

Vande Wiele, R. L., MacDonald, P. C., Bolté, E. and Lieberman, S. (1962). *J. clin. Endocr. Metab.* **22**, 1207.

Van Loon, G. R. (1973). *In* "Frontiers in Neuroendocrinology" (F. W. Ganong and L. Martini, eds), pp. 209–247. University Press, Oxford.

Vecsei, P., Penke, E., Katzy, R. and Baek, L. (1972). *Experientia*, **8**, 1104.

Villee, D. B., Engel, L. L. and Villee, C. A. (1959). *Endocrinology*, **65**, 465.

Villee, D. B., Engel, L. L., Lorning, J. M. and Villee, C. A. (1961). *Endocrinology*, **69**, 354.

Vinson, G. P. and Whitehouse, R. J. (1970). *In* "Advances in Steroid Biochemistry and Pharmacology" (M. H. Briggs, ed.), pp. 163–342. Academic Press, London and New York.

Visser, H. K. A. and Cost, W. S. (1964). *Acta endocr., Copenh.* **47**, 589.

Walker, R. F., Read, G. F. and Riad-Fahmy, D. (1978b). Unpublished data.

Walker, R. F., Riad-Fahmy, D. and Read, G. F. (1978). *Clin. Chem.* **24**, 1460.

Walker, R. F., Read, G. F., Hughes, I. A. and Riad-Fahmy, D. (1979). *Clin. Chem.* **25**, 542.

Ward, M. G. and Engel, L. L. (1964). *J. biol. Chem.* **239**, 3604.

Ward, M. G. and Engel, L. L. (1966). *J. biol. Chem.* **241**, 3147.

Ward, P. J. and Grant, J. K. (1963). *J. Endocr.* **26**, 139.

Watson, R. A. A., Landon, J., Shaw, E. J. and Smith, D. S. (1976). *Clin. chim. Acta*, **73**, 51.

Weiss, L. and Mellinger, R. C. (1970). *J. med. Genet.* **7**, 27.

Weitzman, E. D., Fukushima, D., Nogeire, C., Roffwarg, H., Gallagher, T. F. and Hellman, L. (1971). *J. clin. Endocr. Metab.* **33**, 14.

Weliky, I. and Engel, L. L. (1962). *J. biol. Chem.* **237**, 2089.

Werbin, H., Chaikoff, I. L. and Jones, E. E. (1959). *J. biol. Chem.* **234**, 282.

Werbin, H. and Chaikoff, I. L. (1961). *Arch. biochem. Biophys.* **93**, 476.

Westphal, U. (1970). *In* "Steroid Assay by Protein Binding", Trans 2nd Karolinska Symp. (E. Diczfalusy, ed.), Stockholm, pp. 122–143. Also published as *Acta Endocr., Copenh*, (Suppl. 147).

Westphal, U. (1975). *In* "Handbook of Physiology, Sect. 7, Endocrinology, Vol. VI. Adrenal Gland" (R. O. Greep and E, B. Astwood, eds), pp. 117–125. American Physiological Society, Washington.

Wettstein, A., Kahnt, F. W. and Neher, R. (1955). *In* "Ciba Foundation Colloquium in Endocrinology, Vol. 8: The Human Adrenal Cortex" (G. E. W. Wolstenholme and M. P. Cameron, eds), pp. 170–189, J. and A. Churchill, London.

Wettstein, A. (1959). *In* "Proc. 4th Int. Cong. Biochem., Vienna, 1958", Vol. 4, p. 233. Pergamon Press, Oxford.

Wickings, E. J. (1975). *Horm. Res.* **6**, 78.

Williamson, D. G. and O'Donnell, V. J. (1969). *Biochemistry*, **8**, 1306.

Wilson, A. and Fraser, R. (1971). *J. Endocr.* **51**, 557.

Wilson, A., Mason, P. A. and Fraser, R. (1976). *J. steroid Biochem.* **7**, 611.

Wisdom, G. B. (1976). *Clin. Chem.* **22**, 1243.

Yoffey, J. M. (1955). *In* "Ciba Foundation Colloquia in Endocrinology, Vol. 8: The Human Adrenal Cortex" (G. E. W. Wolstenholme and M. P. Cameron, eds), p. 18. J. and A. Churchill, London.

Youssefnejadian, E. and David, R. (1975). *Clin. Endocr.* **4**, 451.

Youssefnejadian, E., Florensa, E., Collins, W. P. and Sommerville, I. F. (1972). *Steroids*, **20**, 773.

Zurbrugg, R. P. (1975). *In* "Endocrine and Genetic Diseases of Childhood and Adolescence" (L. I. Gardner, ed.), pp. 476–500. W. B. Saunders and Co., Philadelphia.

VI. The Oestrogens

M. J. REED and M. A. F. MURRAY

INTRODUCTION

The last edition of this book was written before the technique of radioimmunoassay had been applied to the measurement of steroids and only

ten references to the levels of oestrogens in the blood of non-pregnant females or males were given. The authors noted that: "a full understanding of the secretion, metabolism and excretion of oestrogens requires a knowledge of oestrogen levels in blood". It will be apparent from the present chapter that there is now much information on the levels of oestrogens in blood. Although synthetic oestrogens are now in widespread use, only naturally occurring oestrogens have been considered in this book. For reviews concerning synthetic oestrogens the articles by Fotherby and James (1972) and Helton and Goldzieher (1977) should be consulted.

In addition to the measurement of oestrogens in blood, studies have also been carried out over the last decade to determine the extent of binding of oestrogens and oestrogen conjugates to plasma proteins. It has also been established that oestrogens interact with target tissues by binding to specific macromolecules called receptors. Oestrogen-cell interactions and the mechanisms by which oestrogens regulate protein synthesis in target tissues although outside the scope of this book, have been fully reviewed (Gorski, Toft, Shyamala, Smith and Notides, 1968; Kellie, 1971; Jensen and DeSombre, 1972; O'Malley and Means, 1974; King and Mainwaring, 1974; Chan and O'Malley, 1976; Clark, Peck, Hardin and Erikson, 1978).

A. SOURCE OF OESTROGENS

1. Origin of Oestrogens

Oestrogens originate in the female by secretion from the ovary, adrenal cortex and during pregnancy from the foetoplacental unit. In the male oestrogens are secreted by the testes and adrenal cortex. In addition to the endocrine secretion of oestrogens, peripheral formation makes an important contribution to oestrogen production, especially in men and post-menopausal women. Although oestrogens had previously been isolated from endocrine glands (see O'Donnel and Preedy, 1967) direct proof of the secretion of a hormone by a gland requires the demonstration of a greater concentration in the venous effluent of the gland than in the arterial or peripheral blood. By the use of modern analytical techniques the glandular secretion of oestrogens has been confirmed (Table 1).

Baird, Uno and Melby (1969) obtained samples of adrenal venous plasma by retrograde catheretization via the femoral vein. The concentration of oestrone in adrenal venous plasma was greater than in peripheral plasma but oestradiol was only detectable in the adrenal venous plasma of one subject who had congenital adrenal hyperplasia. A positive gradient for the concentration of oestrone in adrenal venous plasma versus peripheral levels

Table 1

Endocrine secretion of oestrogens.

Gland	Oestrogen(s) secreted	References
Adrenal	Oestrone	Baird et al. (1969)
Adrenal	Oestrone	Saez et al. (1972)
Adrenal	Oestrone, oestradiol	Yuen et al. (1974)
Ovary	Oestrone, oestradiol	Lloyd et al. (1971)
Ovary	Oestrone, oestradiol	De Jong et al. (1974)
Ovary	Oestrone, oestradiol	Baird and Frazer (1975)
Testis	Oestradiol	Leonard et al. (1971)
Testis	Oestradiol	Jenner et al. (1971)
Testis	Oestradiol	Kelch et al. (1972)
Testis	Oestrone, oestradiol	Longcope et al. (1972)
Testis	Oestradiol	Saez et al. (1972)
Testis	Oestrone, oestradiol	Baird et al. (1973)
Testis	Oestrone, oestradiol	Weinstein et al. (1974)

was also detected by Saez, Morera, Dazord and Bertrand (1972). Secretion of both oestrone and oestradiol by the adrenal cortex, in small but detectable amounts, was demonstrated in normal men by Yuen, Kelch and Jaffe (1974). These authors estimated, however, that the adrenal contribution was less than 4% for oestrone and less than 2% for oestradiol of the reported production rates of these oestrogens.

Although dynamic studies had previously suggested that a proportion of circulating oestrogens in men were derived by testicular secretion (Longcope, Kato and Horton, 1969; Baird, Horton, Longcope and Tait, 1969), it was not until the advent of saturation analysis techniques that the testicular secretion of oestradiol was confirmed in simultaneous reports by Leonard, Flocks and Korenman (1971) and Jenner, Kelch and Grumbach (1971). Other investigations suggested that only oestradiol was secreted by the testes (Saez et al., 1972) but secretion of both oestrone and oestradiol by the testes has been confirmed (Longcope, Widrich and Sawin (1972); Baird, Galbraith, Frazer and Newsam (1973); Weinstein, Kelch, Jenner, Kaplan and Grumbach (1974)). However, the testes appear to secrete 17-hydroxylated steroids rather than the corresponding 17-ketones (Longcope et al., 1972; Saez et al., 1972), with testicular secretion accounting for 25% of oestradiol production (Kelch, Jenner, Weinstein, Kaplan and Grumbach, 1972) but less than 5% of oestrone production in normal men (Weinstein et al., 1974).

Direct measurements of steroids in plasma have confirmed the secretion of oestradiol and oestrone by the ovary (Lloyd, Lobotsky, Baird, McCracken, Weisz, Pupkin, Zanartu and Puga, 1971). These authors measured the concentrations of oestradiol and oestrone in peripheral and ovarian venous plasma, collected from healthy women, on days 7–30 of the menstrual cycle at the time of elective tubal ligation. Although a wide range of values for the concentrations of oestradiol and oestrone in ovarian plasma collected from women at the same stage of the menstrual cycle were found, the overall ratios for the concentrations of oestradiol and oestrone in ovarian compared with peripheral venous plasma were 55 and 7 respectively. As expected, the concentrations of oestradiol and oestrone are higher in venous plasma from the ovary containing a developing follicle or corpus luteum than in the venous plasma from the contralateral ovary (DeJong, Baird and Van der Molen, 1974; Baird and Frazer, 1975). Concentrations of oestradiol and oestrone in ovarian follicular fluid are much greater than in ovarian venous plasma (Baird and Frazer, 1975; McNatty, Baird, Bolton, Chambers, Corker and McLean, 1976). The high concentrations of oestradiol found in follicular fluid may act locally by increasing the sensitivity of granulosa cells of developing follicles to gonadotrophins (Bradbury, 1961; Goldenberg, Vaitukaitis and Ross, 1972), possibly by increasing the number of receptor sites on the granulosa cells for LH (Channing and Kammerman, 1974).

Hormonal changes that occur in post-menopausal women are related to the depletion of primary ovarian follicles (Sherman, West and Korenman, 1976). Although concentrations of oestradiol and oestrone in ovarian plasma from post-menopausal women have been reported as being twice the concentrations found in peripheral plasma (Judd, Judd, Lucas and Yen, 1974) the difference is much less than found in pre-menopausal women (Lloyd et al., 1971) and probably only represents minimal oestrogen secretion.

2. Oestrogen Biosynthesis by the Ovary

The biosynthetic capacity of the human ovary and ovarian components (follicles, corpus luteum and stroma) has been investigated using in vitro techniques. Using follicular cyst linings from human ovaries, Ryan and Smith (1961) first demonstrated the whole sequence of steroid biosynthesis, from acetate to androgens and oestrogens. This and other studies indicated that pregnenolone occupies a central position in the conversion of acetate to androstenedione. The biosynthesis of androstenedione from pregnenolone can occur by two main pathways: the Δ^5 pathway in which pregnenolone is converted to androstenedione via the Δ^5-3β hydroxysteroids, 17α hydroxypregnenolone and dehydroepiandrosterone, and the Δ^4 pathway in which pregnenolone is transformed to androstenedione through the Δ^4-3 keto steroids, progesterone and 17α hydroxyprogesterone. These pathways of androstenedione formations and the conversion of androstenedione to oestrogens are outlined in Fig. 1.

Ryan and Petro (1966) in a later study incubated granulosa and theca cells, obtained from a normal ovary previously stimulated *in vivo* with FSH, separately with [7α-³H] pregnenolone and [4-¹⁴C] progesterone. From this study they concluded that the granulosa cells favoured the

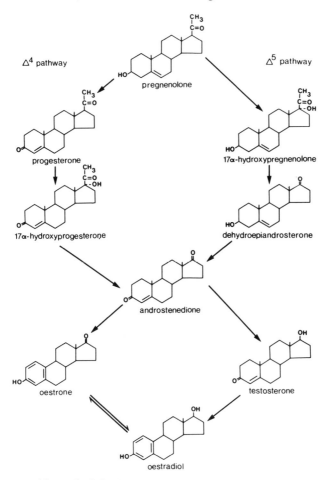

Fig. 1. Oestrogen biosynthesis by the ovary.

production of progesterone by the Δ⁴ pathway while the theca favoured production of androgens and oestrogens by the Δ⁵ pathway. A similar conclusion was arrived at by Somma, Sandor and Lanthier (1969) and Patwardham and Lanthier (1969). However, using follicles obtained from unstimulated ovaries resulted in a much lower capacity to aromatise androgens (Patwardham and Lanthier, 1969).

In vivo perfusion of whole ovaries suggested that dehydroepiandrosterone sulphate could also act as a precursor of ovarian androgens and oestrogens (Oertel, Treiber, Wensel, Knapstein, Wendleberger and Mensel, 1968). Single follicles and fragments of perifollicular stroma obtained from ovaries in the follicular, but not luteal, phase of the menstrual cycle are able to utilize dehydroepiandrosterone sulphate for oestrogen formation (Patwardham and Lanthier, 1972). As considerable sulphatase activity was detected in both follicular and stromal tissue it is likely that hydrolysis of dehydroepiandrosterone sulphate occurred before oestrogen biosynthesis.

From studies carried out on follicular tissue obtained from human ovaries stimulated *in vivo* with gonadotrophins (Ryan and Smith, 1966) and studies with intact Graafian follicles from mares (Younglai and Short, 1970) it is generally assumed that formation of oestrogens occurs predominantly in the thecal cells of the ovarian follicle. However, measurements of oestradiol and progesterone concentrations in human tertiary and Graafian follicles (Kemeter, Salzer, Breitenecker and Friedrich, 1975) lends support to the theory proposed by Falck (1959) that the theca and granulosa cells cooperate functionally in the biosynthesis of oestrogens.

The ability of the corpus luteum to synthesise androgens and oestrogens *in vitro* has been demonstrated and this aspect of oestrogen biosynthesis has been reviewed by Savard (1973). The enzymes of the aromatising system of corpus luteum like the placental aromatase system are concentrated in the microsomal fraction of the tissue homogenate (Arceo and Ryan, 1967). The role of ovarian stroma in the biosynthesis of steroids has also been examined and has the ability to synthesise steroids *in vitro*. Both the Δ^4 and Δ^5 pathways are involved in the synthesis of androstenedione (Rice and Savard, 1966; Leymarie and Savard, 1968) but little, if any, aromatisation occurs in this tissue (Patwardham and Lanthier, 1969). The *in vitro* and *in vivo* synthesis of steroids by the ovary have been fully reviewed (Dorrington, 1977; Baird, 1977).

3. Oestrogen Biosynthesis during Pregnancy

Most of the oestrogen formed during pregnancy is synthesised via 16α-hydroxydehydroepiandrosterone, a different pathway to that used in the non-pregnant state. Oestriol biosynthesis by this neutral (as opposed to phenolic) pathway is largely responsible for the 1000 fold increase in oestrogen production that occurs in pregnancy and is dependent on the placental conversion of androgens that originate mainly in the foetal adrenals. An outline of oestrogen biosynthesis during pregnancy is shown in Fig. 2.

Cholesterol, of which 90% is derived from the material circulation, is converted to pregnenolone and progesterone by placental enzymes (Hellig,

Gattereau, Lefebvre and Bolte, 1970). In the foetus pregnenolone is sulphated and converted to dehydroepiandrosterone sulphate via a 17α-hydroxy-pregnenolone intermediate. Dehydroepiandrosterone sulphate is produced by the foetal adrenal cortex and hydroxylated at the 16α position in the foetal liver. After passing to the placenta dehydroepiandrosterone sulphate and 16α dehydroepiandrosterone sulphate are hydrolysed by a placental sulphatase. Inhibition of placental sulphatase activity has been implicated in a possible mechanism controlling the rate of oestrogen synthesis from conjugated precursors (Townsley, Scheel and Rubin, 1970). After the action of the placental sulphatase, dehydroepiandrosterone and 16α-hydroxy-dehydroepiandrosterone are converted to androstenedione and 16α-hydroxy-androstenedione respectively by a Δ^5 3-ketosteroid isomerase. The resulting Δ^4-3 ketosteroids are converted to oestrogens by the placental aromatising system. The steps involved in the aromatisation mechanism are discussed in the next section.

Although some dehydroepiandrosterone sulphate from the maternal circulation reaches the placenta, the proliferation of the foetal adrenal throughout pregnancy results in a much greater contribution from the foetal

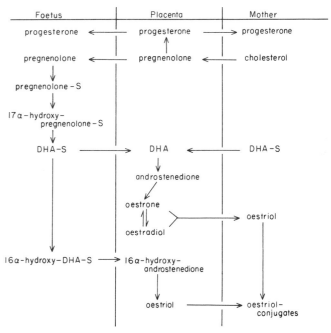

Fig. 2. Oestrogen biosynthesis by the foeto-placental unit during pregnancy (pregnenolone-S = pregnenolone sulphate, DHA = dehydroepiandrosterone and DHA-S = dehydroepiandrosterone-sulphate).

adrenals (Siiteri and MacDonald, 1966). At term more than 90% of the oestriol produced originates from dehydroepiandrosterone sulphate of foetal origin.

The importance of the "neutral" pathway for oestriol formation in pregnancy has been confirmed from the high concentrations of 16α-hydroxy-dehydroepiandrosterone sulphate in umbilical cord blood (Easterling, Summer, Dignam, Frankland and Naftolin, 1966). In addition, by injecting [³H] dehydroepiandrosterone sulphate and [¹⁴C] oestrone sulphate initially into the intact foetoplacental circulation and subsequently into the maternal circulation Kirschner, Wiqvist and Diczfalusy (1966) showed that in the mother urinary oestriol was formed by the phenolic pathway, whereas in the foetus urinary oestriol was derived mainly from dehydroepiandrosterone sulphate.

Although the aromatising system located in the placental microsomes is the main site for the conversion of androgens by the foetoplacental unit, foetal gastro-intestinal tract, liver and skin (Wu, Archer, Flickinger and Touchstone, 1970) and lung, thymus and kidney (Schindler, 1975) are capable of aromatisation. However, the contributions by these tissues are probably negligible compared with the high levels of oestrogen produced by the foetoplacental unit. [¹⁴C] Oestriol has also been isolated from foetal liver extracts after perfusion of [4-¹⁴C] progesterone via the umbilical vein into human foetuses (Taylor, Coutts and MacNaughton, 1974); a possible intermediate being 16α-hydroxy-4-pregnene-3, 20-dione.

The activity of the placental aromatising enzyme system increases during the course of pregnancy but activity is reduced in placental microsomes obtained from toxaemic, diabetic and post-maturity cases (Lehmann, Lauritzen and Schumann, 1973; Laumas, Malkani, Koshti and Hingorami, 1968). In contrast the aromatising capacity of homogenates obtained from cases of intrauterine malnutrition were significantly greater than that of normal term samples and possibly reflects a compensatory mechanism for the decreased placental size which is characteristic of the more severe cases of foetal malnutrition (Sybulski, 1969). For detailed accounts of the experimental procedures used and biosynthesis of oestrogens during pregnancy the following reviews should be consulted: Diczfalusy and Mancuso, 1969; Oakey, 1970; Jeffrey and Klopper, 1970 and Levitz and Young, 1977.

4. Mechanism of Aromatisation

The biosynthesis of oestrogens from C-19 precursors involves the loss of the angular methyl group at C-10 and one each of the hydrogens from C-1 and C-2. Incubation of the 10,000 g supernatant of human term placenta showed that the 1β hydrogen is lost in the conversion of androgens to oestrogens

(Townsley and Brodie, 1968). Hydrogen loss at C-2 in the aromatising process is also highly stereoselective and also involves loss of the β hydrogen (Brodie, Kripalani and Passanza, 1969; Fishman and Guzik, 1969; Fishman, Guzik and Dixon, 1969).

Aromatisation in the ovary also involves the loss of β hydrogens (Townsley and Brodie, 1967). Based on the distribution of tritum in 1α and 2α ^3H testosterone determined by chemical and biochemical means, it was shown that aromatisation of testosterone by human ovarian tissue involves removal of the cis 1β, 2β hydrogens and is therefore the same as the human placental aromatising systems (Spaeth and Osawa, 1974). The stereo-chemistry of the elimination of hydrogen from ring A of circulating androstenedione during the peripheral conversion to oestrogens also proceeds by the same stereo-specific elimination of 1β and 2β hydrogens (Kelly, 1974).

For each mole of oestrogen formed three moles of O_2 and reduced nicotinamide adenine dinucleotide phosphate (NADPH) are required indicating that three mixed function oxidation reactions are involved (Thompson and Siiteri, 1974). This evidence supports a mechanism for aromatisation involving three sequential hydroxylations and a novel mechanism for the conversion of androgens to oestrogens by the placental aromatising complex has recently been proposed by Goto and Fishman (1977) as shown in Fig. 3.

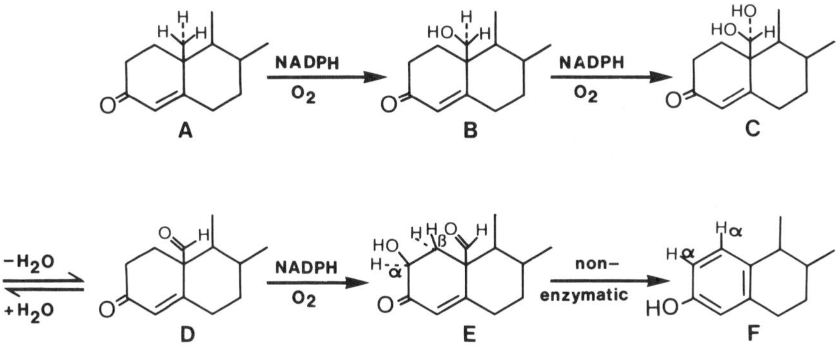

Fig. 3. Mechanism of aromatisation (from Goto and Fishman, 1977 with permission of authors and publisher; copyright 1977 by the American Association for the Advancement of Science).

The first two of the hydroxylations take place on the C-19 methyl group (Meyer, 1955; Wilcox and Engels, 1965) generating the 19-hydroxy intermediate (B) which in turn undergoes a second hydroxylation (C) with subsequent formation of the 19-aldehyde (D) (Akhtar and Skinner, 1968). This compound is the substrate for the final and rate determining step at 2β to give (E) which then rapidly and non-enzymatically rearranges to an oestrogen (Goto and Fishman, 1977). Other mechanisms involving androgen epoxides have also been proposed for the formation of oestrogens (Morand, Williamson, Layne, Lompa-Krzymien and Salvador, 1975). The three successive hydroxylations most likely proceed at the same enzyme site without release of intermediates (Thompson and Siiteri, 1974). During peripheral biosynthesis of oestrone hydroxylation of androstenedione at C-19 and conversion of the resultant 19-hydroxy androstenedione to oestrone occurs at the same site (Kelly, DeLeon and Rizkallah, 1976).

5. Peripheral Formation of Oestrogens

The formation of oestrogens in extra glandular tissues is an important source of oestrogens in women and men (Siiteri and MacDonald, 1973). In pre-menopausal women extraglandular formation of oestrone can account for 10–15% of the total production of oestrone, depending on the phase of the menstrual cycle. In the post-menopausal women most of the oestrone produced is derived from the extraglandular aromatisation of androstenedione (Longcope, 1971; Grodin, Siiteri and MacDonald, 1973).

Both *in vivo* and *in vitro* investigations have been utilised to determine the sites of extraglandular oestrogen formation within the body. Based on the correlations between the conversion of androstenedione to oestrone and body weight, Siiteri and MacDonald (1973) and Rizkallah, Tovell and Kelly (1975) proposed that adipose tissue is an important site for the extraglandular formation of oestrogens in men and women. The ability of adipose tissue to convert androstenedione to oestrogens has been confirmed by *in vitro* studies (Schindler, Ebert and Friedrich, 1972; Nimrod and Ryan, 1975). Fat tissue from cancerous breasts was also able to convert androgens to oestrogens (Nimrod and Ryan, 1975) confirming an earlier tentative report by Jones, Cameron, Griffiths, Gleave and Forrest (1970). Although the aromatising activity found in adipose tissue was low, when the whole mass of body tissue is taken into account, it is possible that several micrograms per day could be produced. Also it is possible that any oestrogen formed may act locally. Bleau, Roberts and Chapdelaine (1974), however, using $[4\text{-}^{14}C]$ andros-tenedione or $[4\text{-}^{14}C]$ testosterone were unable to demonstrate *in vitro* aromatisation using human adipose tissue.

An *in vivo* technique has also been used to investigate the peripheral aromatisation of androgens (Longcope, Pratt, Schneider and Fineberg, 1978). Labelled androstenedione and oestrone or testosterone together with oestradiol were infused into the brachial arm vein. During the infusion blood samples were obtained from the brachial artery, a deep vein draining primarily muscle tissue and a superficial vein draining mainly adipose tissue. Using this technique, Longcope and colleagues found that of the total peripheral aromatisation of androgens to oestrogens, muscle accounted for up to 30% and adipose tissue up to 15%.

Hair follicles also have the ability to convert androgens to oestrogens, although whether hair roots are a significant site of peripheral aromatisation in the human is not known (Schweikert, Milewich and Wilson, 1975).

Cultured human fibroblasts, which can convert androgens to oestrogens, have been used to investigate factors that may be involved in the regulation of aromatisation (Schweikert, Milewich and Wilson, 1976). Aromatisation activity was enhanced with choleragen, theophylline and with concentrations of dexamethazone known to inhibit AMP breakdown, suggesting that the activity of the enzymes involved in aromatisation may be regulated by a cyclic AMP mediated mechanisms.

Although foetal liver is an important site of aromatisation during pregnancy (Mancuso, Dell-Acqua, Eriksson, Wiqvist and Diczfalusy, 1964; Slaunwhite, Karsay, Hollmer, Sandberg and Niswander, 1965; Jungmann, Kot and Schweppe, 1966; Jungmann and Schweppe, 1967) it was thought to lose the ability in adult life. Smuk and Schwers (1977), however, have recently demonstrated the *in vitro* conversion of androstenedione to oestrone and oestradiol by human adult liver, indicating that the aromatising capacity present in human foetal liver has been preserved in the adult. The conversion rate in adult liver was lower than that reported from foetal investigations.

Some tissues from foetal brain also possess aromatising capability. Hypothalamic and limbic tissue, but not frontal cortex, from human foetuses possess aromatisation activity and a specific role for such conversions in these areas of the brain is possible (Naftolin, Ryan and Petro, 1971; Ryan, Naftolin, Reddy, Flores and Petro, 1972).

Aromatisation has also been demonstrated with many animal tissues including rat kidney, adrenals and liver (Frieden, Patkin and Mills, 1968) homogenates of rat mandibular bone (Vittek, Altman, Gordon and Southren, 1974) and the hypothalamus of rats, rabbits and macaque (Ryan *et al.*, 1972). It would therefore appear that the enzyme system responsible for aromatisation is more widely distributed throughout the body than was originally suspected.

B. REGULATION OF OESTROGEN BIOSYNTHESIS

1. In the Female

The ability to measure ovarian steroids and gonadotrophins by radioimmunoassay techniques has made it possible to study the temporal relationships of hormones throughout the menstrual cycle (Ross, Cargille, Lipsett,

Rayford, Marshall, Shott and Rodbard, 1970; Vande Wiele, Bogumil, Dyrenfurth, Ferin, Jewelewicz, Warren, Rizkallah and Mikhail, 1970). Changes in oestrogen secretion throughout the menstrual cycle are regulated by the gonadotrophins, which are synthesised and secreted by the anterior pituitary and exert their biological effect on the ovaries.

It is now established that the neural mechanisms involved in the regulation of oestrogen secretion throughout the menstrual cycle develop gradually over a number of years, starting before the onset of puberty. Levels of serum FSH in female children rise prior to any evidence of secondary sexual development (Angsusingha, Kenny, Nankin and Taylor, 1974). Random fluctuations in serum oestradiol and testosterone concentrations are seen early in puberty and in mid-puberty occasional rhythmic fluctuations in oestrogen secretion occur, marking the appearance of the cyclic variations in hormone levels (Winter and Faiman, 1973). It is possible that these early fluctuations are of sufficient magnitude and duration to induce an LH/FSH peak of ovulatory magnitude. In a prospective longitudinal study where a group of girls aged 8–18 years was studied, a progressive elevation of serum LH, FSH, oestradiol, dehydroepiandrosterone and androstenedione levels occurred during puberty and continued until menarche (Lee, Xenarkis, Winer and Matsenbaugh, 1976).

In the normal adult female, serum FSH levels are relatively high at the time of menstruation due to the low levels of steroids at the end of the preceding luteal phase. The relatively high FSH levels result in follicular growth, and midway through the follicular phase of the menstrual cycle an increase in oestrogen levels can be detected (Fig. 4). Increments in the plasma oestrogen levels are important in the initiation of the midcycle surge of FSH and LH, that results in ovulation. The apparent paradoxical situation of oestradiol, which in most cases exerts a negative feedback on gonadotrophin secretion, exerting a positive feedback at midcycle has been investigated and discussed by Yen and Lein (1976). Towards the end of the luteal phase of the menstrual cycle steroid levels start to decline and a new cycle is initiated. For a full discussion of the control of secretion of gonadotrophins throughout the cycle the publications by Ross et al., 1970, and Vande Wiele et al., 1970, together with Ch. IX, Vol. 1, should be consulted.

Irregularities of the menstrual cycle have also been studied. In subjects with a short luteal phase oestradiol levels are lower than those found in women with normal menstrual cycles (Sherman and Korenman, 1974a) and possibly results from defective follicular maturation due to deficient FSH secretion. Sherman and Korenman (1974b) also studied the hormonal changes throughout the menstrual cycle in six obese subjects who had cycle lengths of 24–157 days. Although serum oestradiol levels fluctuated normally, progesterone levels were significantly reduced when compared to young

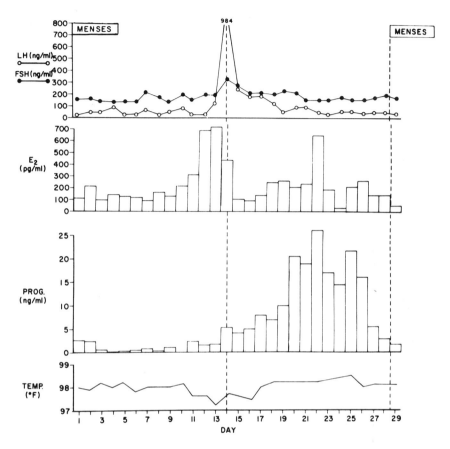

Fig. 4. Simultaneous determinations of LH, FSH, oestradiol (1 pg/ml = 3·67 pmol/l), progesterone (1 ng/ml = 3·18 nmol/l) and basal body temperature in a woman with a normal ovulatory menstrual cycle (from Vande Wiele *et al.*, 1970, with permission of authors and publisher).

healthy women of normal body weight. As women reach the age of 40 years, menstrual irregularities become increasingly common.

2. In Pregnancy

Relatively little is known about the mechanisms controlling oestrogen production during pregnancy. It has been demonstrated that placental and cord blood steroids can inhibit the rate of hydrolysis of the oestrogen precursor, dehydroepiandrosterone sulphate and also the action of the placental 3β hydroxysteroid dehydrogenase enzyme system; these have been suggested as possible mechanisms involved in the regulation of oestrogen biosynthesis during pregnancy (Townsley, Scheel and Rubin, 1970; Townsley, 1975).

The rate of supply of androgen sulphates to the placenta has also been implicated in the control of oestrogen synthesis during pregnancy. There is indirect evidence that the foetal hypothalamic–pituitary–adrenal system is involved in the control of the rate of supply of androgen sulphates to the placenta (Simmer, Dignam, Easterling, Frankland and Naftolin, 1966; Arai, Kiwabara and Okinaga, 1972). In vitro experiments have shown that ACTH and other peptide hormones (HGH and HCSM) can stimulate the production of androgen sulphates by the human foetal adrenal at midgestation without a concomitant stimulation of cortisol biosynthesis (Isherwood and Oakey, 1976). Failure of the foetal adrenal to respond directly to ACTH by increasing cortisol synthesis may be partly responsible for the enlargement of the foetal adrenal gland that occurs in the later stages of pregnancy (Oakey, 1970). Stimulation of the adrenal cortex by ACTH with no inhibitory feedback, could result in increasing quantities of androgen sulphates being made available for placental biosynthesis.

3. In the Male

Regulation of oestrogen formations in the normal adult males has been investigated (Doerr and Pirke, 1974, 1975). Stimulation of the Leydig cells was achieved using HCG which resembles human LH in most of its biological properties while for suppression of Leydig cell functions fluoxymesterone, which is known to suppress LH secretion, was used. Administration of HCG or fluoxymesterone resulted in major changes in plasma oestradiol and testosterone levels, but not of oestrone levels. Administration of dexamethasone, which suppresses adrenocortical secretion, suppressed oestrone levels. A pronounced decrease in testosterone levels after ACTH administration suggested that secretion of testicular hormones is suppressed by ACTH (Doerr and Pirke, 1975). Although it has been suggested that in the male, oestrogens can preferentially suppress FSH secretion, this has not been substantiated (Walsh, Swerdloff and Odell, 1973).

Studies in men have shown that when oestradiol is administered in microgram amounts, plasma levels of LH are suppressed to the same extent as when milligram amounts of testosterone are given. Naftolin et al. (1971) postulated that testosterone may be converted to oestradiol in the brain and have demonstrated the aromatisation of testosterone into oestradiol by brain tissue (see Section A.5). These observations have been used as evidence to suggest that testosterone may be converted to oestradiol in order to exert its biological effect on the hypothalamic–pituitary axis. However, Santen (1975) compared the biological activity of testosterone and oestradiol on the hypothalamic–pituitary axis. Physiologic infusion of testosterone and oestradiol resulted in suppression of LH to a similar mean level, but divergent effects on the pulsatile release of LH were observed. In addition 5α-dihydro-testosterone, which cannot be converted to oestradiol, also suppressed LH secretion. These data therefore suggested that testosterone may not require aromatisation to oestradiol for the inhibition of LH secretion in men.

C. OESTROGEN KINETICS

The production, metabolic clearance rates and interconversions of oestrogens have been determined using isotopically labelled steroids. The production rate (PR) of a hormone is defined as the total rate of *de novo* formation from all sources and includes secretion of hormone by a gland and its formation by peripheral conversion of other secreted precursors (Gurpide, 1975). Production rates can be calculated from the cumulative specific activity of urinary oestrogen metabolites after administration of a dose of labelled oestrogen:

$$PR = \frac{\text{d.p.m. administered}}{\text{specific activity of urinary oestrogen} \times \text{days of urine collection}}$$

(Eqn 1)

As the metabolic clearance rate (MCR) can be defined as the ratio of the rate of irreversible removal of the hormone from the bloodstream to its concentration in peripheral blood (Tait, 1963), the production rate of a hormone can also be calculated by determining the metabolic clearance (MCR) and concentration of endogenous steroid under investigation.

The MCR of a steroid is usually defined as the volume of blood irreversibly cleared of the hormone per unit time (Tait and Burstein, 1964). Metabolic clearance rates can be calculated after a single intravenous injection of radio-labelled tracer or after the infusion of a radiolabelled tracer at a constant rate until a steady state is achieved. The relative merits of each technique have been discussed (Baird, Horton, Longcope and Tait, 1969).

Interconversions between steroids are estimated by measuring the conversion ratio of a precursor to its product ($CR^{PRE-PRO}$) and transfer factors ($[\rho]^{PRE-PRO}$) (Gurpide, MacDonald, Vande Wiele and Lieberman, 1963; Baird et al., 1969; Gurpide, 1975). By infusing an isotopically labelled steroid precursor and measuring the steady state concentrations of labelled product and precursor the conversion ratio can be determined:

$$CR^{PRE-PRO} = \frac{\text{concentration product}}{\text{concentration precursor}}$$

(Eqn 2)

The transfer factor, defined as the fraction of new material entering one pool from all sources that reaches another pool, can be calculated from the conversion ratio (Gurpide et al., 1963; Horton and Tait, 1966):

$$[\rho] = \frac{MCR^{PRO}}{MCR^{PRE}} \times CR^{PRE-PRO} \qquad \text{(Eqn 3)}$$

where MCR^{PRO} = metabolic clearance rate of product and MCR^{PRE} = metabolic clearance rate of precursor.

Alternatively a double isotope technique can be used (Gurpide, Mann and Sandberg, 1964; MacDonald, Rombaut and Siiteri, 1967) to determine the transfer factor from the ratio of isotopes infused and the isotopic ratio of the isolated product. The product hormone can be isolated from blood ($[\rho]_{BB}$) or urine ($[\rho]_{BU}$) but where the urinary metabolite is not identical with the compound in blood different values for rho are usually obtained. This is thought to be due to the further metabolism of the product at the site of conversion, before the product is released into the circulation (Gurpide, 1975).

Several assumptions are made in the derivation of Eqn 1 used to estimate production rates from the specific activity of a urinary metabolite (Laumas, Tait and Tait, 1961; Gurpide, Mann, Vande Wiele and Lieberman, 1962; Gurpide, Angers, Vande Wiele and Lieberman, 1962). The basic assumptions that the isotope tracer should have a metabolic fate identical to that of the endogenous steroid and that the fraction of precursor converted to the product remains constant during the time of urine collection have been challenged with regards to oestrogens (Kelly and Rizkallah, 1973; Rizkallah, Tovel and Kelly, 1975). These authors found large differences in the ratios of urinary oestrogens suggesting that the isotopic tracer had a metabolic fate different to that of the endogenous hormone. However, these studies were carried out in post-menopausal women with endometrial cancer, whereas studies in normal adults and post-menopausal women similar isotopic ratios for urinary oestrogens were found (MacDonald et al., 1967; Grodin et al., 1973). Although variations in the fractional conversion of cortisol occur (Kelly, 1975) the fractional conversion of androstenedione to oestrone was constant (MacDonald et al., 1967).

The ability to obtain a steady-state when determining MCR's for oestrogens by the constant infusion procedure has been challenged (Hembree, Bardin and Lipsett, 1969). In their initial studies to determine the MCR of oestrone and oestradiol, Longcope, Layne and Tait (1968) assumed that a steady-state had been reached after infusion for 2 hr, as free precursor and product concentrations appeared stable. Hembree's group, however, were unable to achieve an isotopic steady-state within a 2 hr period and variations in the concentrations of labelled oestrogens were found even when the infusions were continued for up to 12 hr. Longcope and Tait (1971) validated their earlier results and suggested that variations in posture and hepatic blood flow over a 12 hr period could account for the inability of Hembree to achieve a steady-state when the infusion was continued for 12 hr. In addition, two of the subjects studied by Hembree *et al.* (1969) had metastatic carcinoma. Uptake and retention of oestrogen by the carcinoma could have affected the time required to reach equilibrium in these subjects.

When the production rate of an oestrogen is calculated from the MCR and concentration of endogenous steroid it is important that sufficient samples are taken throughout a 24 hr period to allow accurate estimation of the mean concentration (Hutton, Jacobs, James, Murray and Rippon, 1977). In spite of the possible errors in determining production rates from the specific activity of urinary metabolites or from the MCR and concentration of endogenous hormone the values obtained for production rates of oestrogens are in good agreement (Kirschner and Taylor, 1972). This suggests that these techniques are applicable to the study of oestrogens.

The use of urinary data to estimate transfer factors between metabolically related compounds has a number of theoretical objections (Tait and Horton, 1964; Rizkallah *et al.*, 1975). Where the metabolite in urine is similar to the compound in blood, e.g. DHA and DHAS (Sandberg, Gurpide and Lieberman, 1964) there was good agreement between transfer factors estimated from blood and urinary data. For oestrogens transfer factors estimated from urinary data are usually much greater than those estimated from the isolation of blood borne compounds probably due to the further metabolism or conjugation that can occur before the metabolite passes into the circulation (Gurpide, 1975). Recent studies by MacDonald, however, have suggested that if steroid infusion is continued for a sufficient length of time (e.g. up to 48 hr) then good agreement between transfer factors estimated from blood and urinary data is obtained (Edman, Aiman, Porter and MacDonald, 1978).

1. Production Rates of Oestrogens

(a) Women

The production rates of oestrone, oestradiol, oestriol and oestrone sulphate have been determined in women (Table 2). In the normal menstruating female production of these oestrogens is lowest during the follicular phase increasing 2–6 fold during the luteal phase of the cycle. Highest production rates, as expected, have been found at the time of ovulation (Gurpide *et al.*, 1962; Baird and Frazer, 1974). In post-menopausal women production of oestradiol is greatly reduced while the production rate of oestrone remains similar to that found in the follicular phase of the menstrual cycle (Longcope, 1971; Grodin *et al.*, 1973).

Table 2

Production rates of oestrogens.

Oestrogen	Method[a]	Condition	Production rate (μg/24 hr)	References
FEMALES				
Oestrone	U		44	Macdonald et al. (1967)
(1 μg = 3·70 nmol)	U	Follicular	51 ± 11	Kirschner and Taylor (1972)
	B	Follicular	101 ± 13	Longcope and Williams (1974)
	U	Luteal	178 ± 63	Kirschner and Taylor (1972)
	B	On Oral contraceptive therapy:		
		mestranol + progestion	71 ± 12	Longcope et al. (1974)
		ethynyl oestradiol + progestin	93 ± 12	Longcope et al. (1974)
	B	Post-menopausal	40	Longcope (1971)
	U	Post-menopausal	19 ± 2	Kirschner and Taylor (1972)
	U	Post-menopausal	40	Grodin et al. (1973)
	B	Post-menopausal	38 ± 7	Pratt and Longcope (1978)
	U	Post-menopausal with endometrial cancer:		
		four subjects preoperatively	51	Rizkallah et al. (1975)
		four subjects postoperatively	51	Rizkallah et al. (1975)
	B	Breast cancer	45 ± 7	Pratt and Longcope (1978)
Oestrone sulphate		Early follicular	95	Ruder, Loriaux and Lipsett (1972)
(1 μg = 2·85 nmol)		Early luteal	182	Ruder et al. (1972)
Oestradiol	U	26–38-yr-old	230	Frazer et al. (1967)
(1 μg = 3·67 nmol)	U	42–48-yr-old	260	Frazer et al. (1967)
	U	Follicular	56	Eren, Reynolds, Turner, Schmidt, MacKay, Howard and Preedy (1967)
	U	Follicular	70 ± 23	Kirschner and Taylor (1972)
	B	Follicular	80 ± 11	Longcope and Williams (1974)
	B	Follicular	63	Baird and Frazer (1974)

U	Midcycle	200 and 500	Gurpide et al. (1962)
B	Midcycle	394	Baird and Frazer (1974)
U	Luteal	88	Eren et al. (1967)
U	Luteal	202 ± 150	Kirschner and Taylor (1972)
B	Luteal	337	Baird and Frazer (1974)
	On oral contraceptive therapy:		
B	mestranol + progestin	47 ± 8	Longcope et al. (1974)
	ethynyl oestradiol + progestin	120 ± 22	Longcope et al. (1974)
		6	Longcope (1971)
B	Post-menopausal		
U	Post-menopausal	15 ± 1	Kirschner and Taylor (1972)
B	Post-menopausal	<2 − 15	Ridgway, Longcope and Waloof (1975)
B	Post-menopausal	18 ± 3	Pratt and Longcope (1978)
B	Post-menopausal + breast cancer	16 ± 4	Pratt and Longcope (1978)
U	Cervical cancer – stage 0	570	Frazer et al. (1967)
B	Dysfunctional uterine bleeding	247	Frazer and Baird (1974)
Oestriol			
(1µg = 3·47 nmol)			
B	Follicular	14 ± 2	Flood et al. (1976)
B	Luteal	23 ± 2	Flood et al. (1976)
B	Post-menopausal	5	Flood et al. (1976)
B	Post-menopausal	12 ± 3	Pratt and Longcope (1978)
B	Post-menopausal and breast cancer	12 ± 3	Pratt and Longcope (1978)
MALES			
Oestrone			
U		46 ± 1·1	Crowell, Turner, Schmidt, Howard and Preedy (1967)
U		46	Erens et al. (1967)
U		18	MacDonald et al. (1967)
U		40 ± 12	Kirschner and Taylor (1972)
U	Gynaecomastia	51·6	Kirschner and Taylor (1972)

Table 2—*continued*

Oestrogen	Method[a]	Condition	Production rate	References
Oestrone sulphate	B		77	Ruder *et al.* (1972)
Oestradiol	U		29	Eren *et al.* (1967)
	U	59–74-yr-old	42 ± 12	Kirschner and Taylor (1972)
	B		44 ± 7	Bayard *et al.* (1974)
	B		30–65	Ridgway *et al.* (1975)
	U	Gynaecomastia	64	Kirschner and Taylor (1972)
	B	Hypertrophy of the prostate (54–75-yr-old)	48 ± 5	Bayard *et al.* (1974)
	B	Hyperthyroid	51 ± 8	Ridgway *et al.* (1975)

[a] U = determined from specific activity of a urinary metabolite, B = determined from MCR and endogenous oestrogen concentration.

Investigations by MacDonald *et al.* (1967), Siiteri and MacDonald (1973) and Kirschner and Taylor (1972) have shown that in the menstruating women conversion of androstenedione to oestrone contributes from 10–50% of the amount of oestrone produced, the remainder being derived mainly from the peripheral conversion of oestradiol secreted by the ovary. In the post-menopausal women all the oestrone produced can be accounted for by the peripheral conversion of androstenedione (Grodin, Siiteri and MacDonald, 1973).

Production rates of oestradiol in women taking mestranol or ethynyl oestradiol preparations were within the range found in normal women during the early follicular phase of the menstrual cycle, suggesting that the ovary produces oestrogen even while an individual is receiving oral contraceptive therapy (Longcope, Watson and Williams, 1974).

A significant increase in the production rate of oestradiol was found in women with stage 0 lesions of the cervix (Frazer, Cudmore, Melanson and Morse, 1967). No increase in the production rate of oestradiol was found in women with dysfunctional uterine bleeding, values all being within the normal range (Frazer and Baird, 1974). Measurement of the production rate of oestradiol in ACTH stimulated women with breast cancer, before and after ovariectomy, indicated that the post-menopausal ovaries made no contribution to oestrogen production (Barlow, Emerson and Saxena, 1969). In post-menopausal women with breast cancer production of oestrone and oestriol was similar to that of normal post-menopausal women (Poortman, Thijssen and Schwarz, 1973; Pratt and Longcope, 1978). No elevation in the production rate of oestrone was found in post-menopausal women with endometrial cancer (Rizkallah *et al.*, 1975; Reed, Hutton, Baxendale, James, Jacobs and Fisher, 1979b). Alterations in oestrone production rates have been found, however, in women with various ovarian tumours (MacDonald, Grodin, Edman, Wellios and Siiteri, 1976; Aiman, Nalick, Jacobs, Porter, Edman, Vellios and MacDonald, 1977; Reed, Hutton, Beard, Jacobs and James, 1979a).

(b) Men

The production rates for oestrone and oestradiol are similar in normal males (Table 2). From the limited data available it would appear that the production rate of oestradiol in the male does not decrease with advancing age (Bayard, Louvet, Thijssens, Thouvenot and Boulard, 1974). The origins of oestrogens in men are more complex than in women due to the larger amounts of testosterone available for conversion to oestradiol.

Elevated production rates of oestrone and oestradiol were found in some, but not all, subjects studied with gynaecomastia (Kirschner and Taylor,

1972). No difference was found in the production rate of oestradiol in men aged 59–74 yr with hypertrophy of the prostate, compared to a group of men of similar age (Bayard et al., 1975).

2. Metabolic Clearance Rates of Oestrogens

(a) Normal adults

The metabolic clearance rates for oestrogens have been determined by single injection and constant infusion techniques. Minimal changes in the MCR oestradiol were noted when the mass of oestrogen infused was increased from 17–170 µg/day (62–624 nmol/day). However, when the mass infused was increased to 1440 µg/day (5·3 µmol/day) the MCR oestradiol increased 50% (Hembree, Bardin and Lipsett, 1969).

Although most values reported for MCR's of oestrogens are expressed as litres of plasma/day (or $l/d/m^2$) a significant proportion of oestrone (15–20%) in males and females and oestradiol in males (15%) is associated with red cells (Longcope, Layne and Tait, 1968).

The MCR of oestrone is similar in males and females and greater than the MCR of oestradiol (Table 3). The MCR oestradiol in females is significantly lower than that found in males. These differences can be accounted for by the different affinities of oestradiol and oestrone for SBP and the higher concentrations of SBP found in women.

The phase of the menstrual cycle does not affect the MCR of oestrone, oestradiol or oestriol (Longcope et al., 1968; Baird and Frazer, 1974; Floor, Pratt and Longcope, 1976).

The MCR oestrone and oestradiol decreases by 25% in post-menopausal women compared to a 13% decrease in the MCR of oestriol (Longcope, 1971; Flood et al., 1975) and these decreases occur within three years of the menopause (Hembree et al., 1969). In men aged 59–74 years the MCR oestradiol ($926 \pm 140\,l/d/m^2$) was similar to that found in younger males (Bayard et al., 1975; Longcope et al., 1968; Hembree et al., 1969).

An investigation into the effect of posture on the MCR oestrone showed that changing from a supine to upright position resulted in a 29% decrease in the MCR oestrone (Flood, Hunter, Lloyd and Longcope, 1973).

The conversion ratio of androstenedione to oestrone was also determined in this study, but did not alter with change in posture. As the concentration of endogenous oestrone remained relatively constant during both postural periods, the calculated production rate of oestrone of 56 µg/day (185 nmol/day) decreased to 37 µg/day (137 nmol/day) upon standing. It is possible that more intensive plasma sampling would reveal changes in the endogenous oestrone concentration upon change in posture.

Table 3

Metabolic clearance rates of oestrogens.

Oestrogen	Condition	MCR (M. ± S.E.) 1/24 hr	1/24 hr/m²	References
FEMALES				
Oestrone		2210 ± 120	1320 ± 70	Longcope et al. (1968)
		a3200 ± 170	a1910 ± 100	Longcope et al. (1968)
		1634 ± 183	982 ± 94	Hembree et al. (1969)
		1870 ± 150	1120 ± 80	Longcope and Williams (1974)
	On oral contraceptive therapy:			
	mestranol + progestin	—	1010 ± 60	Longcope et al. (1974)
	ethynyl oestradiol + progestin	—	1180 ± 80	Longcope et al. (1974)
	Post-menopausal	1610 ± 110	1050 ± 70	Longcope (1971)
	Breast cancer	2239	—	Pearlman, Dettertogh, Laumas and Pearlman (1969)
Oestrone Sulphate		146 ± 34	94.1 ± 22	Ruder et al. (1972)
Oestradiol		1350 ± 40	790 ± 20	Longcope et al. (1968)
		a2280 ± 90	a1360 ± 40	Longcope et al. (1968)
		1025 ± 38	614 ± 17	Hembree et al. (1968)
		1202 ± 55	747 ± 30	Baird and Frazer (1974)
		1170 ± 80	740 ± 50	Longcope and Williams (1974)
		1290 ± 40	790 ± 25	Ridgway et al. (1975)
	On oral contraceptive therapy:			
	mestranol + progestin	—	750 ± 60	Longcope et al. (1974)
	ethynyl oestradiol ± progestin	—	1070 ± 60	Longcope et al. (1974)
	Post-menopausal	—	643 ± 42	Hembree et al. (1969)
		910 ± 70	580 ± 30	Longcope (1971)
		940 ± 50	580 ± 20	Ridgway et al. (1974)

Table 3—*continued*

Oestrogen	Condition	MCR (M. ± S.E.) 1/24 hr	1/24 hr/m²	References
	Breast cancer	766	—	Pearlman et al. (1969)
	Dysfunctional uterine bleeding	1198 ± 97		Frazer and Baird (1974)
Oestriol	Follicular	2100 ± 100	1240 ± 40	Flood et al. (1976)
	Luteal	2100 ± 115	1280 ± 65	Flood et al. (1976)
	Post-menopausal	1890 ± 95	1060 ± 35	Flood et al. (1976)
		1960 ± 100	1150 ± 90	Pratt and Longcope (1978)
	Breast cancer	1600 ± 100	950 ± 70	Pratt and Longcope (1978)
MALES				
Oestrone		2570 ± 160	1310 ± 80	Longcope et al. (1968)
		[a]3880 ± 220	[a]1990 ± 120	Longcope et al. (1968)
		2412 ± 258	1168 ± 95	Hembree et al. (1971)
		—	965 ± 70	Longcope and Tait (1971)
		—	1230 ± 150	Flood et al. (1973)
		—	875 ± 120	Flood et al. (1973)
Oestrone sulphate	Supine	167 ± 36	87 ± 21	Ruder et al. (1972)
	Standing	155 ± 15	80 ± 10	Longcope, 1972
Oestradiol		1890 ± 100	990 ± 50	Longcope et al. (1968)
		[a]3060 ± 160	[a]1600 ± 80	Longcope et al. (1968)
		1640 ± 139	827 ± 30	Hembree et al. (1969)
		—	820 ± 40	Longcope and Tait (1971)
		1487	926 ± 140	Bayard et al. (1974)
	Hypertrophy of the prostate	1948	1192 ± 121	Bayard et al. (1974)
	Hyperthyroid	1210 ± 250	650 ± 120	Ridgway et al. (1975)

[a] MCR measured using whole blood.

The metabolic clearance rate of oestrone sulphate is approximately 10% of that found for unconjugated oestrone (Longcope, 1972; Ruder et al., 1972). The extensive binding of oestrone sulphate to serum albumin (Rosenthal et al., 1972) and the possibility that only a small fraction of circulating oestrone sulphate can be metabolised have been suggested in order to explain the low MCR of oestrone sulphate compared to that of oestrone (Longcope, 1972).

(b) In pathological conditions

Alterations in the clearance rates of oestrogens have been studied in few pathological conditions. No difference in the MCR of oestradiol was found in women with dysfunctional uterine bleeding (Frazer and Baird, 1974) and these authors suggested that oestrogen metabolism in women with dysfunctional uterine bleeding was similar to that in normal women.

In male subjects with hyperthyroidism the MCR of oestradiol was significantly reduced and in two post-menopausal women, was at the lower end of the normal range (Ridgway et al., 1975). As thyroid function improved with therapy these changes in the MCR of oestradiol were reversed. In these hyperthyroid subjects a decrease in MCR of oestradiol was accompanied by an increase in the concentration of SBP. However, there was only a poor correlation between the absolute decrease in MCR of oestradiol and increase in SBP concentration. This suggests that factors, other than an increase in SBP concentration, could be involved in causing the decrease in the MCR of oestradiol. As both fat and adipose tissue are involved in oestradiol metabolism (Longcope, Pratt, Schneider and Fineberg, 1976), the decreased mass of tissue found in hyperthyroid subjects could decrease the amount of tissue actively metabolising oestradiol and thus decrease the MCR of oestradiol.

(c) Effect of oral contraceptive therapy on MCR of oestrogens

Administration of oral contraceptives containing ethynyl oestradiol but not mestranol caused an increase in the MCR of oestradiol (Longcope et al., 1974). However, these changes were not permanent and after one year without therapy the MCR's of oestradiol were the same as in normal subjects.

3. Steroid Conversions

(a) Transfer factors

(1) Estimated from hormones in blood ($[\rho]_{BB}$). Transfer factors for the con-

version of androgens to oestrogens and the interconversion of oestrogens have been determined in normal subjects (Table 4). Because of the complexity of these investigations, these values have usually been determined in only a small number of subjects and this should be borne in mind when considering these data.

Table 4

Transfer factors between circulating oestrogen precursors and oestrogens estimated from hormones in blood.

From	To	Female	Male	Reference
		$[\rho]_{BB}$ (%)		
A	E1	0·74	1·35	Longcope, Kato and Horton (1969)
	E1	1·35[a]	—	Grodin et al.(1973)
A	E2	0·07, 0·08	0·07	Longcope et al. (1969)
E1	E2	4·1	5·0	Longcope (1968)
	E1S	—	40·0	Longcope (1972)
	E1S	50·0	67·0	Ruder et al. (1972)
E2	E1	17·3	—	Longcope (1968)
	E1	—	21·0	Longcope and Tait (1971)
	E1S	—	42·0	Longcope (1972)
	E1S	65·0	65·0	Ruder et al. (1972)
E1S	E1	—	15·0	Longcope (1972)
	E1	22·5	12·7	Ruder et al. (1972)
	E2	—	2·2 and 4·4	Longcope et al. (1972)
	E2	1·4		Ruder et al. (1972)
T	E1	—	0·13	Longcope et al. (1969)
	E2	0·15	0·39	Longcope et al. (1969)

[a] Post-menopausal.

Conversion of androstenedione to oestrone and testosterone to oestradiol is more efficient in males than females (Longcope, Kato and Horton, 1969). The higher rates of conversion of androstenedione than testosterone to oestrogens suggests that androstenedione is more readily aromatised than testosterone. In post-menopausal women there is an increase in the efficiency with which androstenedione is converted to oestrone (Grodin et al., 1973) although the mechanism responsible for this increase is not clear.

In the male a significant proportion of the oestradiol entering the blood *de novo* arises as a result of the conversion of testosterone to oestradiol (Baird, Horton, Longcope and Tait, 1968; Kelch, Jenner, Weinstein, Kaplan and Grumbach, 1972). In the female, however, the contribution of testosterone to oestradiol is insignificant due to the low levels of testosterone available for conversion.

Although it is possible that circulating androgens could be aromatised in adrenal or gonadal tissues, the conversion of androstenedione to oestrone, measured by the urinary method, was similar in normal, adrenalectomised and ovariectomised subjects (see Table 5). It is therefore unlikely that conversion occurs in gonadal or adrenal tissues (MacDonald *et al.*, 1967). Both adipose tissue (Nimrod and Ryan, 1975) and adult human liver (Smuk and Schwers, 1977) have the ability to convert androstenedione to oestrone *in vitro*.

In both sexes there is a similar ability to convert oestradiol to oestrone and oestrone to oestradiol (Longcope *et al.*, 1969). However, the values obtained from estimations of hormones isolated from blood are much lower than the transfer factors previously calculated from urinary data (Gurpide *et al.*, 1962; Barlow and Logan, 1966).

Oestrone sulphate is a major circulating oestrogen and interconversion with oestrone and oestradiol have been investigated. Conversion of oestrone and oestradiol to oestrone sulphate is similar and much greater than any other oestrogen interconversions so far examined. Most of the oestrone sulphate entering the circulation is thought to result from conversion of oestrone and oestradiol with little, if any, direct secretion (Longcope, 1972; Ruder *et al.*, 1972). Conversion of oestrone sulphate to oestrone is more efficient than conversion to oestradiol suggesting that tissues capable of the hydrolysis of oestrone sulphate are not efficient at reducing the 17-keto group of oestrone.

(2) *Estimated from urinary metabolites* ($[\rho]_{BU}$). Although there are theoretical objections to the calculation of hormonal interconversion rates from measurements on urinary metabolites, this method has been widely used to investigate the conversion of androstenedione to oestrone in normal and pathological conditions (Table 5).

In normal young adults conversion of androstenedione to oestrone is efficient (MacDonald *et al.*, 1967). The extent of conversion appears to remain constant throughout the menstrual cycle (Kirschner and Taylor, 1972). With advancing age the conversion of androstenedione to oestrone increases and in post-menopausal women extraglandular conversion of androstenedione accounts for the total production of oestrone (Grodin *et al.*, 1973). A significant correlation between $[\rho]_{BU}^{AE1}$ and increasing age has been found in men ($r = 0.86$, $p < 0.001$) and women ($r = 0.62$, $p < 0.001$) by Hemsell, Grodin, Brenner, Siiteri and MacDonald (1974).

A correlation between $[\rho]_{BU}^{AE1}$ and body weight has also been reported (Siiteri and MacDonald, 1973; Rizkallah *et al.*, 1975; Edman and MacDonald, 1978; MacDonald, Edman, Hemsell, Porter and Siiteri, 1978). However, no

Table 5

Transfer factors for androstenedione to oestrone determined by the urinary method.

Condition	$[\rho]_{BU}^{AE1}(\%)$	References
FEMALES		
Normal women	1·3	MacDonald *et al.* (1967)
Follicular	1·2	Kirschner and Taylor (1972)
Luteal	1·1	Kirschner and Taylor (1972)
19–50-yr-old	1·3	Hemsell *et al.* (1974)
Ovariectomised	1·2	MacDonald *et al.* (1967)
Adrenalectomised	1·4	MacDonald *et al.* (1967)
Post-menopausal	2·7	Grodin *et al.* (1973)
Post-menopausal	2·5	Poortman *et al.* (1973)
Post-menopausal	1·7	Hausknecht and Gusberg (1973)
Post-menopausal	1·8	Pelc *et al.* (1978)
Post-menopausal (53-73 y)	2·8	Hemsell *et al.* (1974)
Post-menopausal and obese	3·9	MacDonald *et al.* (1978)
Post-menopausal + breast cancer	2·9	Poortman *et al.* (1973)
Post-menopausal + endometrial cancer	3·1	Hausknecht and Gusberg (1973)
Post-menopausal + endometrial cancer		
Post-menopausal + endometrial cancer and obese	5·1	MacDonald *et al.* (1978)
Post-menopausal + endometrial cancer	2·1	Reed *et al.* (1979b)
Post-menopausal + endometrial hyperplasia and non-endocrine ovarian tumour	3·5	Rizkallah *et al.* (1975)
	1·6	MacDonald *et al.* (1976)
Post-menopausal + endometrial cancer and ovarian thecoma	2·4	Reed *et al.* (1979a)
Post-menopausal + ovarian cystic teratomas	2·9	Aiman *et al.* (1977)
Post-menopausal + bone fractures	1·8	Pelc *et al.* (1978)
MALES		
	1·4	MacDonald *et al.* (1967)
12–45-yr-old	1·5	Hemsell *et al.* (1974)
53–82-yr-old	2·5	Hemsell *et al.* (1974)

correlation between $[\rho]_{BU}^{AE1}$ and age or between $[\rho]_{BU}^{AE1}$ and weight was found in a group of post-menopausal women studied by Pelc, Marshall, Guha, Khan and Nordin (1978).

Since the demonstration in post-menopausal women that oestrone is derived solely from the extraglandular conversion of androstenedione (Grodin *et al.*, 1973) investigations have been carried out to examine the relationship between $[\rho]_{BU}^{AE1}$ and a number of pathological conditions.

A significant difference between the extent of conversion of androstenedione to oestrone in subjects with and without endometrial cancer was found by Hausknecht and Gusberg (1973) but this was not confirmed by MacDonald *et al.* (1978) and Reed *et al.* (1979b). Whereas MacDonald *et al.* (1978) and Reed *et al.* (1979b) gave the weights of the subjects studied. Hausknecht and Gusberg (1973) did not. It is therefore possible that the significant difference found by Hausknecht and Gusberg could have resulted from differences in weight of the two groups studied.

Similar studies carried out in normal post-menopausal women and women with breast cancer and oesteoporosis have failed to reveal any differences in the extent of the conversion of androstenedione to oestrone (Poortman *et al.*, 1973; Pelc *et al.*, 1978). In post-menopausal women with various ovarian tumours, although alterations in the production rate of oestrone have been found, the extent of conversion of androstenedione to oestrone was within the normal limits (MacDonald *et al.*, 1976; Aiman *et al.*, 1977; Reed *et al.*, 1979a).

Although most studies carried out in women with pathological conditions have failed to reveal an increase in the conversion of androstenedione to oestrone, increased rates of conversion have been found in some male subjects with gynaecomastia (Kirschner and Taylor, 1972). Severe feminisation in a prepubertal boy was also shown to result from an increase in the extent of the conversion of androstenedione to oestrone (Hemsell, Edman, Marks, Siiteri and MacDonald, 1977).

(b) Conversion ratios

In other investigations conversion ratios (CR) have been measured. The CR values obtained in these studies are shown in Table 6. The conversion ratios for testosterone to oestradiol, testosterone to oestrone and androstenedione to oestrone were significantly higher in males than in females but there was no sexual difference in the contribution of androstenedione to oestradiol (Olivo, Vittek, Southren, Gordon and Raffi, 1973). These results confirmed the earlier observations of Longcope *et al.* (1969) that the conversion of androstenedione to oestrogens was greater than that of testosterone with androstenedione and testosterone being converted preferentially to oestrone and oestradiol respectively.

In subjects with hyperthyroidism a significant increase in the conversion of androstenedione and testosterone to oestrone in men and women and of androstenedione to oestradiol in men occurred (Southren, Olivo, Gordon, Vittek, Brenner and Raffi, 1974). From these CR values, theoretical transfer constants were calculated with $[\rho]^{TE2}$ equal to 0·9% and $[\rho]^{AE2}$ equal to 0·6% in male subjects. In spontaneous hyperthyroidism the increased plasma oestrogen levels often seen would therefore appear to result from increased

Table 6

Conversion ratios.

	From	To	CR (%)	References
FEMALES				
Normal women	A	E1	0·99 ± 0·052	Olivo et al. (1973)
	A	E2	0·21 ± 0·037	Olivo et al. (1973)
	E2	E1	10·5 ± 1·0	Baird and Frazer (1974)
	T	E1	0·07 ± 0·009	Olivo et al. (1973)
	T	E2	0·125 ± 0·017	Olivo et al. (1973)
Post-menopausal women	A	E1	1·8 ± 0·07	Canalog et al. (1977)
	A	E2	0·24 ± 0·07	Canalog et al. (1977)
Pathological conditions: dysfunctional uterine bleeding	E2	E1	8·9 ± 1·0	Frazer and Baird (1974)
Hyperthyroidism	T	E1	0·70 ± 0·15	Southren et al. (1974)
	T	E2	0·16 ± 0·01	Southren et al. (1974)
Endometrial cancer	A	E1	2·6 ± 0·5	Canalog et al. (1977)
	A	E2	0·23 ± 0·3	Canalog et al. (1977)
MALES				
Normal men	A	E1	2·1 ± 0·33	Olivo et al. (1973)
	A	E2	0·2 ± 0·02	Olivo et al. (1973)
	T	E1	0·12 ± 0·009	Olivo et al. (1973)
	T	E2	0·27 ± 0·040	Olivo et al. (1973)
Hyperthyroidism	T	E1	0·72 ± 0·23	Southren et al. (1974)
	T	E2	0·30 ± 0·03	Southren et al. (1974)

peripheral conversion from androgens rather than from increased secretion.

In other pathological conditions no alteration in conversion ratios of androgen to oestrogens in women with endometrial cancer (Canalog, Sall, Gordon and Southren, 1977) or of oestradiol to oestrone in women with dysfunctional uterine bleeding were found (Frazer and Baird, 1974).

D. METABOLISM OF OESTROGENS

Studies of oestrogen metabolism have established that hydroxylation can occur at aromatic positions 2 and 4 and aliphatic carbon atoms 6, 7, 11, 14, 15, 16 and 18; some of these transformations are outlined in Fig. 5. Oestradiol and oestrone are interconvertible by an oestradiol 17β dehydrogenase. Oestrone, or oestrone sulphate, has a central position in the metabolism of the oestrogen molecule and is probably the main substrate for further

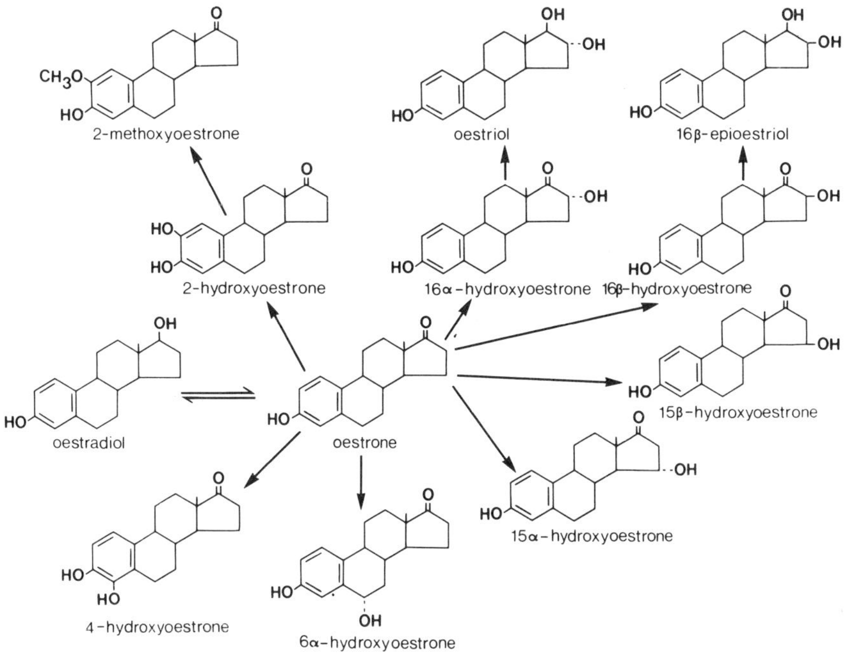

Fig. 5. Metabolism of oestrogens.

biotransformations (Fishman, Bradlow and Gallagher, 1960; Fishman, Bradlow, Zumoff, Hellman and Gallagher, 1961; Fishman, Goldberg, Rosenfeld, Zumoff, Hellman and Gallagher, 1969).

The formation of 2-hydroxy and 2-methoxy oestrogens is now known to be a major metabolic pathway for oestrogen metabolism. The ability of the human to form C-2 substituted oestrogens was first demonstrated by Kraychy and Gallagher (1957a). Both Kraychy and Gallagher (1957b) and Engel, Baggett and Carter (1957) isolated 2-methoxyoestrone from urine after administration of [16-14C] oestradiol to women. Kraychy and Gallagher (1957b) suggested that the formation of 2-methoxyoestrone probably involved 2-hydroxyoestrone and this was confirmed by Fishman, Cox and Gallagher (1960). These authors isolated 2-hydroxyoestrone from the urine of men after the administration of [16-14C] oestradiol. Administration of a mixture of [6,7-3H] oestradiol and [16-14C] oestrone showed that oestrone, rather than oestradiol was the substrate for ring A hydroxylation (Fishman, Bradlow and Gallagher, 1960).

As oestrone sulphate had been implicated as a major intermediate in the oxidative metabolism of oestradiol (Fishman and Hellman, 1972) the role of oestrone sulphate in the formation of catechol oestrogens was investigated by the simultaneous administration of [6,7, ^{3}H] oestrone-sulphate and oestrone [^{35}S]sulphate to men (Fishman, Yoshizawa and Hellman, 1973). Whereas 2-methoxyoestrone-sulphate and oestrone-sulphate isolated from urine exhibited similar ^{3}H:^{35}S ratios and about 23% of the radioactive sulphur isotope was retained in these compounds, in contrast the sulphur content of excreted 2-hydroxyoestrone monosulphate was much lower. From this study in man and *in vitro* studies carried out with rat liver (Miyasaki, Yoshizawa and Fishman, 1969) a mechanism for the formation of catechol oestrogens in man was proposed in which oestrone sulphate was the substrate from which 2-methoxyoestrone sulphate was derived without prior hydrolysis. As shown in Fig. 6, Fishman *et al.* (1973) postulated that

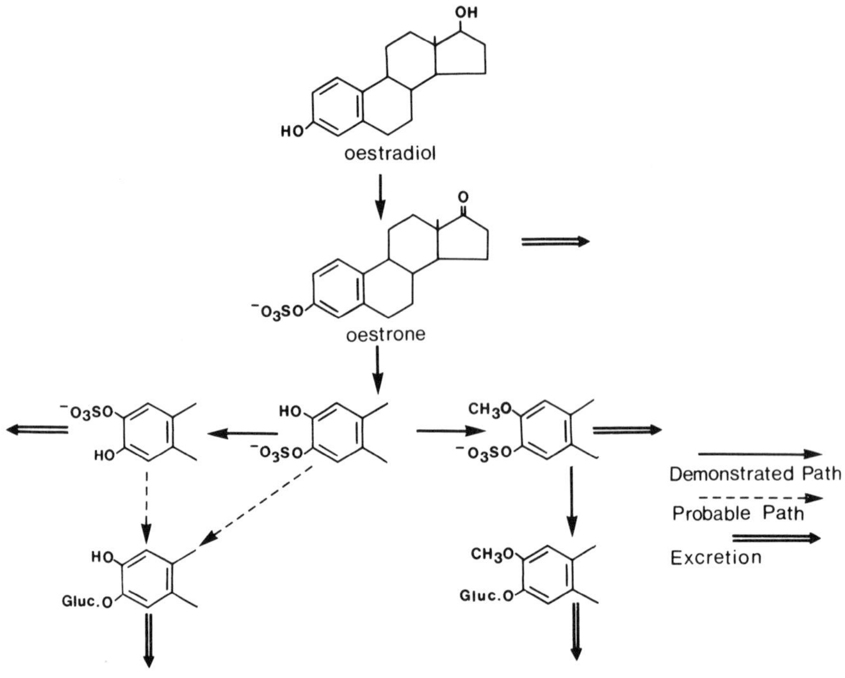

Fig. 6. Biosynthesis and subsequent fate of catechol oestrogens in man (from Fishman *et al.*, 1973 with permission of authors and publisher).

oestradiol is transformed into oestrone sulphate, part of which is then hydroxylated at C-2 to 2-hydroxyoestrone-3-sulphate. The latter compound is then partially *O*-methylated to 2-methoxyoestrone-3-sulphate which is excreted as such or is transconjugated to the 3-glucuronide.

However, the formation of catechol oestrogens by this pathway does not explain the finding that although oestrone-3-sulphate is the principal intermediate postulated in the formation of catechol oestrogens, 2-hydroxy-oestrone-2-sulphate is the predominant conjugate found in urine and no 2-hydroxyoestrone-3-sulphate has been isolated from urine.

The results of a comparative study into the *in vivo* and *in vitro* metabolism of oestradiol and 2-hydroxyoestradiol in man and by human liver has also questioned the pathway proposed by Fishman *et al.* (1973). Ball, Farthman and Knuppen (1976) were only able to detect 2-hydroxyoestrone-2-sulphate and no 2-hydroxyoestrone-3-sulphate when [4-^{14}C] oestradiol was incubated with human liver. When oestrone sulphate was used as the substrate much less catechol oestrogen conjugate were formed than when incubations with oestradiol were carried out.

The further metabolism of methoxyoestrogens has also been the subject of a number of investigations. Following the intravenous administration of the two isomeric monomethyl ethers of 2-hydroxyoestrone to humans, Yoshizawa and Fishman (1970) found that apart from conjugation both compounds were excreted in an essentially unchanged form. In contrast, after the oral administration of 2 and 4-methyoxyoestrones, Ball, Stuben-rauch and Knuppen (1977) found these compounds were extensively metabolised. Besides conjugation and 17β oxido-reduction quantitatively the most significant metabolic reaction consisted in the O-demethylation of the orally administered monomethyl ethers. This finding that methoxy-oestrogens when orally administered to human subjects are converted to a high extent to the corresponding catechol oestrogens should facilitate further investigations into the effects of catechol oestrogens in the human.

The physiological role of catechol oestrogens has been investigated. Although O-methylation of oestrogens is an important pathway of oestrogen metabolism it is the main pathway for adrenaline and noradrenaline metabolism in man. Enzymatic methylation and biological inactivation of these neurotransmitters is strongly inhibited by 2-hydroxyoestrogens (Ball, Knuppen, Haupt and Breuer, 1972) and the possibility that 2-hydroxy-oestrogens might be involved in the regulation of blood pressure under normal and pathological conditions has been suggested. Recently the presence of a potent C-2 hydroxylase has been shown in central tissue obtained from the human foetus (Fishman, Naftolin, Davies, Ryan and Petro, 1976). Catechol oestrogens also bind to the hypothalamic cytosol receptor (Fishman and Norton, 1975) and rat uterine cytosol receptors (Martucci and Fishman, 1976) and has provided evidence suggesting that catechol oestrogens may act as a naturally occurring antioestrogen having an important role in the modulation of oestrogenic activity of the female sex hormone.

Although hydroxylation at aromatic position 2 of the oestrogen molecule is a major metabolic pathway in humans, hydroxylation at the alternative carbon atom ortho to the phenolic hydroxyl group, i.e. position 4 also occurs (Williams, Longcope and Williams, 1974). [4-^{3}H] Oestradiol admixed with [4-^{14}C] oestradiol was injected intravenously into a male and female subject to assess the involvement of position 4 in the oxidative metabolism of oestradiol. 4-Hydroxyoestrone was identified in the urine of both subjects by a reverse isotope dilution procedure. Hydroxylation at position 4 accounted for 1·1% and 0·5% of the [4-^{14}C] oestradiol dose administered to the female and male respectively. The biological potency of 4-hydroxy-oestradiol was greater than that of 2-hydroxyoestradiol as measured by the induction of uterine growth in 21 day old mice and ovariectomised rats.

Oestrogen metabolites hydroxylated at the 6α position were isolated after incubation of oestrone and oestradiol with adult human liver tissue (Breuer, Knuppen and Haupt, 1966). 6α Hydroxylated metabolites were also identified after incubation with liver tissue from a human foetus at 11 weeks of gestation (Thorsen and Støa, 1965) and also from placental perfusions carried out in the fifth to sixth month of pregnancy (Alonso and Troen, 1966). 6α-Hydroxy-oestrone has also been isolated from human pregnancy urine (Knuppen, Haupt and Breuer, 1966b).

Although the main site for the metabolism of oestrogens has been generally considered to be the liver, the adrenal gland may also play an important role in the metabolism of oestrogens. The in vitro metabolism of oestrone and oestradiol by human adrenal tissue (Knuppen, Haupt and Breuer, 1965) and ox adrenal tissue (Knuppen, Haupt and Breuer, 1967), results in hydroxyl-ation at several positions of the oestrogen molecule.

Luukainen and Adlercreutz (1965) demonstrated the presence of an additional oestradiol-like compound in the phenolic fractions of extracts from late pregnancy urine. Mass spectral analysis of derivatives of the compound showed the presence of an additional double bond and the steroid was identified as 11-dehydro-oestradiol-17α. 11-Dehydro-oestradiol-17α was always detectable in samples of late pregnancy urine and enzyme hydrolysed extracts of pregnancy urine contained as much 11-dehydro-oestradiol-17α as oestradiol-17β. The origin and physiological significance of 11-dehydro-oestradiol-17α remains unresolved.

Although 14α-hydroxyoestrone has so far not been identified from human pregnancy urine, human placental tissue does have the ability to form 14α-hydroxyoestrone from 14α hydroxyandrost-4-ene 3, 17-dione by aromatisation (Knuppen et al., 1967).

15α-Hydroxy and 15β-hydroxyoestrone metabolites have been isolated from human pregnancy urine (Knuppen, Haupt and Breuer, 1965; Knuppen, Haupt and Breuer, 1966a). Breuer et al. (1966) identified 15α-hydroxy oestradiol after incubation of oestradiol with human liver slices. Human adrenal tissue (Knuppen *et al.*, 1965) and liver of a previable foetus perfused with oestrone or oestradiol (Schwers, Eriksson, Wiqvist and Diczfalusy, 1965), also have the ability to hydroxylate oestrogens at this position. 15α-Hydroxyoestradiol has also been isolated from enzymatically hydrolysed late pregnancy urine and concentrations in late pregnancy urine ranged from 15–100 μg/24 hr (52–347 nmol/24 hr) (Knuppen and Breuer, 1967). The possibility that 15α-hydroxyoestradiol was secreted by the foetus to the mother and subsequently eliminated in urine was suggested by Lisboa, Goebelsman and Diczfalusy (1967).

When 15α hydroxyoestradiol was given to two pregnant women it was excreted in urine conjugated predominantly at C-15 with *N*-acetylglucosamide (NAG) or as the double 3-sulphate-15 NAG conjugate (Jirku, Kadner and Levitz, 1972). Simultaneous infusion of 15α-hydroxyoestradiol intravenously and into the renal artery suggested that 15α-hydroxyoestradiol was conjugated with NAG in the kidney (Nagatomi, Osawa, Kirdani and Sandberg, 1973).

A major metabolite of 15α-hydroxyoestradiol is 15α-hydroxyoestriol (oestetrol). The structure of oestetrol was first proposed by Hagen, Barr and Diczfalusy (1965). These authors injected $[4\text{-}^{14}C]$ oestradiol into three infants with multiple malformations and found that quantitatively the major metabolite was an hydroxylation product more polar than 2-hydroxyoestriol and suggested that its structure was oestetrol. In a study of the foetal and maternal metabolism of oestradiol by an isotope dilution procedure, it was concluded that oestetrol was synthesised by the foetus but not by the mother (Gurpide, Schwers, Welch, Vande Wiele and Lieberman, 1966). As in the foetal organism the liver is the site of 15α- and 16α-hydroxylations, oestetrol is thought to be a specific product of the foetal liver (Lisboa, Simonitsch, Roth, Hagen and Diczfalusy, 1967).

Oestetrol can apparently be formed from oestradiol or oestriol as when $[4\text{-}^{14}C]$ oestradiol and $[6,7\text{-}^{3}H]$ oestriol were administered intravenously to a human anencephalic, oestetrol was formed from both substrates. This demonstrates that the presence of an hydroxyl group at C-16 of the oestrogen structure does not prevent subsequent hydroxylation at C-15 (Hagen, 1970). A neutral pathway for the formation of oestetrol is also possible as it has been demonstrated that 15α-hydroxyandrostenedione can be aromatised to 15α-hydroxyoestrone (Stern, Givner and Solomon, 1968).

Oestetrol has not been detected in the urine of non-pregnant adults. The failure of oestetrol to be detected in the urine of non-pregnant adult urine could be due to its further metabolism to other products. However, this does not appear to be the case as when oestetrol was administered to adults it was rapidly and completely excreted. Therefore, it would appear that oestetrol is not formed in the adult (Fishman, 1970).

Although it has been suggested that the presence of oestetrol in late pregnancy urine could be a useful indicator of foetal viability further investigations are required to confirm their value in normal and abnormal pregnancies (Taylor and Shackleton, 1978).

Hydroxylation at C-16 with subsequent reduction to oestriol is one of the main pathways for the metabolism of oestrone (Fishman *et al.*, 1969). Details of 16-hydroxylated oestrogen metabolites were given in the last edition of this book. For a more detailed description of oestrogen metabolic pathways, reviews by the following authors should be consulted: Breuer (1962); Gallagher *et al.* (1966); Adlercreutz (1970); Breuer and Nocke-Finck (1974) and Gelbke, Ball and Knuppen (1977).

The rate and pathways by which oestrogens are metabolised in the human appears to be dependent on the sex and body weight of an individual. In addition, abnormal thyroid or liver function can lead to alterations in oestrogen metabolism.

The metabolism of oestradiol differs in normal adult females and males (Fishman, Boyar and Hellman, 1972). The rate and extent of oxidation of $[17\alpha\text{-}^3H]$ oestradiol was measured by following the appearance of tritiated water into the body water pool. Although there was an initial rapid stage of 5–10 min common to both sexes, subsequent oxidation was much slower in males than in females. The total amount of oestradiol oxidised in females (86%) was much greater than in males (54%). As noted by these authors, the conversion of oestradiol to oestrone was much higher than suggested from transfer constant determinations. It is possible that extensive transformations of plasma oestrone serves to diminish the concentration of free oestrone in plasma and hence decrease the oestradiol to oestrone transfer factor.

Increasing body weight was found to result in an increase in 16α-hydroxylase activity and a decrease in 2-hydroxylase activity (Fishman, Boyar and Hellman, 1975). Oestrogen metabolism is also altered in subjects with liver disease (Adlercreutz, 1970) and an increase in 16α-hydroxylase activity with a corresponding decrease in the excretion of 2-methoxyoestrone was found in subjects with cirrhosis of the liver (Zumoff, Fishman, Gallagher and Hellman, 1968). Low thyroid hormone levels also favour an increase in 16α-hydroxylase activity whereas 2-hydroxylase activity is increased when thyroid levels are elevated (Fishman, Hellman, Zumoff and Gallagher, 1965).

As oestrogens circulate in blood and are excreted in urine mainly conjugated with sulphuric and glucuronic acid, an awareness of the role of conjugates in the overall metabolism of oestrogens has resulted in an increasing number of investigations of their metabolism.

Oestrone sulphate is an important circulatory oestrogen and could be the source of other oestrogen metabolites (Fishman *et al.*, 1969). When doubly labelled [6,7-^{3}H] oestrone [^{35}S] sulphate was administered to a woman, 20% of the dose was excreted in urine within 24 hr mainly as oestrogen glucuronides (Oertel, Menzel and Hullen, 1969). However, some sulphate conjugated steroids were also detected in urine and included oestrone-3-sulphate (E_1-3-S), oestradiol-3-sulphate (E_2-3-S), oestriol-3-sulphate (E_3-3-S) and oestriol-3-17 disulphate (E_3-3-17 diS). The isotopic ratio of urinary oestrogen sulphates was much higher than the injected material indicating that hydrolysis and resulphurylation of liberated oestrogens had occurred. In plasma the isotopic ratio of sulphate conjugates was unchanged compared to the injected dose. Doubly labelled [6,7-^{3}H] oestrone [^{35}S] sulphate was also administered to a woman with a bile fistula by Jirku and Levitz (1969). Almost 70% of the tritum dose was recovered in urine with the remainder recovered in bile. Corresponding values for the excretion of ^{35}S in urine and bile were 64 and 3% respectively. Glucuronide conjugates were again predominant in urine while sulpho-glucuronides were identified in bile and urine.

In a comparative study of the metabolism of oestrone and oestrone sulphate, Fishman and Hellman (1975) injected [^{14}C] oestrone and [^{3}H] oestrone sulphate into a 37-yr-old woman. The metabolism of oestrone differed from that of oestrone sulphate. Products of oestrone sulphate were excreted more rapidly and to a greater extent than the co-administered oestrone. Oestrone was converted to oestrone glucuronide (E_1-G) and oestradiol glucuronide (E_2-G) to a greater extent than oestrone sulphate. However, all other metabolites isolated had identical isotopic ratios and Fishman and Hellman (1975) suggested that their rate of biosynthesis was slow compared to oestrone–oestrone sulphate interconversion, and therefore only occurs after equilibrium of oestrone and oestrone sulphate.

Incubation of [6,7-^{3}H] oestradiol with adult liver tissue showed that 51–76% of the tritiated material identified consisted of E_1-3-S or E_2-3-S with only minor amounts of glucuronides formed (Hobkirk, Mellar and Nilsen, 1975). It would therefore appear that the liver favours sulphurylation as a conjugating mechanism for oestradiol and oestrone. Oestradiol was, however, converted to a small but definite extent (<0.1-5.0%) to oestrone-3-glucuronide (E_1-3-G), oestradiol-3-glucuronide (E_2-3-G) and oestradiol-17-glucuronide (E_2-17-G) by human kidney homogenate in the presence of uridine diphosphoglucuronic acid (Hobkirk, Green, Nilsen and Jennings, 1974). The kidney homogenate was also capable of directly dehydrogenating E_2-3-G and E_2-3-S to their respective 17-keto forms. The interconversion of oestradiol and oestrone while conjugated with glucuronic acid was also demonstrated by Roy and Slaunwhite (1969) using an oestradiol 17β-dehydrogenase obtained from placental tissue. The ability of oestrone-3-glucuronide and oestradiol-3-glucuronide to interconvert without prior removal of the glucuronic acid moiety has also been demonstrated *in vivo* (Hobkirk and Nilsen, 1970).

The possibility that conjugates of oestradiol may be formed prior to the conversion of oestradiol to oestrone was suggested by Hobkirk and Nilsen (1974). Within 10 min of administration of $[6,7\text{-}^3\text{H}]$ oestradiol, E_2-17-G and, to a lesser extent E_2-3-G were excreted in urine in the absence of E_1-3-G.

When ^{14}C oestradiol and ^3H oestradiol-17-glucuronide were administered simultaneously, 2-methoxyoestrone, oestrone and oestradiol glucuronides were produced to a greater extent from the injected conjugate than from the free steroid (Hobkirk and Nilsen, 1969). As the extent of 16 hydroxylation of the E_2 17-conjugate was small these authors suggested that the presence of a glucuronic acid residue at C-17 appears to decrease the degree of metabolism in ring D of the steroid nucleus. Metabolism of oestrogens conjugated at C-3 with glucuronic acid differs from that of C-17 glucuronides and glucuronic acid esterified at C-3 of oestrone or oestradiol is much less liable to be removed than when esterified at C-17 (Hobkirk and Nilsen, 1969).

Oestrogens and their conjugates undergo an enterohepatic circulation to a much greater extent than neutral steroids although the physiological significance of the enterohepatic circulation remains obscure (Adlercreutz and Luukainen, 1967). Conjugation of oestrogens with glucuronic acid at C-3 probably occurs in the gastro-intestinal tract. When oestradiol 17-glucuronide (E_2-17-G) was administered intravenously, E_2-17-G and E_2-3-16 diG were initially excreted in urine. After a time lag of about 6 hr, E_1-3-G and E_2-3-G were predominantly excreted in urine, the lag being due to the delivery of conjugates to the intestines via the bile in the form of E_2-3S-17G (Musey, Green and Hobkirk, 1972). Thus metabolism of E_2-17-G to urinary E_1-3-G and E_2-3-G appears to occur in the intestine from biliary E_2-3S-17G via deconjugation and partial conversion of oestradiol to oestrone before or after reconjugation with endogenous glucuronic acid at C-3. The enterohepatic circulation of metabolites was thought to account for a similar delay in the excretion of oestriol-3-glucuronide after administration of oestriol-3-sulphate-16 glucuronide or oestriol-16-glucuronide (Levitz and Katz, 1968).

Oestrogen glucuronides are cleared from the circulation at a greater rate than oestrogen sulphates (Young, Jirku, Kadner and Levitz, 1976). These authors found that E_3-3S-16G and E_3-3S were the predominant conjugates in the plasma of pregnant subjects whereas E_3-16G was the predominant urinary conjugate. These differences in the renal handling of oestriol conjugates may be partly explained in terms of the relative binding of each oestriol conjugate to serum proteins (Goebelsmann, Chen, Saga, Nakamura and Jaffe, 1973).

E. PROTEIN BINDING

Oestrogens circulate in blood mainly bound to plasma proteins with only a small fraction (1–3%) present in an unbound state. In human blood oestrogens are mainly bound to albumin and to a sex steroid binding protein (SBP). The non-specific binding of oestrogens to cortisol binding globulin (CBG), α1-acid glycoprotein (AAG) and association with erythrocytes, have also been reported (Doe and Seal, 1963; Kerkay and Westphal, 1968; Longcope, Layne and Tait, 1968).

Plasma proteins form dissociable complexes with the oestrogens in blood and it is the fraction of steroid present in an unbound state that is thought to be biologically active. It is generally accepted that steroids enter cells by passive diffusion and that oestrogen responsive tissues contain cellular receptors which bind oestrogens. Therefore interactions of oestrogens with intracellular receptors will depend not only on the binding of the oestrogen to its receptor but also on the amount of unbound hormone that is available for entry into target tissues.

Evidence that steroids bound to plasma proteins are biologically inactive originated from observations on cortisol bound to CBG (Robertson, Stiefel and Laidlow, 1959; Slaunwhite, Lockie, Back and Sandberg, 1962) and progesterone bound to AAG (Westphal and Forbes, 1973). It has now been demonstrated that the biological activity of testosterone (Mowszowicz, Kahn and Dray, 1970; Lasnitski and Franklin, 1972; Mercier-Bodard, Marchut, Perrot, Picard, Baulieu and Roben, 1976) and oestradiol (Ferin, Tempone, Zimmering and Vande Wiele, 1969; Whitaker and Oakey, 1972; Raynaud, 1973) is related to the unbound rather than the protein bound concentration in plasma.

Investigation of the binding of oestrogens to plasma proteins commenced soon after the isolation of the first oestrogenic hormones, and the early studies on the binding of oestrogens to plasma proteins have been reviewed (Sandberg, Slaunwhite and Antoniades, 1957; Sandberg, Rosenthal, Schneider and Slaunwhite, 1966). These original investigations, together with the solubility determinations of steroids in albumin (Eik-Nes, Schellman, Lumry and Samuels, 1954) suggested that albumin could account for all the binding of oestrogens in plasma, although Bruenelli (1935) reported that oestrogen binding activity was associated with a globulin fraction. Since these early investigations, the presence in plasma of a glycoprotein with a high specificity but low capacity for oestradiol has been demonstrated.

The work of Daughaday (1958) first suggested the presence of a specific protein that bound testosterone with a high affinity, but the presence of a specific protein that bound oestradiol was first shown by Rosenbaum,

L

Christy and Kelly (1966). Although it is now generally accepted that the specific binding protein for oestradiol is a β globulin the specific binding of oestradiol to an $\alpha2$ globulin has also been reported (Barlow, MacLaren and Pothier, 1969). It is now apparent that the specific sex binding β globulin in plasma that binds oestradiol is the same as that which binds testosterone (Pearlman and Fong, 1968; Van Baelen, Heyns, Schonne and De Moor, 1968; Murphy, 1968).

1. The Role of Protein Binding of Oestrogens

The increased solubility of steroids in aqueous media when associated with serum albumin (Eik-Nes et al., 1954) originally led to the suggestion that plasma proteins were involved in the transport of steroids. However, as most steroids are soluble in water at their physiological concentrations a transport function does not seem likely. The possibility that protein binding could have a storage and buffer function was suggested by Daughaday (1959). Thus binding of steroids to plasma proteins could make them available by dissociation, yet protect them from metabolism and excretion. It is known that the binding of steroids to plasma proteins reduces their metabolic clearance rate (Tait and Burstein, 1964) and protects them from enzymic oxidation (Geisthonel and Breuer, 1971).

As SBP binds oestradiol and testosterone, Burke and Anderson (1972) from in vitro observations suggested that SBP could be involved in the regulation of oestrogen-androgen balance, and possible objections to their hypothesis have been fully discussed (Anderson, 1974; Ridgway, Longcope and Maloof, 1975; Anderson, 1976). The ability of SBP to decrease the penetration of testosterone, and alter the metabolism of testosterone by hyperplastic human prostate tissue, suggests that SBP may also be involved in a control mechanism for the uptake and metabolism of steroids by target organs (Mercier-Bodard et al., 1976).

The binding of steroids to plasma proteins may also direct steroids towards organs with protein-permeable vascular beds (Keller, Richardson and Yates, 1969). Oestradiol increases the retention and accumulation of albumin by the rat uterus (Peterson and Spaziani, 1971). As albumin bound oestrogen is also presumably retained it has been suggested that the accumulation of bound oestrogen may establish levels of total oestrogen in the rat uterus above that in the systemic circulation (Clark, Peck, Schrader and O'Malley, 1976).

2. Binding Characteristics for Oestrogens and Plasma Proteins

The association of oestrogens with plasma proteins involves the formation of non-covalent dissociable bonds presumably by Van der Waals forces and hydrogen bonding (Burton and Westphal, 1972). The free energies of these bonds are low $(25 \text{ kJ}_\text{M}^{-1}$, King and Mainwaring, 1974) and allow rapid association and dissociation to occur (Dixon, 1968). The affinity of oestrogens for albumin is much weaker than for the specific sex binding β globulin. The apparent equilibrium constants for the association of oestradiol with SBP and albumin at 37° are of the order 10^9 M^{-1} and 10^4 M^{-1} respectively (Burke and Anderson, 1972). Some oestrogen conjugates also circulate in plasma mainly bound to albumin. For the sulphate conjugates of oestrone and oestradiol albumin has a group of primary binding sites $(K_A \sim 10^6 \text{ M}^{-1})$ and a larger number of secondary binding sites $(K_A \sim 10^4 \text{ M}^{-1})$, Rosenthal, Pietrzak, Slaunwhite and Sandberg (1972); Rosenthal, Ludwig, Pietrzak and Sandberg (1975).

The binding of oestradiol to SBP is not as strong as that of testosterone and this is reflected in their dissociation rate constants from SBP which at 0° are 0.054 min^{-1} for testosterone and 0.21 min^{-1} for oestradiol (Heyns and De Moor, 1971). Investigations of the specificity of SBP have shown that a 17β hydroxyl group is a necessary characteristic for binding to SBP (Vermeulen and Verdonck, 1968; Kato and Horton, 1968; Murphy, 1970). A detailed review of the physicochemical properties of SBP has recently been published (Heyns, 1977).

F. MEASUREMENT OF OESTROGENS

1. General Procedures

(a) Introduction

There have been considerable advances in the methods available for the measurement of hormones in blood in the last decade. The important development has been that of protein binding and especially immunological methods, enabling accurate measurements to be made of hormones that are present at very low concentrations in blood. Suitable methods of reliable sensitivity and specificity for the low concentrations of oestrogens in plasma, especially from males and post-menopausal females, were not available until this time and such data were therefore scarce.

As the earlier methods of measurement of oestrogens have been amply covered in the previous edition of "Hormones in Blood" (O'Donnell and Preedy, 1967), only the recent use of such procedures will be mentioned here and most emphasis given to those methods currently employed in human (and animal) endocrinology. The term plasma will be used throughout but is synonymous with serum in this context as measurements in either medium yield identical results.

The three classical oestrogens, oestrone, oestradiol-17β and oestriol will be discussed first followed by some mention of those conjugates and metabolites of physiological and clinical interest.

(b) Criteria for assessing methods and procedures

The theoretical aspects of assay methods (including those suitable for the measurement of oestrogens) and the determination of their reliability criteria, have been amply covered by several authors (Borth, 1952, 1957; Ekins and Newman, 1970; Reeves and Calhoun, 1970). Briefly the important criteria for any assay of clinical value are that it should be accurate, precise, sensitive and specific. In addition there should be a good recovery of the sample under investigation through any purification steps carried out prior to assay.

(c) Extraction of oestrogens from blood samples

Most circulating oestrogens, whether unconjugated or conjugated, are associated with plasma proteins and bound to these with varying degrees of affinity (Slaunwhite, Lockie, Back and Sandberg, 1962). Therefore in any method for measuring ostrogens, all protein binding should be abolished. Preliminary extraction with an organic solvent breaks the weak binding to plasma proteins, but conjugates are not extracted into non-polar solvents (Onikki and Aldercreutz, 1973). For oestrone and oestradiol-17β a simple extraction method of shaking the plasma sample with hexane, diethyl ether or a combination of the two is satisfactory when a measurement of the plasma total oestrone or oestradiol is required. Since 85% of the plasma total oestriol is conjugated, a preliminary acid or enzyme hydrolysis step is required prior to extraction with, for example, diethyl ether.

When selecting a method for the extraction of oestrogens (or any steroid) from plasma there are two main requirements. These are to obtain as high a recovery as possible of the compound under investigation whilst at the same time extracting as little as possible of extraneous materials (including other steroids). When the end point of an assay is very specific and sensitive for the hormone under investigation, the extraction of other steroids is of less importance. With low endogenous plasma levels in the picogram range, as with oestrogens, it is very important that a good recovery (at least 80%) of added oestrogen through the extraction (and purification) procedure is obtained. Addition of the radioactive form of the steroid under investigation to the biological specimen, and measurement of radioactivity after extraction, can correct for incomplete removal of steroid from the sample. Providing the radioactive and endogenous forms behave similarly during extraction, this technique obviates the need for quantitative extraction. Even with the simple radioimmunoassay methods currently in use where no purification stage is employed (p. 311) it is important to monitor losses due to extraction. Solvents such as diethyl ether that are commonly used produce in general a recovery of 75–85% of added radioactive oestrogen. Individual recoveries should nevertheless still be monitored as there is a considerable variation between samples and this can make quite a difference to the estimation of low oestrogen levels. Where the endogenous oestrogen level is high as for example in late pregnancy plasma, it is not necessary to monitor losses in this way as the differences at the picogram level are not important.

(d) Radioactive labelling of oestrogens

Oestrogens are usually labelled with ^{3}H or ^{14}C in stable positions in rings A or B. Tritium labelled oestrogens are usually of much higher specific activities (up to 100 Ci/mmol or more) than ^{14}C labelled oestrogens (about 50 mCi/mmol). Consequently ^{3}H is the radioactive isotope of choice and it can be readily measured with the appropriate instrumentation (for example windowless gas flow counter or more usually a scintillation counter). The possibility of utilising radioactive iodine derivatives for steroid hormones has been investigated (Niswender and Midgley, 1970), as these have very high specific activities enabling reliable counting statistics to be obtained using a gamma counter in considerably less time and with less expense than with liquid scintillation methods. There are, however, certain limitations to the use of radioactive iodines for labelling steroids. Because of the high specific activity of these isotopes, the number of iodine atoms that can be introduced into a particular molecule without modifying its radiochemical reactivity is limited. The radioactive iodines are also highly electronegative atoms and significantly alter the net charge of the molecules into which they are incorporated. In addition the relatively large size of the iodine atom (larger than ring A of the steroid molecule) would interfere with the steric fit of antibody binding sites in current radioimmunoassay methods. Therefore although radioiodinated steroids can be used in radioimmunoassays where relative displacement of the tracer is the important factor, tritiated steroids must be used to determine recoveries of individual samples as these labelled molecules are structurally and chemically similar to the unlabelled form. Although as many as four atoms of ^{3}H can be incorporated into a steroid molecule, thus producing a tritiated steroid of high specific activity, these molecules are rather unstable and therefore less acceptable for use in routine assays than either the lower specific activity tritiated molecule with two atoms of tritium, or the iodinated conjugate.

Since it is known that steroids of high specific activity undergo self-radiation decomposition, especially when stored in the dry state, certain precautions are necessary when using radioactive oestrogens for the measurement of stable oestrogens. In addition oestrogens, whether stable or radioactive, undergo decomposition in dilute solution and radiochemical purity cannot be assumed. It is important, therefore, to check the homogeneity of the radioactive sample by subjecting it to at least one separation procedure (for example thin-layer, paper or column partition chromatography) before use. Commercially prepared radioisotopes undergo stringent tests before dispatch for radionuclidic, radiochemical and chemical purity and the specific activity is determined directly from measurements of the radioactivity and mass of the sample. However, as stated above, the purity of the sample should always be tested on receipt and at regular intervals throughout its period of use. Storage of the labelled compound should be at the lowest molar specific activity acceptable in the experiments. If stored as dilute solutions in benzene these should be kept at room temperature. If stored in ethanol or aqueous solutions these are best kept at 2–4°. A sensible precaution is to purchase only the minimum amount required as labelled compounds are most stable in unopened containers.

As stated above, chromatography of radioactive oestrogens is a good method of checking the purity of the sample, the discrete area of radioactivity being eluted and either rechromatographed if considered necessary, or dissolved in the appropriate solute for storage and use. Irrespective of the solvent system used, pure radioactive oestrogen will run parallel to pure standard oestrogen and the area of radioactivity on the chromatogram should correspond to the area of the chromatogram representing the stable oestrogen. Therefore with a radioactive sample of proven purity, the unlabelled oestrogen to be used as a reference standard can also be checked for purity. Similarly plasmas or urine extracts containing endogenous oestrogens can be run in parallel lanes to a radioactive sample and the corresponding area to the oestrogen under investigation eluted.

(e) Purification of samples prior to assay

Specificity of the older quantitative methods of determination was in general dependent upon the efficiency of the steps employed to eliminate interfering material rather than the final detection procedure. With the advent of immunological techniques and specific antisera the final detection is the most important stage and the more time consuming purification steps can be eliminated. This is a great advantage as these steps (for example thin-layer or gas-liquid chromatography) themselves often caused blank problems. Furthermore the use of additional purification steps necessitates the presence of the hormone in high concentrations (for example in pregnancy plasma) or very extensive preliminary purification of biological extracts.

2. Assay Techniques

(a) Bioassay

Biological assay methods were used extensively before the advent of chemical methods of greater sensitivity and specificity. Hence as there has been little change in this field since these bioassay methods for oestrogens and their limitations were reviewed by Emmens (1939, 1947, 1950) and Loraine (1958), the reader is referred to these reports and to the section in the previous edition of "Hormones in Blood" (p. 126–129).

Probably the most useful role for bioassay at the present time is for determining the oestrogenic "potency" of newly discovered oestrogens as described by Loraine (1958).

(b) Chemical and physiochemical methods

The details of these methods used up to 1966 have been extensively reviewed in the previous edition of this book (O'Donnell and Preedy, 1966). The most suitable analytical methods in use prior to the development of protein binding and immunological methods, used fluorimetry, isotope dilution or gas-liquid chromatography (GLC) (Wotiz, Charransol and Smith, 1967; Baird, 1968; Zmigrod, Ladany and Lindner, 1970; Cooper, Coyle and Mills, 1971; Loraine and Bell, 1971). The main disadvantages of all these procedures for routine use were that they are all relatively complex procedures requiring large volumes of plasma and did not permit the assay of a large number of samples at one time.

Nachtigall, Bassett, Hogsander, Slagle and Levitz (1966), developed a rapid fluorimetric method for pregnancy oestriol without prior chromatography. This method obviated some of the difficulties of previous fluorimetric methods being less extensive and requiring only 1 ml of plasma. It has been used in more recent studies by Taylor, Hagerman, Betz, Williams and Grey (1970); Rado, Deans and Townsley, 1970, and Edwards, Diver, Davies and Hipkin (1976). A similar method requiring only 0·2 ml of plasma was used by Miklosi, Biggs, Selvage, Canning and Lythal (1975). All these methods are rapid and reliable with good precision and accuracy and are suitable for routine use on samples where the oestrogen content is high. However, quenching is always an important problem in fluorescence procedures and may produce unreasonably low values. Meticulous cleaning of glassware and heating to 540° (to destroy organic impurities) reduces the interference (Kushinsky and Paul, 1969).

Baird (1968) developed a double-isotope derivative method suitable for the estimation of oestrone and oestradiol-17β in human peripheral blood.

The phenolic extract of blood was reacted with ^{35}S p-iodobenzene sulphonyl chloride (pipsyl chloride) and the derivatives purified by four chromatographic and the two additional derivative steps. This method allowed for the measurement of oestrogens in amounts less than 1 ng/plasma sample (10 ml) with accuracy and precision. The sensitivity of such double-isotope derivative methods is limited by the specific activities of the isotopes and the degree of specificity that can be obtained. Radioactive derivatives formed from other substances than the steroid under investigation must be separated completely from the steroid derivative, hence the need for extensive chromatography and further derivative formation. High losses therefore occur so that only about 10% of the steroid under investigation is present in the final sample used for counting. The use of ^{35}S (specific activity up to 200 mC/mmol) for the radioactive indicator enables the mass of the indicator to remain below that of the steroid measured whilst reducing the statistical error in a reasonable counting time to below 5%. The addition of oestrone and oestradiol-17β labelled with tritium as indicator prior to extraction allowed for all losses during extraction, purification and derivative formation to be calculated. With the inclusion of all the necessary chromatographic steps, this method was rather time consuming as only eight samples for both oestrone and oestradiol could be analysed by one technician in five working days. This could be shortened by one day for samples containing more than 5 ng of the steroids as the acetylation and last paper chromatogram could then be omitted.

The most sensitive of these older methods were the GLC methods using electron capture detection of oestrogen heptafluorobutyrates (Wotiz et al., 1967; Exley and Feder, 1967). However, oestrogen heptafluorobutyrates suffer from the great disadvantage that they are unstable and can not be separated by paper or thin-layer chromatography and this inefficient separation from interfering substances leads to loss of specificity. The iodomethyl-dimethyl-silyl ether of oestradiol-17β is two to three times more sensitive than the respective heptafluorobutyrate but it too is not stable on TLC. However, hydroxyetherification of the phenolic hydroxyl group prior to iodomethyl silation leads to a more stable derivative. This method was used to advantage by Exley and Dutton (1969) in developing a method of suitable specifications to check the accuracy of the recently developed protein binding method for oestradiol (Corker and Exley, 1969).

Prior to 1969, therefore, the development of techniques of sufficient sensitivity to enable quantitative determinations to be performed on small volumes of plasma or other biological fluids, were greatly needed. The development of protein binding and immunological methods of steroid determination supplied this need.

(c) Protein binding methods

The term saturation analysis was proposed by Barakat and Ekins (1961) to describe the general analytical method relying on progressive saturation by a test compound of a specific binding reagent. The binding reagents most commonly used are specific proteins such as "transport" proteins in the blood, receptor proteins in target tissue, or antibodies directed against the substances being investigated. The initial demonstrations of the feasibility of this method of assay were those of Ekins (1960) who used plasma binding proteins for thyroid hormones to measure serum thyroxine, and of Yalow and Berson (1960) who used anti-insulin antibodies (formed after insulin treatment in man) to measure plasma immunoreactive insulin. The latter authors soon demonstrated the value of their method for use on a clinical basis as did Murphy, Engleberg and Pattee (1963) and Murphy (1964), when they published a method and its application for the first steroid (corticoids) assay using the technique of competitive protein binding.

Rosenbaum, Christy and Kelly (1966) and Tavernetti, Rosenbaum, Kelly, Christy and Roginsky (1967) gave clear evidence that oestradiol was bound to the same β-globulin- sex-hormone-binding globulin (SHBG)—which had been shown to bind testosterone (Chen, Mills and Bartter, 1961; Mercier, Alfsen and Baulieu, 1966). Murphy (1968) in parallel studies of testosterone and oestradiol, showed that SHBG had the greatest affinity for testosterone but that oestradiol was a strong competitor for the binding sites. Murphy demonstrated that because of the high affinity of SHBG for both of these hormones it could be used in competitive binding assays for testosterone and oestradiol. A 17β-hydroxyl group appears to be the requirement for binding to SHBG, therefore of the three classical oestrogens, oestradiol is the only one to bind and methods utilising this binding protein cannot be used for the measurement of oestrone or oestriol.

Methods using SHBG as the binding protein therefore demonstrate limited specificity due to the large number of steroids (with 17β-hydroxyl groups) that are bound. The relative affinity of the compound under study and efficient separation from interfering compounds is obviously important. Mayes and Nugent (1970) developed a competitive protein binding method for oestradiol-17β utilising SHBG and purification was carried out by solvent partition, paper chromatography and TLC. Such methods were not widely used for oestradiol assays, partly due to the limited specificity but also because Jensen (1958) and Jensen and Jacobsen (1960) had demonstrated the presence of a highly specific oestrogen receptor in uterine tissue which led to the development of oestrogen assays using a uterine cytosol extract as the binding agent.

Korenman (1968) demonstrated that there was a specific oestrogen binding macromolecule in the high speed supernatant from a pregnant rabbit uterus and illustrated the high molecular weight and steroid specificity of this material. The relative *in vitro* binding potencies using oestradiol as 100% were oestrone 23%, oestriol 17% and diethylstilboestrol 256%. This report was also the first demonstration that an intracellular binding protein could be used for a sensitive, specific and relatively precise hormone assay. Several methods utilising this rabbit uterine cytosol were then developed for oestradiol (Corker and Exley, 1969; Korenman, Perrin and McCallum, 1969; Ahmed and Mester, 1973; Pratt, Van der Lundèn, Doorenbos and Woldring, 1974), for oestrone (Tulchinsky and Korenman, 1970; Nagai and Longcope, 1971) and for oestriol (Corker and Naftolin, 1971). Purification of plasma extracts was most usually carried out by means of alumina TLC or celite column chromatography and separation of bound from free hormone with dextran coated charcoal. All these methods demonstrated increased sensitivity (5–25 pg) and specificity over older methods. Blank values were lower due to the decrease in the number of purification steps required and smaller plasma samples could be used. Although rabbit uterine cytosol was the most frequently used binding protein, Shutt and Cox (1973) developed a competitive protein binding technique suitable for the measurement of oestrone, oestradiol-17β, oestradiol-17α and oestriol using sheep uterine cytosol as binding reagent. These authors had previously demonstrated that sheep uterine cytosol had the advantage over rabbit uterine cytosol in its high stability on storage at $-10°$. The specificity of this fraction for use in oestrogen assays has also been well defined (Shutt, 1969; Shutt and Cox, 1972). Corker and Exley (1970) overcame the disadvantage of the instability of the rabbit uterine cytosol by freeze-drying the material whereupon it remained stable for periods of at least six months.

(d) Radioimmunoassay

A further development of the basic principle of saturation analysis is the radioimmunoassay (RIA) utilising an antiserum to the hormone under investigation as the binding reagent. Such methods have greatly facilitated the measurement of oestrogens at the low levels at which they occur in blood and are the methods in widest use at the present time. The binding affinity of oestrogens is greater for the rabbit uterine cytosol fraction than it is for artificially produced antisera, but other substances such as diethylstilboestrol and clomiphene can also bind to the uterine cytosol fraction and therefore, the specificity is less. Due to this non-specificity of the protein it is always necessary to include a chromatographic step in the assay to eliminate any possible interfering material. However, when an antiserum is specific for the substance under investigation, it is no longer necessary to perform extensive preliminary purification of the sample. Since chromatography is a time-consuming step and is also liable to increase the blank problems of an assay, its elimination from a method is obviously an advantage in the development of rapid and sensitive methods for laboratory and clinical use.

Although the classical studies of Landsteiner (1946) were the start of the development of radioimmunoassays, the initial introduction of these methods for oestrogens was not until 1969 (Jaing and Ryan, 1969; Mikhail, Wu, Ferin and Vande Wiele, 1970). In these methods oestradiol-17β-succinyl-BSA was used as an antigen to produce antibodies to oestradiol-17β. Although the sensitivity and accuracy of these assays were good, the antisera produced in this way have a high cross-reactivity with the other major oestrogens that would be present in substantial amounts in the blood sample. This meant that a chromatographic step was still always necessary, as shown by Abraham, Odell, Edwards and Purdy (1970) in comparing three methods. Chromatography and its associated radioimmunoassayable contamination can be avoided by the use of Girard's reagent to separate oestrone from oestradiol (Kushinsky and Anderson, 1974). The reason for the lack of specificity of these antibodies is that the site of conjugation of the antigen is through the functional hydroxyl group at C-17. It can be improved by utilising a different antigen. If the two characteristic hydroxyl groups of oestradiol (C-3 and C-17) are used as the site of conjugation, several workers have shown that the antisera elicited will then have a high cross-reaction with oestradiol-17α, oestrone and oestriol (Exley, Johnson and Dean, 1971; Lindner, Perel, Friedlander and Zeitlin, 1972; Cameron and Jones, 1972; Kuss and Gobel, 1972). These authors showed that a highly specific antiserum for oestradiol-17β could be obtained by using the hapten oestradiol-17β-6-(O-carboxymethyl) oxime-BSA and methods utilising antisera conjugated at position 6 of the steroid molecule are currently in use for oestrone, oestradiol and oestriol. They are simple rapid methods and have been validated for use without chromatography (Exley and Choo, 1974; Korenman, Stevens, Carpenter, Robb, Niswender and Sherman, 1974; Jurjens, Pratt and Woldring, 1975; Aso, Guerro, Cekan and Diczfalusy, 1975; Chew and Ratnam, 1976; Wilson, John, Groom, Pierrepoint and Griffiths, 1977; Katagiri, Stanczyl and Goebelsman, 1974; Hull, Monro, Morgan and Murray, 1979). Exley et al. (1971) demonstrated that the only significant cross-reaction (77–140%) of the C-6-keto-oestradiol antisera is with 6-keto-oestradiol-17β. Such C-6 substituted steroids although known to be present as urinary metabolites were thought not to be present in any significant amount in plasma. However, Bolton and Rutherford (1976) measured both 6-keto-oestradiol-17β and oestradiol-17β in plasma samples from normal men, women in the luteal phase of the menstrual cycle and samples collected from women during pregnancy. They used an oestradiol-17β-6-(O-carboxy-methyl)-oxime-BSA antiserum with a 200% cross-section with 6-keto-oestradiol-17β. Measurable amounts of 6-keto-oestradiol were found only in late pregnancy and using their antiserum these levels would contribute up to 5% of the apparent oestradiol-17β concentration. However, as in testing several antisera to oestradiol-17β conjugates linked via the 6 position, they had found cross-reactions ranging from 150–500%. It is clearly important, therefore, especially when such antisera are to be used for pregnancy samples, that an antiserum with a relatively low cross-reaction with 6-keto-oestradiol is used. LH-20 column chromatography, a widely used purification procedure did not separate oestradiol-17β from its 6-keto metabolite showing that such interference is not limited to those assays avoiding chromatography. Celite column chromatography, as used by Bolton and Rutherford (1976) will separate oestradiol-17β from 6-keto-oestradiol-17β.

Wright, Robinson, Collins and Preedy (1973) showed that whilst separating oestrone from oestradiol, LH20 chromatography did not separate either of these from their naturally occurring metabolites such as 2-methoxy-oestradiol-17β, 2-methoxy oestrone, oestradiol-17α, 2-hydroxy oestrone, 16-keto oestrone, 16-keto oestradiol-17β, 16α-hydroxy oestrone and 16β-hydroxy oestrone. Although substantial interference was therefore possible, they found that there was an insignificant difference in the values obtained for oestrone and oestradiol measured in normal men and non-pregnant women when they compared their RIA with a fluorimetric method and other identification procedures. Linder, Desfosses and Emiliozzi (1977) prepared antisera to both oestrone and oestradiol using immunogens with a C-15 linkage. With such antisera the cross-reaction to the metabolites mentioned above (with the exception of 16α-hydroxy oestrone) was so greatly reduced as to be insignificant. However, for both antisera, oestrogens substituted on C-16 presented important cross-reactions which can probably be ascribed to the proximity of the steroids linkage at C-15. Thus antisera to oestrone or oestradiol-17β-15-carboxymethyl derivatives can only be used for oestrone or oestradiol RIA when cross-reaction with oestriol is not important.

Therefore at the present time it would appear that the most suitable antisera to use in RIA of oestrone, oestradiol and oestriol are those with a C-6 linkage which have the lowest cross-reactions with possible interfering substances. Using such antisera it is possible to set up simple assays involving only prior extraction of the plasma sample. Chromatography of plasma extracts is, however, still used in methods utilising these specific antisera, when it is desired to separate the various oestrogen fractions for individual measurement within the same plasma sample. This is most often the case with pregnancy plasma samples (De Hertogh, Thomas, Bietlot, Van der

Heyden and Ferin, 1975).

The lack of specificity of the oestradiol-17β-succinyl-BSA antiserum has been employed to advantage by several authors to measure oestrone, oestradiol-17α and oestriol in the same plasma sample using the one antiserum (Mikhail *et al.*, 1970; Wu and Lundy, 1971; Robertson, Smeaton and Durnford, 1972; Cohen and Cohen, 1974; Antonipillai and Murphy, 1977). Similarly Loriaux, Ruder, Knals and Lipsett (1972) measured oestrone sulphate, oestrone, oestradiol and oestriol levels in human pregnancy plasma using an antiserum generated against oestrone-17β-oxime-BSA. Tulchinsky (1973) measured the placental secretion of unconjugated oestrone, oestradiol and oestriol into the foetal circulation using a method involving two chromatographic systems which yielded oestrone, oestradiol and oestriol fractions with less than 1% cross-contamination. This enabled him to use an oestriol antiserum, that had 140% cross-reaction with oestrone and 160% cross-reaction with oestradiol, as the binding agent for all three oestrogens.

(1) Liquid phase immunological methods. The methods in general use at the present time (including those referred to above) are simple liquid phase methods. Briefly the following steps are taken. The plasma sample to which tritium labelled oestrogen has been added (to monitor recovery) is extracted with a solvent such as diethyl-ether. The extract is dried and redissolved in a small volume of buffer (for example phosphate buffer pH 7·0–7·4). From this extract one aliquot is removed to a scintillation mixture, counted in a beta counter and the loss through the extraction procedure estimated. A further aliquot of the ether extract is taken for RIA. To these aliquots, antiserum at the appropriate dilution (in assay buffer) and tritiated oestrogen in buffer are added and incubation carried out either at room temperature or at 4° depending on the optimum conditions for the assay. After equilibration the chosen solution for separating bound from free hormone (see p. 314) is added. The free or bound fraction (depending on the separation procedure) is then removed to a scintillation mixture and counted. A set of standards covering the range required by the method are assayed in exactly the same way and at the same time as the unknown samples. Thus a direct comparison can be made between the samples and the known standards and the amount of oestrogen present in a given volume of plasma can be calculated.

Such assay procedures are extremely quick and many plasma samples can be measured in one batch which is a great advantage especially for routine clinical laboratories. These methods also lend themselves well to automation.

(2) Solid phase immunological methods. Solid phase antibody systems for oestrogens (oestradiol-17β) were introduced by Abraham (1969) using antibody-coated polystyrene tubes and such methods were used by some authors (Exley *et al.*, 1971). Mikhail *et al.* (1970) used a solid phase system

for oestrone and oestradiol utilising a polymerised antiserum to oestradiol-17β prepared using ethyl chloroformate and Moore and Axelrod (1972) developed a solid phase RIA using enzacryl AA. Further discussion of these techniques is in the following section on separation techniques.

(3) *Choice of assay system.* Exley and Choo (1974) tested the specificity of an antiserum to oestrone raised against oestrone-6-(O-carboxymethyl)-oxime BSA conjugate, using four different RIA systems. They showed that the specificity of the antiserum to cross-reacting steroid varied according to the method used. Therefore the choice of RIA technique should be made on the basis that the highest specificity to cross-reacting steroids is obtained for the type of specimen to be examined.

(4) *Separation techniques.* A wide variety of methods have been employed for the separation of free from protein/antibody bound steroid hormones. For the three classical oestrogens these include: (i) dextran coated charcoal (DCC) (Wu and Lundy, 1971; Abraham, Hopper, Tulchinsky, Swerdloff and Odell, 1971; Exley and Choo, 1974; Cohen and Cohen, 1974; De Hertogh *et al.*, 1975; Jurjens *et al.*, 1975; Doerr, 1976; Hay and Lorscheider, 1976; (ii) solid phase (Abraham, 1969; Mikhail *et al.*, 1970; Exley *et al.*, 1971; Moore and Axelrod, 1972); (iii) double antibody (Niswender and Midgley, 1969; Exley and Choo, 1974); (iv) polyethylene glycol (PEG) (Schiller and Brammall, 1974) and (v) ammonium sulphate (Hull *et al.*, 1979).

Of all the methods DCC has been the most widely used. It is a simple, rapid, precise and inexpensive method to use. With this method, however, incubation conditions and timing are critical based on the dissociation constants of the antiserum, because although theoretically the charcoal adsorbs the free hormone, antibody-bound hormone may also be removed from the solution under certain conditions. This is partly due to the association of hormone from the antibody during the separation procedure and may also be due to some protein "absorption" to the charcoal although the addition of dextran should prevent the latter. The timing and validity of this procedure must be verified for each new antiserum and once determined for a certain batch size, the number of samples should not be increased above this level without the inclusion of additional standard curves. Once all the criteria have been satisfied for a particular assay system and antiserum, then this is a very convenient and reproducible method. The problems associated with the stripping of antiserum-bound steroid may be partially overcome by the use of charcoal-gelatin discs instead of DCC solution (Saba, 1976). Some simplification to the RIA may also be afforded by this method as, after shaking the discs in the RIA tubes for the required length of time, they are removed and scintillation fluid added directly to the tubes.

Solid phase methods include the dry coating of plastic tubes with antisera

(Abraham, 1969) or polymerising antisera using ethyl chloroformate (Mikhail *et al.*, 1970) or enzacryl AA (Moore and Axelrod, 1972). The theoretical advantages of all these methods are that several time-consuming and error-producing steps can be eliminated by having in one unit the antibody, the tracer activity and the means of separating bound from un-bound fractions (centrifugation). The specific limitations of such methods, however, are that they require routine and reproducible coupling of high affinity antibody to solid supports whilst retaining antibody affinity and specificity. For example, binding of antibodies to polystyrene surfaces may partially fractionate the antisera so that certain fractions bind in preference to others. Also with the enzacryl AA method, the preparation of water insoluble antibodies by diazotisation may slightly alter the configuration of some of the active sites of the original antibodies.

Double antibody methods have also not been widely used due to the long incubation times required (16 hr compared with 10 min for DCC). In addition the second antibody is very expensive compared with charcoal, ammonium sulphate or PEG.

Ammonium sulphate although not as widely used as DCC has the advantage that it is more stable and therefore less time dependent than charcoal. Larger batches of samples can therefore be assayed using only one set of standards. The choice between this method and DCC is probably one of personal preference.

Recently PEG has come into use for separation of free from antibody-bound hormone. The original publication (Desbuquois and Aurbach, 1971) described its use in the RIA of polypeptide hormones, but these authors suggested its applicability for small molecular weight compounds. Barrett and Cohen (1972) and Van Orden and Farley (1973) demonstrated the use of PEG for non-polypeptide compounds and Schiller and Brammall (1974) developed a precise, accurate and reliable assay for oestradiol-17β with PEG as the separation technique. PEG precipitates only antibody-bound hormone therefore two important advantages are achieved using this method of separation. Firstly, timing of the separation procedure is unimportant, there being no evidence of any dissociation of the antibody/steroid complex for several hours after the initial precipitation. Secondly, PEG precipitation is dependent only upon the globulin characteristic of the antibody and not its binding properties, therefore similar optimum conditions can be expected when establishing assays with different antisera. In addition the homogeneity of the solution enables easier and more precise pipetting and is suitable for use with automatic dispensers. This may well be the method of choice in the future as it is also inexpensive and solutions once prepared can be kept for several weeks at 4°.

(e) *Non-protein bound oestrogens*

Although several *in vitro* methods have been used to measure the unbound steroid fraction in plasma, *in vitro* studies do not necessarily represent *in vivo* steroid-protein interactions in plasma. However, it is usually accepted that the *in vitro* experiments are a general reflection of *in vivo* conditions (Forest, Rivarola and Migeon, 1968).

The fraction of steroid bound to plasma proteins depends on several factors including the concentrations of binding proteins, the number of binding sites on the protein, the concentration of steroid hormone and the association constants between protein and steroid. Unbound oestrogen levels are usually low and below the limits of sensitivity of available assay techniques and so indirect methods have been employed to distinguish bound from free forms. As yet there is no general agreement about the method or conditions that should be used to measure the fraction of unbound steroid in plasma. Therefore, the three methods in common use will be considered and their relative merits discussed.

(*1*) *Equilibrium dialysis.* According to Westphal (1971) equilibrium dialysis is the method of choice for the characterisation of all steroid–protein interactions as equilibrium dialysis does not alter the dynamic equilibrium that exists between the steroid and protein. Methods for the determination of the unbound fraction of steroids in plasma by equilibrium dialysis have been described in detail (Slaunwhite, 1960; Westphal, 1969).

Using dialysis bags, 12–24 hr are normally required to attain equilibrium. However, the introduction of dialysis cells has greatly reduced the time needed to reach equilibrium (Weder, Schildknecht and Kesselring, 1971; Weder, Schildknecht, Lutz and Kesselring, 1974; Hutton, Murray, Reed, Jacobs and James, 1978).

Both diluted and undiluted plasma have been used to determine the unbound fraction of oestradiol in plasma at 37° by equilibrium dialysis (Chopra, Abraham, Chopra, Solomon and Odell, 1972; Chopra, Tulchinsky and Greenway, 1973; Kley, Bartmann and Kruskemper, 1977). The use of diluted plasma has been advocated by Vermeulen, Stoica and Verdonck (1971) to reduce errors caused by impurities in radiolabelled tracers. Calculation of the unbound steroid fraction in undiluted plasma from determinations made with diluted plasma requires caution. Chopra and colleagues (1972, 1973) applied a constant correction factor to the value obtained with diluted plasma, calculated according to Slaunwhite (1960). However, when individual dialysis bags were weighed before and after dialysis, increases in the plasma volume ranged from 3–20% (Kley *et al.*, 1977). Therefore, the use of a constant correction factor can give rise to erroneous results. An alternative procedure has been used by Vermeulen et al. (1971). Knowing the concentration of steroid and albumin in plasma the unbound concentration of testosterone in undiluted plasma was calculated after equilibrium dialysis of diluted plasma. Thus the possible error in deriving the unbound fraction of a steroid in undiluted plasma by simply dividing the unbound fraction obtained in diluted plasma by the dilution factor was avoided. Non-specific binding of steroids by albumin can be eliminated by dialysing plasma against an equivalent concentration of albumin (Vermeulen and Verdonck, 1968).

(2) *Ultrafiltration.* The use of equilibrium dialysis to study steroid–protein interactions at room temperature or 37° has been questioned by Sandberg et al. (1966). These authors suggested that at 37° some proteins could slowly denature under the experimental conditions used and favour ultrafiltration for experiments at 37°. Ultrafiltration has the disadvantage that the total protein concentration increases as the ultrafiltration is removed. However, if less than 10% of the volume is filtered, the error introduced is negligible (Westphal, 1971). Ultrafiltration does have the advantage that undiluted plasma can be used without the problems encountered when equilibrium dialysis is used. The all glass apparatus of Toribara (Toribara, 1953; Toribara, Terepka and Dewey, 1957) in which fluid is expressed through the semipermeable membrane by centrifugal force has been used to study interaction of oestrogen conjugates with plasma proteins (Rosenthal et al., 1972; Rosenthal et al., 1975).

(3) *Steady state gel filtration (SSGF).* Another method used to determine the unbound fraction of a steroid in plasma that meets the requirements of maintaining a thermodynamic equilibrium is SSGF (Burke, 1969). This method, originally used to measure unbound levels of cortisol in plasma, has been used to determine unbound levels of testosterone and oestradiol simultaneously in undiluted plasma (Fisher, Anderson and Burke, 1974). The main objection to this method, that it requires a large volume of plasma (8 ml) to maintain a steady state, has now been overcome. By using microcolumns, only a small volume of plasma (0·5–1·0 ml) is required to maintain a steady state (Greenstein, Puig-Duran and Franklin, 1977).

(4) *Measurement of SBP.* The concentration of SBP in plasma is an important determinant of the level of unbound oestradiol in plasma and has been measured indirectly by many methods. These include equilibrium dialysis (Tavernetti, Rosenbaum, Kelly, Christy and Roginsky, 1967; Forest et al., 1968), radioligand assay (Tulchinsky and Chopra, 1974), selective precipitation (Rosner, 1972), poly-acrylamide gel electrophoresis (Corvol, Chrambach, Rodbard and Bardin, 1971), equilibrium partition in an aqueous phase (Shanbhag, Södergård, Carstensen and Albertsson, 1973) and affinity chromatography (Ratajczak and Hahnel, 1976). These and other methods have recently been reviewed (Anderson, 1974; Heyns, 1977).

(f) Oestrogen conjugates and metabolites

(1) Conjugates. The major conjugating oestrogen in blood is oestrone sulphate and has been identified by several groups of workers (Smith and Hagerman, 1965; Brown and Smyth, 1971; Lordiaux, Ruder and Lipsett, 1971).

To date there are no published RIA methods for the measurement of blood levels of oestrone sulphate although Sanyaolu, Eccles and Oakey (1976) reported on the preparation of two different antisera to oestrone sulphate using antigens prepared by linking BSA through an *O*-carboxy methyl oxime group at C-6 or C-17. Although some binding and some degree of specificity was achieved, neither antiserum was suitable for use in the development of a RIA at that time. Prior hydrolysis is therefore still a necessary step in the measurement of oestrone sulphate and current methods used are based on that of Hawkins and Oakey (1974). This involves the extraction of free oestrogens with ether, the oestrone sulphate in the residual plasma being solvolysed and the oestrone liberated is isolated using TLC and reduced to oestradiol-17β. A competitive protein binding assay using the rabbit uterine cytosol system is then carried out.

Apart from oestrone sulphate the measurement of other monoconjugates and diconjugates of oestrogens with glucuronic and sulphuric acid have in general been confined to their measurement in pregnancy where they are of considerable physiological importance (Smith and Hagerman, 1965). The older methods for the estimation of oestrogen conjugates have been amply described in the previous edition of this book (p. 158 *et seq.*).

Recently various workers have developed more rapid methods for some of these conjugates. For example Levitz, Kadner and Young (1976) measured oestriol-16-sulphate and oestriol-3-16-disulphate in maternal serum, cord serum and amniotic fluid at delivery in human pregnancies. The conjugates were separated and purified by sequential chromatography on alumina, celite and sephadex LH-20 and each conjugate hydrolysed with an enzyme preparation rich in 16-sulphatase, phenol sulphatase and β-glucuronidase activity. The released oestriol from these fractions was then estimated by RIA using an anti-oestriol-6 (*O*-carboxymethyl)-oxime serum.

Antisera to some oestrogen conjugates have been developed. Dipietro (1976) reported a rapid RIA for oestriol-16α-(β-D-glucuronide) suitable for use in 10,000 fold dilution of pregnancy urine. Immunogens in which oestriol glucuronide hapten is linked through positions 2 or 4 of ring A of the oestriol molecule to BSA or agarose gel were used. The resultant antibody had less than 1% cross-reactions with all other conjugated and unconjugated oestrogens tested and good linear correlation was obtained for this RIA with a routine colorimetric method, separating and measuring free oestriol after hydrolysis. Sugar, Alexander, Dessy and Schwers (1977) described a specific RIA for oestriol-16-glucuronide suitable for quick, reliable measurement of urinary oestriol-16-glucuronide in high risk pregnancies. The antiserum used had very low cross-reactions with other conjugated and unconjugated oestrogens and the specificity of the method was good for the measurement of oestriol-glucuronide in urine and amniotic fluid without hydrolysis, extraction or purification, requiring only dilution of the crude sample. However, specificity was not adequate for the measurement of oestriol-16-glucuronide in pregnancy plasma which apparently contains material interfering with the RIA at dilutions of less than 1/100. However, this may be possible in the future when new antisera are developed.

(2) *Catechol oestrogens.* The catechol oestrogens are very unstable and may often be destroyed to a considerable extent by extremely mild methods of isolation (Fishman, 1963). Although it was not possible to estimate losses before formation of the free compound because the site and type of conjugation was not known, Fishman showed that once the metabolite had been cleaved from its conjugate, there was a steady and progressive loss of this compound using such mild treatment as enzymatic hydrolysis, separation by countercurrent distribution or acetylation at room temperature. Use of Girard's reagent T to separate 2-hydroxyoestrone from oestradiol was also damaging. Such separation methods had been used by Givner, Bauld and Vagi (1960) in the quantitative determination of 2-methoxyoestrone. Hence as a result of this instability, the development of methods of measurement of these metabolites, in blood especially, has been very slow. Various methods for urine are available including countercurrent distribution, column partition chromatography, double isotope derivative and GLC (Fishman, 1963; Hobkirk and Nilsen, 1963; Hellman, Fishman, Zumoff, Cassouto and Gallagher, 1967; Zumoff, Fishman, Cassouto, Gallagher and Hellman, 1968; Ball, Gelbke and Knuppen, 1976). The double isotope and gas chromatographic techniques are highly specific, accurate and precise but all methods are extremely complicated and laborious and not, therefore, suitable for routine clinical use. They have, however, helped to provide reliable data on the concentrations of the different metabolites.

One drawback to the development of simple methods is the absence of commercially available radioactive forms of the catechol oestrogens. The compound under investigation must therefore be labelled in the laboratory. Marks and Hecker (1967) reported a simple and rapid method for the preparation of 2-hydroxy [4-^{14}C] oestrone by hydroxylation of [4-^{14}C] oestrone with rat liver microsomes, and this has been the method most usually used in recent studies (Ball *et al.*, 1975; Yoshizawa and Fishman, 1971).

Because of the labile nature of the catechol oestrogens early attempts to quantitate 2-substituted oestrogens concentrated on measurement of the corresponding monomethylethers (Givner *et al.*, 1960; Wotiz and Chattoraj, 1964; Adlercreutz and Luukkainen, 1968). Yoshizawa and Fishman (1971) described a radioimmunoassay for 2-hydroxyoestrone in plasma and reported that concentrations of 2-hydroxyoestrone are similar to those of oestrone and oestradiol.

With the development of methods which prevent the oxidative decomposition of catechol oestrogen during purification procedures (Gelbke and Knuppen, 1972) it became possible to measure levels of catechol oestrogens in urine. During pregnancy 2-hydroxyoestrone is excreted to a greater extent than 2-hydroxyoestradiol or 2-hydroxyoestriol (Gelbke and Knuppen, 1976). Using a highly sensitive and specific double isotope derivative assay method Ball, Gelbke and Knuppen (1975) found that excretion of 2-hydroxyoestrone is similar to that of oestriol throughout the menstrual cycle. Recently a radioimmunoassay for urinary catechol oestrogens has been developed (Chattoraj, Fanous, Cecchini and Lowe, 1978), in which ascorbic acid was incorporated into the buffer solution to eliminate the problem of oxidative decomposition. The results obtained by radioimmunoassay confirmed those previously obtained by other methods (see p. 335).

(3) *15α-Hydroxyoestriol.* 15α-Hydroxyoestriol (oestetrol) is an oestrogen the estimation of which in pregnancy studies may offer some advantage over that of oestriol or HPL in the assessment of foetal jeopardy. As a result there have been several methods for its measurement in plasma published in recent years. Kaplan and Hreshchyshyn (1973) used a rapid GLC method for the quantitation of oestetrol in molar pregnancies, but most of the recent methods are RIA. These are all in general simple, rapid and sensitive methods requiring no purification (chromatographic) stage and have good accuracy, precision and specificity. Fishman and Guzik (1972) and Korda, Challis, Anderson and Turnbull (1975) both used an antiserum to 15α-hydroxy-oestriol-3-(O-carboxymethyl) oxime-BSA. The only significant cross-reaction was with oestriol (2·5%) but as levels of unconjugated oestriol in late pregnancy are only three to four times higher than oestetrol, this cross-reaction would only give a 10% overestimation of oestetrol levels. A slight modification of Fishman and Guzik's method was used by Tulchinsky, Frigoletto, Ryan and Fishman (1975) in their assessment of the use of plasma oestetrol measurements as an index of foetal well-being. Kundu and Grant (1976) produced an antiserum to 6-oxo-oestetrol-6(carboxymethyl) oxime-BSA and this enabled them to set up an assay with a sensitivity of 50 pg (164 fmol) per tube (167 pg/ml—0·55 nmol/l) and greater specificity than previous methods which probably accounts for the lower values obtained. However, Giebenhain, Tagatz and Gurpide (1972) had used column chromatographic spearation before RIA and therefore might have achieved even better specificity,

but levels found were higher than those of Kundu and Grant (1976).

G. OESTROGEN CONCENTRATIONS

1. The Classical Oestrogens

(a) Puberty

There are several good reviews on the hormonal changes associated with normal and abnormal puberty (Bierich, 1975; Marshall, 1975; Swerdloff and Odell, 1975; Escobar, Rivarola and Bergada, 1976).

Jenner, Kelch, Kaplan and Grumbach (1972) were the first to study the change of oestradiol levels during puberty in the female. They found that although there was a significant correlation of plasma oestradiol concentrations with both bone age and chronological age, the best correlation was that with clinical evaluation of sexual development, a finding confirmed by Gupta, Altemasio and Reef (1975). Saez, Morera and Bertrand (1973) also reported on both oestrone and oestradiol levels before puberty and more extensive studies were reported by Bidlingmaier, Wagner-Barnack, Butenandt and Knorr (1973). This latter study which was in agreement with the previous one showed levels of both oestrone and oestradiol of between 30–50 ng/100 ml (1·1–1·8 nmol/l) in neonates shortly after birth, these levels falling within a few days to 0·5–1·5 ng/100 ml (18·6–55·1 pmol/l). This is the normal range of levels for both sexes up to seven years. Plasma(oestrone) levels rise earlier in girls than in boys before puberty and the increase of oestradiol follows the onset of puberty. In boys the increase of oestrogen levels (particularly oestrone) is due to the peripheral conversion of androgens the concentration of which is increasing at this time. Boys reach adult oestrogen levels in Tanner's stage IV of puberty whereas in stage V, girls still have lower oestrogen levels than boys. Thus the ratio of oestrone or oestradiol to testosterone, which pre-pubertally is similar in both sexes, increases in the female and decreases in the male with the progression of puberty. Girls also demonstrate a steep increment in the standard deviations for oestrogen values as sexual maturation progresses (between stage IV and V) probably reflecting the onset of cyclical activity (Gupta *et al.*, 1975). Lee and Migeon (1975) studying puberty in boys, including measurements of oestrone and oestradiol, obtained very similar results to all the above authors. Boyar, Wu, Roffwarg, Kapen, Weitzman, Hellman and Finkelstein (1976) measured oestradiol levels in samples collected every 20 min over 24 hr from pubertal, premenarchial girls whose sleep was monitored polygraphically. They found a definite circadian variation of oestradiol with the highest values occurring during the day

(14.00–16.00 hr) and the lowest value during sleep when gonadotrophin secretion was augmented.

(*1*) *Precocious puberty*. Precocious puberty occurs in both sexes and is usually constitutional or familial. Pathological causes include various tumour conditions (for example hypothalamic, gonadal, adrenal). Increased levels of oestradiol, much higher than would be expected for the chronological age of the patient, but consistent with the stage of puberty reached, are observed in iso-sexual precocious puberty of constitutional or hypothalamic types and that caused by ovarian or testicular tumours.

(*2*) *Delayed puberty*. In both sexes, delayed puberty of the constitutional type is the most common but in all types oestradiol levels are low or low–normal. In the male, Klinefelter's syndrome is associated with oestrone and oestradiol levels that are normal or increased (Federman, 1967; Kley *et al.*, 1976).

(b) Adult female

A strict comparison of oestrone and oestradiol levels reported in the menstruating female is often difficult to make, due to the fact that measurements are often grouped according to the phase of the cycle and there is a relatively wide range at any stage. In addition, Kletzky, Nakamura, Thorneycroft and Mishell (1975) have shown that the distribution of oestradiol levels at any stage of the cycle is not normal (Gaussian) but log-normal. They presented a direct graphical estimation of values with a useful clinical range which includes the mean and 95% confidence limits.

The basic cyclical pattern of oestrone and oestradiol levels is well known, the lowest levels occurring at the beginning and end of the cycle with a progressive increase after day 6 to the ovulatory peak. The ovulatory peak of oestradiol always precedes the LH peak but the exact separation of the two in time is variable as also are the peak levels attained and the duration of the rise (Abraham, Odell, Swerdloff and Hopper, 1972). The levels of oestrone and oestradiol in the follicular and luteal phases are very similar, but peak oestradiol levels always exceed those of oestrone (Tulchinsky and Korenman, 1970). These latter authors also found a distinct diurnal variation for oestrone but not for oestradiol. Certainly for any one individual, the true mean oestrogen level is best reflected by the mean of several measurements taken at frequent intervals throughout the day.

There have been many reports of oestrone and oestradiol throughout the menstrual cycle so the few given in Table 7 are representative rather than comprehensive. For a detailed bibliography (1962–1970) of hormonal levels throughout the menstrual cycle see Anon, 1971.

Studies of oestriol in plasma have largely been limited to pregnant females.

Table 7

Plasma oestrone and oestradiol levels (ng/100 ml) in the normal menstrual cycle[a].

Follicular phase		Mid-cycle		Luteal phase		References
Oestrone	Oestradiol	Oestrone	Oestradiol	Oestrone	Oestradiol	
5·7	6·4	—	—	11·1	19·6	Baird (1968)
4·0	2·9	17·0	31·8	12·1	19·1	Baird and Guevara (1969)
—	6·3	—	33·2	—	14·3	Corker and Exley (1969)
—	—	33·8	51·3	—	—	Mikhail et al. (1970)
—	1–10	—	14–77	—	19–34	Dufau et al. (1970)
7·9	—	—	—	10·7	—	Tulchinsky and Korenman (1970)
2·9	3·1	8·1	19·4	8·9	16·3	Kim et al. (1974)
5·2	5·8	—	—	—	—	De Vane et al. (1975)

[a] Oestrone: 1 ng/100 ml = 37·0 pmol/l; oestradiol 1 ng/100 ml = 36·7 pmol/l.

In the non-pregnant human female Wu and Lundy (1971) reported oestriol levels of 2·9 ± 0·9 ng/100 ml (101 ± 37 pmol/l) in the early follicular and late luteal phase. Dignam, Parlow, Coyotupa, Honda, Hiroi, Kinoshita and Kushinsky (1974) reported much higher values for oestriol rising to a maximum of 83 ng/100 ml (2·9 nmol/l). Peaks of oestriol were coincident with those of the gonadotrophins and as expected in the light of the biochemical role of oestrone as a precursor for oestriol, were preceded by peaks of oestrone and oestradiol. Their reported levels for oestrone and oestradiol (presumably as the sulphates) were also higher than those reported by other workers. This is probably partly due to their less sensitive assay technique. Rotti, Stevens, Watson and Longcope (1975) using a specific oestriol antiserum along with a partition purification step, reported levels of 0·79 ± 0·06 ng/100 ml (27·4 ± 2·1 pmol/l) and 1·11 ± 0·008 ng/100 ml (38·5 ± 0·3 pmol/l) in the follicular and luteal phases respectively. For some other reported values see Table 8.

The data available for oestrogen levels after treatment with steroid contraceptives in the adult menstruating female, suggest that those steroid contraceptives that block ovulation, decrease the production of oestrone,

Table 8

Plasma oestriol levels (ng/100 ml) in non-pregnant women[a].

Follicular phase	Luteal phase	Mid-cycle	References
Mean level 2·0 (r 0–7·5)	Stage of cycle not stated		Cedard et al. (1970)
Mean level <1·0	Stage of cycle not stated		Loriaux et al. (1972)
2·9	2·9	—	Wu and Lundy (1971)
—	12·0	15·0	Powell and Stevens (1973)
—	—	83·0	Dignam et al. (1974)
0·76	1·1	—	Rotti et al. (1975)
0·70	1·1	—	Flood et al. (1976)

[a] Oestriol 1 ng/100 ml = 34·7 pmol/l.

oestradiol and androstenedione by the ovary. Weisz, Lloyd, Lobotsky, Pupkin, Zanartu and Puga (1973) measured oestrogens and androgens in ovarian and peripheral venous plasma in normal women and those treated with either intramuscular medroxyprogesterone, oral chlormadinone or oral ethynodiol diacetate with mestranol. Oestradiol was low in those on contraceptive therapy compared with controls for both ovarian venous plasma 2·5–777·0 ng/100 ml (0·09–28·2 nmol/l) and 7·0–4064 ng/100 ml (0·03–14·9 μmol/l) respectively, and peripheral venous plasma <0·5–12·46 ng/ 100 ml (<0·02–0·46 nmol/l) and 2·3–34·7 ng/100 ml (0·08–1·3 nmol/l) respectively. Oestrone in ovarian vein plasma was in the lower part of the normal range for those on contraceptive therapy compared with normals, 7·0– 102 ng/100ml (0·3–3·8 nmol/l) and 8·9–378·1 ng/100 ml (0·3–14·0 nmol/l) respectively, and in peripheral vein plasma it was below the mean normal range of 1·35–47·0 ng/100 ml (0·05–1·7 nmol/l).

The reason for the smaller relative decrease in oestrone values than in oestradiol values is probably due to increased adrenal secretion of oestrone or peripheral conversion of adrenal androstenedione. This study also suggested that there was a greater suppression of both gonadotrophin and ovarian steroid levels using the combined ethynodiol diacetate with mestranol. The characteristic cyclical pattern of oestrogen secretion is also abolished by oral contraceptives (England et al., 1974). Rotti et al. (1974) measured oestriol concentrations in women taking oral contraceptives and they found the mean level of 7·6 ± 1·5 ng100ml (263 ± 52 pmol/l) to be no different from those of women in the follicular phase of the cycle.

(1) Infertility. There has been a great deal of work carried out into the investigation of male and female infertility (Marshall, 1975; Jacobs, Hull,

Murray and Franks, 1975).

Female infertility may be due to any number of causes including such conditions as the polycystic ovarian syndrome (PCO), anorexia nervosa, pituitary tumour and various genetical and anatomical disorders. The follicular cyst fluid content of oestradiol is low, but plasma levels comparable, in PCO and normal subjects. Plasma oestrone levels are, however, higher than normal (De Vane, Czekala, Judd and Yen, 1975) suggesting adrenal involvement as androstenedione, testosterone, DHA sulphate and LH are also increased.

Oestradiol levels are also low in patients with anorexia nervosa and correspond well with clinical evaluation of deoestrogenisation (Jacobs et al., 1975).

Oestrone and oestradiol levels are low in patients with hyperprolactinaemia with or without galactorrhoea, but these measurements are of no clinical value without the measurement of prolactin levels (Jacobs, Franks, Murray, Hull, Steele and Nabarro, 1976).

(c) Pregnancy

Urinary oestriol measurements have for many years been the accepted method for assessing foetal growth and well-being. Their usefulness may be limited in some clinical situations due to the time taken for collection of 24 hr urine specimens and the incompleteness of some specimens presented to the laboratory. Oestriol determinations in amniotic fluid have been suggested (Schindler and Herrman, 1966; Biggs, Klopper and Wilson, 1969) but this has limitations due to the variable amount of fluid available and the inconvenience to the patient. Thus many workers have been measuring oestriol levels in blood using a variety of assay techniques. Taylor et al. (1970), Macourt, Corker and Naftolin (1971) and Hull (1976) have compared the use of total plasma oestriol determinations as a substitute for urinary oestrogen measurements and all concluded that similar, but more accurate and valuable results could be obtained from plasma assays. Plasma levels of oestriol by various methods have been compared by Masson (1973) and Table 9 gives a comparison of the levels of unconjugated oestriol in the pregnant female, by some of the many workers in this field.

The general pattern of oestrogen changes through pregnancy is for oestrone, oestradiol and oestriol to remain fairly low for the first trimester, oestrone and oestradiol rising first followed by oestriol at the 10th week. All oestrogens increase regularly to the end of pregnancy with oestriol showing a biphasic increase. After the 12th week the increase of oestriol is steeper than that of oestrone or oestradiol whereas from the 18th to the 30th week, the increase in oestriol is again steeper than oestrone or oestradiol. Therefore

Table 9

Plasma oestrogen levels (ng/ml) in normal pregnancy[a].

Period of gestation	Oestrone	Oestradiol	Oestriol	References
First trimester	0·5–8·0	1·0–5·0	<1·0	
28 wk	3·0–16·0	12·0–19·0	3·0–6·0 (wk 30)	Cohen and Cohen (1974)
39 wk	4·4–27·0	10·0–39·0	8·5–16·0	
5–6 wk	0·4	0·5	0·6	
11–12 wk	1·0	2·0	0·2	
17–18 wk	3·1	4·8	1·8	De Hertogh et al. (1975)
27–28 wk	5·6	11·6	5·4	
39–40 wk	7·2	17·3	14·7	
16 wk	—	—	1·4	Tulchinsky and Korenman
Term	—	15·0	11·1	(1971)
Term	12·2	35·1	14·2	Wu and Lundy (1971)
Term	10·5	18·1	9·7	Cohen et al. (1972)
Term	—	—	13·9	Gorwill and Sarda (1977)
31–40 wk	—	24·9	—	Sibulski and Maughan (1972)
34–40 wk	—	21·9	—	Munson et al. (1970)
30 wk	—	19·0	—	
35 wk	—	22·4	—	Chew and Ratnam (1976)
40 wk	—	31·6	—	

[a] Oestrone 1 ng/ml = 3·70 nmol/l, oestradiol 1 ng/ml = 3·67 nmol/l, oestriol 1 ng/ml = 3·47 nmol/l.

the ratio of oestradiol to oestriol tends to decrease from week 20 to week 40 of gestation (Tulchinsky and Abraham, 1971; Cohen and Cohen, 1974; De Hertogh et al., 1975). This steep surge in unconjugated oestriol levels occurs at about 35–36 weeks (Sakakini, Buster and Killam, 1977) and these authors have shown that it can be used as an indicator of normal pregnancy. The gestational age at birth, as determined by careful neonatal examination, agreed with the age predicted by the oestriol surge within ± one week. Hay and Lorscheider (1976) have demonstrated a positive correlation between infant birth weight and the oestriol value during the last week of normal pregnancy, prior to the onset of labour. Although unconjugated oestriol (being produced by the placenta) is the theoretical choice for assessing foetal well-being (Hull, 1975; Hull and Chard, 1976), it has been suggested that oestradiol levels may better reflect foetoplacental function when growth retardation is complicated by certain congenital abnormalities, including those involving the foetal kidney (Sybulski, Asswad and Maughan, 1976). The observations on the changes of oestradiol levels that take place before the onset of labour have been more contradictory than for oestriol. No consistent change in the concentration of unconjugated oestradiol in relation to labour was found by Tulchinsky, Hobel, Yeager and Marshall (1972) or Shaaban and Klopper (1973). Turnbull, Patten, Flint, Keirse, Jeremy and Anderson (1974), however, demonstrated a marked rise in oestradiol levels during the five weeks preceding labour. In contrast Chew and Ratnam (1976) demonstrated a linear increase in mean oestradiol levels during this same five week period reaching a plateau during the last two weeks.

There is also some disagreement as to the degree and timing of diurnal variations in pregnancy oestrogens. Selinger and Levitz (1969) observed a diurnal variation of total plasma oestriol in pregnant women and this was the first report of a steroid hormone predominantly of foetal origin showing such a variation. There were significantly lower results of oestriol at 16.30 hr and the average 08.00 hr value was lower than the 21.30 hr value. Samples were only collected at these times and not at more frequent intervals. Townsley, Rubin, Grannis, Gartmann and Crystle (1973) showed that there was a more significant diurnal variation for oestradiol (00.00 hr values greater than 12.00 hr values) than for oestriol which had a less marked rhythm, although the daytime mean (08.00–12.00–16.00 hr) was significantly greater than the night-time mean (20.00–00.00–04.00 hr). Similar results were obtained by Munson, Yanone and Mueller (1972). Goebel and Kuss (1974), however, observed a circadian rhythm of unconjugated oestriol with the lowest levels at 08.00 hr and the highest at 20.00 hr during which time oestriol levels increased by an average of 31%. Total plasma oestriol values were at one time measured in preference to unconjugated oestriol levels as it was thought that there was a greater individual fluctuation of unconjugated oestriol levels throughout the day, making clinical interpretation on one or a few samples difficult (Klopper and Shaaban, 1974). However, Hull et al. (1979) demonstrated that the degree of individual fluctuation of plasma unconjugated oestriol concentrations was no greater than for the other oestrogens, thus confirming its choice in obstetric practice.

(d) Post-menopausal female

At the extremes of reproductive life, there is characteristically a wide variability in cycle length. This was first reported by Treloar, Boynton, Benn and Brown (1967) and further substantiated by Sherman and Korenman (1975). Treloar et al. (1967) showed that it was particularly the five to seven years after the menarche and the six to eight years before the menopause during which the cycle length was irregular. There was also a gradual decrease of two to three days in mean cycle length with increasing age. The menopausal transition was studied in more detail by Sherman, West and Korenman (1976) and this gave further support to their previous hypothesis that there was an ovarian regulatory hormone (an inhibin) exerting a negative feedback control over FSH secretion. As the number of ovarian follicles diminished with advancing years so the inhibin and consequently its control over FSH secretion would be reduced. Hence the amount of oestradiol secreted by the ovary is almost insignificant after the menopause (Judd, Judd, Lucas and Yen, 1974), and oestrone becomes quantitatively the dominant of the three classical oestrogens circulating in the blood (Edman and MacDonald, 1976). In fact the ovary is responsible for only a very small amount of the circulating oestrone, oestradiol and oestriol. Oestrone is derived predominantly from the peripheral conversion of androstenedione (MacDonald, Rombaut and Siiteri, 1967), oestradiol from peripheral conversion of testosterone, and oestriol as a metabolite of oestrone and oestradiol (Siiteri and MacDonald, 1973).

As levels of these oestrogens are very low in post-menopausal women's plasma it is only recently that techniques of measurement have been suitably specific and sensitive to allow such studies to be carried out. Table 10 gives some of the levels reported recently. Whether the menopause has occurred naturally or as a result of castration, there does not appear to be any significant difference in the oestrone and oestradiol levels observed (Baird and Guevera, 1969; Radar, Flickinger, DeVilla, Mikula and Mikhail, 1973; Vermeulen, 1976; Hutton, Jacobs, James, Murray and Rippon, 1977). Chakravarti, Collins, Forcast, Newton, Oram and Studd (1976) studied a series of women grouped with respect to the number of years since the menopause. They found that both oestrone and oestradiol remained consistently low for 10 years after the menopause, having fallen to about 20% of their pre-menopausal values within a year of the menopause. Between 10–20 years after the menopause they found a further significant reduction in oestrone levels and a corresponding increase in oestradiol levels to the lower end of the normal range for females of reproductive age. No explanation was given for this finding. The levels they found for oestrone (0·92–2·4 ng/100 ml; 34–89 pmol/l) and oestradiol (1·3–2·1 ng/100 ml; 48–77 pmol/l) are lower than most other reports, see Table 10.

There have been only a very few reports of oestriol levels in post-menopausal women since the development of oestriol radioimmunoassay has in general been directed towards measurement of levels during pregnancy. Such assays are not usually of sufficient sensitivity to measure the low levels in post-menopausal women. However, Flood, Pratt and Longcope (1976) reported values of 0·3–1·1 ng/100 ml (11–38 pmol/l) in post-menopausal women and similar levels were reported by Rose, Fern, Liskowski and

Table 10

Plasma oestrone and oestradiol levels (ng/100 ml) in post-menopausal women aged 40–90 years[a].

Oestrone	Oestradiol	References
7·1	1·3	Baird and Guevara (1969)
4·0	—	Tulchinsky and Korenman (1970)
2·5	0·7	Longcope (1971)
2·2	0·5	Nagai and Longcope (1971)
4·1	1·3	Radar et al. (1973)
—	1·1	Korenman et al. (1974)
4·2	3·4	Yen et al. (1975)
4·9	2·0	Vermeulen (1976)
2·9	1·2	Judd et al. (1976)
5·4	3·4	Hutton et al. (1978)

[a] Oestrone 1 ng/100 ml = 37·0 pmol/l, oestradiol 1 ng/100 ml = 36/7 pmol/l.

Milbrath (1977) in post-menopausal women treated with Premarin.

In cases of premature menopause oestrogen levels are the same as those observed after the normal menopause (Jacobs and Murray, 1976).

(e) Adult male

Plasma levels of oestrone and oestradiol in normal men tend to be in the same range as those observed during the follicular phase of the menstrual cycle in women (Table 11). As with the levels observed in post-menopausal women, oestrone tends to be three times higher than oestradiol in men (Baird and Guevara, 1969). There appears to be an increase in oestrone levels with age in male senescence (Nagai and Longcope, 1971; Kley, Nieschlag, Bidlingmaier and Krüskemper, 1974; Korenman et al., 1974; Doerr, 1976). Also Pirke and Doerr (1973), Kley et al. (1974) and Rubens, Dhont and Vermeulen (1974) have shown that oestradiol also increases with age in men. One hypothesis for explaining this increase is that of an increased blood production rate of oestrone and oestradiol due to an increased peripheral aromatisation of plasma androgens.

Oestradiol levels are normal in male infertility due to germ cell damage and low when there is secondary testicular failure due to hypothalamic and pituitary disease (Marshall, 1975).

Gynaecomastia in the male is frequently seen at puberty and is associated

Table 11

Plasma oestrone and oestradiol levels (ng/100 ml) in men aged 20–60 years[a].

Oestrone	Oestradiol	References
5·7	1·9	Baird and Guevara (1969)
7·4	1·7	Mikhail *et al.* (1970)
6·2	—	Tulchinsky and Korenman (1971)
3·0	2·6	Nagai and Longcope (1971)
—	2·0–6·8	Onikki and Aldercreutz (1973)
—	1·2–3·5	Doerr (1973)
—	4·6	Wu *et al.* (1973)
3·0	—	Ichii *et al.* (1974)
—	2·1	Korenman *et al.* (1974)
2·8	—	Doerr (1976)

[a] Oestrone 1 ng/100 ml = 37·0 pmol/l, oestradiol 1 ng/100 ml = 36·7 pmol/l.

with a transient rise in oestradiol levels. Gynaecomastia may also occur at other times of life in association with a variety of different disorders in which oestrogen levels are not useful for diagnosis.

2. Non-protein Bound Oestrogens

(a) Physiological conditions

(*1*) *Birth to puberty.* Changes in the concentrations of oestrogens and the percentage of unbound oestradiol that occur between birth and puberty have been investigated by Radfar, Ansusingha and Kenny (1976). The unbound concentration of oestradiol decreased rapidly during the first 72 hr after birth, although the percentage of unbound oestradiol remained constant. Two weeks after birth, the percentage of unbound oestradiol had decreased, presumably due to the increase in SBP concentrations that occur in the first few weeks of life (Tulchinsky and Chopra, 1973; Forest, Cathiard and Bertrand, 1973).

In pre-pubertal children (0–8 yr) there was no difference in the percentage unbound plasma oestradiol of boys and girls although the unbound concentration in girls from this age group was three times that of boys. During puberty, the percentage of unbound oestradiol increased in boys and girls during stages II and III of adolescence. In boys a further increase in the percentage of unbound oestradiol occurred during stages IV and V of adolescence but no further increase occurred in girls. This sex difference may be due to the opposing effects of oestrogens and androgens on SBP synthesis by the liver during adolescence.

(2) *Normal adults.* There are relatively few reports of the percentage of unbound oestradiol and concentration of unbound oestradiol in plasma of normal adult men and women (Table 12). Where the percentage of unbound oestradiol has been measured in men and women, levels in men are marginally higher than in women (Chopra *et al.*, 1973; Fisher *et al.*, 1974). The sexual difference in the percentage of unbound oestradiol is less than found for testosterone (Chopra *et al.*, 1973; Fisher *et al.*, 1974). Although the concentration of SBP in adult women is greater than in men, the affinity of oestradiol for SBP is lower than that of testosterone (Vermeulen, Verdonck, Van Der Straeten and Orie, 1969; Rosner, 1972; Burke and Anderson, 1972; Shanbhag *et al.*, 1973).

In women no marked variations in SBP have been found throughout the menstrual cycle (Pearlman, Crepy and Murphy, 1967; Anderson, 1974) and the percentage of unbound oestradiol remains constant throughout the menstrual cycle (Wu, Motohashi, Abdel-Rahman, Flickinger and Mikhail, 1976). The concentration of unbound oestradiol reflected changes in the concentration of unconjugated plasma oestradiol throughout the menstrual cycle and ranged from 100 pg/100 ml (3·67 pmol/l) during the follicular phase to 500 pg/100 ml (18·3 pmol/l) at the mid-cycle peak (Wu *et al.*, 1976). Similar results for the concentration of unbound oestradiol throughout the menstrual cycle were also obtained by Stahl, Dorner, Rohde and Schott (1976).

An increase of SBP occurs in men with ageing (Vermeulen, Rubens and Verdonck, 1972; Pirke and Doerr, 1973) and the percentage of unbound oestradiol is lower in older men (Rubens, Dhont and Vermeulen, 1974; Pirke and Doerr, 1975).

(b) *Pathological conditions*

Alterations in the circulating levels of unbound oestradiol have been found in a number of pathological conditions (Table 13). In male subjects with hyperthyroidism due to Graves' disease, the concentrations of unbound oestradiol were determined in order to evaluate the role of oestrogens in the onset of gynaecomastia which is frequently associated with this condition (Chopra *et al.*, 1972). The percentage of unbound oestradiol in subjects with Graves' disease was significantly lower than found in normal males although the concentration of unbound oestradiol was above the normal range. The possibility that alterations in unbound oestradiol and testosterone levels may

Table 12

Non-protein bound oestradiol in normal men and women.

Age	Males Percentage unbound	Concentration unbound (pg/100 ml)[a]	Females Percentage unbound	Concentration unbound (pg/100 ml)[a]	References
	2·10 ± 0·06	54·9 ± 4·12	1·47 ± 0·11	144 ± 34·9	Chopra et al. (1973)
	1·79 ± 0·08	—	1·49 ± 0·10	—	Fisher et al. (1974)
<50	1·96	25·9	—	—	Rubens et al. (1974)
>65	1·29	28·1	—	—	Rubens et al. (1974)
22–61	2·49	42·4	—	—	Pirke and Doerr (1975)
67–93	2·31	55·7	—	—	Pirke and Doerr (1975)
	—	—	1·39	—	Radfar et al. (1976)
	—	—	2·21 ± 0·04	—	Wu et al. (1976)
	—	44·0	—	98·0	Kley et al. (1977)
	—	55·0 ± 1·5	—	158·3 ± 12·4	Speight et al. (1977)

[a] 1 pg/100 ml = 36·7 fmol/l.

Table 13

Non-protein bound oestradiol in pathological conditions.

Condition	Patient (P) or control (C)	Sex	Percentage unbound	Concentration unbound (pg/100 ml)[a]	References
Graves' disease	P	M	2·23 ± 0·16	106·8 ± 14·4	Chopra et al. (1972)
	C	M	4·25 ± 0·13	91·5 ± 9·4	
Liver disease	P	M	—	52 ± 18	Galvao-Teles et al. (1972)
	C	M	—	58	
Liver disease	P	M	2·54 ± 0·14	122 ± 18·0	Chopra et al. (1973)
	C	M	2·10 ± 0·06	54·9 ± 4·12	
Hirsutism and amenorrhoea	P	F	1·94 ± 0·15	81 ± 13·0	Tulchinsky and Chopra (1974)
	C	F	1·47 ± 0·11	172 ± 16·0	
Hirsutism	P	F	1·55 ± 0·28	—	Fisher et al. (1974)
	C	F	1·49 ± 0·35	—	

[a] 1 pg/100 ml = 36·7 fmol/l.

M

result from a direct effect on the liver by thyroid hormones and consequent rise in SBP levels has been discussed (Anderson, 1974).

Gynaecomastia, together with testicular atrophy, also occurs in subjects with liver disease (Galvao-Teles, Anderson, Burke, Marshall, Corker, Brown and Clark, 1973; Chopra, Tulchinsky and Greenway, 1973). No difference in the unbound concentration of oestradiol was found in men with liver disease by Galvao-Teles *et al.* (1973). These authors suggested that this could be accounted for by an increase in SBP and a decrease in albumin concentrations that occurs in men with liver disease. In contrast Chopra *et al.* (1973) found that the percentage of unbound oestradiol was 20% higher in subjects with liver disease. Total and unbound concentrations of oestradiol were also significantly higher than found in normal males. Although different techniques were used to determine the unbound fraction of oestradiol, the reason for this discrepancy is not clear.

As alterations in the balance of unbound hormones might be implicated in hirsutism, levels of unbound oestradiol and testosterone have been measured in hirsute women (Tulchinsky and Chopra, 1974; Fisher *et al.*, 1974). Again, different techniques were used to measure the unbound fraction of oestradiol by these groups and there are some discrepancies in the results. No significant difference in the percentage of unbound oestradiol in hirsute and normal women was found by Fisher *et al.* (1974) whereas a highly significant difference was found by Tulchinsky and Chopra (1974). Despite the higher unbound fraction of oestradiol found by the later authors in hirsute women, concentrations of unbound oestradiol were only half those found in normal women during the follicular phase of the menstrual cycle. In both studies, however, the percentage of unbound testosterone was greater in hirsute than normal women suggesting that it is the alteration in the relative levels of unbound oestradiol and testosterone that are important in hirsutism.

(c) Effect of hormone treatment

In addition to alterations in the unbound level of oestradiol found in pathological conditions administration of hormones can cause changes in the level of unbound oestradiol. Some oral contraceptives are known to increase the concentration of SBP (van Kamnen, Thijssen, Rademaker and Schwarz, 1975; Briggs, 1975) and a decrease in the percentage of unbound oestradiol has been reported in women receiving oestrogen therapy (Fisher *et al.*, 1974; Kley *et al.*, 1977). In post-menopausal women hormone replacement therapy with ethynyloestradiol resulted in a much greater reduction in the percentage of unbound oestradiol and oestrone than "natural" oestrogen therapy (Hutton *et al.*, 1978).

3. Conjugates and Metabolites

(a) Oestrogen sulphates

As stated earlier, oestrone sulphate is probably the most abundant oestrogen in plasma, oestrone and oestradiol concentrations being approximately one-fifth to one-tenth the oestrone sulphate levels (Loriaux et al., 1971). It has not been widely investigated at the present time due to the lack of a simple RIA for its measurement in blood. The levels found by some authors are given in Table 14.

Levels of oestrone sulphate and oestradiol sulphate have recently been measured in eight normal women throughout the menstrual cycle (Nunez, Aedo, Landgren, Cekan and Diczfalusy, 1977). Both oestrone sulphate and oestradiol sulphate displayed a marked cyclic pattern similar to that of the unconjugated oestrogens (Fig. 7). The mean levels of oestrone sulphate were 10–15 times higher than that of oestrone whereas those of oestradiol sulphate were 1–4 times lower than those of oestradiol.

The recently identified conjugates such as the 16-sulphates of oestriol which comprise less than 1% of the total oestriol are apparently present in blood at concentrations too low to be of diagnostic value in human pregnancy. Any measurements made have been in urine, amniotic fluid or breast cyst fluid (Levitz et al., 1976; Dipietro, 1976; Manikanguly and Levitz, 1977; Sugar et al., 1977).

(b) Catechol oestrogen

The only report to date of blood levels of either 2-hydroxyoestrone or 2-methoxyoestrone is that of Yoshizawa and Fishman (1971) in their description of a RIA for 2-hydroxyoestrone. The levels of 2-hydroxyoestrone they report are very similar to levels that would be expected for oestradiol. The range of values they found in ng/100 ml are as follows: young men 2·8–3·9 (0·10–0·14 nmol/l), young women 10·8–29·5 (0·4–1·0 nmol/l), late pregnancy (third trimester) 120–360 (4·2–12·6 nmol/l) and post-menopausal women 2·4–7·2 (0·08—0·25 nmol/l).

(c) Oestetrol

Values for oestetrol at various stages of pregnancy are given in Table 15. Fishman and Guzik (1972) found that it could not be demonstrated in male or non-pregnant female plasma. This is in agreement with the observation that oestetrol is derived mainly from metabolism, in the foetal liver, of placental oestrone or oestradiol (Schwers, Eriksson, Wiqvist and Diczfalusy, 1965).

Table 14

Plasma oestrone sulphate levels (ng/100 ml)[a].

Female						
Pool	Follicular phase	Luteal phase	Mid-cycle	Pregnancy	Male	References
—	46·7	89·1	—	—	33·0	Loriaux *et al.* (1971)
—	—	—	334·0	—	—	Brown and Smyth (1971)
188·0	20–120	50–230	308·0	—	71·6	Hawkins and Oakey (1974)
—	—	—	—	—	46·0	Ruder *et al.* (1972)
—	—	—	—	5000	—	Touchstone and Murawec (1965)

[a] 1 ng/100 ml = 28·5 pmol/l

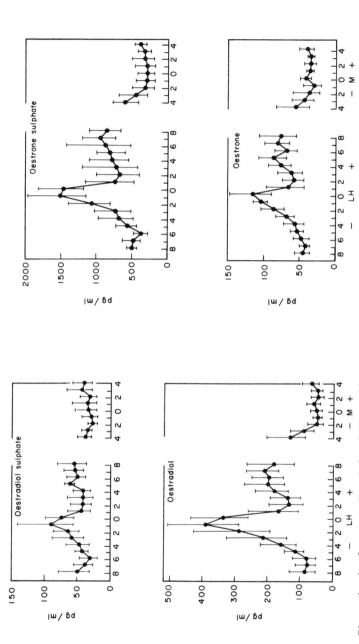

Fig. 7. Plasma levels of oestrone (1 pg/ml = 3·70 pmol/l), oestrone sulphate (1 pg/ml = 2·85 pmol/l), oestradiol (1 pg/ml = 3·67 pmol/l) and oestradiol sulphate (1 pg/ml = 2·83 pmol/l) throughout the menstrual cycle (from Nunez *et al.*, 1977 with permission of authors and publisher).

4. In Tissues

In spite of extensive data on the levels of oestrogens in plasma in various physiological conditions there is only limited information about oestrogen concentrations in human tissues. The concentrations of oestrone and oestradiol in endometrium from normal menstruating women (Guerro, Landgren, Montiel, Cekan and Diczfalusy, 1975) and oestradiol in myometrium of pregnant subjects (Batra, 1976; Batra and Bengtsson, 1978) have been measured (Table 16).

Table 15

Plasma oestetrol levels (ng/ml) in pregnant women[a].

Period of gestation	Oestetrol	References
Up to 18 wk	UD < 0·5	
20–28 wk	0·2	Tulchinsky et al. (1975)
Term	1·2	
20–28 wk	2·0	
34 wk	3·0	Korda et al. (1975)
Term	4·5–5·0	
Third trimester	1·0–4·0	Fishman and Guzik (1972)
Third trimester	0·2–1·0	Kundu and Grant (1976)
Term	2·2	Giebenhain et al. (1972)

[a] 1 ng/ml = 3·28 nmol/l.

The concentration of oestrone and oestradiol in endometrium (ng/100 g wet weight) were significantly higher than those in plasma in both the proliferative and secretory phase of the menstrual cycle. The concentration of oestradiol decreased in secretory phase endometrium whereas the concentration of oestrone remained constant. There was no clear correlation between endometrial and plasma levels of oestradiol.

In myometrium obtained from mid-term pregnant subjects oestradiol concentrations were lower, but not significantly different from plasma concentrations (Batra and Bengtsson, 1978). At term concentrations of oestradiol in plasma were significantly greater than the concentration in myometrium. A reduced oestradiol binding capacity as a result of a progesterone induced decrease in tissue oestradiol receptors (Batra, 1976) or greater binding of oestradiol to plasma proteins with advancing pregnancy may account for the low myometrial oestradiol concentrations at term.

Table 16

Oestrogens in uterine tissue.

	Tissue (ng/100 g)	Plasma[a] (ng/100 ml)	Tissue/plasma ratio
Endometrium from non-pregnant subjects			
Proliferative			
Oestrone	29·6	6·2	4·8
Oestradiol	119·0	11·9	10·0
Secretory			
Oestrone	27·5	8·0	3·4
Oestradiol	50·5	13·5	3·8
Myometrium from pregnant subjects			
Mid-term			
Oestradiol	160·0	290·0	0·55
Term			
Oestradiol	320·0	2222·0	0·14

[a] Oestrone 1 ng/100 ml = 37·0 pmol/l, oestradiol 1 ng/100 ml = 36·7 pmol/l.

CONCLUSION

The development of analytical methods that have enabled the concentrations of the classical oestrogens in blood to be measured has resulted in a major advance in our understanding of the role of these oestrogens in normal and pathological conditions. However, information regarding the many other oestrogens and oestrogen conjugates in blood is still limited.

The development of radioimmunoassay techniques has been responsible for major advances in the field of endocrinology but does have some inherent disadvantages in requiring radioactive material and expensive counting equipment (Jeffocate, 1977). Methods have been developed in which the enzymeimmunoassay principle has been applied to the measurement of plasma oestradiol and oestriol using the enzyme horse radish peroxidase as a label for the antigen, instead of a radioactive label as used in radio-immunoassay (Van Weeman and Schuurs, 1972; Ven Hell, Bosch, Brands, Van Weemen and Schuurs, 1976). Although further development of the enzymeimmunoassay techniques, especially with respect to improvements in sensitivity are required (Numazawa, Haryu, Kurosaka and Nambara, 1977), it is possible that enzymeimmunoassay could supersede radioimmuno-assay on the counts of cost, simplicity, speed and ease of automation (Exley and Abuknesha, 1977).

The development of assays to measure the cytoplasmic oestrogen receptor concentration in oestrogen target tissues and hormone responsive neoplasms has been another important advance in the study of oestrogens in recent years (Gorski et al., 1968; Jensen and De Sombre, 1972; O'Malley and Means, 1974; Chan and O'Malley, 1976). Initial attempts to predict the response of subjects with breast cancer to therapy on the basis of oestrogen receptor concentration, however, have not been as successful as originally expected (Braunsberg, 1977). Improvements in oestrogen receptor assay methodology, together with the measurement of progesterone receptors, also present in some neoplasms, may increase the prognostic value of receptor estimations (McGuire, Howitz, Zava, Garola and Chamness, 1978). Finally, studies which combine measurement of plasma oestrogen concentration with tissue concentrations of oestrogen and oestrogen receptor should be of great interest in both normal and pathological conditions.

REFERENCES

Abraham, G. E. (1969). J. clin. Endocr. Metab. 29, 866.
Abraham, G. E., Hopper, K., Tulchinsky, D., Swerdloff, R. S. and Odell, W. D. (1971). Anal. Lett. 4, 19.
Abraham, G. E., Odell, W. D., Edwards, R. and Purdy, J. M. (1970). Acta endocr., Copenh. 147 (Suppl.), 332.
Abraham, G. E., Odell. W. D., Swerdloff, R. S. and Hopper, K. (1972). J. clin. Endocr. Metab. 34, 312.
Adlercreutz, H. (1970). J. Endocr. 46, 126.
Adlercreutz, H. and Luukkainen, T. (1967). Acta endocr., Copenh. 124 (Suppl.), 101.
Adlercreutz, H. and Luukkainen, T. (1968). "Gas Phase Chromatography of Steroids" pp. 115–149. Springer-Verlag, Berlin, Heidelberg and New York.
Ahmed, J. and Mester, J. (1973). Clin. chim. Acta, 48, 37.
Aiman, J., Nalick, R. H., Jacobs, A., Porter, J. C., Edman, C. D., Vellios, F. and MacDonald, P. C. (1977). Obstet. Gynec. 49, 695.
Akhtar, M. and Skinner, S. J. M. (1968). Biochem. J. 109, 318.
Alonso, C. and Troen, P. (1966). Biochemistry, 5, 337.
Anderson, D. C. (1974). Clin Endocr. 3, 69.
Anderson, D. C. (1976). "The Endocrine Function of the Human Ovary." Academic Press, New York and London.
Angsusingha, K., Kenny, F. M., Nanhin, H. R. and Taylor, F. H. (1974). J. clin. Endocr. Metab. 39, 63.
Anon. (1971). Bibliog. Reprod. 17, 293.
Antonipillai, I. and Murphy, B. E. P. (1977). Br. J. Obstet. Gynaec. 84, 179.
Arai, K., Kuwabara, Y. and Okinaga, S. (1972). Am. J. Obstet. Gynec. 113, 316.
Arceo, R. B. and Ryan, K. J. (1967). Acta endocr., Copenh. 56, 225.
Aso, T., Guerro, R., Cekan, Z. and Diczfalusy, E. (1975). Clin. Endocr. 4, 173.
Baird, D. T. (1968). J. clin. Endocr. Metab. 28, 244.
Baird, D. T. (1977). "The Ovary" Vol. 3, p. 305. Academic Press, New York and London.

Baird, D. T. and Frazer, I. S. (1974). *J. clin. Endocr. Metab.* **38**, 1009.
Baird, D. T. and Frazer, I. S. (1975). *Clin. Endocr.* **4**, 259.
Baird, D. T. and Guevera, A. (1969). *J. clin. Endocr. Metab.* **29**, 149.
Baird, D. T., Uno, A. and Melby, J. C. (1969). *J. clin. Endocr. Metab.* **45**, 135.
Baird, D. T., Galbraith, A., Frazer, I. S. and Newsam, J. E. (1973). *J. Endocr.* **57**, 285.
Baird, D. T., Horton, R., Longcope, C. and Tait, J. F. (1968). *Perspect. Biol. Med.* **11**, 384.
Baird, D. T., Horton, R., Longcope, C. and Tait, J. F. (1969). *Recent Prog. Horm. Res.* **25**, 611.
Ball, P., Farthmann, E. and Knuppen, R. (1976). *J. Steroid Biochem.* **7**, 139.
Ball, P., Gelbke, H. P. and Knuppen, R. (1975). *J. clin. Endocr. Metab.* **40**, 406.
Ball, P., Knuppen, R., Haupt, M. and Breuer, H. (1972). *J. clin. Endocr. Metab.* **34**, 736.
Ball, P., Stubenrauch, G. and Knuppen, R. (1977). *J. Steroid Biochem.* **8**, 989.
Barakat, R. M. and Ekins, R. P. (1961). *Lancet,* **ii**, 25.
Barlow, J. J. and Logan, C. M. (1966). *Steroids,* **7**, 309.
Barlow, J. J., Emerson, K. and Saxena, B. N. (1969). *New Engl. J. Med.* **280**, 633.
Barlow, J. J., Maclaren, J. A. and Pothier, L. (1969). *J. clin. Endocr. Metab.* **29**, 767.
Barrett, M. J. and Cohen, P. S. (1972). *Clin. Chem.* **18**, 1339.
Batra, S. (1976). *Endocrinology,* **99**, 1178.
Batra, S. and Bengtsson, L. P. (1978). *J. clin. Endocr. Metab.* **46**, 622.
Bayard, F., Louvet, J. P., Thijssens, J. L., Thouvenot, J. P. and Boulard, C. (1974). *Ann. Endocr.* **35**, 563.
Bidlingmaier, F., Wagner-Barnack, M., Butenandt, O. and Knorr, D. (1973). *Pediat. Res.* **7**, 901.
Bierich, J. R. (1975). *Clin. Endocr. Metab.* **4**, 1.
Biggs, J. S., Klopper, A. and Wilson, G. B. (1969). *J. Endocr.* **44**, 579.
Bleau, G., Roberts, K. D. and Chapdelaine, A. (1974). *J. clin. Endocr. Metab.* **39**, 236.
Bolton, A. E. and Rutherford, F. J. (1976). *J. Steroid Biochem.* **7**, 71.
Borth, L. (1952). *Ciba Fdn. Collq. Endocr.* **2**, 45.
Borth, R. (1957). *Vit. Horm.* **15**, 259.
Boyar, R. M., Wu, R. H. K., Roffwarg, H., Kapen, S., Weitzman, E. D., Hellman, L. and Finkelstein, J. W. (1976). *J. clin. Endocr. Metab.* **43**, 1418.
Bradbury, J. T. (1961). *Endocrinology,* **68**, 115.
Braunsberg, H. (1977). *La Ricerca Clin. Lab.* **7**, 47.
Breuer, H. (1962). *Vit. Horm.* **20**, 285.
Breuer, H. and Nocke-Finck, L. (1974). "Clinical Biochemistry, Principles and Methods", p. 790. Walter de Gruyter, Berlin.
Breuer, H., Knuppen, R. and Haupt, M. (1966). *Nature, Lond.* **212**, 76.
Briggs, M. H. (1975). *Contraception,* **12**, 149.
Brodie, H. J., Kripalani, K. J. and Possanja, G. (1969). *J. Am. Chem. Soc.* **91**, 1291.
Brown, J. B. and Smyth, B. J. (1971). *J. Reprod. Fertil.* **24**, 142.
Bruenelli, B. (1935). *Arch. int. Pharmacodynie,* **49**, 262.
Burke, C. W. (1969). *Biochim. biophys. Acta,* **176**, 403.
Burke, C. W. and Anderson, D. C. (1972). *Nature, Lond.* **240**, 38.
Burke, C. W. and Beardwell, C. G. (1973). *Quart. J. Med.* **42**, 175.
Burton, R. M. and Westphal, U. (1972). *Metabolism,* **21**, 253.
Cameron, E. H. D. and Jones, D. A. (1972). *Steroids,* **20**, 737.
Canalog, A., Sall, S., Gordon, G. G. and Southren, A. L. (1977). *Am. J. Obstet. Gynec.* **129**, 553.
Cedard, L., Mosse, A. and Klotz, H. P. (1970). *Ann. Endocr.* **31**, 453.

Chakravarti, S., Collins, W. P., Newton, J. R., Oram, D. H. and Studd, J. W. W. (1976). *Br. med. J.* **2**, 784.

Chan, L. and O'Malley, B. (1976). *New Engl. J. Med.* **294**, 1322, 1372, 1430.

Channing, C. P. and Kammerman, S. (1974). *Biol. Reprod.* **10**, 179.

Chattoraj, S. C., Fanous, A. S., Cecchini, D. and Lowe, E. W. (1978). *Steroids*, **31**, 375.

Chen, P. S., Mills, I. H. and Bartter, F. C. (1961). *J. Endocr.* **23**, 129.

Chew, P. C. T. and Ratnam, S. S. (1976). *J. Endocr.* **71**, 267.

Chopra, I. J. and Tulchinsky, D. (1974). *J. clin. Endocr. Metab.* **38**, 269.

Chopra, I. J., Tulchinsky, D. and Greenway, F. L. (1973). *Ann. int. Med.* **79**, 198.

Chopra, I. J., Abraham, G. E., Chopra, U., Solomon, D. H. and Odell, W. D. (1972). *New. Engl. J. Med.* **286**, 124.

Clark, J. H., Peck, E. J., Hardin, J. W. and Eriksson, H. (1978). "Receptors and Hormone Action", Vol. 2. Academic Press, New York and London.

Clark, J. H., Peck, E. J., Schrader, W. T. and O'Malley, B. W. (1976). *Meth. Cancer Res.* **12**, 367.

Cohen, M. and Cohen, H. (1974). *Am. J. Obstet. Gynec.* **118**, 200.

Cohen, M., Cohen, H., Saez, J. M., Bertrand, J. and Dumont, M. (1972). 8th Int. Congr. Clin. Chem., Copenhagen, 2380 A.

Cooper, W., Coyle, M. G. and Mills, J. A. (1971). *J. Endocr.* **51**, 447.

Cope, C. L. and Hurlock, B. (1954). *Clin. Sci.* **13**, 69.

Corker, C. S. and Exley, D. (1969). *J. Endocr.* **43**, xxx.

Corker, C. S. and Exley, D. (1970). *Steroids*, **15**, 469.

Corker, C. S. and Naftolin, F. (1971). *J. Obstet. Gynaec. Br. Cwlth*, **78**, 330.

Corvol, P. L., Chrambach, A., Rodbard, D. and Bardin, C. W. (1971). *J. biol. Chem.* **246**, 3435.

Crowell, G. C., Turner, M. E., Schmidt, F. H., Howard, C. M. and Preedy, J. R. K. (1967). *J. clin. Endocr. Metab.* **27**, 807.

Daughaday, W. H. (1958). *J. clin. Invest.* **37**, 511.

Daughaday, W. H. (1959). *Physiol. Rev.* **39**, 885.

Davies, I. J., Naftolin, F., Ryan, K. J., Fishman, J. and Siu, J. (1975). *Endocrinology*, **97**, 554.

DeHertogh, R., Thomas, K., Bietlot, Y., Vanderheyden, I. and Ferin, J. (1975). *J. clin. Endocr. Metab.* **40**, 93.

De Jong, F. H., Baird, D. T. and Van der Molen, H. J. (1974). *Acta endocr., Copenh.* **77**, 575.

Desbuquois, B. and Aurbach, G. D. (1971). *J. clin. Endocr. Metab.* **33**, 732.

DeVane, G. W., Czekala, N. M., Judd, H. L. and Yen, S. S. C. (1975). *Am. J. Obstet. Gynec.* **121**, 496.

Diczfalusy, E. and Mancuso, S. (1969). "Foetus and Placenta", p. 191. Blackwell Scientific Publications, Oxford.

Dignam, W. J., Parlow, A. F., Coyotupa, J., Honda, K., Hiroi, M., Kinoshita, K. and Kushinsky, S. (1974). *Obstet. Gynec.* **43**, 484.

Dipietro, D. L. (1976). *Am. J. Obstet. Gynec.* **125**, 841.

Dixon, P. F. (1968). *J. Endocr.* **40**, 457.

Doe, R. P. and Seal, U. S. (1963). *J. clin. Invest.* **42**, 929.

Doerr, P. (1973). *Acta endocr., Copenh.* **72**, 330.

Doerr, P. (1976). *Acta endocr., Copenh.* **81**, 655.

Doerr, P. and Pirke, K. M. (1974). *Acta endocr., Copenh.* **75**, 617.

Doerr, P. and Pirke, K. M. (1975). *Acta endocr., Copenh.* **78**, 531.

Dorrington, J. H. (1977). "The Ovary", Vol. 3, p. 359. Academic Press, New York and London.

Easterling, W. E., Simmer, H. H., Dignam, W. J., Frankland, M. V. and Naftolin, F. (1966). *Steroids*, **8**, 157.

Edman, C. D. and MacDonald, P. C. (1976). "Endocrine Function of the Human Ovary", p. 135. Academic Press, London and New York.

Edman, C. D. and MacDonald, P. C. (1978). *Am. J. Obstet. Gynec.* **130**, 456.

Edman, C. D., Aiman, E. J., Porter, J. C. and MacDonald, P. C. (1978). *Am. J. Obstet. Gynec.* **130**, 439.

Edwards, R. P., Diver, M. J., Davis, J. C. and Hipkin, L. J. (1976). *Br. J. Obstet. Gynaec.* **83**, 229.

Eik-Nes, K., Schellman, J. A., Lumry, R. and Samuels, L. T. (1954). *J. biol. Chem.* **206**, 411.

Ekins, R. P. (1960). *Clin. chim. Acta*, **5**, 453.

Ekins, R. P. and Newman, B. (1970). *Acta endocr., Copenh.*, **147** (Suppl.) 11.

Emmens, C. W. (1939). Spec. Rep. Ser., Med. Res. Counc., London.

Emmens, C. W. (1947). *J. Endocr.* **5**, 170.

Emmens, C. W. (1950). "Hormone Assay", p. 391. Academic Press, London and New York.

Engel, L. L., Baggett, B. and Carter, P. (1957). *Endocrinology*, **61**, 113.

Eren, S., Reynolds, G. H., Turner, M. E., Schmidt, F. H., Mackay, J. H., Howard, C. M. and Preedy, J. R. K. (1967). *J. clin. Endocr. Metab.* **27**, 819.

Escobar, M. E., Rivarola, M. A. and Bergada, C. (1976). *Acta endocr., Copenh.* **81**, 351.

Exley, D. and Abuknesha, R. (1977). *FEBS Lett.* **79**, 301.

Exley, D. and Choo, Q. L. (1974). *J. steroid Biochem.* **5**, 497.

Exley, D. and Dutton, A. (1969). *Steroids*, **14**, 575.

Exley, D. and Feder, H. H. (1967). *Acta endocr., Copenh.* **119** (Suppl.) 100.

Exley, D., Johnson, M. W. and Dean, P. D. G. (1971). *Steroids*, **18**, 605.

Falck, B. (1959). *Acta physiol. Scand.* **47** (Suppl.), 163.

Federman, D. D. (1967). "Abnormal Sexual Development." W. B. Saunders, London.

Ferin, M., Tempone, A., Zimmering, P. E. and Vande Wiele, R. L. (1969). *Endocrinology*, **85**, 1070.

Fisher, R. A., Anderson, D. C. and Burke, C. W. (1974). *Steroids*, **24**, 809.

Fishman, J. (1963). *J. clin. Endocr. Metab.* **23**, 207.

Fishman, J. (1970). *J. clin. Endocr. Metab.* **31**, 436.

Fishman, J. and Guzik, H. (1969). *J. Am. chem. Soc.* **91**, 2805.

Fishman, J. and Guzik, H. (1972). *J. clin. Endocr. Metab.* **35**, 892.

Fishman, J. and Hellman, L. (1973). *J. clin. Endocr. Metab.* **36**, 160.

Fishman, J. and Norton, B. (1975). *Endocrinology*, **96**, 1054.

Fishman, J., Boyar, R. M. and Hellman, L. (1972). *J. clin. Endocr. Metab.* **34**, 989.

Fishman, J., Boyar, R. M. and Hellman, L. (1975). *J. clin. Endocr. Metab.* **41**, 989.

Fishman, J., Bradlow, H. L. and Gallagher, T. F. (1960). *J. biol. Chem.* **235**, 3104.

Fishman, J., Bradlow, H. L., Zumoff, B., Hellman, L. and Gallagher, T. F. (1961). *Acta endocr., Copenh.* **37**, 57.

Fishman, J., Cox, R. I. and Gallagher, T. F. (1960). *Arch. Biochem. Biophys.* **90**, 318.

Fishman, J., Goldberg, S., Rosenfeld, R. S., Zumoff, B., Hellman, L. and Gallagher, T. F. (1969). *J. clin. Endocr. Metab.* **29**, 41.

Fishman, J., Guzik, H. and Dixon, D. (1969). *Biochemistry*, **8**, 4304.

Fishman, J. Hellman, L., Zumoff, B. and Gallagher, T. F. (1965). *J. clin. Endocr.*

Metab. **25**, 365.

Fishman, J., Naftolin, F., Davies, I. J., Ryan, K. J. and Petro, Z. (1976). *J. clin. Endocr. Metab.* **42**, 177.

Fishman, J., Yoshizawa, I. and Hellman L. (1973). *Steroids,* **22**, 401.

Flood, C., Pratt, J. H. and Longcope, C. (1976). *J. clin. Endocr. Metab.* **42**, 1.

Flood, C., Hunter, S. A., Lloyd, C. A. and Longcope, C. (1973). *J. clin. Endocr. Metab.* **36**, 1180.

Fotherby, K. and James, F. (1972) *Adv. Steroid Biochem. Pharmac.* **3**, 67.

Forest, M. G., Cathiard, A. M. and Bertrand, J. A. (1973). *J. clin. Endocr. Metab.* **36**, 1132.

Forest, M. G., Rivarola, M. A. and Migeon, C. J. (1968). *Steroids,* **12**, 323.

Fraser, I. S. and Baird, D. T. (1974). *J. clin. Endocr. Metab.* **39**, 564.

Fraser, R. C., Cudmore, D. C., Melanson, J. and Morse, W. I. (1967). *Am. J. Obstet. Gynec.* **98**, 509.

Frieden, E. H., Patkin, J. K. and Mills, M. (1968). *Proc. Soc. exp. Biol. Med.* **129**, 606.

Gallagher, T. F., Fukushima, D. K., Shunsaku, N., Fishman, J., Bradlow, H. L., Cassouto, J., Zumoff, B. and Hellman, L. (1966). *Rec. Prog. Horm. Res.* **22**, 283.

Galvao-Teles, A., Anderson, D. C., Burke, C. W., Marshall, J. C., Corker, C. S., Brown, R. L. and Clark, M. L. (1973). *Lancet,* **i**, 173.

Geisthonel, W. and Breuer, H. (1971). *Hoppe-Seyler's Z. physiol. Chem.* **352**, 1206.

Gelbke, H. P. and Knuppen, R. (1972). *J. Chromat.* **71**, 465.

Gelbke, H. P. and Knuppen, R. (1976). *J. steroid Biochem.* **7**, 457.

Gelbke, H. P., Ball, P. and Knuppen, R. (1977). *Adv. steroid Biochem. Pharmac.* **6**, 81.

Giebenhain, M. E., Tagatz, G. E. and Gurpide, E. (1972). *J. steroid Biochem.* **3**, 707.

Givner, M. L., Bauld, W. S. and Vagi, K. (1960). *Biochem. J.* **77**, 406.

Goebel, R. and Kuss, E. (1974). *J. clin. Endocr. Metab.* **39**, 969.

Goebelsmann, U., Chen, L.-C., Saga, M., Nakamura, R. M. and Jaffe, R. B. (1973). *Acta endocr., Copenh.* **74**, 592.

Goldenberg, R. L., Vaitukaitis, J. L. and Ross, G. T. (1972). *Endocrinology,* **90**, 1492.

Gorski, J., Toft, D., Shyamala, G., Smith, D. and Notides, A. (1968). *Rec. Prog. horm. Res.* **24**, 45.

Gorwill, R. H. and Sarda, I. R. (1977). *Am. J. Obstet. Gynec.* **127**, 17.

Goto, J. and Fishman, J. (1977). *Science,* **195**, 80.

Greenstein, B. D., Puig-Duran, E. and Franklin, M. (1977). *Steroids,* **30**, 331.

Grodin, J. M., Siiteri, P. K. and MacDonald, P. C. (1973). *J. clin. Endocr. Metab.* **36**, 207.

Guerro, R., Landgren, B.-M., Montiel, R., Cekan, Z. and Diczfalusy, E. (1975). *Contraception,* **11**, 169.

Gupta, D., Altemasio, A. and Raaf, S. (1975). *J. clin. Endocr. Metab.* **40**, 636.

Gurpide, E. (1975). "Tracer Methods in Hormone Research." Springer-Verlag: Berlin, Heidelberg and New York.

Gurpide, E., Mann, J. and Sandberg, E. (1964). *Biochemistry,* **3**, 1250.

Gurpide, E., Angers, M., Vande Wiele, L. and Liberman, S. (1962), *J. clin. Endocr. Metab.* **22**, 935.

Gurpide, E., MacDonald, P. C., Vande Wiele, R. and Lieberman, S. (1963). *J. clin. Endocr. Metab.* **23**, 346.

Gurpide, E., Wann, J., Van de Wiele, L. and Lieberman, S. (1962). *Acta endocr., Copenh.* **39**, 213.

Gurpide, E., Schwers, J., Welch, M. T., Van de Wiele, R. L. and Lieberman, S. (1966). *J. clin. Endocr. Metab.* **26**, 1355.

Hagen, A. A. (1970). *J. clin. Endocr. Metab.* **30**, 763.
Hagen, A. A., Barr, M. and Diczfalusy, E. (1965). *Acta endocr., Copenh.* **49**, 207.
Hausknecht, R. U. and Gusberg, S. B. (1973). *Am. J. Obstet. Gynec.* **116**, 981.
Hawkins, R. A. and Oakey, R. E. (1974). *J. Endocr.* **60**, 3.
Hay, D. M. and Lorscheider, F. L. (1976). *Br. J. Obstet. Gynaec.* **83**, 118.
Hellig, H., Gattereau, D., Lefebvre, Y. and Bolté, E. (1970). *J. clin. Endocr. Metab.* **30**, 624.
Hellman, L., Fishman, J., Zumoff, B., Cassouto, J. and Gallagher, T. F. (1967). *J. clin. Endocr. Metab.* **23**, 274.
Helton, E. D. and Goldzieher, J. W. (1977). *Contraception,* **15**, 255.
Hembree, W. C., Bardin, C. W. and Lipsett, M. B. (1969). *J. clin. Invest.* **48**, 1809.
Hemsell, D. L., Edman, C. D., Marks, J. F., Siiteri, P. K. and MacDonald, P. C. (1977). *J. clin. Invest.* **60**, 455.
Hemsell, D. L., Grodin, J. M., Brenner, P. F., Siiteri, P. K. and MacDonald, P. C. (1974). *J. clin. Endocr. Metab.* **38**, 476.
Heyns, W. (1977). *Adv. Steroid Biochem. Pharmac.* **6**, 59.
Heyns, W. and DeMoor, P. (1971). *J. clin. Endocr. Metab.* **32**, 147.
Hobkirk, R. and Nilsen, M. (1963). *J. clin. Endocr. Metab.* **23**, 274.
Hobkirk, R. and Nilsen, M. (1969a). *Steroids,* **13**, 679.
Hobkirk, R. and Nilsen, M. (1969b). *Steroids,* **14**, 533.
Hobkirk, R. and Nilsen, M. (1970). *Steroids,* **15**, 649.
Hobkirk, R. and Nilsen, M. (1974). *J. steroid Biochem.* **5**, 15.
Hobkirk, R., Mellor, J. D. and Nilsen, M. (1975). *Can. J. Biochem.* **53**, 903.
Hobkirk, R., Green, R. N., Nilsen, M. and Jennings, B. A. (1974). *Can. J. Biochem.* **52**, 15.
Horton, R. and Tait, J. F. (1966). *J. clin. Invest.* **45**, 301.
Hull, M. G. R. (1975). *Bibliogr. Reprod.* **26**, 1, 111.
Hull, M. G. R. (1976). *J. perinat. Med.* **4**, 137.
Hull, M. G. R. and Chard, T. (1976). "Foetal Physiology and Medicine", p. 371. W. B. Saunders, London.
Hull, M. G. R., Monro, P. P., Morgan, R. J. M. and Murray, M. A. F. (1979). *Clin. Endocr.* **11**, 179.
Hutton, J. D., Jacobs, H. S., James, V. H. T., Murray, M. A. F. and Rippon, A. E. (1977). *J. Endocr.* **73**, 25P.
Hutton, J. D., Murray, M. A. F., Jacobs, H. S. and James, V. H. T. (1978). *Lancet,* **i**, 678.
Hutton, J. D., Murray, M. A. F., Reed, M. J., Jacobs, H. S. and James, V. H. T. (1978). "Endometrial Cancer and Related Topics." Balliere-Tindall, London.
Ichii, S., Forchielli, E., Perloff, W. H. and Dorfmann, R. E. (1963). *Anal. Biochem.* **5**, 422.
Isherwood, D. M. and Oakey, R. E. (1976). *J. Endocr.* **68**, 321.
Jacobs, H. S., Franks, S., Murray, M. A. F., Hull, M. G. R., Steele, S. J. and Nabarro, J. D. N. (1976). *Clin. Endocr.* **5**, 439.
Jacobs, H. S., Hull, M. G. R., Murray, M. A. F. and Franks, S. (1975). *Hormone Res.* **6**, 268.
Jacobs, H. S. and Murray, M. A. F. (1976). "The Management of the Menopause and Post-menopausal Years", p. 359. MTP Press, Lancaster, UK.
Jaing, N. S. and Ryan, R. J. (1969). *Proc. Mayo Clin.* **44**, 461.
Jeffcoate, S. L. (1977) *J. Reprod. Fert.* **51**, 267.
Jeffrey, J. and Klopper, A. (1970). *Adv. Steroid Biochem. Pharmac.* **2**, 71.

Jenner, M. R., Kelch, R. P. and Grumbach, M. M. (1971). Prog. Endocr. Soc. 53rd Meet.
Jenner, M. R., Kelch, R. P., Kaplan, S. L. and Grumbach, M. M. (1972). *J. clin. Endocr. Metab.* **34**, 521.
Jensen, E. V. (1958). *Proc. 4th Int. Cong. Biochem.* **15**, 9, 120A.
Jensen, E. V. and Jacobson, H. I. (1960). "Biological Activities of Steroids in Relation to Cancer", p. 161. Academic Press, New York and London.
Jensen, E. V. and DeSombre, E. R. (1972). *Ann. Rev. Biochem.* **41**, 203.
Jirku, H. and Levitz, M. (1969). *J. clin. Endocr. Metab.* **29**, 615.
Jirku, H., Kadner, S. and Levitz, M. (1972). *Steroids,* **19**, 519.
Jones, D., Cameron, E. H. D., Griffiths, K., Gleave, E. N. and Forrest, A. P. M. (1970). *Biochem. J.* **116**, 919.
Judd, H. L., Judd, G. E., Lucas, W. E. and Yen, S. S. C. (1974). *J. clin. Endocr. Metab.* **39**, 1020.
Judd, H. L., Lucas, W. E. and Yen, S. S. C. (1976). *J. clin. Endocr. Metab.* **43**, 272.
Jungmann, R. A. and Schweppe, J. S. (1967). *J. clin. Endocr. Metab.* **27**, 1151.
Jungmann, R. A., Kot, E. and Schweppe, J. S. (1966). *Steroids,* **8**, 977.
Jurjens, H., Pratt, J. J. and Woldring, M. G. (1975). *J. clin. Endocr. Metab.* **40**, 19.
Kaplan, H. G. and Hreshchyshyn, M. M. (1973). *Am. J. Obstet. Gynec.* **115**, 803.
Katagiri, H., Stanczyl, F. Z. and Goebelsman, U. (1974). *Steroids,* **24**, 225.
Kato, T. and Horton, R. (1968). *J. clin. Endocr. Metab.* **28**, 1160.
Kelch, R. P., Jenner, M. R., Weinstein, R., Kaplan, S. L. and Grumbach, M. M. (1972). *J. clin. Invest.* **51**, 824.
Kellie, A. E. (1971). *Ann. Rev. Pharmac.* **11**, 97.
Keller, N., Richardson, W. I. and Yates, F. E. (1969). *Endocrinology,* **84**, 49.
Kelly, W. G. (1970). *Steroids,* **16**, 579.
Kelly, W. G. (1974). *Endocrinology,* **95**, 308.
Kelly, W. G. and Rizkallah, T. H. (1973). *J. clin. Endocr. Metab.* **36**, 196.
Kelly, W. G., DeLeon, O. and Rizkallah, T. H. (1976). *J. clin. Endocr. Metab.* **43**, 190.
Kemeter, P., Salzer, H., Breitenecker, G. and Friedrich, F. (1975). *Acta endocr., Copenh.* **80**, 686.
Kerkay, J. and Westphal, U. (1968). *Biochem. biophys. Acta,* **170**, 324.
King, R. J. B. and Mainwaring, W. I. P. (1974). "Steroid-Cell Interactions", p. 190. Butterworths, London.
Kirschner, M. A. and Taylor, J. P. (1972). *J. clin. Endocr. Metab.* **35**, 513.
Kirschner, M. A., Wiquist, N. and Diczfalusy, E. (1966). *Acta endocr., Copenh.* **53**, 584.
Kletzky, O. A., Nakamura, R. M., Thorneycroft, I. H. and Mishell, D. R. (1975). *Am. J. Obstet. Gynec.* **121**, 688.
Kley, H. K., Bartman, E. and Krüskemper, H. L. (1977). *Acta endocr., Copenh.* **85**, 209.
Kley, H. K., Nieschlag, E., Bidlingmaier, F. and Krüskemper, H. L. (1974). *Hormone Metab. Res.* **6**, 213.
Klopper, A. and Shaaban, M. M. (1974). *Obstet, Gynec.* **44**, 187.
Knuppen, R. and Breuer, H. (1967). *Hoppe-Seyler's Z. physiol. Chem.* **348**, 581.
Knuppen, R. and Breuer, H. (1968). *Hoppe-Seyler's Z. physiol. Chem.* **349**, 8.
Knuppen, R., Haupt, M. and Breuer, H. (1965a). *J. Endocr.* **33**, 529.
Knuppen, R., Haupt, O. and Breuer, H. (1965b). *Biochem. J.* **96**, 330.
Knuppen, R., Haupt, O. and Breuer, H. (1966a). *Steroids,* **8**, 403.
Knuppen, R., Haupt, O. and Breuer, H. (1966b). *Biochem. J.* **101**, 397.

Knuppen, R., Haupt, O. and Breuer, H. (1967). *Biochem. J.* **105**, 971.

Korda, A. R., Challis, J. J., Anderson, A. B. M. and Turnbull, A. C. (1975). *Br. J. Obstet. Gynaec.* **82**, 882.

Korenman, S. G. (1968). *J. clin. Endocr. Metab.* **28**, 127.

Korenman, S. G., Perrin, L. E. and McCallum, T. P. (1969). *J. clin. Endocr. Metab.* **29**, 879.

Korenman, S. G., Stevens, R. H., Carpenter, L. A., Robb, M., Niswender, G. D. and Sherman, B. M. (1974). *J. clin. Endocr. Metab.* **38**, 718.

Kraychy, S. and Gallagher, T. F. (1957a). *J. Am. Chem. Soc.* **79**, 754.

Kraychy, S. and Gallagher, T. F. (1957b). *J. biol. Chem.* **229**, 519.

Kundu, N. and Grant, M. (1976). *Steroids,* **27**, 785.

Kushinsky, S. and Anderson, M. (1974). *Steroids,* **23**, 535.

Kushinsky, S. and Paul, W. (1969). *Anal. Biochem.* **30**, 435.

Kuss, E. and Goebel, R. (1972). *Steroids,* **19**, 509.

Landsteiner, K. (1976). "The Specificity of Serological Reactions". Harvard University Press, Cambridge, MA.

Lasnitski, I. and Franklin, H. R. (1972). *J. Endocr.* **54**, 333.

Laumas, K. R., Tait, J. F. and Tait, S. A. S. (1961). *Acta endocr., Copenh.* **36**, 265.

Laumas, K. R., Malkani, P. K., Koshti, G. S. and Hingorani, V. (1968). *Am. J. Obstet. Gynec.* **101**, 1062.

Lee, P. A. and Migeon, C. J. (1975). *J. clin. Endocr. Metab.* **41**, 556.

Lee, P. A., Xenakis, T., Winer, J. and Matsenbaugh, S. (1976). *J. clin. Endocr. Metab.* **43**, 775.

Lehmann, W. D., Lauritzen, C. and Schumann, R. (1973). *Acta endocr., Copenh.* **73**, 771.

Leonard, J. M., Flocks, R. H. and Korenman, S. G. (1971). *Prog. Endocr. Soc. 53rd Meet.* Abst. 113.

Levitz, M. and Katz, J. (1968). *J. clin. Endocr. Metab.* **28**, 862.

Levitz, M. and Young, B. K. (1977). *Vit. Horm.* **35**, 109.

Levitz, M., Kadner, S. and Young, B. K. (1976). *Steroids,* **27**, 287.

Leymarie, P. and Savard, K. (1968). *J. clin. Endocr. Metab.* **28**, 1547.

Linder, M., Desfosses, B. and Emiliozzi, R. (1977). *Steroids,* **29**, 161.

Lindner, H. R., Perel, E., Friedlander, A. and Zeitlin, A. (1972). *Steroids,* **19**, 357.

Lisboa, B. P., Goebelsman, U. and Diczfalusy, E. (1967). *Acta endocr., Copenh.* **54**, 467.

Lloyd, C. W., Lobotsky, J., Baird, D. T., McCracken, J. A., Weisz, J., Pupkin, M., Zanartu, J. and Puga, J. (1971). *J. clin. Endocr. Metab.* **32**, 155.

Longcope, C. (1971). *Am. J. Obstet. Gynec.* **111**, 778.

Longcope, C. and Williams, K. I. H. (1974). *J. clin. Endocr. Metab.* **38**, 602.

Longcope, C., Kato, T. and Horton, R. (1969). *J. clin. Invest.* **48**, 2191.

Longcope, C., Layne, D. S. and Tait, J. F. (1968). *J. clin. Invest.* **47**, 93.

Longcope, C., Watson, D. and Williams, K. I. H. (1974). *Steroids,* **24**, 15.

Longcope, C., Widrich, W. and Sawin, C. T. (1972). *Steroids,* **20**, 439.

Longcope, C., Pratt, J. H., Schneider, S. H. and Fineberg, S. E. (1976). *J. clin. Endocr. Metab.* **43**, 1134.

Longcope, C., Pratt, J. H., Schneider, S. H. and Fineberg, S. E. (1978). *J. clin. Endocr. Metab.* **46**, 146.

Loraine, J. A. (1958). "Clinical Application of Hormone Assay". E. S. Livingstone, Edinburgh.

Loraine, J. A. and Bell, E. T. (1971). "Hormone Assays and their Clinical Appli-

348   M. J. REED AND M. A. F. MURRAY

cation", 3rd edition. E. S. Livingstone, Edinburgh and London.
Loriaux, D. L., Ruder, H. J. and Lipsett, M. B. (1971). *Steroids,* **18,** 463.
Loriaux, D. L., Ruder, H. J. and Lipsett, M. B. (1972). *J. clin. Endocr. Metab.* **35,** 887.
Luukkainen, T. and Adlercreutz, H. (1965). *Biochem. biophys. Acta,* **107,** 579.
MacDonald, P. C., Rombaut, R. P. and Siiteri, P. K. (1967). *J. clin. Endocr. Metab.* **27,** 1103.
MacDonald, P. C., Edman, C. D., Hemsell, D. L., Porter, J. C. and Siiteri, P. K. (1978). *Am. J. Obstet. Gynec.* **130,** 488.
MacDonald, P. C., Grodin, J. M., Edman, C. D., Vellios, F. and Siiteri, P. K. (1976). *Obstet. Gynec.* **47,** 644.
Macourt, D., Corker, C. S. and Naftolin, F. (1971). *J. Obstet. Gynaec. Br. Cwlth.* **78,** 335.
McGuire, W. L., Horwitz, K. B., Zava, D. T., Garola, R. E. and Chamness, G. C. (1978). *Metabolism,* **27,** 487.
McNatty, K. P., Baird, D. T., Bolton, A., Chambers, P., Corker, C. S. and McLean, H. (1976). *J. Endocr.* **71,** 77.
Mancuso, S., Dell-Acqua, S., Eriksson, G., Wiqvist, N. and Diczfalusy, E. (1964). *Steroids,* **5,** 183.
Manikanguly, U. R. and Levitz, M. (1977). *J. clin. Endocr. Metab.* **45,** 429.
Marks, F. and Hecker, E. (1967). *Biochem. biophys. Acta,* **144,** 690.
Marshall, J. C. (1975). *Clin. Endocr. Metab.* **4,** 1.
Martucci, C. and Fishman, J. (1976). *Steroids,* **27,** 325.
Masson, G. M. (1973). *J. Endocr.* **54,** 245.
Mayes, D. and Nugent, C. A. (1970). *Steroids,* **15,** 389.
Mercier, C., Alfsen, A. and Baulieu, E.-E. (1966). *Excerpta Med. Int. Cong. Ser.* **101,** 212.
Mercier-Bodard, C., Marchut, M., Perrot, M., Picard, M.-T., Baulieu, E.-E., and Robel, P. (1976). *J. clin. Endocr. Metab.* **43,** 374.
Meyer, A. S. (1955). *Biochim. biophys. Acta,* **17,** 441.
Mikhail, G., Wu, C. H., Ferin, M. and Van de Wiele, R. L. (1970). *Steroids,* **15,** 333.
Miklosi, S., Biggs, J. S. G., Selvage, N., Canning, J. and Lythal, G. (1975). *Steroids,* **26,** 671.
Miyazaki, M., Yoshizawa, I. and Fishman, J. (1969). *Biochemistry,* **8,** 1669.
Moore, P. H. and Axelrod, L. R. (1972). *Steroids,* **20,** 199.
Morand, P., Williamson, D. G., Layne, D. S., Lompa-Krzymien, L. and Salvador, J. (1975). *Biochemistry,* **14,** 635.
Mowszowicz, I., Kahn, D. and Dray, F. (1970). *J. clin. Endocr. Metab.* **31,** 584.
Munson, A. K., Mueller, J. R. and Yannone, M. E. (1970). *Am. J. Obstet. Gynec.* **108,** 340.
Munson, A. K., Yanone, M. E. and Mueller, J. R. (1972). *Acta endocr., Copenh.* **69,** 410.
Murphy, B. E. P. (1964). *Nature, Lond.* **201,** 679.
Murphy, B. E. P. (1968). *Can. J. Biochem.* **46,** 299.
Murphy, B. E. P. (1970). *Steroids,* **16,** 791.
Murphy, B. E. P., Engleberg, W. and Pattee, C. J. (1963). *J. clin. Endocr. Metab.* **23,** 293.
Musey, P. I., Green, R. N. and Hobkirk, R. (1972). *J. clin. Endocr. Metab.* **35,** 448.
Nachtigall, L., Bassett, M., Hogsander, U., Slagle, S. and Levitz, M. (1966). *J. clin. Endocr. Metab.* **26,** 941.

Naftolin, F., Ryan, K. J. and Petro, Z. (1971). *J. clin. Endocr. Metab.* **33**, 368.

Nagai, N. and Longcope, C. (1971). *Steroids,* **17**, 631.

Nagatomi, K., Osawa, Y., Kirdani, R. Y. and Sandberg, A. A. (1973). *J. clin. Endocr. Metab.* **37**, 887.

Nimrod, A. and Ryan, K. J. (1975). *J. clin. Endocr. Metab.* **40**, 367.

Niswender, G. D. and Midgley, A. R. (1969). Proc. 51st Meet. Endocr. Soc. 22 A.

Niswender, G. D. and Midgley, A. R. (1970). "Immunological Methods in Steroid Determination", p. 149. Appleton Century Crofts, New York.

Numazawa, M., Haryu, A., Kurosaka, K. and Nambara, T. (1977). *FEBS Lett.* **79**, 396.

Nunez, M., Aedo, A.-R., Landgren, B.-M., Cekan, S. Z. and Diczfalusy, E. (1977). *Acta endocr., Copenh.* **86**, 621.

Oakey, R. E. (1970). *Vit. Horm.* **28**, 1.

O'Donnell, V. J. and Preedy, J. R. K. (1966). "Hormones in Blood", p. 109, 2nd edition. Academic Press, London and New York.

Oertel, G. W., Menzel, P. and Hullen, B. (1969). *Hoppe-Seyler's Z. physiol. Chem.* **350**, 755.

Oertel, G. W., Treiber, L., Wensel, D., Knapstein, P., Wendleberger, F. and Mensel, P. (1968). *Experientia,* **24**, 607.

Olivo, J., Vittek, J., Southren, A. L., Gordon, G. G. and Rafii, F. (1973). *J. clin. Endocr. Metab.* **36**, 153.

O'Malley, B. W. and Means, A. R. (1974). *Science,* **183**, 610.

Onikki, S. and Aldercreutz, H. (1973). *J. Steroid Biochem.* **4**, 633.

Patwardhan, V. V. and Lanthier, A. (1969). *J. clin. Endocr. Metab.* **29**, 1335.

Patwardhan, V. V. and Lanthier, A. (1972). *Steroids,* **20**, 761.

Payne, A., Kelch, R. D., Musich, S. S. and Halpern, M. E. (1976). *J. clin. Endocr. Metab.* **42**, 1081.

Pearlman, W. H. and Fong, I. F. F. (1968). *Fed. Proc.* **27** (Abst.), 624.

Pearlman, W. H., Crepy, O. and Murphy, O. (1967). *J. clin. Endocr. Metab.* **27**, 1012.

Pearlman, W. H., De Hertogh, R., Laumas, K. R. and Pearlman, M. R. (1969). *J. clin. Endocr. Metab.* **29**, 707.

Pelc, B., Marshall, D. H., Guha, P., Khan, M. Y. and Nordin, B. E. C. (1978). *Clin. Sci. mol. Med.* **54**, 125.

Peterson, R. P. and Spaziani, E. (1971). *Endocrinology,* **89**, 1280.

Pirke, K. M. and Doerr, P. (1973). *Acta endocr., Copenh.* **74**, 792.

Pirke, K. M. and Doerr, P. (1975). *Acta endocr., Copenh.* **80**, 171.

Poortman, J., Thijssen, J. H. H. and Schwarz, F. (1973). *J. clin. Endocr. Metab.* **37**, 101.

Powell, J. E. and Stevens, V. C. (1973). *Clin. Chem.* **19**, 210.

Pratt, J. H. and Longcope, C. (1978). *J. clin. Endocr. Metab.* **46**, 44.

Pratt, J. J., Van der Lunden, G., Doorenbos, H. and Woldring, M. G. (1974). *Clin. chim. Acta,* **50**, 137.

Rader, M. D., Flickinger, G. L., De Villa, G. O., Mikula, J. J. and Mikhail, G. (1973). *Am. J. Obstet. Gynec.* **116**, 1069.

Radfar, N., Ansusingha, K. and Kenny, F. M. (1976). *J. Pediat.* **89**, 719.

Rado, A., Deans, C. D. and Townsley, J. D. (1970). *J. clin. Endocr. Metab.* **30**, 497.

Ratajczak, T. and Hähnel, R. (1976). *Clin. chim. Acta,* **73**, 379.

Raynaud, J.-P. (1973). *Steroids,* **21**, 249.

Reed, M. J., Hutton, J. D., Beard, R. W., Jacobs, H. S. and James, V. H. T. (1979a) *Clin. Endocr.* **11**, 141.

Reed, M. J., Hutton, J. D., Baxendale, P. M., James, V. H. T., Jacobs, H. S. and Fisher, R. P. (1979b) *J. Steroid Biochem.* **11**, 905.

Reeves, B. D. and Calhoun, D. W. (1970). *Acta endocr., Copenh.* **147** (Suppl.), 61.

Ridgway, E. C., Longcope, C. and Maloof, F. (1975). *J. clin. Endocr. Metab.* **41**, 491.

Rice, B. F. and Savard, K. (1966). *J. clin. Endocr. Metab.* **26**, 593.

Rizkallah, T. H., Tovel, H. M. M. and Kelly, W. G. (1975). *J. clin. Endocr. Metab.* **40**, 1045.

Robertson, H. A., Smeaton, T. C. and Durnford, R. (1972). *Steroids,* **20**, 651.

Robertson, M. E., Stiefel, M. and Laidlow, J. C. (1959). *J. clin. Endocr. Metab.* **19**, 1381.

Rose, D. P., Fern, M., Liskowski, L. and Milbrath, J. R. (1977). *Am. J. Obstet. Gynec.* **49**, 80.

Rosenbaum, W., Christy, N. P. and Kelly, W. G. (1966). *J. clin. Endocr. Metab.* **26**, 1399.

Rosenthal, H. E., Ludwig, G. A., Pietrzak, E. and Sandberg, A. A. (1975). *J. clin. Endocr. Metab.* **41**, 1144.

Rosenthal, H. E., Pietrzak, E., Slaunwhite, W. R. and Sandberg, A. A. (1972). *J. clin. Endocr. Metab.* **34**, 805.

Rosner, W. (1972). *J. clin. Endocr. Metab.* **34**, 983.

Ross, G. T., Cargille, C. M., Lipsett, M. B., Rayford, P. L., Marshall, J. R., Strott, C. A. and Rodbard, D. (1970). *Rec. Prog. Horm. Res.* **26**, 1.

Rotti, K., Stevens, J., Watson, D. and Longcope, C. (1975). *Steroids,* **25**, 807.

Rowe, P. H., Cook, I. F. and Dean, P. D. G. (1973). *Ster. Lip. Res.* **4**, 24.

Rubens, R., Dhont, M. and Vermeulen, A. (1974). *J. clin. Endocr. Metab.* **39**, 40.

Ruder, H. J., Loriaux, L. and Lipsett, M. B. (1972). *J. clin. Invest.* **51**, 1020.

Ryan, K. J. and Petro, Z. (1966). *J. clin. Endocr. Metab.* **26**, 46.

Ryan, K. J. and Smith, O. W. (1961). *J. biol. Chem.* **236**, 705.

Ryan, K. J., Naftolin, F., Reddy, V., Flores, F. and Petro, Z. (1972). *Am. J. Obstet. Gynec.* **114**, 454.

Saba, N. (1976). *J. Endocr.* **70**, 141.

Saez, J. M., Morera, A. M. and Bertrand, J. (1972). 4th Int. Cong. Endocr. Abst.

Saez, J. M., Morera, A. M., Dazord, A. and Bertrand, J. (1972). *J. Endocr.* **55**, 41.

Sakakini, J., Buster, J. E. and Killam, A. P. (1977). *Am. J. Obstet. Gynec.* **127**, 452.

Sandberg, A. A., Slaunwhite, W. R. and Antoniades, H. N. (1957). *Rec. Prog. Horm. Res.* **13**, 209.

Sandberg, A. A., Rosenthal, H., Schneider, S. L. and Slaunwhite, W. R. (1966). "Steroid Dynamics", p.111. Academic Press, New York and London.

Sandberg, E., Gurpide, E. and Lieberman, S. (1964). *Biochemistry,* **3**, 1256.

Santen, R. J. (1975). *J. clin. Invest.* **56**, 1555.

Sanyaolu, A. A., Eccles, S. S. and Oakey, R. E. (1976). *J. Endocr.* **69**, 11 P.

Savard, K. (1973). *Biol. Reprod.* **8**, 183.

Schiller, H. S. and Brammal, M. A. (1974). *Steroids,* **24**, 665.

Schindler, A. E. (1975). *Am. J. Obstet. Gynec.* **123**, 251.

Schindler, A. E. and Hermann, W. L. (1966). *Am. J. Obstet. Gynec.* **95**, 301.

Schindler, A. E., Ebert, A. and Friedrich, E. (1972). *J. clin. Endocr. Metab.* **35**, 627.

Schweikert, H. U., Milewhich, L. and Wilson, J. D. (1975). *J. clin. Endocr. Metab.* **40**, 413.

Schweikert, H. U., Milewich, L. and Wilson, J. D. (1976). *J. clin. Endocr. Metab.* **43**, 785.

Schwers, J., Eriksson, G., Wiqvist, N. and Diczfalusy, E. (1965). *Biochim. biophys.*

Acta, **100**, 313.

Selinger, M. and Levitz, M. (1969). *J. clin. Endocr. Metab.* **29**, 995.

Shaaban, M.M. and Klopper, A. (1973). *J. Obstet. Gynaec. Br. Cwlth,* **80**, 210.

Shanbhag, V. P., Södergård, R., Carstensen, H. and Albertsson, P. Å. (1973). *J. Steroid Biochem.* **4**, 537.

Sherins, R. J. and Loriaux, D. L. (1973). *J. clin. Endocr. Metab.* **36**, 886.

Sherman, B. M. and Korenman, S. G. (1974a). *J. clin. Endocr. Metab.* **38**, 89.

Sherman, B. M. and Korenman, S. G. (1974b). *J. clin. Endocr. Metab.* **39**, 145.

Sherman, B. M. and Korenman, S. G. (1975). *J. clin. Invest.* **55**, 699.

Sherman, B. M., West, J. H. and Korenman, S. G. (1976). *J. clin. Endocr. Metab.* **42**, 629.

Shutt, D. A. (1969). *Steroids,* **13**, 69.

Shutt, D. A. and Cox, R. I. (1972). *J. Endocr.* **52**, 299.

Shutt, D. A. and Cox, R. I. (1973). *Steroids,* **21**, 565.

Siiteri, P. K. and MacDonald, P. C. (1966). *J. clin. Endocr. Metab.* **26**, 751.

Siiteri, P. K. and MacDonald, P. C. (1973). "Handbook of Physiology—Section 7, Endocrinology", Vol. II, p. 615. American Physiological Society, Washington, DC.

Simmer, H. H., Dignam, J., Easterling, W. E., Frankland, M. V. and Naftolin, F. (1966). *Steroids,* **8**, 179.

Slaunwhite, W. R. (1960). "Hormones in Human Plasma", p. 478. Little, Brown, Boston.

Slaunwhite, W. R., Lockie, G. N., Back, N. and Sandberg, A. A. (1962). *Science,* **135**, 1062.

Slaunwhite, W. R., Karsay, M. A., Hollmer, A., Sandberg, A. A. and Niswander, K. (1965). *Steroids,* **6** (Suppl II), 211.

Smith, O. W. and Hagerman, D. D. (1965). *J. clin. Endocr. Metab.* **25**, 732.

Smuk, M. and Schwers, J. (1977). *J. clin. Endocr. Metab.* **45**, 1009.

Somma, M., Sandor, T. and Lanthier, A. (1969). *J. clin. Endocr. Metab.* **29**, 457.

Southren, A. L., Olivo, J., Gordon, G. G., Vittek, J., Breuer, J., and Rafii, F. (1974). *J. clin. Endocr. Metab.* **38**, 207.

Spaeth, D. G. and Osawa, Y. (1974). *J. clin. Endocr. Metab.* **38**, 783.

Speight, A., Hancock, K. W. and Oakey, R. E. (1977). *J. Endocr.* **73**, 23 P.

Stahl, F., Dorner, G., Rohde, W. and Schott, G. (1976). *Endokinologie,* **68**, 112.

Stern, M., Givner, N. and Solomon, S. (1968). *Endocrinology,* **83**, 348.

Stewart-Bently, M., Odell, W. and Horton, R. (1974). *J. clin. Endocr. Metab.* **38**, 545.

Sugar, J., Alexander, S., Dessy, C. and Schwers, J. (1977). *J. clin. Endocr. Metab.* **45**, 945.

Swerdloff, R. S. and Odell, W. D. (1975). *Postgrad. med. J.* **51**, 200.

Sybulski, S. (1969). *Am. J. Obstet. Gynec.* **105**, 1055.

Sybulski, S. and Maughan, G. B. (1972). *Am. J. Obstet. Gynec.* **113**, 310.

Sybulski, S., Asswad, A. and Maughan, G. B. (1976). *Am. J. Obstet. Gynec.* **125**, 864.

Tait, J. F. (1963). *J. clin. Endocr. Metab.* **23**, 1285.

Tait, J. F. and Burstein, S. (1964). "The Hormones", Vol. 5, p. 441. Academic Press, New York and London.

Tait, J. F. and Horton, R. (1966). "Steroid Dynamics", p. 393. Academic Press, New York and London.

Tavernetti, R. R., Rosenbaum, W., Kelly, W. G., Christy, N. P. and Roginsky, N. S. (1967). *J. clin. Endocr. Metab.* **27**, 920.

Taylor, E. S., Hagerman, D. D., Betz, G., Williams, K. L. and Grey, P. A. (1970).

Am. J. Obstet. Gynec. **108**, 868.

Taylor, N. F. and Shackleton, C. H. L. (1978). *Ann. clin. Biochem.* **15**, 1.

Taylor, T., Coutts, J. R. T. and MacNaughton, M. C. (1974). *Acta endocr., Copenh.* **75**, 595.

Thompson, E. A. and Siiteri, P. K. (1974). *J. biol. Chem.* **249**, 5364.

Thosen, T. and Støa, K. F. (1965). *Acta endocr., Copenh.* **100** (Suppl.), Abst. 83.

Toribara, T. Y. (1953). *Anal. Chem.* **25**, 1286.

Toribara, T. Y., Terepka, A. R. and Dewey, P. A. (1957). *J. clin. Invest.* **36**, 738.

Touchstone, J. C. and Murawec, T. (1965). *Biochemistry*, **4**, 1612.

Townsley, J. D. (1975). *Acta endocr., Copenh.* **79**, 740.

Townsley, J. D. and Brodie, H. J. (1967). *Biochem. biophys. Acta*, **144**, 440.

Townsley, J. D. and Brodie, H. J. (1968). *Biochemistry*, **7**, 33.

Townsley, J. D., Scheel, D. A. and Rubin, E. J. (1970). *J. clin. Endocr. Metab.* **31**, 670.

Townsley, J. D., Rubin, N. H., Grannis, G. F., Gartman, L. J. and Crystle, C. D. (1973). *J. clin. Endocr. Metab.* **36**, 289.

Treolar, A. E., Boynton, R. E., Benn, B. G. and Brown, B. W. (1967). *Int. J. Fertil.* **12**, 77.

Tulchinsky, D. (1973). *J. clin. Endocr. Metab.* **36**, 1079.

Tulchinsky, D. Abraham, G. E. (1971). *J. clin. Endocr. Metab.* **33**, 775.

Tulchinsky, D. and Chopra, I. J. (1973). *J. clin. Endocr. Metab.* **37**, 873.

Tulchinsky, D. and Chopra, I. J. (1974). *J. clin. Endocr. Metab.* **39**, 164.

Tulchinsky, D. and Korenman, S. G. (1970). *J. clin. Endocr. Metab.* **31**, 76.

Tulchinsky, S. G. and Korenman, S. G. (1971). *J. clin. Invest.* **50**, 1490.

Tulchinsky, D., Frigoletto, F. D., Ryan, K. J. and Fishman, J. (1975). *J. clin. Endocr. Metab.* **40**, 560.

Tulchinsky, D., Hobel, C. J., Yeager, E. and Marshall, J. R. (1972). *Am. J. Obstet. Gynec.* **112**, 1095.

Turnbull, A. C., Patten, P. T., Flint, A. P. F., Keirse, M. J., Jeremy, J. Y. and Anderson, A. B. M. (1974). *Lancet*, **i**, 101.

Van Baelen, H., Heyns, W., Schonne, E. and De Moor, P. (1968). *Ann. Endocr.* **29**, 153.

Van Hell, H., Bosch, A. M. G., Brands, J. A. M., Van Weemen, B. K. and Schuurs, A. H. W. M. (1976). *Z. Anal. Chem.* **279**, 143.

Van Kamnen, E., Thijssen, J. H. H., Rademaker, B. and Schwarz, F. (1975). *Contraception*, **11**, 53.

Van Orden, D. E. and Farley, D. B. (1973). *Prostaglandins*, **4**, 247.

Vande Wiele, R. L., Bogumil, J., Dyrenfurth, I., Ferin, M., Jewelewicz, R., Warren, M., Rizkallah, T. and Mikhail, G. (1970). *Rec. Prog. Horm. Res.* **26**, 63.

Vermeulen, A. (1976). *J. clin. Endocr. Metab.* **42**, 247.

Vermeulen, A. and Verdonck, L. (1968). *Steroids*, **11**, 609.

Vermeulen, A., Stoica, T. and Verdonk, L. (1971). *J. clin. Endocr. Metab.* **33**, 759.

Vermeulen, A., Rubens, R. and Verdonck, L. (1972). *J. clin. Endocr. Metab.* **34**, 730.

Vermeulen, A., Verdonck, L., Van der Straeten, M. and Orie, N. (1969). *J. clin. Endocr. Metab.* **29**, 1470.

Vittek, J. K., Gordon, G. G. and Southren, A. L. (1974). *Endocrinology*, **94**, 325.

Walsh, P. C., Swerdloff, R. S. and Odell, W. D. (1973). *Acta endocr., Copenh.* **74**, 449.

Weder, H. G., Schildknecht, J. and Kesselring, P. (1971). *Am. Lab.* **10**, 15.

Weder, H. G., Schildknecht, J., Lutz, R. A. and Kesselring, P. (1974). *Eur. J. Biochem.* **42**, 475.

Weinstein, R. L., Kelch, R. P., Jenner, M. R., Kaplan, S. L. and Grumbach, M. M.

(1974). *J. clin. Invest.* **53**, 1.

Weisz, J., Lloyd, C. W., Lobotsky, J., Pupkin, M., Zanortu, J. and Puga, J. (1973). *J. clin. Endocr. Metab.* **37**, 254.

Westphal, U. (1969). "Methods in Enzymology", Vol. 15, pp. 761–796. Academic Press, London and New York.

Westphal, U. (1971). "Steroid-Protein Interactions." Springer-Verlag, Berlin, Heidelberg and New York.

Westphal, U. and Forbes, T. R. (1963). *Endocrinology,* **73**, 504.

Whitaker, E. M. and Oakey, R. E. (1972). *Steroids,* **20**, 295.

Wilcox, R. B. and Engels, L. L. (1965). *Steroids,* **6** (Suppl. II), 249.

Williams, J. G., Longcope, C. and Williams, K. I. H. (1974). *Steroids,* **24**, 687.

Wilson, D. W., John, B. M., Groom, G. V., Pierrepoint, C. G. and Griffiths, K. (1977). *J. Endocr.* **74**, 503.

Winter, J. S. D. and Faiman, C. (1973). *J. clin. Endocr. Metab.* **37**, 714.

Wotiz, H. H. and Chattoraj, S. C. (1964). *Anal. Chem.* **36**, 1466.

Wotiz, H. H., Charransol, G. and Smith, I. N. (1967). *Steroids,* **10**, 127.

Wright, K., Robinson, H., Collins, D. C. and Preedy, J. R. K. (1973). *J. clin. Endocr. Metab.* **36**, 165.

Wu, C. H. and Lundy, L. E. (1971). *Steroids,* **18**, 91.

Wu, C. H., Flickinger, G. L., Archer, D. F. and Touchstone, J. C. (1970). *Am. J. Obstet. Gynec.* **107**, 313.

Wu., C. H., Motohashi, T., Abdel-Rahman, H. A., Flickinger, G. L. and Mikhail, G. (1976). *J. clin. Endocr. Metab.* **43**, 436.

Yalow, R. S. and Berson, S. A. (1960). *J. clin. Invest.* **39**, 1157.

Yen, S. S. C. and Lein, A. (1976). *Am. J. Obstet. Gynec.* **126**, 942.

Yen, S. S. C., Martin, P. L., Burnier, A. M., Czekala, N. M., Greaney, M. C. and Callantine, M. R. (1975). *J. clin. Endocr. Metab.* **40**, 518.

Yoshizawa, I. and Fishman, J. (1970). *J. clin. Endocr. Metab.* **31**, 324.

Yoshizawa, I. and Fishman, J. (1971). *J. clin. Endocr. Metab.* **32**, 3.

Young, B. K., Jirku, H., Kadner, S. and Levitz, M. (1976). *Am. J. Obstet. Gynec.* **126**, 38.

Younghai, E. V. and Short, R. V. (1969). *J. Endocr.* **47**, 321.

Yuen, B. H., Kelch, R. P. and Jaffe, R. B. (1974). *Acta endocr., Copenh.* **76**, 117.

Zmigrod, A., Ladany, S. and Lindner, H. R. (1970). *Steroids,* **15**, 635.

Zucconi, G., Lisboa, B. P., Simonitsch, E., Roth, L., Hagan, A. A. and Diczfalusy, E. (1967). *Acta endocr., Copenh.* **56**, 413.

Zumoff, B., Fishman, J., Gallagher, T. F. and Hellman, L. (1968). *J. clin. Invest.* **47**, 20.

Zumoff, B., Fishman, J., Cassouto, J., Gallagher, T. F. and Hellman, L. (1968). *J. clin. Endocr. Metab.* **28**, 937.

VII. The Androgens

A. VERMEULEN

INTRODUCTION

Androgens can be defined as substances that induce, regulate and maintain differentiation, development and function of the male reproductive tract and male sex characteristics such as to permit adequate reproduction. The role of androgens in females is less well defined; they increase libido and are necessary for growth of clitoris, pubic and axillary hair and development of sebaceous glands; in excessive amounts they cause virilisation. They also have general metabolic effects on skin, skeletal and muscle tissue which have as a common denominator the anabolic effect of these compounds, causing increased protein formation.

The principal circulating androgens in man are testosterone (T), 5α-androstan-17β-ol-3-one or dihydrotestosterone (DHT), 5α-androstane-3α, 17β-diol (androstanediol), androstenedione, dehydroepiandrosterone (DHEA) and its sulphate (DHEA-S) and androst-5-ene-3β,17β-diol (androstenediol). Of all these, by far the most potent androgens are testosterone and dihydrotestosterone. Although the relative potency of the androgens depends upon the assay system used, the other natural androgens have only a fraction of the potency of testosterone.

A. BIOSYNTHESIS OF ANDROGENS

Androgens are secreted by the testis, the ovary and the adrenal cortex; moreover, biologically active androgens (testosterone and dihydrotestosterone) are formed from weakly active precursors in peripheral tissues from where they may escape into the circulation.

From available evidence it appears that the pathways of androgen synthesis are fundamentally similar in both gonads and adrenal cortex (Dorfman and Ungar, 1965). The common precursor to all androgens in the three glands appears to be cholesterol. Both the gonads and the adrenal cortex have the capacity to synthesise cholesterol from acetate (Menon, Dorfman and Forchielli, 1965), although cholesterol is partly taken up as such from the blood stream. There is some evidence that there exists a direct bypass to pregnenolone not involving cholesterol, via zymosterol or desmosterol (Hall, 1964; Shimizu and Gut, 1965).

1. Testes

The testes have the ability to synthesise cholesterol from acetate whereas the ability to take up cholesterol from the bloodstream, in contrast to the adrenal glands, seems to be limited (Morris and Chaikoff, 1959; Hall, Irby and De Kretser, 1969). After dihydroxylation of cholesterol to 20,22 di-hydroxycholesterol, a desmolase splits off the side chain, yielding pregnenolone. Two biosynthetic pathways for the synthesis of testosterone are available: the Δ5 pathway (Neher and Wettstein, 1960) via 17-hydroxypregnenolone, dehydroepiandrosterone and androst-5-ene-$3\beta,17\beta$-diol, and the Δ4-pathway (Slaunwhite and Samuels, 1956), via progesterone, 17-hydroxyprogesterone and androstenedione; transition from the Δ5 to the Δ4-pathway at each level seems possible, however (Fig. 1).

The relative importance of both pathways in man is difficult to evaluate, although some recent data suggest the Δ5-pathway to be the more important (Yanaihara and Troen, 1972; Vihko and Ruokonen, 1974); it seems, however, that whatever route is used, androstenedione is an important intermediate, the androstenediol pathway accounting probably only for a minor (less than 1%) fraction of testosterone biosynthesis (Chapdelaine and Lanthier, 1966). Although T is also quantitatively the most important androgen secreted by the testes, the Leydig cells being practically the only source of T in men, about 30% of plasma androstenedione has a testicular origin (Longcope, 1973), either by direct secretion (Eik-Nes, 1970; Baird, Uno and Melby, 1969), or indirectly by peripheral conversion of T. Moreover, small quantities of DHT (Fiorelli, Borelli, Forti, Gonnelli, Pazzagli and Serio, 1976; Pazzagli, Borrelli, Forti and Serio, 1976) contributing up to 50% of plasma DHT (Saez, Forest, Morera and Bertrand, 1971) are secreted as such by the testes. As far as androstanediol is concerned, it would appear from plasma levels (Kinouchi and Horton, 1974a, b), metabolic clearance rate (Bird, Choong, Knight and Clark, 1974) and conversion rates, that most, if not all, originate from peripheral conversion of T and DHT (Mahoudeau, Bardin and Lipsett, 1971). Finally, the testes secrete substantial amounts of DHEA (Laatikainen, Laitinen and Vihko, 1971) and are the main source of androstenediol in men (Demisch, Magnet, Neubauer and Schöffling, 1973).

The Leydig cells are almost the unique source of androgens secreted by the testes although there is some evidence that the seminiferous tubules produce some androgens, mainly DHT, from C_{19} steroids but not from cholesterol (Christensen and Mason, 1965; Dufau, De Kretser and Hudson, 1971), probably essentially for local use (Lacy, 1973; Bartke, Croft and Dallerio, 1975).

2. Ovary

As stated above, the biosynthetic pathways of androgens in the ovary are similar to those in the testes. The quantitatively major androgen secreted by the ovaries is androstenedione (Horton, Romanoff and Walker, 1966),

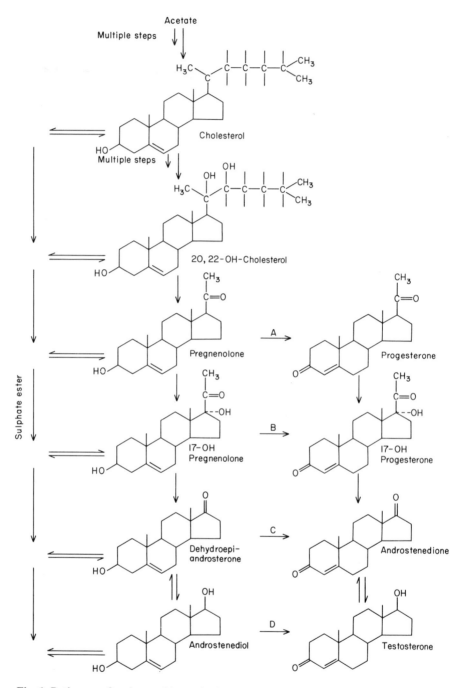

Fig. 1. Pathways of androgen biosynthesis. Routes A and B indicate the pathways of androstenedione and testosterone synthesis from C_{21} steroid precursors; routes C and D from C_{19} steroid precursors.

but the ovary secretes also minute quantities of T (Horton *et al.*, 1966) and small amounts of DHEA (Gandy and Peterson, 1968; Mikhail, 1970). The normal ovary probably does not secrete DHEA-S (Rivarola, Saez, Jones and Jones, 1967), however.

Little is known concerning the type of cell(s) secreting androgens, but it is generally believed that the stromal cells are the major ovarian source of androgens (Savard, Marsh and Rice, 1965; Marsh, Savard and Lemaire, 1976), although all three compartments (follicle, corpus luteum and stroma) secrete androgens (Baird, 1976).

3. Adrenal Cortex

Androgens of the adrenal cortex probably originate mainly from the zona reticularis. Quantitatively by far the most important androgens secreted by the adrenal cortex in adults are DHEA and DHEA-S (Baulieu, 1962; Wieland, De Courcy, Levy, Zala and Hirschman, 1965). The latter arises mainly from sulphation of DHEA, although a minor fraction may arise via sulphated precursors of the $\Delta 5$ pathway, from cholesterol sulphate (Calvin, Van de Wiele and Lieberman, 1964a, b). The possibility that some DHEA might be formed by a pathway independent of pregnenolone, via 17,20 dihydroxy-cholesterol cannot be excluded (Shimizu, 1965), The adrenal cortex is also the main source of plasma androstenedione (Wieland *et al.*, 1965); it does not appear that under physiological conditions it secretes significant amounts of T, although Kirschner and Bardin (1972) suggest that in women it might secrete from 0–30% of total T secreted. Androstenediol on the other hand is probably secreted as such by the adrenal cortex and the testes (Rosenfield and Otto, 1972; Demisch, Magnet, Neubauer and Schöffling, 1973) although substantial amounts arise from peripheral conversion of DHEA (Poortman, Andriesse, Agema, Donker, Mulder and Thyssen, 1977). 11β-hydroxyandrostenedione, a steroid of unknown physiological significance, is also secreted by the adrenal cortex (Jeanloz, Levy, Jacobsen, Hechter, Schenker and Pincus, 1953; Pincus and Romanoff, 1955).

During foetal life the adrenal cortex, which develops from the mesonephros, consists essentially of a foetal X-zone, which is almost devoid of $\Delta 4,5$ isomerase 3β-hydroxysteroid-dehydrogenase activity. Hence the foetal adrenal secretes large amounts of DHEA and DHEA-S which in the foetal liver and adrenal cortex, are largely converted to 16α-hydroxy-dehydro-epiandrosterone sulphate; these $\Delta 5$-androgens function as precursors of oestrogens in the placenta.

From the earliest time of gestation, high activity of adrenal 17-hydroxylase has been demonstrated *in vitro*, whereas 11- and 21-hydroxylase appear after the 8–10th week (Villee, Engib, Loring and Villee, 1961).

The main differences in steroid biosynthesis between foetal and adult adrenal glands can be summarised as follows:

(i)   low 3β-hydroxysteroid dehydrogenase activity, favouring the secretion of $\Delta5$ steroids over those of the $\Delta4$-series;

(ii) high sulphurylating activity;

(iii) high 16-hydroxylating activity.

Near term, the foetal zone regresses and the definitive zone of the adrenal cortex develops.

B. REGULATION OF ANDROGEN BIOSYNTHESIS AND SECRETION

1. Factors Regulating Foetal Androgen Secretion

Androgen secretion by the foetal testes starts at 6–8 weeks of foetal life, simultaneously with sexual differentiation, reaches a maximum between the 11th and the 18th week, followed by a progressive decline during the second half of pregnancy (Reyes, Winter and Faiman, 1973; Reyes, Boroditsky, Winter and Faiman, 1974; Abramovich, Baker and Neal, 1974). This early testicular secretion seems to be under the control of placental chorionic gonadotrophin (hCG). Indeed, although testicular androgens are necessary to induce the development of Wolffian structures and later for masculinisation of external genitalia and derivatives of the urogenital sinus, genitals never fail to differentiate normally in anencephalic or apituitary infants. The situation changes, however, during the second half of pregnancy, when foetal pituitary LH appears to be the stimulus of T secretion; hence in anencephalics, testes, penis, and scrotum are often hypoplastic at birth (Grumbach and Kaplan, 1973).

No evidence is available for an active androgen secretion by the foetal ovaries (Reyes *et al.*, 1974).

The foetal adrenal cortex on the other hand secretes large quantities of DHEA. There is some evidence that during early foetal life the X-zone of the adrenal cortex is under the control not of adrenocorticotrophin (ACTH), but of a related polypeptide, the corticotrophin-like intermediate polypeptide (CLIP), a polypeptide which in man is not secreted during post-natal life, but is secreted by animals that possess an intermediate lobe in the hypophysis (Rees, 1977; Silman, Chard, Lowry, Mullen, Smith and Young, 1977). It has been suggested that CLIP stimulates $\Delta5$-steroid bio-synthesis. In the second half of gestation (Silman *et al.*, 1977), and during post-natal life, ACTH is known to stimulate secretion of DHEA, DHEA-S, androstenedione and androstenediol by the adrenal cortex.

2. Factors Regulating Androgen Secretion in Adults

(a) Testes

Androgen secretion by the Leydig cells, which are the only cells having an LH receptor (Catt, Dufau and Tsuruhara, 1972), is under the control of pituitary LH secretion, although experimental evidence supports a synergistic effect of FSH (Johnson and Ewing, 1971; Odell and Swerdloff, 1974), which can be explained by the fact that the Leydig cells have a small number of FSH receptors (Catt and Dufau, 1973). Chorionic gonadotrophin binds to the LH receptors of the Leydig cells (Kirschner, Lipsett and Collins, 1965; Rivarola, Saez, Meyer, Jenkins and Migeon, 1966) and both hCG and LH behave similarly at the cellular level. Although it is generally accepted that the LH effects are mediated largely via cAMP, the classical second messenger, at low levels of LH stimulation no increase in cAMP with increasing testosterone synthesis could be observed, indicating that another mechanism may be operating (Catt and Dufau, 1973). However, small changes in cAMP levels might occur within the cell which are not detectable with the methods available; that this may be the case is suggested by the fact that theophylline increases testosterone release by low levels of HCG, but is without effect on detectable cAMP (Catt and Dufau, 1973). LH appears to act at the 20α-hydroxylation level, stimulating the conversion of cholesterol into 20α-hydroxy cholesterol (Forchielli, Dorfman, Ichii and Ménon, 1965).

The testicular secretion inhibits, by a negative feedback mechanism, gonadotrophin secretion directly at the pituitary and indirectly, via LH-RH inhibition, at the hypothalamic level. The feedback is not effected by T itself, but prior local transformation to oestradiol in the hypothalamus and to either DHT or androstanediol at the pituitary level is required (Zanisi, Motta and Martini, 1974). However, recent evidence indicates that T itself is responsible for part of the feedback effect (Marynick, Sherins, Pita and Lipsett, 1977).

LH stimulation of the testes causes an increase not only in T secretion (Kirschner et al., 1965) but also DHT (Mahoudeau, Valcke and Bricaire, 1975; Vermeulen and Verdonck, 1976a), androstenedione, DHEA (Chapdelaine, MacDonald, Gonzales, Gurpide, Van de Wiele and Lieberman, 1965), and androstenediol (Weinstein, Kelch, Jenner, Kaplan and Grumbach, 1974; Pirke, Doerr, Sintermann and Vogt, 1977) secretion are stimulated.

In rodents, prolactin appears to increase the number of LH receptors on the Leydig cells and hence to potentiate the LH effects (Bartke et al., 1975). In the human, however, results are controversial as some experimental data (Rubin, Poland and Tower, 1976) seem to indicate that also in men prolactin might potentiate the LH effects on androgen secretion, whereas clinical evidence shows that hyperprolactinemia induces both hypogonadism and low androgen secretion; the latter becomes normal under the influence of dopaminergic drugs (bromocriptine) which inhibit prolactin secretion. It is possible that prolactin is required by the Leydig cells for optimal androgen secretion, whereas excess prolactin might block the LH sensitivity.

Androgen secretion may also be influenced by factors acting locally at the Leydig cell level. Data obtained by Sholiton, Srivastava and Taylor (1976) suggest that oestrogens affect directly Leydig cell function; the latter were shown by Mulder, Van Beurden-Lamers, Brinkmann, Mechielsen and Van der Molen (1974) to possess oestrogen receptors.

Finally, the Leydig cell sensitivity for LH may change with nutritional state (Smith, Chetri, Johanson, Radfar and Migeon, 1975), testicular blood flow (Eik-Nes, 1964) and probably many other factors.

(b) Ovaries

As mentioned earlier the interstitial tissue (stroma) is the main source of ovarian androgens, but follicles and corpus luteum also secrete androstene-dione (Savard et al., 1965; Baird et al., 1977). Androstenedione and T blood levels are higher around ovulation, when LH levels are high, than during the rest of the cycle, suggesting a stimulatory effect of LH on ovarian androgen secretion (Judd and Yen, 1973; Abraham, 1974; Vermeulen, Vandeweghe, Rubens, Comhaire and Verdonck, 1974). Although DHEA levels do not show similar cyclical variations, HCG has nevertheless been shown to stimulate ovarian DHEA secretion (Vermeulen, 1976b).

(c) Adrenals

Adrenal androgen secretion occurs synchronously with cortisol secretion (Rosenfield, 1971; Vermeulen, 1976b) and since ACTH increases DHEA, DHEA-S and androstenedione (Rivarola et al., 1966) secretion, whereas administered glucocorticoids lead to a diminished secretion of these steroids (Kirschner et al., 1965), it is evident that ACTH is the main regulator of adrenal androgen secretion. Nevertheless, based on the increase in adrenal androgen secretion in prepuberty (adrenarche) and on the decrease in androgen secretion in elderly persons (Gandy and Peterson, 1968; Vermeulen, 1976b; Vermeulen and Verdonck, 1976a), without any concomitant changes in cortisol secretion, the existence of a separate adrenal androgen stimulating hormone has been postulated. Up to now, however, the existence and nature of the postulated hormone remain hypothetical.

Prolactin seems to influence adrenal androgen secretion, as in patients with a prolactinoma (Bassi, Giusti, Borsi, Cattaneo, Gianotti, Forti, Pazzagli,

Vigiani and Serio, 1977) or pharmacologically-induced hyperprolactinaemia (Vermeulen, Suy and Rubens, 1977) DHEA and DHEA-S plasma levels and secretion are generally increased; ACTH appears, however, to be necessary for prolactin to exert this effect (Vermeulen and Ando, 1978). The physiologic significance, if any, and the mechanism of this prolactin effect remains to be elucidated.

C. MECHANISM OF ACTION OF ANDROGENS

The mechanism of action of androgens is essentially similar to that of other steroid hormones. Androgen-sensitive tissues are characterised by the presence of androgen receptors that can bind both DHT and T (Anderson and Liao, 1968; Fang, Anderson and Liao, 1969; Bruchowski and Wilson, 1968a, b). Whereas like other steroid hormones, androgens enter passively (or aided by an active mechanism) (King and Mainwaring, 1974) all cells, and are eventually metabolised, in target organs, generally after enzymatic transformation to DHT (Anderson and Liao, 1968; Bruchowski and Wilson, 1968a, b), they interact with the cytosol receptor which is converted to an activated form (Liao and Fang, 1969; Little, Szendro, Teran, Hughes and Jungblut, 1975) for translocation into the cell nucleus. There the steroid-activated receptor complex associates with the acceptor site on the chromatin (Loeb and Wilson, 1966; Mangan, Neal and Williams, 1968) enhancing genetic transcription and stimulating synthesis of all types of RNA (Davies and Griffith, 1973), and subsequently formation of protein. The steps beyond RNA synthesis are still poorly understood. Not all effects of androgens seem to involve the receptor system, however: induction of the glycolytic enzymes by androgens for example seems to involve cAMP (Mainwaring, 1975).

As at least in some target tissues, biological activity of T requires local prior reduction to DHT, whereas in other tissues transformation to oestrogens may be required, it has been suggested that T is a prohormone.

However, several observations seem to indicate that some hormonal effects are effected by T itself. Indeed, differentiation of the Wolffian duct under the influence of testicular androgen occurs at a time when a 5α-reductase is still absent, whereas in 5α-reductase deficiency, spermatogenesis, which is androgen-dependent, is nevertheless normal. Similarly, growth of muscle appears to be T-mediated, as is psychosexual orientation. Moreover, in some organs, formation of DHT may be important only during periods of maximum growth (Imperato McGinley and Peterson, 1976). On the other hand, induction of haem synthesis requires formation of 5β-reduced metabolites (Valladares and Mingnell, 1975).

As the expression of at least most of the androgenic effects requires the presence of androgen receptors, the question arises whether androgens such as androstenedione or DHEA are active *per se* or whether they require prior transformation to T or DHT. Because of the very low affinity of the androgen receptors for these steroids, evidence at the present time favours the hypothesis of the necessity for prior transformation to T. It is highly improbable that there are separate androgen receptors for DHEA or androstenedione for example, because in the testicular feminisation syndrome, characterised by the absence of the DHT receptor (Bardin, Bullock, Sherins, Mowszowicz and Blackburn, 1973) no virilisation occurs despite normal DHEA and androstenedione levels.

On the other hand, the virilisation of the female foetus observed in $\Delta 5$-isomerase-3β hydroxysteroid-dehydrogenase deficiency is difficult to explain, if prior transformation to T is required for virilising activity, unless we accept an enzyme deficiency which is limited to some tissues only (Schneider, Genel, Bongiovanni, Goldman and Rosenfield, 1975). Recent evidence suggests, however, that in various tissues of the same animal, there are different receptor proteins for various steroids related to androgens (for review see Liang, Tymoczko, Chan, Hung and Liao, 1977).

D. METABOLISM OF ANDROGENS

1. Peripheral Interconversion

Once secreted into the general circulation, androgens are taken up by the cells where they undergo metabolic transformation and degradation. During these metabolic processes biologically highly active intermediates may be formed, part of which may escape into the general circulation. This escape will be the more important when the metabolising tissue is devoid of further catabolising or conjugating enzymes.

For example in the prostrate, rich in 5α-reductase but poor in further catabolising enzymes, T is metabolised to DHT, which escapes partially into the general circulation, whereas in the liver, which is also rich in 5α-reductase, further metabolism occurs immediately and relatively little DHT will escape into the general circulation.

The ratio of the plasma concentration of product appearing in the blood, to the plasma concentration of precursor is called the blood conversion ratio ($CR_{BB}^{Pro-Pre}$), whereas the product of this CR and the ratio of the metabolic clearance rate (MCR) of the product to that of the precursor is called the transfer constant: it determines the fraction of the precursor produced per unit of time and circulating in the blood, converted to circulating product (Horton and Tait, 1966).

T is readily converted to DHT and in fact in females most plasma DHT derives from peripheral conversion of T and androstenedione (Table 1); in the male on the other hand DHT is also secreted as such by the testes, but peripheral transformation accounts nevertheless for at least 50% of plasma DHT (Mahoudeau et al., 1971; Ito and Horton, 1971; Saez et al., 1972; Ishimaru, Pages and Horton, 1977). Androstenedione and T are also readily interconvertible; in the female 60% of plasma T is derived from peripheral conversion of androstenedione (Horton and Tait, 1966) whereas in males this represents only a minor fraction of plasma T. Plasma androstanediol probably is derived almost exclusively from peripheral conversion of T or DHT (Mahoudeau et al., 1971).

Plasma DHEA-S, quantitatively a major steroid secreted by the adrenal cortex, is converted peripherally to DHEA, which partially escapes into the circulation. Virtually all tissues, except during foetal life, contain steroid sulphatase. DHEA may be converted to blood androstenedione and T, although it is a poor precursor of the latter (Horton and Tait, 1967), to DHEA-S (60%) and to androstenediol of which one-third of total production would originate from DHEA (Poortman et al., 1977).

Androst-5-ene-$3\beta,17\beta$-diol may also be converted to plasma T, but due on the one hand to its relatively low concentration in plasma, and to the low conversion rate ($CR_{BB}^{D5diol \rightarrow T} = 0.01-0.02$) it does not seem to be a major precursor of T in women (Kirschner, Sinhamahapatra, Zucker, Loriaux and Nieschlag, 1973).

The site of this peripheral conversion with escape into the blood has been the subject of few studies, probably due to the difficulty of the experimental approach of the problem. However, from studies of Horton et al. (1966) and of Rivarola, Singleton and Migeon (1967), it appears that the liver contributes little to the overall blood conversion rates of androgens, which represent largely conversion occurring in extraplanchnic tissues (Baird, Horton, Longcope and Tait, 1969; Ishimaru, Edmiston, Pages and Horton, 1978). T and androstenedione are also converted to oestradiol and oestrone respectively. The mean conversion rates are estimated at 0.18% for $CR_{BB}^{T \rightarrow oestradiol}$ (Longcope, Kato and Horton, 1969) and at ca 1.3% for $CR_{BB}^{\Delta 4 \rightarrow oestrone}$ (Longcope et al., 1969; Grodin, Siiteri and MacDonald, 1973) in males and at 0.05% and 0.7–1% respectively in young females. There is good evidence that this conversion occurs in fat tissue (Siiteri and MacDonald, 1973) and muscle (Longcope, Pratt, Schneider and Fineberg, 1978). An increase of this conversion rate with weight has been reported (Siiteri and MacDonald, 1973); according to Hemsell, Grodin, Brenner, Siiteri and MacDonald (1974) the conversion also increases with age. During pregnancy DHEA-S and 16-hydroxydehydroepiandrosterone sulphate are converted

N

Table 1

Blood conversion rates and transfer constants (values are as per cent of precursor).

Steroid	Blood conversion rate		Transfer constant		References
	Males	Females	Males	Females	
T → androstenedione	2–3·2	2·8–3·4 3·3 ± 1·4	4·6–7·6	6·6–8·0 7·8 ± 2·3	Tait and Horton (1966) Abraham et al. (1969)
Androstenedione → T	13·3 (6·2–24·0)	15·5 ± 4·1 11·1 ± 2·0	5·4 (2·6–10·0) 6·2–12·6	6·5 (5·0–9·4) 4·3–4·5 5·0 ± 1·7	Tait and Horton (1966) Rivarola et al. (1966) Abraham et al. (1969)
T → DHT	5·6 ± 0·6 6·6 ± 1·4 2·8 ± 0·3	3·5 ± 0·4 – 1·6 ± 0·5	3·9 ± 1·0 4·7 ± 2·6	1·7 ± 0·6	Ito and Horton (1971) Mahoudeau et al. (1971) Saez et al. (1972)
T → androstanediol			2·3	0·6	Kinouchi and Horton (1974)
androstenedione → DHT	8·3 ± 0·8		2·6 ± 0·9		Mahoudeau et al. (1971)
Androstanediol → DHT	50 ± 18	68 ± 12			Bird et al. (1974)
DHT → androstanediol	15·3 ± 5·9	4·4 ± 0·5	43	22	Mahoudeau et al. (1971) Kinouchi and Horton (1974)
DHEA → T			0·6 ± 0·1	0·9 ± 0·05 0·4 ± 0·05	Horton and Tait (1967) Kirschner et al. (1973)
DHEA → androstenedione			7·5 ± 1·9	4·2 ± 1·2 4·5 ± 1·9	Kirschner et al. (1973) Horton and Tait (1967)
DHEA → DHEA-S				60	Poortman et al. (1977)
DHEA-S → DHEA				15	Poortman et al. (1977)

Reaction				Reference
DHEA → androstenediol			4	Poortman et al. (1977)
			2·7 ± 0·5	Kirschner et al. (1973)
DHEA → androstenediol-S			56	Portman et al. (1977)
DHEA-S → androstenediol-S			9·7	Portman et al. (1977)
Androstenediol → T		1–2	2·3 ± 0·2	Kirschner et al. (1973)
Androstenediol → DHEA	6 ± 3	5 ± 2		Bird et al. (1976)
Androstenediol → androstenediol-S			6	Portman et al. (1977)
Androstenediol → DHEA-S			40	Portman et al. (1977)

to a large extent into oestrogen by the placenta (Bolte, Mancuso, Eriksson, Wiqvist and Diczfalusy, 1964; MacDonald and Siiteri, 1965). In the non-pregnant woman this conversion has not been demonstrated although oestrogenic effects have been observed after DHEA-S administration (Drucker, Blumberg, Gandy, David and Verde, 1972).

2. Degradative Metabolism

The overall metabolism of androgens, as measured by the metabolic clearance rate (MCR), is very rapid when compared to the metabolism of corticosteroids (Table 2). This MCR seems to be related to the specific binding of the androgens to sex hormone binding globulin (SHBG) (Baird et al., 1969b). Indeed, androstenedione and DHEA which are not specifically bound have a high MCR, whereas T, DHT and androstanediol have a lower MCR; moreover, there exists a linear relationship between the free T or DHT fraction and MCR (Vermeulen, Verdonck, Van der Straeten and Orie, 1969; Vermeulen, Rubens and Verdonck, 1972). DHEA-S on the other hand has a very low MCR of ca 15 1/24 hr (Sandberg, Gurpide and Lieberman, 1964; Gant, Hutchinson, Siiteri and MacDonald, 1971; Wang, Bulbrook, Sneddon and Hamilton, 1967; Oseko, Yoshimi, Fukase and Kono, 1974).

In as far as the MCR of androstenedione and DHEA are higher than the hepatic plasma flow, it is evident that extrahepatic tissues metabolise these steroids extensively. The mean hepatic extraction of androstenedione, i.e. the fraction entering the liver which is metabolised irreversibly in the liver, was estimated at 82% by Rivarola et al. (1967); for T this value was 44% whereas Kinouchi and Horton (1974b) observed an hepatic extraction of 76% for androstanediol, surprising in the view of its high affinity for SHBG. However, the hepatic extraction of T formed from androstenedione in the liver was much higher, 75–83% (Horton and Tait, 1960). Also when androstenedione was infused through a nasogastric tube, Horton and Tait (1966) found very little T to appear in the circulation notwithstanding efficient conversion.

These results suggest that the SHBG-bound T fraction is not readily extracted by the liver. As to the relative importance of the overall extrahepatic metabolism of T, Baird et al. (1969b) calculated that in males about 30–35% should occur extrahepatically but only about 10% in women; for androstene-dione it was calculated that about 50% would be metabolised extrahepatic-ally. Degradative metabolism of androgens involves mainly saturation of ring A to 5α and 5β-androstanes and reduction of the 3-oxo group, whereas the major metabolic pathway involves the oxidation of the 17β-hydroxyl group. After reduction of ring A, androgen metabolites are conjugated,

Table 2

Metabolic clearance rate (l/24 hr) of androgens (M. ± S.D.).

Steroid	Males	Females	References
T	1020–1240	765–995	Horton and Tait (1966)
	1179 ± 284	545 ± 103	Southren et al. (1968)
		828 ± 232	Abraham et al. (1969)
	1030 ± 141	—	Mahoudeau et al. (1971)
	(545 ± 68 l/m²		
	516 ± 108 l/m²	304 ± 53 l/m²	Saez et al. (1972)
Androstenedione	2430 ± 373	2234 ± 383	Horton and Tait (1966)
		1886 ± 228	Abraham et al. (1969)
	2073 ± 112		Mahoudeau et al. (1971)
	(1098 ± 44 l/m²)		
DHT	652 ± 34	314 ± 64	Ito and Horton (1971)
	745 ± 125	274 ± 92	Bird and Clark (1972)
	(394 ± 63 l/m²)	(167 ± 47 l/m²)	
	634 ± 190 l	243 ± 65	Mahoudeau et al. (1971)
	(336 ± 105 l/m²)	(153 ± 40 l/m²)	
	391 ± 71 l/m²	209 ± 45 l/m²	Saez et al. (1972)
Androstanediol	1767 ± 492	1297 ± 219	Kinouchi et al. (1974)
	1371 ± 262	1021 ± 166	Bird et al. (1974)
	(727 ± 117 l/m²)	(616 ± 87 l/m²)	
		754	Poortman et al. (1977)
		(449 l/m²)	
Androstenediol		584 ± 44	Kirschner et al. (1973)
	1311 ± 67	858 ± 63	Bird et al. (1976)
DHEA	1750 ± 221	1535 ± 213	Horton and Tait (1967)
		2017	Poortman et al. (1977)
		(1195 l/m²)	
		1510 ± 192	Kirschner et al. (1973)
DHEA-S		22	Wang et al. (1967)
	8–10		Sandberg et al. (1964)
		23	Poortman et al. (1977)
		(13·61 l/m²)	
		13·6 ± 8.1	Oseko et al. (1974)

essentially in the liver, with glucuronic or, to a lesser extent, with sulphuric acid. This increases the polarity of the metabolites, makes them more water-soluble and possibly facilitates urinary excretion.

Urinary clearance of androgen glucuronosides approaches the glomerular filtration rate of the kidneys; hence the concentration of these glucuronosides in plasma is extremely low. The clearance of androgen sulphates is much lower and although androsterone sulphate is a minor testosterone metabolite when compared to the glucuronoside, plasma levels are much higher. The steroid glucuronosides are probably filtered through the glomerulus, whereas the sulphates would be secreted by the renal tubule (Bongiovanni and Eberlein, 1957; Kellie and Smith, 1957; Cox and Kellie, 1965). Unconjugated androgen metabolites, present in minute concentration in plasma, may be partly conjugated with glucuronic acid in the kidney (Cohn and Hume, 1960). Finally androgen sulphates are partly (*ca* 15%) excreted in the bile of which 80% is reabsorbed in the gut (Baulieu *et al.*, 1965). After i.v. injection of radioactively labelled T or androstenedione, almost all radioactivity appears in the urine within 48 hr (Sandberg and Slaunwhite, 1956). Nevertheless in some subjects excretion of metabolites appears to be significantly lower, without apparent cause. Approximately 10% of radioactivity is recovered in the bile, of which half is reabsorbed (Martin, Loriaux and Farnham, 1965).

Androsterone and aetiocholanolone are quantitatively the most important metabolites of T, corresponding to *ca* 60% of urinary metabolites. In young males 5α-metabolites are more important than 5β-metabolites; in women 5β-metabolites predominate slightly over the 5α-metabolites (Baulieu, Robel and Mauvais-Jarvis, 1963). Besides this 17-oxo metabolic pathway, there exists a quantitatively less important 17β-hydroxyl pathway giving rise to 5α and 5β-androstane-$3\alpha,17\beta$-diols, which together represent about 4% of T metabolites in males and *ca* 2% in women (Baulieu and Mauvais-Jarvis, 1964a). Although these metabolites might arise by reduction of androsterone and aetiocholanolone respectively, the major metabolic route is probably by direct reduction of testosterone (17β-hydroxyl pathway) (Fig. 2).

The androstanediols when injected intravenously undergo in turn oxidation of the 17β-hydroxyl group. This is in contradiction with the observation by Kuttenn and Mauvais-Jarvis (1975) that urinary excretion of $3\alpha,5\alpha$-androstanediol corresponds roughly to the blood production rate. Possibly this is purely coincidental, metabolism of plasma androstanediol being eventually compensated by hepatic formation of androstanediol, directly conjugated without entering the circulation as free steroid. Other minor metabolites of T are derivatives hydroxylated at C-1, C-6 and C-16 (Schubert, Weinberger and Frankenberg, 1964); certain pharmacological agents that act as enzyme inducers (barbiturates, phenytoin, phenylbutazone) may increase the relative importance of these metabolites (Conney, Kuntzmann and Jacobson, 1966).

The origin of urinary 17α-testosterone (epitestosterone) is still contro-

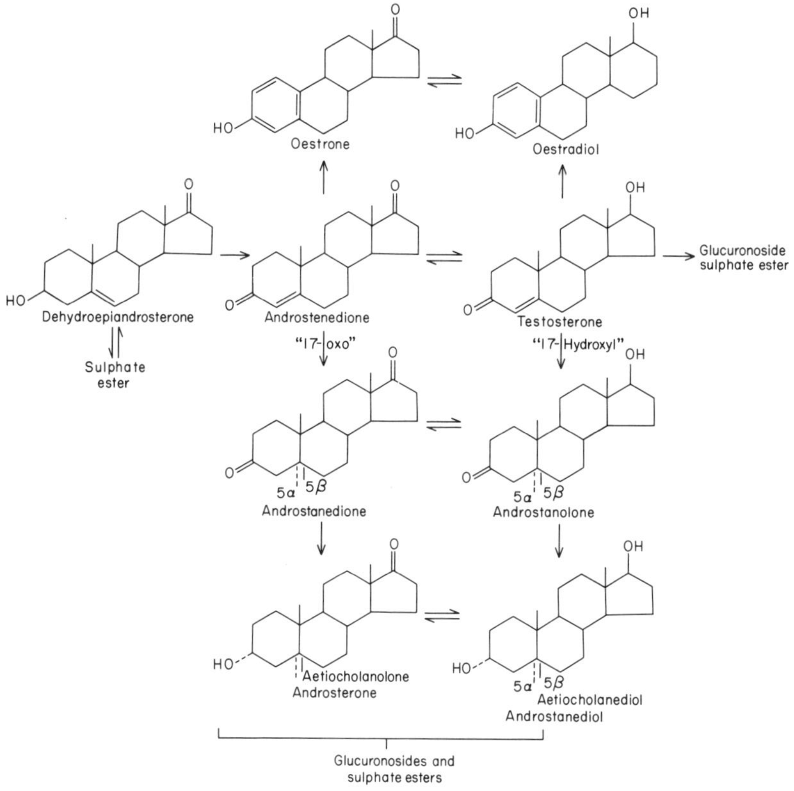

Fig. 2. The major peripheral interconversions of the androgens and their metabolism in the body are illustrated, with emphasis upon the degradative metabolism of these steroids via the "17-oxo" and "17-hydroxyl" pathways.

versial; the most logical precursor appears to be androstenedione although this has been questioned (Dray, 1966; Korenman, Wilson and Lipsett, 1964). A small fraction of testosterone is conjugated as such with glucuronic acid. At first sight unexpectedly, testosterone glucuronoside is not a unique metabolite of plasma testosterone, since androstenedione is also converted to testosterone-glucuronoside in the liver and in women or hypogonadal males androstenedione may be a major precursor of this conjugate (Korenman and Lipsett, 1964). It is possible that testosterone-glucuronoside undergoes direct metabolism to ring A-saturated glucuronosides (Robel, Emiliozzi and Baulieu, 1966). Testosterone sulphate has been isolated from the urine (Dessypris, Drosdowski, McNiven and Dorfman, 1960) but whether this results from peripheral T metabolism (Saez, Bertrand and Migeon, 1971) or only from direct secretion (Laatikainen, Laitinen and Vihko, 1969; Dessypris, 1975) is unclear. The metabolism of androstenedione follows similar pathways to the metabolism of T and it is generally considered that also quantitatively the metabolites are almost identical. However, the androstanediols appear to be quantitatively significantly less important (2% in males and 1% in females) (Baulieu and Mauvais-Jarvis, 1964b).

DHEA-S may be excreted as such, it may be metabolised to androstenediol sulphate and to hydroxylated metabolites (Baulieu, Corpéchot, Dray, Emiliozzi, Leveau, Mauvais-Jarvis and Robel, 1963), or it may be hydrolysed to DHEA which, after glucuronosidation may be excreted as such or which is further metabolised to androstenedione, androsterone and etiocholanolone (Mauvais Jarvis and Baulieu, 1965). DHEA is also conjugated with either sulphuric or glucuronic acid, either without prior metabolism or after metabolism to androsterone and etiocholanolone.

E. ANDROGENS IN BLOOD

1. Physical State

Androgens in plasma are largely bound to plasma proteins. Albumin has a high capacity and generally a low affinity for all androgens: this binding is generally called non-specific binding. For all practical purposes this binding is a linear function of the albumin concentration and within physiological limits independent of steroid concentration.

Where DHEA, DHEA-S and androstenedione are almost exclusively bound to plasma albumin, T, DHT and androstanediol are not only non-specifically bound to albumin, but besides to a specific, high affinity but low capacity, binding β-globulin, variously called testosterone-oestradiol binding globulin or sex hormone binding globulin (SHBG) (Mercier, Alfsen and Baulieu, 1966; Pearlman and Crépy, 1966). The approximate affinity constants of this protein for the various 17β-hydroxyandrogens are given in Table 3. The binding capacity of the protein is estimated at $3–5 \times 10^{-8}$M in adult males and at $6–7.5 \times 10^{-8}$M in women (Vermeulen and Verdonck, 1967, 1968; Vermeulen et al., 1969; Rosner, 1972).

Transcortin, or corticosteroid-binding globulin is a low capacity α-globulin, which, at 37° has a low binding affinity for T (1.5×10^{6}M^{-1}): hence transcortin-bound T varies between 0.5 and 2 times the free T fraction (Vermeulen, Stoïca and Verdonck, 1971).

Table 3

Association constants of plasma androgens at 37°.

	Albumin (M^{-1})	SHBG (M^{-1})
T	$3\cdot6 \times 10^4$	8×10^8
DHT	$6\cdot5 \times 10^4$	10×10^8
Androstanediol	18×10^4	$6\cdot5 \times 10^8$
Androstenediol	4×10^5	$7\cdot2 \times 10^8$
DHEA	$3\cdot8 \times 10^4$	—
DHEA-S	2×10^5	—

The α1-acid glycoprotein (AAG) has a large binding capacity ($1 \times 10^{-5}\text{M}$) but at 37° a low binding affinity ($2\cdot4 \times 10^5\text{M}^{-1}$) for T (Kirkay and Westphal, 1968): hence AAG-bound T will correspond roughly to twice the free fraction. Although the latter two proteins probably exhibit some affinity for the other androgens, no data concerning their binding are available; this binding appears to be of minor physiological significance.

In normal males the free T fraction corresponds to about 2% of the total T level, whereas in normal women this value is about 1% (Vermeulen and Verdonck, 1967, 1968; Vermeulen et al., 1971). Due to the higher association constant of SHBG for DHT and androstanediol (Vermeulen and Verdonck, 1968) the free fraction of these androgens is slightly lower than that of T. There is good evidence that only the non-specifically bound androgen fraction is biologically active. Indeed, the metabolic clearance rate of T and DHT parallels the non-specifically bound fraction (Vermeulen et al., 1969; Southren, Gordon, Tochimoto, Olivo, Sherman, Pinzon, 1969; Vermeulen et al., 1972b). Mowszowicz, Kahn and Dray (1970) showed that SHBG inhibits the aromatisation of T by placental microsomes in vitro, whereas Lasnitski and Franklin (1971) showed that T uptake by prostate explants is inhibited by SHBG. Finally, clinical experience reveals that androgenic activity parallels much better the free T concentration than total T (Vermeulen et al., 1969; Rosenfeld, Hellman, Roffwarg, Weitzman, Fukushima and Gallagher, 1971; Dray, Sebaoun, Delzan, Ledru and Mowszowicz, 1968).

2. Androgen Secretion From Foetal Life Until Senescence

(a) Males

(1) During foetal life and in newborn. Under the influence of placental chorionic gonadotrophin, the foetal testes start to secrete androgens between the 6th and 8th week of foetal life. Plasma levels of T in 9–25 week foetuses vary between 40 and 580 ng/dl (1·4 and 20·1 nmol/l), significantly higher than in females (<20–130 ng/dl; <0·7–4·5 nmol/l) with highest values, some of these within the normal adult male range, between 11 and 17 weeks. After 17 weeks of age, T levels decline to levels indistinguishable from those observed in female foetuses (Reyes et al., 1973, 1974; Abramovich et al., 1974). As mentioned earlier, during the second half of gestation, testicular secretion appears to be under the control of foetal pituitary LH. Between days 80–160 foetal serum LH levels are in the castrated adult range, decreasing afterwards until delivery. After the 24th week the feedback mechanism becomes functional and progressively more sensitive to sex steroids.

At birth, plasma T levels in the male are in the low adult range (ca 300 ng/100 ml; 10·4 nmol/l) (Forest, Cathiard and Bertrand, 1973). They decrease rapidly during the first week of life to about 30 ng/100 ml (1·04 nmol/l), followed by an increase to levels as high as 300 ng/100 ml (10·4 nmol/l) lasting for 30–60 days. This is followed by a gradual decrease until the seventh month, when levels of about 7–10 ng/100 ml (0·24–0·35 nmol/l) are reached, which will be maintained until puberty (Forest, Cathiard, Bourgeois and Genoud, 1974; Forest, Sizonenko, Cathiard and Bertrand, 1974; Winter, Hughes, Reyes and Faiman, 1976).

Little is known concerning the secretion of the other androgens by the testes during foetal life. DHEA-S and 16α-OHDHEA-S are the major circulating steroids in the human foetus (Simmer, Easterling, Pion and Dignam, 1964; Colas, Heirichs and Tatum, 1964); They have probably mainly an adrenal origin. At birth, plasma androstenedione levels in cord (ca 100 ng/dl; 3·5 nmol/l) and peripheral (ca 185 ng/dl; 6·5 nmol/l) blood, are similar in both sexes; after birth there occurs a rapid decrease in these levels (at 5 day: 28 ± 12 ng/dl (0·89 ± 0·42 nmol/l)) (Forest and Cathiard, 1971; Forest and Bertrand, 1975) followed by a moderate increase between days 10 and 30 (44 ± 18 ng/dl; 1·54 ± 0·63 nmol/l); after the first month of life, androstenedione levels decrease again to about 10 ± 3 ng/dl (0·35 ± 0·10 nmol/l) after 6 months, levels which are maintained until the adrenarche.

There is no sex difference of DHEA levels in either cord (m̄ ca 600 ng/dl (20·8 nmol/l)) or peripheral blood (m̄ 920 ng/dl (31·9 nmol/l)) but the levels in the latter are significantly higher than in the former (De Peretti and Forest, 1976). Levels decrease rapidly during the first year of life to reach a nadir of *ca* 25 ng/dl (0·87 nmol/l), which is maintained from age 1–6 yr (de Peretti and Forest, 1976).

Plasma DHEA-S levels which are similar in both sexes, and slightly higher in arterial than in venous cord blood (Simmer *et al.*, 1964; Laatikainen and Peltonen, 1975) follow a similar pattern, with a birth level of 130 ± 50 µg/dl (3·07 ± 1·18 µmol/l). After age 1 until age 6, levels are below 10 µg/dl (0·25 µmol/l) (Turnipseed, Bentley and Reynolds, 1976; Hooper and Yen, 1975; Bertrand, De Peretti and Forest, 1977).

Whereas at birth the SHBG capacity is extremely low, resulting in a very high free T fraction of about 3% (August, Tkachuk and Grumbach, 1969; Forest and Bertrand, 1975) by the second week of life SHBG capacity has increased to about $1·5 \times 10^{-7}$M in both sexes and will remain at this level until puberty; the free T fraction is therefore small (0·7%). Due to this increase in SHBG capacity, the free T concentration, which at birth is *ca* 10 ng/100 ml (350 pmol/l), is only 1·5 ng/100 ml (52 pmol/l) during the post-natal testosterone peak, and from the sixth month until puberty it is only ±0·1 ng/100 ml (±3·5 pmol/l) (Vermeulen, 1977).

Whether the high neonatal androgen levels play a role in the differentiation of neural structures controlling adult sexual behaviour remains to be shown. In man, unlike some other animal species (Forest, 1975) they do not seem to be responsible for imprinting the male pattern of gonadotrophin release. Indeed, in girls with congenital adrenal hyperplasia, after corticosteroid therapy, cyclical gonadotrophin release occurs; moreover, in testicular feminisation, due to absence of androgen receptors and hence androgen impregnation, oestrogens do not have a stimulating effect on gonadotrophin release (Van Look, Hunter, Corker and Baird, 1977).

(*2*) *Adrenarche.* From the sixth month of life, androgen plasma levels remain extremely low, similar in both sexes, until age 6–8, when a rapid increase in DHEA, DHEA-S and androstenedione levels occurs. This is attributable to increased androgen secretion by the adrenal cortex without concomitant increase in cortisol secretion and without activation of gonadal secretion. The mechanism and significance of this adrenarche (Sizonenko and Paunier, 1975; Forest, 1975; Korth-Schutz, Levine and New, 1976) remain unknown; the existence of an adrenal androgen stimulation hormone has been postulated (Mills, 1968; Gupta, 1975). During these prepubertal years the androstenedione levels are higher than plasma T levels.

(*3*) *At puberty.* At puberty, characterised by a decrease of the sensitivity of the hypothalamic mechanism for the sex hormone feedback, gonadotrophin levels increase and sleep-associated LH discharges occur (Boyar, Rosenfeld, Knapen, Finkelstein, Roffwarg, Weizman and Hellman, 1974), stimulating fibroblast differentiation to Leydig cells and androgen secretion. The latter increases slowly two years before the onset of pubic hair growth, the first clinical sign of puberty. Ultimately, the feedback threshold becoming higher than the threshold of stimulation of secondary sex organs, puberty starts, generally between age 10 and 14. Plasma T and DHT (Gupta, McCafferty and Rager, 1972) as well as androstanediol levels (Klemm, Liebich and Gupta, 1976) increase rapidly and within three to four years, at pubertal stage 5, adult levels are reached. Androstenedione, DHEA and DHEA-S levels increase also (Hopper and Yen, 1975), adult levels being reached already at pubertal stage 3. In parallel with the increase in T levels, SHBG capacity decreases to a mean adult level of 4×10^{-8}M: hence the free T concentration increases even more than total T levels (Vermeulen et al., 1971) (Table 4).

Table 4

Plasma testosterone levels (ng/dl)[a] in relation to pubertal stage in boys.

Pubertal stage	Testosterone	Apparent free testosterone	SHBG (10^{-8}M)
P1 (n = 23)	23 (10–45)	0·15 (0·06–0·36)	14·8 (11·2–17·2)
P2 (n = 53)	83 (47–157)	0·89 (0·51–1·53)	11·3 (10·1–12·7)
P3 (n = 42)	173 (118–278)	2·4 (1·4–4·0)	7·6 (6·4–8·9)
P4 (n = 14)	409 (228–658)	6·0 (3·0–11·8)	6·7 (4·5–8·7)
P5	632 (325–1025)	9·4 (5·5–20·0)	5·2 (4·8–5·6)

[a] 1 ng/dl testosterone = 34·7 pmol/l.

(4) *In adults.* In 20–50-yr-old adults, T concentration varies between 280 and 1200 ng, M. *ca* 650 ng/100 ml (9·7 and 41·7 nmol/1, M. *ca* 22·6 nmol/1) with a mean T/DHT ratio of *ca* 10 (Vermeulen, 1977); androstanediol levels vary between 5 and 25 ng, M. 15 ng/dl (170–860 pmol/1, M. 514 pmol/1), (Kinouchi and Horton, 1974a; Barberia, Pages and Horton, 1976), androstenedione between 50–150 ng/dl, M. 120 ng/dl (1·7–5·2 nmol/1, M. 4·2 nmol/1), DHEA between 350 and 700 ng, M. 400 ng/dl (12·2 and 24·3 nmol/1, M. 13·9 nmol/1), and DHEA-S between 80 and 150 µg/dl (1·9 and 3·5 µmol/1)

(expressed as DHEA). Adult androstenediol levels finally vary between 20 and 180 ng/dl, M. = ±100 ng/dl (0·7 and 6·2 nmol/1, M = 3·4 nmol/1) (Rosenfield and Otto, 1972; Demisch *et al.*, 1973; Bird, Morrow, Fukumoto, Marcellus and Clark, 1976; Pirke *et al.*, 1977).

The mean blood production rates (BPR) in adult males age 20–50 yr are 6 mg/24 hr (20·8 μmol/24 hr) for T (Horton and Tait, 1966), 300 μg (1·0 μmol) for DHT (Ito and Horton, 1971), 2–3 mg (7·0–10·5 μmol) for androstenedione (Horton and Tait, 1966), 7 mg (24·3 μmol) for DHEA (Horton and Tait, 1967) and 8 mg (18·8 μmol) for DHEA-S (MacDonald, Chapdelaine, Gonzales, Gurpide, Van de Wiele and Lieberman, 1965). Androstanediol production is *ca* 225 μg (0·8 μmol)/24 hr (Kinouchi and Horton, 1974b), whereas BPR of androstenediol is *ca* 1 mg (3·5 μmol) (Demisch *et al.*, 1973; Poortman *et al.*, 1977; Bird *et al.*, 1976).

Plasma T levels start to decrease during the sixth to seventh decade of life and during the ninth decade, mean T levels are only *ca* 250 ng/dl (8·7 nmol/l); interindividual variations are, however, very important, with some nonagenarians having T levels well within the range of normal young men, others, however, having T levels hardly higher than levels observed in women (Vermeulen *et al.*, 1971, 1972b) (Table 5).

Table 5

Plasma testosterone levels (ng/dl)[a] in males at different ages (M ± S.D.).

Age	Testosterone	Apparent free testosterone	% Free testosterone
20–30	669 ± 192	10·3 ± 3·5	2·09 ± 0·45
30–40	593 ± 196	12·7 ± 4·8	2·08 ± 0·63
40–50	561 ± 129	9·7 ± 3·4	1·77 ± 0·70
50–60	555 ± 196	8·6 ± 3·2	1·48 ± 0·44
60–70	412 ± 200	5·8 ± 3·1	1·52 ± 0·42
70–80	310 ± 178	4·1 ± 3·2	1·26 ± 0·36
80	234 ± 127	2·6 ± 1·3	1·10 ± 0·40

[a] 1 ng/dl testosterone = 34·7 pmol/l.

As a consequence of a progressive increase of SHBG capacity with age the free T concentration starts to decline earlier (Table 5) with, however, again important individual variations (Vermeulen *et al.*, 1971, 1972). Also DHT

(Vermeulen and Verdonck, 1976a) and probably androstanediol levels decrease, but the decrease is much less important than for T levels.

An important decrease with age is also observed in DHEA (Vermeulen and Verdonck, 1976a; Serio, Cattaneo, Borrelli, Gonnelli, Pazzagli, Forti, Fiorelli, Gianotti and Giusti, 1977) and DHEA-S levels (Gandy and Peterson, 1968), whereas androstenedione levels remain largely unaffected by age (Vermeulen and Verdonck, 1976a) although Pirke *et al.* (1977) observed also for this steroid as well as for androstenediol levels a decrease in plasma levels in aging males. In parallel with the age-dependent increase in SHBG binding capacity, the MCR of T and DHT decreases, and hence the blood production rate of both steroids decreases even more than plasma levels (Kent and Acone, 1966; Vermeulen *et al.*, 1972b).

(5) *Physiological factors affecting plasma androgen levels in males.* The testes, as well as the adrenal cortex, show secretory episodes. For Leydig cells, the frequency of these episodes is about one to two pulses in 6 hr, resulting in transitory spikes of T levels (Naftolin, Judd and Yen, 1973) preceded 1–2 hr earlier by an LH spike, although only one-third of LH spikes are followed by a T spike. These spikes may double the basal T levels. Due to the short half-life of testosterone these elevated levels persist only for a very short period.

Androstenedione and DHEA are secreted synchronously with the pulses of cortisol secretion (Rosenfield *et al.*, 1971); hence their plasma levels show also pulsatile variations. Similar pulses in plasma levels are not observed for DHEA-S, probably a consequence of the large pool.

Plasma androgen levels show also circadian variations with maximum levels in the early morning (06·00 hr) and minimum in the late evening (22.00–24.00 hr). The amplitude for T is *ca* 25% (Dray, Reinberg and Sebaoun, 1965; Southren, Tochimoto, Carmody and Isurugi, 1965), for androstenedione and DHEA *ca* 40–50% (Vermeulen and Verdonck, 1976a, b). The circadian variations of DHEA-S plasma levels are minimal (Rosenfeld, Rosenberg, Fukushima and Hellman, 1975). Plasma T levels show also seasonal variations: Reinberg, Lagoguey, Chauffournier and Cesselin (1975), reported higher levels in October–November than in spring, with a shift in the peak from 08·00 hr in spring to 14.00 hr in November.

The influence of age on plasma levels has already been discussed earlier. ACTH stimulation (Rivarola, Saez, Meyer, Senkins and Migeon, 1966; Beitins, Bayard, Kowarski and Migeon, 1973; Irvine, Toft, Wilson, Fraser, Young, Hunter, Ismail and Burger, 1974) as well as stress (Aono, Kurachi, Miyata, Nakasima, Koshiyama, Uozumi and Matsumoto, 1976; Kreuz, Roso and Jennings, 1972) cause a decrease in plasma T levels, but an increase in androstenedione and DHEA levels. Also after exhausting physical exercises (Vermeulen, 1973; Dessypris, Kuoppasalmi and Adlercreutz,

1976) decreased T levels are found. The mechanism of this decrease in T levels in stress is still poorly understood; it has been suggested that the increase in plasma cortisol levels might be responsible (Doerr et al., 1976) and that cortisol might inhibit the nocturnal rise of testosterone. However, this decrease occurs also after short term ACTH stimulation during the day (Vermeulen and Verdonck, 1976a, b), and we observed that a pyrogen-induced decrease in T levels persists when a rise in cortisol levels is prevented by administration of an antipyretic. A decrease in testicular blood flow remains a possible mechanism (Eik Nes, 1964). On the other hand elevated corticosteroid levels, either of endogenous (Smals, Kloppenborg and Benraad, 1977) or exogenous origin (Doerr and Pirke, 1976) appear to lower plasma T levels.

(b) Females

(1) During foetal life and in newborn. Few data are available concerning androgen levels in the female foetus, but Reyes et al. (1974) reported that between 9 and 25 weeks plasma T levels vary between less than 20 and 130 ng/dl, significantly lower than in males; they probably reflect placental and foetal liver testosterone production. The foetal adrenal cortex probably secretes equivalent amounts of $\Delta 5$-steroids in both sexes.

At birth cord (25 ng/dl) (0·87 nmol/l) and peripheral (ca 15 ng/dl) (0·52 nmol/l) plasma T levels in the female are much lower than in the male (Forest et al., 1974a, b), the difference being attributable to testicular secretion. They decrease rapidly after the first 2 weeks of life and remain constant throughout the first year of life (7 ± 3 ng/dl) (0·24 ± 0·10 nmol/l) until prepuberty. The SHBG capacity follows a similar evolution as in the male neonate: low at birth, followed within a few days by a rapid increase.

Androstenedione levels at birth are similar in both sexes, with peripheral blood levels (175 ± 75 ng/dl) (6·1 ± 2·6 nmol/l) significantly higher than cord levels (95 ng/dl) (3·3 nmol/l); they decrease rapidly during the first week of life (ca 30 ng/dl) (1·0 nmol/l) and in contrast to levels in males, continue to decrease, albeit more slowly, to reach a mean level of about 10 ng/dl (0·3 nmol/l) after one to two months, a level which is maintained until prepuberty. DHEA and DHEA-S levels, and their evolution during childhood, are similar in both sexes.

(2) Adrenarche. As in the boy, adrenal androgen secretion increases at age 6–10 (adrenarche), plasma levels being similar to values in boys (Sizonenko and Paunier, 1975; De Peretti and Forest, 1976; Forest, 1975; Korth-Schutz et al., 1976).

(3) At puberty. At puberty, ovarian secretion is stimulated progressively and ovarian androgen secretion contributes significantly to plasma androgen

levels. Whereas at age 8, the mean androstenedione level is *ca* 25 ng/dl
(0·9 nmol/l), it is *ca* 40 ng/dl (1·4 nmol/l) at age 10, 75 ng/dl (2·6 nmol/l) at
age 12 and 140 ng/dl (4·9 nmol/l) at age 14 (Collu and Ducharme, 1975).
T levels increase progressively and in parallel to adult levels (*ca* 35 ng/dl)
(*ca* 1·2 nmol/l).

(4) *Reproductive life.* Plasma androgens during reproductive life show
not only nycthemeral variations comparable to variations in the male, but
moreover cyclical variations, T and androstenedione levels being highest
during the periovulatory period (Judd and Yen, 1973, Abraham, 1974,
Vermeulen and Verdonck, 1976). DHEA and DHEA-S levels on the other
hand do not show any significant cyclical variations (Vermeulen and Verdonck, 1976a, b). As the observed variations in plasma levels persist after
adrenalectomy or dexamethasone suppression of adenocortical function
(Abraham and Chakmakjian, 1973; Kim, Hosseinian and Dupon, 1974;
Kim, Rosenfield and Dupon, 1976) it is evident that they are the consequence
of variations in ovarian secretion. Normal androgen levels during the
menstrual cycle are given in Table 6. The concentration of SHBG in women is
higher than in men; as a consequence the free T fraction is only *ca* 1%; hence
also the MCR of T, DHT and androstanediol is lower than in males, even
when expressed in $1/m^2/24$ hr (Table 2).

Table 6

Androgen levels (ng/dl) in women during the menstrual cycle
(M. ± S. D.; values expressed as DHEA).

Steroid	Follicular phase	Midcycle (LH peak ± 2day)	Luteal phase
T[a]	34 ± 5	42 ± 7	38 ± 6
DHT[b]	23 ± 4	26 ± 4	24 ± 4
Androstenedione[c]	142 ± 66	220 ± 45	120 ± 24
DHEA[a]	550 ± 90	550 ± 74	520 ± 66
DHEA-S (µg/dl)[d]	89 ± 36	88 ± 30	82 ± 39
Androstenediol[b]	73 ± 12	75 ± 8	68 ± 13

[a] 1 ng/dl = 34·7 pmol/l.
[b] 1 ng/dl = 34·4 pmol/l.
[c] 1 ng/dl = 34·9 pmol/l.
[d] 1 µg/dl = 34·7 nmol/l.

The mean blood production rate of T in women of reproductive age is *ca* 300 µg (1·0 µmol) (Horton and Tait, 1966; Southren *et al.*, 1965; Southren, Gordon, Tochimoto, Pinzon, Lane and Stypulkowski, 1967; Saez *et al.*, 1972), of DHT 50 µg–75 µg/24 hr (0·2–0·3 µmol/24 hr) (Saez *et al.*, 1972; Ito and Horton, 1974; Mahoudeau *et al.*, 1971), of androstanediol *ca* 35 µg/day (0·1 µmol/day) (Kinouchi and Horton, 1974b), of androstenedione 2–4 mg/24 hr (7–14 µmol) (Horton and Tait, 1966; Rivarola *et al.*, 1966; Abraham, Lobotsky and Lloyd, 1969). DHEA and DHEA-S blood production rates are similar (*ca* 7 mg/24 hr) (24·3 µmol/24 hr) to values observed in males (Horton and Tait, 1967).

(5) *Menopause.* After the menopause, androgen levels are significantly lower than during reproductive age. Although this is partly a consequence of a decreased androgen secretion by the ovaries, adrenal DHEA and DHEA-S secretion decrease with age, and whereas T and androstenedione levels remain constant in post-menopausal women, levels of DHEA and its sulphate continue to decrease with age (Vermeulen, 1976b; Vermeulen *et al.*, 1978).

(6) *Pregnancy.* During pregnancy T levels increase moderately (Mizuno, Lobotsky, Lloyd, Kobayashi and Murasawa, 1968; Tyler, Newton and Callens, 1975; Diez D'aux and Murphy, 1974), but due to the important increase in SHBG levels, the free T concentration is lower than in non-pregnant women (Vermeulen *et al.*, 1971; Vermeulen, 1973). Androstenedione levels increase to a plateau of about 300 ng/dl (10·5 nmol/l) (Mizuno *et al.*, 1968) with highest level at delivery, whereas both DHEA and DHEA-S levels decrease during pregnancy (Gandy, 1970; Nieschlag, Walk and Schindler, 1974), although the production of both DHEA and DHEA-S is increased; indeed the MCR of DHEA-S is much higher during pregnancy due to utilisation by the placenta for oestrogen formation (Gant *et al.*, 1971). Some androgen levels obtained during pregnancy are given in Table 7.

In amniotic fluid T as well as A levels are higher in male foetuses than in females (Robinson, Judd, Young, Jones and Yenn, 1977; Zondek, Mansfield and Zondek, 1977; Younglai, 1972); the same applies to venous cord blood.

(7) *Physiological factors affecting plasma androgen levels in females.* Except for testosterone, androgens show nycthemeral variations with an amplitude similar to that in males. In the peri-ovulatory period, androgen levels are significantly higher than during the rest of the cycle, probably due to stimulation by LH of androgen secretion by the ovary. Stress causes an increase of adrenal androgen secretion; it can be assumed that levels attained may be similar to values found after a i.v. injection of ACTH.

Table 7

Plasma androgen levels (ng/dl) during pregnancy (M. ± s.D.; for conversion factors see Table 6).

Week of pregnancy	T	% free T	Free T concentration	SHBC cap. (10^{-8} M)	Androstene-dione	DHT	DHEA	DHEA-S (μg/dl)
5–10 (n = 6)	45 ± 10	0·60 ± 0·02	0·40 ± 0·03	18 ± 1	227 ± 57	33 ± 6		
11–20 (n = 20)	65 ± 20	0·40 ± 0·17	0·25 ± 0·12	34 ± 15	237 ± 50	34 ± 8	334 ± 148	76 ± 39
21–30 (n = 11)	72 ± 31	0·37 ± 0·18	0·29 ± 0·07	39 ± 15	271 ± 76	37·8 ± 15		
30–term (n = 8)	56 ± 22	0·39 ± 0·21	0·24 ± 0·15	45 ± 21	282 ± 78	43 ± 12		

F. PHARMACOLOGICAL FACTORS AFFECTING
ANDROGEN LEVELS

1. Males

Chorionic gonadotrophin in a dose of 1500–5000 u/d for three days or longer doubles basal T and DHT levels and production rates (Kirschner *et al.*, 1965; Rivarola *et al.*, 1966; Vermeulen, 1968), increases androstenedione levels by about 50% and androstenediol levels by about 75%; in elderly males the relative increase is similar, but the absolute increase is lower than in younger males. As expected, as they have an almost exclusive adrenal origin, DHEA and DHEA-S levels remain uninfluenced by HCG stimulation (Rubens, Dhont and Vermeulen, 1974; Vermeulen and Verdonck, 1976a; Pirke *et al.*, 1977). In pre-pubertal boys as well as in hypogonadotropic hypogonadism a more prolonged stimulation with HCG may be required before maximal elevation of T levels is obtained (Vermeulen, 1974).

LH-RH in a continuous infusion causes a 50% elevation of T (and oestradiol) levels about 6 hr after the start of the infusion (Kley, Wiegelmann, Nieschlag, Solbach, Zimmerman and Krüskemper, 1974).

Androgens, both natural and synthetic, produce a dose-related fall in LH and in T secretion (Lipsett, Wilson, Kirschner, Korenman, Fishman, Sarfaty and Bardin, 1966). This effect is also observed with synthetic non-aromatisable anabolic steroids and androgens (DHT), although the latter are not as efficient as T (Davis, Lipsett and Korenman, 1965; Lipsett *et al.*, 1966; Sherins and Loriaux, 1973).

Testosterone administered in a pharmacological dose orally is largely inactivated by the liver. Nevertheless, 1–3% escapes hepatic metabolism and after a single dose of 100–200 mg by mouth, a significant increase in T levels, lasting for 8–12 hr, may be observed (Vermeulen, 1976c). This escape and increase in T levels is more important in women and hypogonadic males than in normal men (Johnsen, Bennett and Jensen, 1974; Vermeulen, 1976b, c; Føgh, Corker, McLean, Bruunshuus-Petersen, Philip and Skakke-baek, 1978), and Nieschlag, Cuppers and Wickings (1977) did not even observe any increase in normal men. Oral testosterone appears to induce hepatic drug-metabolising enzymes including those metabolising testosterone (Johnsen, Kampmann, Bennett and Schønau-Jørgensen, 1976).

Oestrogens cause a decrease in LH and in T levels (Stewart-Bentley, Odell and Horton, 1974) even when infused in physiological doses. Moreover, as oestrogen receptors have been found in Leydig cells (Mulder *et al.*, 1974), it is possible that by a direct effect they modulate Leydig cell functions.

Moreover, oestrogens increase SHBG levels, decrease the free T fraction and MCR and also influence T metabolism (Clark, Carson, DeLory, Clemow and Bird, 1973; Mauvais Jarvis, Bercovici and Floch, 1964).

Progestogens also inhibit LH secretion and hence plasma T levels decrease; as they decrease SHBG and increase 5α-hepatic reductase activity, MCR of T increases (Gordon, Southren, Tochimoto, Olivo, Altman, Rand and Lemberger, 1970).

Cyproterone acetate, a potent progestogen, inhibits LH secretion and decreases plasma T levels; this substance, however, also inhibits ACTH secretion in children and hence adrenal androstenedione, DHEA and DHEA-S secretion (Girard and Baumann, 1977); moreover, by competing for T receptors, it has an anti-androgen effect.

Antioestrogens by their competing effect for the hypothalamic receptor, cause LH-RH release, resulting in increased T levels. After short term (10 day) use of the antioestrogen tamoxifen (20 mg/day), the increase in T levels is moderate (ca 40%) but in long term use (one month or more), T levels are almost doubled. A similar effect is seen with Clomiphene at a dose of 100–150 mg/day (Vermeulen and Comhaire, 1978). The antiandrogen, cyproterone, also causes LH-RH release resulting in increased T levels.

Corticosteroids cause a decrease of plasma T levels by abolishing or flattening the nocturnal rise in testosterone (Doerr and Pirke, 1976).

Spironolactone inhibits testicular cytochrome P 450 and hence T biosynthesis (Menard, Stripp and Gillette, 1974), and secretion (Dymling, Nilsson and Hökfelt, 1972) but by interfering with receptor binding it has also a peripheral anti-androgenic action (Bonne and Raynaud, 1974; Corvol, Michaud, Menard, Freifeld and Mahoudeau, 1975).

Metyrapone causes within 2–8 hr of administration, a decrease of T and an increase of androstenedione levels; these effects may be secondary to increased ACTH secretion (Nilsson and Hökfelt, 1971).

Ethanol abuse lowers plasma T levels significantly (Van Thiel, Gavaler, Lester and Goodman, 1975), decreases SHBG levels, increases hepatic 5α-reductase activity and the MCR of testosterone. Blood production rate of T is, however, decreased (Gordon, Altman, Southren, Rubin and Lieber, 1976). Huttunen, Härkönen, Niskanen, Leino and Ylikahri (1976) on the other hand observed normal T levels in chronic alcoholics.

The influence of drug addiction on plasma androgen levels is controversial. Azizi, Vagenakis, Ingbar and Braverman (1973), as well as Mendelson, Mendelson and Patel (1975) observed decreased T levels in heroin and methadon addicts, which returned, however, to normal during protracted abstinence (Mendelson and Mello, 1975). Cushman (1973) found no influence of these drugs on plasma T levels. Marihuana does not seem to affect Leydig cell function (Mendelson, Kuehnle, Ellingboe and Babor, 1974).

Anti-epileptic drugs (phenylhydantoins) increase SHBG capacity and, indirectly, T levels (Bäckström and Södergård, 1977).

Barbiturates, although increasing hydroxylation of T, affect neither T levels nor MCR (Southren, Gordon, Tochimoto, Krikun and Krieger, 1969).

Corticosteroids (dexamethasone) have been claimed to inhibit testicular T biosynthesis. By blocking ACTH secretion they cause a significant decrease in androstenedione, DHEA and DHEA-S levels.

Lithium therapy has been claimed to lower plasma T levels by Sanchez, Murthy, Mehta, Shreeve and Singh (1974), but this could not be confirmed by Sheard, Marini and Giddings (1977).

Adrenaline was reported by Levin, Lloyd, Lobotsky and Friedreich (1967) to decrease T plasma levels and production rates without affecting the MCR.

2. Females

ACTH in women causes an important increase in androstenedione, DHEA and, after prolonged stimulation, of DHEA-S plasma levels. T levels increase slightly via peripheral conversion of adrenal prohormones (Vermeulen, 1976b).

Dexamethasone, by blocking ACTH secretion, causes a decrease of androstenedione, DHEA-S, androstenediol, and indirectly of T levels (Abraham and Chakmakjian, 1973; Kim et al., 1974, 1976) (Table 8).

Triamcinolone-acetonide in a dose of 25 mg inhibits ovulation by hypo-thalamic suppression and possibly by a direct effect on the ovary: hence the cyclical variations in androgen levels disappear (Cunningham, Goldzieher, de la Pena and Oliver, 1978).

Oestrogens alone are poor suppressants of LH and hence of ovarian androgen secretion (Givens, Andersen, Wiser, Umstot and Fish, 1976; Kirschner, Bardin, Hembree and Ross, 1970). They are claimed to inhibit adrenal Δ4,5-isomerase-3β-hydroxysteroid-dehydrogenase which might lead to increased secretion of Δ5-steroids accompanied by a decrease of the secretion of androstenedione.

Progestagens, either alone (Vermeulen, Dhondt, Thiery and Vande-kerckhove, 1976) or in combination with oestrogens, cause better suppression of ovarian androgen secretion when given for at least three weeks (Givens, Andersen, Wiser, Umstot and Fish, 1976).

Progestagens are reported to inhibit tissue 5α-reductase (Mauvais Jarvis, Charransol and Bobas-Masson, 1973); hence a decrease in DHT and androstanediol levels may be expected although no data have been reported so far.

hCG in a dose of 5000 u/day for five days during the luteal phase of the

Table 8

Influence of dexamethasone (3×1 mg dd. -5 day) on plasma androgens (ng/dl; M. $\pm$ s.D.; for conversion factors see Table 6).

	Basal values			Dexamethasone treatment		
	F	M	L	F	M	L
T	34 ± 5	42 ± 7	38 ± 6	20 ± 3	22 ± 4	20 ± 4
DHT	23 ± 4	26 ± 4	24 ± 4	10 ± 3	12 ± 4	13 ± 3
Androstenedione	142 ± 66	220 ± 45	120 ± 24	93 ± 20	120 ± 12	75 ± 14
DHEA	550 ± 90	550 ± 74	520 ± 66	85 ± 22	80 ± 16	91 ± 18
DHEA-S (μg/dl)	89 ± 36	88 ± 30	82 ± 39	35 ± 5	35 ± 10	34 ± 5
Androstenediol	73 ± 12	75 ± 8	68 ± 13	15 ± 14	17 ± 4	16 ± 3

F = Follicular phase; M = midcycle (LH peak $\pm$ 2 day); L = luteal phase.

cycle and in post-menopausal women, eventually causes a moderate increase in plasma androgens (Table 9).

Metyrapone has an effect similar to ACTH, whereas cyproterone acetate inhibits LH (Petry, Mauss, Rausch-Strooman and Vermeulen, 1972) and ACTH (Girard and Baumann, 1975) secretion and hence lowers both ovarian and adrenal androgen secretion.

G. ANDROGEN EXCESS

Androgen excess in the female leads to virilisation. This is characterised by seborrhea and hirsutism (which often is the only sign of virilisation), clitoral hypertrophy, deepening of the voice, bitemporal balding and male body build. In some cases, hirsutism, i.e. increased growth of terminal hair in the face, the extremities or the body with male distribution of pubic hair, may occur in the presence of normal androgen levels. As antiandrogen treatment may result in regression of this hirsutism, an increased sensitivity of the tissues for androgens may be a cause of virilisation. The source of the excessive androgen levels may be the adrenal, the ovary or both, either directly or by way of secretion of precursors converted peripherally in active androgens.

In males, androgen excess will rarely cause clinical symptoms except in infants and children where the androgen excess may cause rapid development of growth, muscle development and bone maturation as well as development of secondary sex characteristics, causing the syndrome of constitutional sexual precocity and precocious pseudopuberty.

1. Adrenal Androgen Excess

(a) Congenital adrenal hyperplasia

This group of inherited disorders of cortisol synthesis is the commonest cause of congenital virilisation; it is due to an enzyme block in the biosynthetic chain leading from cholesterol to cortisol. In girls it causes foetal masculinisation and pseudohermaphroditism; in boys it may lead to constitutional sexual precocity and later to precocious puberty. Three enzymatic defects lead to excessive androgen secretion: 21-hydroxylase, 11-hydroxylase and the $\Delta 4,5$ isomerase-3β-hydroxysteroid-dehydrogenase deficiency.

The 21-hydroxylase deficiency is by far the most frequent variety. It leads to an increased secretion of 17-hydroxyprogesterone with moderately increased testosterone and androstenedione levels (Degenhart, Visser, Wilmink and Exley, 1966; McKenna, Jennings, Liddle and Burr, 1976).

T and androstenedione production rates are manyfold increased in the untreated state, further increased after ACTH stimulation and markedly suppressed by dexamethasone; the increased T production is the consequence of the conversion of secreted androstenedione (Horton and Frasier, 1967).

The 11-hydroxylase deficiency occurs much less frequently; it leads to an increased secretion of 11-deoxycortisol and deoxycorticosterone (the cause of hypertension) and indirectly to increased androgen secretion. Like the 21-hydroxylase deficiency it causes masculinisation of the female foetus with pseudohermaphroditism. Few data are available concerning androgen levels. Sizonenko, Schindler, Kohlberg and Paunier (1972) reported two girls with testosterone-like substances in the normal adult male range whereas Jänne, Perheentupa, Viinikka and Vihko (1975) reported a 16-yr-old girl with normal plasma T levels.

The least frequent variety is the $\Delta 4,5$ isomerase-3β-hydroxysteroid dehydrogenase deficiency. Here there exists a block in the formation of $\Delta 4$-steroids leading in males to incomplete virilisation at birth, with often perineoscrotal hypospadias; the defect is less pronounced at the testicular level and at puberty T levels may be almost normal (Schneider et al., 1975). Plasma levels of DHEA and its sulphate are greatly increased (Parks, Bermudez, Anast, Bongiovanni and New, 1971; Jänne, Perheentuppa, Viinikka and Vihko, 1974; Rosenfield, Barmach de Niepomicsze, Kenny and Genel, 1974). In girls this enzyme defect causes less pronounced virilisation than either the 21- or the 11-hydroxylase deficiency.

(b) Cushing's syndrome

Cushing's syndrome is the consequence of excessive plasma corticosteroid levels. In women, some manifestations of androgen excess (hirsutism, amenorrhea) nearly always accompany this hypercortisolism, although they are generally mild. In women with Cushing's syndrome due to bilateral adrenal hyperplasia, androgen levels, including testosterone, are generally elevated, a consequence of direct adrenal secretion but probably mainly of peripheral conversion of androstenedione (Dignam, Pion, Lamb & Simmer, 1964; Smals, Kloppenborg and Benraad, 1977); in men, however, T levels are generally moderately decreased (Smals et al., 1977).

(c) Adrenal tumours

Adrenal tumours causing Cushing's syndrome give androgen levels rather similar to those observed in adrenal hyperplasia except for the carcinomas which often but not always cause a considerable increase in DHEA and DHEA-S secretion (Bardin, Lipsett and French, 1968).

Virilising adrenal tumours are very rare and are biochemically characterised by increased T, androstenedione, DHEA and DHEA-S production, the latter being often enormously increased in adrenal carcinoma (Baulieu, 1962; Saez, Rivarola and Migeon, 1967). Virilising adenomata generally secrete androstenedione and testosterone (Werk, Sholiton and Kaleis, 1973; Larson, Vander Laan, Judd and McCullough, 1976), in which case urinary excretion of 17-oxosteroids is generally normal or moderately increased, but testosterone glucuronide excretion is high; occasionally DHEA-S appears to be secreted (Leichter and Daughaday, 1974), in which case 17-oxosteroid excretion may be extremely high. Some of these adenomata are LH-dependent, oestrogen administration resulting in a decrease of plasma LH and testosterone (Werk *et al.*, 1973; Larson *et al.*, 1976; Lipsett, 1973). This gonadotrophin dependence suggests that some of these tumours might have a testicular origin (Larson *et al.*, 1976).

(d) Prolactinoma

In patients with prolactinoma and in chronic pharmacologically induced hyperprolactinemia (Bassi *et al.*, 1977; Vermeulen *et al.*, 1977; Vermeulen and Ando, 1978) increased DHEA and DHEA-S plasma levels and secretion have been observed. These appear to have an adrenal origin. This stimulation of DHEA-S secretion occurs only in the presence of ACTH. It is suggested that prolactin might interfere with the $\Delta4,5$-isomerase-3β-hydroxysteroid dehydrogenase activity.

2. Ovarian Androgen Excess

(a) Virilising ovarian tumours

Masculinising ovarian tumours are rare. Essentially, the following histological types may produce virilisation: arrhenoblastoma, hilus-cell (Leydig cell) tumour, adrenal-like tumours (luteoma or masculinovoblastoma), gynandroblastoma and thecoma.

The histogenesis of these tumours is still highly controversial and based on studies of the normal ovary. Arrhenoblastomas are considered to be derived from the rete ovarii (Meyer, 1931); hilar cell tumours (Leydig cell tumours) strongly resemble the interstitial cells of the testes, whereas adrenal rest tumours would derive from adrenal-like cells found in the ovary, probably a consequence of the common embryonic origin of adrenal and ovary. These tumours may secrete important amounts of androgens, mainly androstenedione and/or T. Plasma T levels in excess of 200 ng/dl (7·0 nmol/l) in women are practically always associated with either an adrenal or an ovarian androgen-secreting tumour (Finkelstein, Forchielli and Dorfman, 1961; Dignam *et al.*, 1964; Coppage and Cooner, 1965).

LH-dependence of androgen levels does not prove an ovarian origin, as several LH-responsive adrenal tumours have been described (Werk *et al.*, 1973; Larson *et al.*, 1976; Lipsett, 1973; Givens, Andersen, Wiser, Coleman and Fish, 1974).

17-Oxosteroid excretion is generally only moderately increased or even normal, a consequence of the fact that generally secretion of DHEA and DHEA-S, the main precursors of urinary 17-oxosteroids, is normal and that moderate increases in plasma T levels, which may cause marked virilisation, have only a slight effect on urinary 17-oxosteroid excretion.

(b) *Polycystic ovary syndrome (PCO)*

Stein and Leventhal (1935) described a syndrome characterised by oligo-menorrhea, hirsutism and obesity, together with palpable enlarged poly-cystic ovaries. Stein (1964), with 34 years experience, found only 108 patients that satisfied these criteria, and when one adheres to his strict criteria, the Stein-Leventhal syndrome is rare. This precise clinical entity has since, however, disappeared, the name Stein-Leventhal syndrome being used indis-criminatingly for a variety of disorders characterised by various combinations of some or all of the symptoms originally described by Stein and Leventhal (1935). The finding of enlarged polycystic ovaries with a thickened ovarian capsule is no longer considered to be obligatory as not all polycystic ovaries with the typical hyperplasia of the theca interna appear to be enlarged; hirsutism is present in only half of the patients; obesity is a common but not a consistent finding; anovulatory oligomenorrhea is a diagnostic criterion but sometimes only a luteal phase deficiency can be detected, and, rarely, even regular ovulatory menses occur!

In the view of the vague delineation of the syndrome, it is not surprising that there does not appear to exist a common pathogenetic mechanism. In the majority of patients with PCO syndrome, moderately increased androgen plasma levels (androstenedione, T. DHEA, singly or in combination) and production rates are found (Greenblatt and Mahesh, 1976; Horton and Neisler, 1968; Bardin and Lipsett, 1967).

The increase in T production (M: 1·2 mg compared with 0·23 mg in normals; Bardin and Lipsett, 1967) is the cause of increased T levels, but also of a decrease in SHBG levels (Dray *et al.*, 1968; Southren *et al.*, 1969; Vermeulen *et al.*, 1969; Rosenfield, Ehrlich and Cleary, 1972; Judd, Rigg, Anderson and Yen, 1976), resulting in an increased MCR (Bardin and Lipsett, 1967). Mahesh and Greenblatt (1962) on the basis of excessive DHEA concentrations in ovarian tissue and ovarian vein blood, have suggested as primary patho-genetic mechanism the existence of a block of the $\Delta4,5$ isomerase 3β-hydroxy-steroid-dehydrogenase. However, the most commonly observed abnormality is an increase in plasma androstenedione levels and production rates (Bardin and Lipsett, 1967; Horton and Neisler, 1968; Baird, Corker, Davidson, Hunter, Michie and Van Look, 1977). LH levels are also generally increased, whereas oestrogen levels are normal or even increased (Jeffcoate, Brooks, London, Smith, Spathis and Prunty, 1968), especially oestrone, probably a consequence of the conversion of androstenedione. It has been suggested that these increased LH levels might constitute the primary pathology in PCO (Yen, Vela and Rankin, 1970; Patton, Berger, Thompson, Chang, Grimes and Taylor, 1975; Scaglia, Medina, Gual, Cabeza and Perez-Palacios, 1976); others, however, believe that the increased LH levels are secondary to excessive and prolonged extraglandular production of oestrone from androstenedione (Baird *et al.*, 1977) exerting a positive feedback on LH secretion; indeed lowering of androstenedione levels by whatever means, has often resulted in resumption of normal ovulatory cycles.

Besides an increased ovarian androgen secretion, adrenal androgen secretion may also be increased (Bardin, Hembree and Lipsett, 1968; Greenblatt and Mahesh, 1976; Horton and Neisler, 1968). It is known that hyperandrogenism due to adrenal androgen secretion may lead to pathological findings indistinguishable from PCO (Greenblatt and Mahesh, 1976). As there is some evidence that when endogenous LH levels are increased in cases of PCO, the response of androgen levels to HCG may be absent (Givens *et al.*, 1976a), the detection of the origin of the excessive androgen secretion is still further complicated. Wedge resection often results only in a very temporary (three days) decrease of androstenedione levels, sometimes with perhaps a persistent reduction in T secretion (Judd *et al.* 1976).

In patients with ovarian hyperthecosis (diffuse luteinisation of the ovarian stroma), the ovaries may secrete important amounts of T, approaching the production rate in males (Bardin, Lipsett, Edgcomb and Marshall, 1967) sometimes causing severe virilisation.

(c) *Idiopathic hirsutism*

In a large group of patients with isolated hirsutism, eventually accompanied with obesity and oligo- or amenorrhea, moderately increased androgen levels and production rates are observed, without any clear-cut enzymatic (congenital adrenal hyperplasia) or anatomical abnormality (adrenal or ovarian tumour) being found. This group is often called idiopathic hirsutism, although dysfunctional hirsutism would be a better name, idiopathic hirsutism being reserved for those cases of hirsutism in which no increased androgen levels are found; the latter comprises about 5–10% of cases of hirsutism.

It is remarkable that often plasma T and/or DHT levels are normal, whereas the levels of their precursors (androstenedione, DHEA, DHEA-S, androstenediol) are significantly increased. Abraham, Maroulis, Buster, Chang and Marschall (1976) in a group of 59 women with various degrees of hirsutism, found T levels increased in 53%, DHT in 72%, DHEA-S levels in 75%, DHEA in 41% and androstenedione in 41%. In seven (12%) all five parameters were increased, in 15 cases four parameters were increased whereas in only one case was a single parameter (T) increased. In all subjects studied at least one of the androgen levels was elevated. It should be stressed that androgens are secreted episodically, and that concentrations may vary within a wide range over a short period; moreover plasma levels show important nycthemeral variations. Hence several plasma samples should be taken over the 24 hr to evaluate the androgenic state of an individual.

When total T or DHT plasma levels are normal, determination of the free androgen fraction may show an elevation of the biologically active androgen concentration (Dray et al., 1968; Vermeulen et al., 1969; Southren et al., 1969). The site of the increased androgen secretion is generally deduced from the response of the hormone levels to dexamethasone suppression and to HCG stimulation; alternatively they may be determined from venous catheterisation studies. The results of the suppression and stimulation tests should, however, be interpreted cautiously. Tumours generally do not respond, but ovarian androgen secretion may be partly dexamethasone-suppressible. Moreover the existence of an ACTH-independent adrenal androgen secretion has been postulated (Kirschner and Jacobs, 1971; Kirschner et al., 1973; Kirschner, Zucker and Jespersen, 1976; Givens, Andersen, Ragland, Wiser and Umstot, 1975).

Catheterisation studies are also subject to criticism, the approach being complex and the assumptions underlying the interpretation of the results, being not necessarily correct.

Most studies suggest that increased peripheral conversion of precursors alone does not explain the increased T levels in hirsutism and postulate an increased glandular secretion (Bardin and Lipsett, 1967; Kirschner et al., 1973); nevertheless studies in the author's laboratory suggest that an increased conversion may be responsible for part of the increased androgen level, as the peripheral conversion of T to plasma DHT was observed to be a function of the free T fraction.

In a small group of cases of idiopathic hirsutism normal free androgen levels and production rates are found, which suggest an increased sensitivity of the target tissues for androgens as a cause of virilisation. This could be a consequence of an increased number of androgen receptors or of increased enzymatic activities at the target level. As most of the biological effects of T require its prior reduction to DHT, one can imagine that an increased local transformation to DHT might account for the hirsutism, and in as far as DHT is not necessarily an end metabolite appearing in plasma, this might not show up in peripheral plasma levels. Mauvais-Jarvis *et al.* (1973) have suggested that urinary androstanediol excretion might be a good parameter of this androgen formation at the target level. Even when the source of the increased androgen level has been detected, the physiopathological mechanism underlying this androgen secretion remains to be elucidated.

Except in cases where a tumour or a congenital adrenal hyperplasia can be detected, the physiopathological mechanism remains largely hypothetical. Even if one accepts increased ovarian androstenedione secretion leading to high oestrone levels, with secondary increased LH secretion to be the responsible mechanism in the PCO syndrome, the reason for the primarily increased androstenedione secretion remains to be elucidated. Since the excessive adrenal androgen secretion is unaccompanied by increased cortisol secretion, one has to postulate either an enzyme defect in the biosynthetic chain from cholesterol to cortisol or inhibition of one of the enzymes by an unknown factor.

As to an enzyme defect as cause of increased androgen secretion in idiopathic hirsutism, Newmark, Dluhy, Williams, Pochi and Rose (1977) conclude that there is a partial 11- and/or 21-hydroxylase defect in 13 out of 31 hirsute women, whereas Fleetwood *et al.* (1974) on the basis of pregnanetriol excretion values during combined ACTH and metyrapone administration found evidence for a partial 21-hydroxylase deficiency in eight out of ten hirsute patients. Data of Maroulis, Manlimos, Garza and Abraham (1976), on the other hand, suggest that even a minor 11-hydroxylase deficiency is not a common occurrence in patients with hirsutism, and Anderson, Child and Bu'lock (1977) consider that only one out of 35 to 44 hirsute women might have a heterozygous 21-hydroxylase deficiency. The question may moreover be raised whether, with the methodology used at present, it is possible to detect heterozygous carriers. Indeed Childs, Grumbach and Van Wyck (1956); Hall, Smith and Harkness (1970) as well as Bongiovanni (1971) found that even in parents of children with CAH, who are obligatory heterozygotes for the enzyme defect, a significantly greater increase of 17 OH-progesterone and 21-deoxycortisol secretion on ACTH stimulation compared with controls is not always observed.

As to inhibitors of certain enzyme activities, no such factor has been identified so far. However, because of the increased adrenal DHEA and DHEA-S secretion in patients with prolactinoma and other hyperprolactinaemic states (Bassi *et al.*, 1977; Vermeulen *et al.*, 1977; Vermeulen and Ando, 1978), prolactin might be an inhibitor of the $\Delta4,5$ isomerase-3β-hydroxysteroid dehydrogenase system. Although intermittently increased prolactin levels have been reported in many cases of hirsutism (Schneider, Bohnet and Mühlenstedt, 1977) and in PCO (Jaffee, Russell, Longcope and Vaitukaitis, 1978), further studies are necessary to ascertain the role, if any, of prolactin in hirsutism.

H. ANDROGEN DEFICIENCY

As androgens are substances that induce, regulate and maintain differentiation, development and function of the male reproduction tract and male sex characteristics, it is evident that the consequences of androgen deficiency will be different whether it occurs before or after completion of sexual differentiation. Moreover, as androgens have also anabolic effects, androgen deficiency will in addition be characterised by lack of muscle development, delayed closing of epiphyseal growth lines, and eventually decrease in bone mass. As the role of androgens in females is poorly understood, deficiency states will be only evident in males.

1. Congenital Adrenal Deficiency

Androgens are not necessary for the differentiation of the gonadal primordium into a testis. They are, however, necessary for the differentiation of the Wolffian duct, urogenital sinus tubercles and labioscrotal swellings. Hence, inadequate levels of, or insensitivity of the tissues to androgens during the foetal period of sexual differentiation will lead to atrophic epididymis, ductus deferens and seminal vesicles, whereas the structures derived from the genital tubercle and sinus will develop in the female direction. Gonads will, however, be differentiated in the male direction and the Müllerian structures will regress normally except in pure XY gonadal dysgenesis (Swyer syndrome) where no Müllerian inhibiting factor is formed.

(a) Enzyme deficiencies

Four enzyme defects may lead to androgen deficiency: 17-hydroxylase; 17,20 desmolase (lyase); $\Delta4,5$ isomerase-3β-hydroxysteroid dehydrogenase and 17β-hydroxysteroid dehydrogenase (17-oxoreductase) deficiency. In $\Delta4,5$ isomerase-3β-hydroxysteroid deficiency there exists a block in the formation of $\Delta4$-steroids and hence testosterone, leading in males to incomplete virilisation at birth often with perineoscrotal hypospadias. The defect is generally less pronounced at the testicular than at the adrenal level and at puberty testosterone levels may be almost normal (Schneider et al., 1975). Plasma levels of $\Delta5$-steroids (DHEA, 17-hydroxy-pregnenolone and pregnenolone and their sulphates) are greatly increased (Parks et al., 1971;

Jänne *et al.*, 1974, 1975; Rosenfield *et al.*, 1974).

In 17-hydroxylase deficiency, both androgen and oestrogen biosynthesis are impaired (Biglieri, Hirson and Brust, 1966) both in the gonads and in the adrenals and the phenotype is female. As the synthesis and secretion of deoxycorticosterone is increased, there exists hypertension and hypokalaemic alkalosis.

In the extremely rare 17-20-lyase deficiency (Zachman, Völlmin, Hamilton and Prader, 1972) neither androgens nor oestrogens are formed; again the phenotype is female.

In the 17-oxosteroid reductase deficiency, the final step in testosterone biosynthesis, reduction of androstenedione to T, is impaired: hence androstenedione levels and production rates are extremely high (Saez, de Peretti, Morera, David and Bertrand, 1971; Tourniaire, Audi, Parera, Loras, Blum, Castelnovo and Forest, 1976).

(b) Defects of androgen action

After entering the target cell, testosterone is generally enzymatically reduced to DHT, which subsequently combines with the androgen receptor. Absence or decrease of androgen receptors is the cause of the testicular feminisation syndrome (Bardin *et al.*, 1973). In the complete syndrome the phenotype is completely female. Testes are found in the inguinal canal or in the labia majora; development of sexual and axillary hair is completely absent, notwithstanding high male testosterone levels. The SHBG capacity is increased, the free T fraction is decreased but the free T concentration is nearly normal, whereas the MCR is in the female range (Southren *et al.*, 1965). As a consequence of the unresponsiveness to androgens of the hypothalamus, gonadotropin levels are moderately increased, notwithstanding high oestradiol levels.

In the incomplete syndrome (incomplete pseudohermaphroditism type I; Wilson, Harrod, Goldstein, Hemsell and MacDonald, 1974) the receptor is present but in reduced quantity. Various names have been associated with this syndrome, e.g. Reifenstein, Gilbert Dreyfus and Rosewater. The clinical picture is characterised by a variable degree of scrotal malfusion, with hypospadias, diminished facial and axillary hair and more or less pronounced eunuchoid proportions. Plasma T and LH levels vary from normal to high.

In the steroid 5α-reductase deficiency (type II incomplete male pseudohermaphroditism) syndrome, target tissues lack the ability to form DHT and organs that need DHT for differentiation, i.e. organs derived from the urogenital sinus and tubercle will not differentiate in the male direction (Imperato McGinley, Guerrero, Gauthier and Peterson, 1974). Plasma T

levels are normal but DHT levels are extremely low, whereas in the urine
5β-metabolites dominate largely over 5α-metabolites.

(c) Klinefelter's syndrome

Although Leydig cell hyperplasia is regularly found in Klinefelter's syndrome,
T levels are generally decreased or in the low normal range (Lipsett, Davis,
Wilson and Canfield, 1965; Lipsett et al., 1966; Smals, Kloppenborg and
Benraad, 1975; Raboch, Neuwirth and Starka, 1975; Wang, Baker, Burger,
de Kretser and Hudson, 1975); moreover, the response to HCG stimulation
is generally impaired (Smals, Kloppenborg and Benraad, 1974; Steward-
Bentley and Horton, 1973).

2. Acquired Androgen Deficiency

In Leydig cell hypoplasia, presenting as a phenotypic female, T and
androstenedione levels are low, and the response to HCG extremely weak
(Brown, Markland and Dehner, 1978; Berthezenc, Forest, Grimaud,
Claessen and Mornex, 1976). Similarly in anorchia, T levels are low, in the
prepubertal range, and do not increase upon HCG stimulation (Aynsley,
Green, Zachmann, Illig, Rampirii and Prader, 1976; Vermeulen, 1973).

It is evident that in all cases of either primary or secondary hypogonadism,
plasma T levels, free T concentration (Vermeulen et al., 1971) and T production
rates are decreased. It is not possible to discuss these conditions at length, it
suffices to mention that in secondary pituitary hypogonadism, prolonged
HCG stimulation causes a normal increase in T levels, whereas in primary
gonadal insufficiency the response to HCG is decreased.

In adenocortical insufficiency, DHEA and DHEA-S levels are extremely
low, whereas in women androstenedione and T levels are also lower than
normal (Abraham and Chakmakjian, 1973).

I. PLASMA ANDROGENS IN NON-ENDOCRINE DISEASES

1. Hyperthyroidism

Dray, Sebaoun, Mowszowicz, Delzan, Dergez and Dreyfus (1967) reported
that in hyperthyroidism T levels are greatly increased in both males and
females, a consequence of an increased SHBG capacity. These results have
since been confirmed by several authors. As a consequence of this increase
in SHBG, with a decreased free fraction but normal free T concentration,
the MCR of T is decreased. The blood production rate of T is, however,

normal (Gordon, Southren, Tochimoto, Rand and Olivo, 1969; Vermeulen *et al.*, 1969; Chopra and Tulchinsky, 1974). The peripheral conversion of androstenedione to oestrone is increased, as is the conversion of oestrone to oestradiol, the conversion of T to oestradiol being normal; as a consequence the oestradiol levels are increased, as is the free oestradiol/T ratio (Chopra and Tulchinsky, 1974; Southren, Olivo, Gordon, Vittek, Brener and Rafii, 1974; Vermeulen, 1976a).

2. Cirrhosis of the Liver

Most authors have found low plasma T levels (Southren, Gordon, Olivo, Rafii and Rosenthal, 1973; Chopra, Tulchinsky and Greenway, 1973; Kley, Nieschlag, Wiegelmann, Solbach and Krüskemper, 1975; Van Thiel, Lester and Sherins, 1974; Galvao Teles, Anderson, Burke and Marshall, 1973) as well as increased SHBG levels and T binding in cirrhotics (Breuer, Schneider and Breuer, 1970; Rosenbaum, Christy and Kelly, 1966; Rosenfield, 1971) but others (Baker, Dulmanis, Hudson, Paulsen, Purcell and Woinarski, 1972; Kley *et al.*, 1975) observed variable levels of SHBG. Androstenedione levels are elevated (Kley *et al.*, 1975; Vermeulen *et al.*, 1972a) and its conversion to oestrone and oestradiol appears to be significantly increased with variable oestradiol levels (Vermeulen *et al.*, 1972a; Vermeulen, 1976a; Gordon, Olivo, Rafii and Southren, 1975). The ratio of oestradiol to testosterone is generally elevated (Chopra, Tulchinsky and Greenway, 1973; Vermeulen *et al.*, 1972a; Baker, Burger, de Kretser, Dulmanis, Hudson, O'Connor, Paulsen, Purcell, Rennie, Seach, Taft and Wang, 1976). Kley, Nieschlag and Krüskemper (1975) reported a decreased response of T secretion to HCG stimulation.

3. Renal Insufficiency

In terminal renal insufficiency T levels are generally decreased (Chen, Vidt, Zorn, Hallberg and Wieland, (1970), MCR is increased and BPR is low (Corvol, Bertagna and Bedrossian, 1974). LH levels are generally high, supporting a primary testicular origin of the low T levels (Chen *et al.*, 1970). The response to HCG stimulation is often subnormal (Stewart, Bentley, Gans and Horton, 1974; Rager, Bundschu and Gupta, 1975; Lim and Fang, 1975). Bundschu, Rager, Heller, Hayduk, Pfeiffer, Lüders and Liebau (1976) reported high DHT and androstanediol levels in these patients.

o

J. ANALYTICAL METHODS

1. Androgens in Blood

Early analytical methods, based upon fluorimetry (Finkelstein *et al.*, 1961) or gas-liquid chromatography with electron capture detection (Brownie, Van der Molen, Nishizawa and Eik-Nes, 1964; Vermeulen, 1967) used for the determination of androgens in plasma are now largely of historical interest only. Even double isotope derivative methods (Hudson, Coghlan, Dulmanis, Wintour and Ekkel, 1963; Riondel, Tait, Gut, Tait, Jaochim and Little, 1963; Burger, Ken and Kellie, 1964) which for a long time have been considered as reference methods, are now outdated. The same applies to competitive protein-binding methods using plasma SHBG (Horton, Kato and Sherins, 1967), which are now replaced by the more specific and more sensitive radioimmunological methods (Furuyama, Mayes and Nugent, 1968).

For testosterone the most frequently used antibodies have been obtained by the immunisation of rabbits with either testosterone-3-carboxy methyl-oxime-bovine serum albumin (testosterone-3CMO-BSA) (Furuyama *et al.*, 1970; Ismail, Niswender and Midgley, 1972; Kinouchi, Pages and Horton, 1973) or testosterone-11-CMO-BSA (Joyce, Fahmy and Hillier, 1975).

So far no completely specific antibody against testosterone has been obtained. All methods require therefore prior extraction of steroids from plasma with an organic solvent, generally diethylether or dichloromethane. Most testosterone antibodies cross-react with dihydrotestosterone, but the affinity for the latter is generally less than 60% of the affinity for testosterone. Since DHT concentration in males is only *ca* one-tenth of the testosterone concentration and as T and DHT levels generally vary in parallel, for clinical purposes RIA of T may be performed on the crude extract, the value obtained being little higher than the true T concentration. With this technique the so called "17β-hydroxyandrogens" are determined.

In women, however, DHT levels are about two-thirds of T levels and considering the low concentration of the latter and that in crude extracts other non-steroid substances may interact with the antibody, a chromatographic purification of the extract prior to RIA is essential to obtain sufficient specificity. The same applies to plasma samples from prepubertal or hypogonadal males. This chromatographic purification may involve a column chromatography on LH 20 (Murphy, 1970), florisil (Abraham, Manlimos, Solis and Wickman, 1975), or alumina (Furuyama *et al.*, 1968), thin-layer chromatography on silica-gel (Nieschlag and Loriaux, 1972), or paper chromatography, in fact any system which separates T from DHT.

DHT after adequate prepurification of the extract is generally determined with the same antibody used for T (Coyotypa, Parlow and Abraham, 1972). Alternatively an antibody raised against a DHT conjugate may be used, but again complete specificity has not yet been obtained (Bauminger, Kohen, Lindner and Weinstein, 1974; Condom and Desfosses, 1977) and in view of the much higher T concentrations, separation of T from DHT remains necessary before performing RIA.

Androstenedione in plasma is generally measured using a specific antibody obtained against androstenedione-6-CMO-BSA (Judd and Yenn, 1973; Vermeulen *et al.*, 1976), prepurification of the extract being generally required.

The same applies for androstanediol; however, in view of the very low concentration of the steroid in male and even more so in female plasma, more extensive purification of the extract is generally necessary in order to obtain a specific determination (Kinouchi and Horton, 1974).

Dehydroepiandrosterone is usually measured using an antibody raised either against DHEA-17-CMO-BSA (Nieschlag, Loriaux and Lipsett, 1972; Hopper and Yen, 1975), or against DHEA-7-CMO-BSA (Rosenfeld, Rosenberg and Hellman, 1975a). The latter antibody has been used on unextracted plasma (Rosenfeld *et al.*, 1975b).

DHEA-S is measured as such, using an antibody raised against DHEA-3-hemisuccinate-BSA (Buster and Abraham, 1972). In the view of the high concentration of DHEA-S (three orders of magnitude higher than the other plasma androgens) DHEA-S may be determined on a crude plasma extract or even on unextracted plasma (Buster and Abraham, 1972). Alternatively the sulphate may be solvolysed (Andre and James, 1973; Sekihara, Ohsawa and Ibayashi, 1972; Nieschlag *et al.*, 1972) and the free DHEA measured as usual; correction for free DHEA present in plasma is not necessary in view of the great difference in concentration between DHEA and its sulphate.

Androst-5-ene-3β-17β-diol may be measured using an antibody against DHEA-17-CMO-BSA (Loriaux and Lipsett, 1972) after adequate chromatographic separation from DHEA, or a specific antibody raised against androst-5-ene-3β-17β-diol coupled in position 16 may be used (Pirke, 1977). In view of the high affinity of SHBG for this steroid it has also been measured by CPB, using diluted plasma as source of binding protein (Rosenfield and Otto, 1972; Demisch *et al.*, 1973).

Free androsterone has rarely been measured in plasma but Gandy and Peterson (1968) described a double isotope dilution technique, and a RIA has been described (Youssefnejadian, Collins and Sommerville, 1970). Androsterone sulphate as well as epiandrosterone sulphate have been measured together with DHEA-S after solvolysis followed by paper-chromatography and a micro-Zimmerman reaction (Oertel and Eik-Nes,

1961; Oertel and Kaiser, 1962; Eberlein, 1963; De Neve and Vermeulen, 1965), and more recently by gas-liquid chromatography (Sandberg, Ahmed, Zachmann and Cleveland, 1965; Panicucci, 1966) eventually coupled with mass spectrometry (GLC-MS; Vihko, 1966). The latter technique, which has also been applied to other androgens (Dehennin, Reiffsteck and Scholler, 1974) is at present probably the most specific, albeit highly sophisticated method. Although applicable with difficulty to routine measurement of plasma steroids, it is an excellent tool for checking the specificity and accuracy of other methods. By judicious use of GLC-MS several steroids can be measured in a single plasma sample, adequate techniques having been described (Abraham *et al.*, 1975; Apter, Yänne, Karvonen and Vihko, 1976; Hammond, Ruokonen, Kontturi, Koskela and Vihko, 1977). Space does not permit discussion at length of the respective advantages and disadvantages of different methods nor to give detailed descriptions of the methodology for which the reader should consult the original publications.

2. Measurement of Production, Conversion and Secretion Rates

Plasma levels of a steroid are the momentary resultant of secretion in blood by the endocrine glands and peripheral converting tissues on the one hand, distribution in the cells and extracellular fluid, metabolism and excretion on the other hand. Changes in any of these determinants will result in changes in plasma steroid levels and as some of these changes may occur very rapidly (steroid secretion for example occurs often episodically and changes in metabolism may occur by change in hepatic blood flow, a consequence of digestion or changes in posture), it is evident that a single determination of plasma steroid levels may give a false impression of the real hormonal state of the individual over 24 hr. This may be obviated by taking multiple samples over 24 hr, eventually by a continuous sampling of blood over 24 hr using a microwithdrawal pump (Kowarski, Thompson, Migeon and Blizzard, 1971). The latter procedure, however, is not very convenient for the patient. Measuring blood production and secretion rates may give a more exact idea of the amount of hormone being actually secreted in the blood over 24 hr. Two different methods may be used for measuring production rates. The urinary method measures the dilution of a tracer amount of labelled steroid in the pool, by determining the cumulative specific activity of an unique urinary metabolite of that steroid (Pearlman, Pearlman and Rakoff, 1954).

It is not appropriate here to discuss at length all requirements for obtaining results reflecting the real production rate. An excellent review of these is available (Tait and Burstein, 1964).

Although testosterone-glucuronide at first sight might be expected to be a unique urinary metabolite of T, and hence its cumulative specific activity would permit calculation of the T production rate. Korenman and Lipsett (1964) have shown that T produced peripherally from precursors such as androstenedione or DHEA is conjugated before entering the plasma pool; hence part of the urinary testosterone glucuronoside does not derive from plasma T and the specific activity of the urinary testosterone glucuronoside is too low, resulting in an overestimation of the T-production rate. The error is especially important in women and hypogonadal males, where peripheral formation of testosterone glucuronoside from precursors is not negligible relative to circulating T; in normal adult males the error remains small. As no other urinary metabolite appears to be a unique metabolite of any of the androgens circulating in blood, the urinary isotope dilution method is not suited for the determination of androgen secretion rates.

In the other method, the clearance rate of labelled hormone from the plasma is determined (Tait, Little, Tait and Flood, 1962). The clearance rate multiplied by the plasma concentration of the hormone gives the blood production rate per unit of time. The latter is the sum of the hormone secreted as such by the endocrine glands and the hormone arising from peripheral conversion of precursors and secreted into the blood. If all precursors are known, the contribution of the latter can be calculated by determining the blood conversion rates and transfer constants, obtained by (simultaneous) infusion of differently labelled precursors. The blood production rate minus the contribution of precursors yields the secretion rate of the steroids (Horton and Tait, 1966). Two techniques may be used for measuring the metabolic clearance rate: the single intravenous injection of labelled steroid and the continuous infusion technique (Tait, 1963) of which the latter is conceptualisticly the more satisfying. This metabolic clearance is generally obtained over a period of 2–4 hr. As both plasma steroid hormone concentration and MCR vary over the nycthemer, production rates obtained cannot be extrapolated over 24 hr. Variations in plasma levels over the nycthemer may be compensated by using the mean plasma level obtained from samples taken every 4–6 hr. Variations in MCR (which in part may be the cause of variations in plasma levels) cannot at present be compensated for. The blood production rate obtained therefore is only an approximation of the real production rate. Excellent reviews of the problems involved in measuring MCR and conversion rates can be found in Tait (1963), Tait and Burstein (1964), Tait and Horton (1966) and Baird et al. (1969).

3. Dynamic Exploration of Androgen Secretion

With the restrictions mentioned above, dynamic tests may be used to deter- mine the source of increased androgen secretion, mainly in the female. In the male, the HCG stimulation test is sometimes performed, essentially for evaluating Leydig cell reserve in Klinefelter's syndrome or for excluding anorchia in bilateral cryptorchidism; absence of increase of plasma T levels confirms the absence of Leydig cell tissue.

(a) Dexamethasone suppression test

Whereas overnight suppression with 1 mg of dexamethasone is a satisfactory screening test to evaluate the suppressibility of cortisol secretion, a longer period of dexamethasone administration is required to suppress adrenal androgen secretion. This is probably related to the long half-life of DHEA-S. Although maximal depression of androgen levels may. not be obtained within this period, five days of adrenal suppression with 3 mg of dexamethasone, with determination of plasma levels at days five and six, permits an evaluation of the adrenal contribution to androgen levels. A correct interpretation of the results requires, however, knowledge of postdexamethasone androgen levels in normal women. As during dexamethasone treatment, cyclical variations in women persist (Abraham and Chakmakjian, 1973; Kim et al., 1974, 1976; Abraham, 1974), results should be interpreted in relation to the menstrual cycle (Table 8).

(b) ACTH stimulation test

The value of the ACTH test for exploring the source of androgen secretion is rather limited and results difficult to interpret (Demisch et al., 1975; Ettinger, Van Werder, Thenaers and Forsham, 1971; Givens et al., 1975). In both males (Vermeulen and Verdonck, 1976a) and females (Vermeulen, 1976b) ACTH causes increases in androgen levels, although in men it decreases T levels. A supranormal reaction, which might point to an adrenal origin of the androgen excess, is difficult to evaluate because of the wide range of normal responses.

(c) HCG stimulation under dexamethasone suppression

This test is used in women to evaluate the role of the ovary in androgen secretion; the test is based on the stimulation by HCG of ovarian androgen secretion, dexamethasone suppression being used to eliminate variations in adrenal androgen secretion.

The test is generally performed with the dexamethasone suppression test: dexamethasone at a dose of 3 mg/day is continued for an additional five days, 5000 uHCG being administered each day; plasma levels are determined on the fourth and fifth day of HCG stimulation. Because of the danger of eliciting a hyperstimulation syndrome in women with ovulatory cycles, the test is best performed during the luteal phase. Few data obtained in normal women are available for comparison which makes interpretation of the results the more difficult. Most data in the literature moreover concern only urinary 17-oxosteroids and testosterone-glucuronide excretion (Lopez, Migeon and Jones, 1967; Jayle, Scholler, Mauvais-Jarvis and Szper, 1962). Data concerning plasma androgens in normal women obtained in our laboratory are given in Table 9. An increase of T levels by more than 25 ng/dl, of DHT by more than 7 ng/dl or of androstenedione by more than 100 ng/dl is considered pathological. A supranormal elevation of androgen levels would indicate an ovarian origin, but Ettinger et al. (1971) in eight patients with proven Stein-Leventhal syndrome found such a response in only four. This may perhaps be the consequence of the fact that in PCO, endogenous LH levels are often already increased (Givens et al., 1976a).

Table 9

Effect of dexamethasone suppression and HCG stimulation (5 × 5000 u) on plasma androgens (ng/dl) in women (for conversion factors see Table 6).

	Luteal phase (n = 6)		Postmenopausal ovary (n = 10)	
	DX	DX + HCG	DX	DX + HCG
T	27 ± 4	48 ± 5	20 ± 6	35 ± 9
DHT	13 ± 3	17 ± 2	< 5	—
Androstenedione	75 ± 14	161 ± 21	27 ± 4	30 ± 6
DHEA	91 ± 18	105 ± 12	57 ± 16	95 ± 30
DHEA-S (μg/dl)	34 ± 3	35 ± 12	15 ± 2	27 ± 1
Androstenediol	16 ± 3	16 ± 4	—	—

(d) Combined oestrogen-progestogen oral contraception suppression (OCS) test

In as far as combined or progestational contraceptives inhibit LH secretion, androgen levels during their use will reflect essentially adrenal androgen secretion. However, it should be realised that these drugs suppress only LH-dependent androgen secretion, and that ovarian androgen secretion during the follicular phase, for example, is largely LH-independent. Moreover, as the oestrogen component increases SHBG capacity, this will tend to increase 17β-hydroxysteroid levels.

Oestrogens alone are ineffective, as oestradiol is a poor LH suppressant (Kirschner et al., 1970). Givens et al. (1976) showed that the pituitary–ovarian axis is slower to suppress than the pituitary–adrenal axis, and they suggest that the pill should be given for at least three weeks before evaluating the ovarian contribution to androgen levels.

Values observed for four normal women during combined oral contraceptive use are given in Table 10. The pitfalls and difficulties in correctly interpreting the suppression and stimulation tests have been discussed earlier.

Table 10

Influence of oral contraception[a] on plasma androgens (ng/dl; M. ± S. D.; for conversion factors see Table 6).

	Follicular phase	Periovular phase LH peak ± 2 day	Luteal phase	During contraceptive (Mean of cycle)
T	34 ± 5	42 ± 7	38 ± 6	34 ± 4
DHT	23 ± 4	26 ± 4	24 ± 4	13 ± 4
Androstenedione	144 ± 66	220 ± 45	120 ± 24	138 ± 18
DHEA	550 ± 90	550 ± 74	520 ± 66	459 ± 67
DHEA-S (µg/dl)	89 ± 36	88 ± 30	82 ± 39	79 ± 7
Androstenediol	73 ± 12	75 ± 8	68 ± 13	65 ± 13

[a] Combined 75 µg mestranol and 5 mg norethindrone.

4. Catheterisation of Adrenal and Ovarian Veins

Analysis of the effluents of the endocrine glands permits a direct estimation of their contribution to the plasma hormone levels (Kirschner and Jacobs, 1971). For steroids with a complex origin, such as androgens in females (ovarian and adrenal secretion plus peripheral conversion) the method requires: measurement of the BPR of the androgens studied, determination of the conversion rate of all precursors, and estimation of blood flow of either adrenals or ovaries in order to evaluate either adrenal or ovarian androgen secretion rate.

It is not surprising that this complex approach is subject to many possible errors. In order to be able to calculate the contribution of the ovaries and the adrenals respectively to the blood production rate, we have to assume that the catheterisation is not stressful to the patient, that the ratio of androgen to cortisol secretion is a constant, that cortisol secretion is *ca* 10 mg/m^2/24 hr and that the conversion rate of androgen precursors is identical in all subjects. Using this method Kirschner *et al.* (1976) concluded in 42 out of 44 women studied the source of excessive androgen levels were the ovaries; the results, however, were often in contradiction to the dexamethasone suppression test.

REFERENCES

Abraham, G. E. (1974). *J. clin. Endocr. Metab.* **39**, 340.
Abraham, G. E. and Chakmakjian, Z. H. (1973). *J. clin. Endocr. Metab.* **35**, 581.
Abraham, G. E., Lobotsky, S. and Lloyd, C. W. (1969). *J. clin. Invest.* **48**, 696.
Abraham, G. E., Manlimos, F. S., Solis, M. and Wickman, A. C. (1975). *Clin. Biochem.* **8**, 374.
Abraham, G. E., Maroulis, G. B., Buster, J. E., Chang, R. S. and Marshall, J. R. (1976). *Obstet. Gynec.* **47**, 395.
Abramovich, D. R., Baker, T. G. and Neal, P. (1974). *J. Endocr.* **60**, 179.
Anderson, D. C., Child, D. F. and Bu'lock, D. E. (1977). *In* "The Endocrine Function of the Human Adrenal Cortex". Int. Symp. Florence, p. 45.
Anderson, K. M. and Liao, S. (1968). *Nature, Lond.* **219**, 777.
Andre, C. M. and James, V. H. T. (1973). *Clin. chim. Acta*, **43**, 295.
Aono, T., Kurachi, T., Miyata, M., Nakasima, A., Koshiyama, K., Uozumi, T. and Matsumoto, K. (1976). *J. clin. Endocr. Metab.* **42**, 144.
Apter, D. O., Jänne, O., Karvonen, P. and Vihko, R. (1976). *Clin. Chem.* **22**, 32.
August, G. P., Tkachuk, M. and Grumbach, M. M. (1969). *J. clin. Endocr. Metab.* **29**, 891.
Aynsley-Green, A., Zachmann, M., Illig, R., Rampini, S. and Prader, A. (1976). *Clin. Endocr.* **5**, 381.
Azizi, F., Vagenakis, A., Longcope, C., Ingbar, S. H. and Braverman, L.E. (1973). *Steroids*, **22**, 467.
Bäckström, T. and Södergard, R. (1977). *Acta endocr.* **85** (Suppl. 212), 42.
Baird, D. T. (1976). *In* "The Endocrine Function of the Human Ovary" (V. H. T. James, M. Serio and G. Giusti, eds). Academic Press, London and New York.
Baird, D. T., Uno, A. and Melby, J. C. (1969). *J. Endocr.* **45**, 135.
Baird, D. T., Horton, R., Longcope, C. and Tait, J. F. (1969b). *Rec. Prog. Horm. Res.* **25**, 615.
Baird, D. T., Corker, C. S., Davidson, D. W., Hunter, W. M., Michie, E. A. and Van Look, P. F. A. (1977). *J. clin. Endocr. Metab.* **45**, 798.
Baker, H. W. G., Dulmanis, A., Hudson, B., Paulsen, H. C., Purcell, M. and Woinarski, S. (1972). 4th Int. Cong. Endocr. Int. Cong. Ser. 252, Abst. 327. Excerpta Medica Foundation, Amsterdam.
Baker, H. W. G., Burger, H. G., de Kretser, D. M., Dulmanis, A., Hudson, B., O'Connor, S., Paulsen, C. A., Purcell, M., Rennie, G., Seach, C. S., Taft, H. P. and Wang, C. (1976). *Q. J. Med.* **XLV**, 145.
Barberia, S., Pages, L. and Horton, R. (1976). *Fert. Steril.* **27**, 1101.
Bardin, C. W. and Lipsett, M. B. (1967). *J. clin. Invest.* **46**, 891.
Bardin, C. W., Hembree, W. C. and Lipsett, M. B. (1968). *J. clin. Endocr. Metab.* **28**, 1300.
Bardin, C. W., Lipsett, M. B. and French, A. (1968). *J. clin. Endocr. Metab.* **28**, 215.
Bardin, C. W., Lipsett, M. B., Edgcomb, J. H. and Marshall, J. R. (1967). *J. clin. Endocr. Metab.* **277**, 399.

Bardin, C. W., Bullock, L. P., Sherins, R. M., Mowszowicz, I. and Blackburn, W. R. (1973). *Rec. Prog. Horm. Res.* **29**, 65.

Bartke, A., Croft, B. T. and Dallerio, S. (1975). *Endocrinology,* **75**, 1601.

Bassi, F., Giusti, G., Borsi, L., Cattaneo, S., Gianotti, P., Fosti, G., Pazzagli, M., Vigiani, C. and Serio, M. (1977). *Clin. Endocr.* **6**, 5.

Baulieu, E. E. (1962). *J. clin. Endocr. Metab.* **22**, 501.

Baulieu, E. E. and Mauvais-Jarvis, P. (1964a). *J. biol. Chem.* **239**, 1569.

Baulieu, E. E. and Mauvais-Jarvis, P. (1964b). *J. biol. Chem.* **239**, 1578.

Baulieu, E. E., Robel, P. and Mauvais-Jarvis, P. (1963). *C. r. Acad. Sc.* **256**, 1016.

Baulieu, E. E., Corpéchot, C., Dray, F., Emiliozzi, R., Lebeau, M. C., Mauvais-Jarvis, P. and Robel, P. (1965). *Rec. Prog. Horm. Res.* **21**, 411.

Bauminger, Kohen, T., Lindner, H. R. and Weinstein, A. (1974). *Steroids,* **24**, 477.

Beitins, I. Z., Bayard, F., Kowarski, A. and Migeon, C. J. (1973). *Steroids,* **21**, 553.

Berthezène, F., Forest, M. G., Grimaud, S. A., Claustrat, B. and Mornex, R. (1976). *New Engl. J. Med.* **295**, 969.

Bertrand, J., De Peretti, E. and Forest, M. G. (1977). *In* "The Endocrine Function of the Human Adrenal Cortex". Int. Symp. Florence, p. 26.

Biglieri, E. G., Hirson, M. A. and Brust, N. (1966). *J. clin. Invest.* **45**, 1946.

Bird, C. E. and Clark, A. F. (1972). *J. clin. Endocr. Metab.* **34**, 467.

Bird, C. E., Choong, A., Knight, L. and Clark, A. F. (1974). *J. clin. Endocr. Metab.* **38**, 372.

Bird, C. E., Morrow, L., Fukumoto, L., Marcellus, S. and Clark, A. F. (1976). *J. clin. Endocr. Metab.* **43**, 1317.

Bolté, E., Mancuso, S., Eriksson, G., Wiqvist, N. and Diczfalusy, E. (1969). *Acta endocr, Copenh.* **45**, 576.

Bongiovanni, A. M. (1977). *In* "The Endocrine Function of Human Adrenal Cortex". Int. Symp. Florence, p. 31.

Bongiovanni, A. M. and Eberlein, W. R. (1957). *J. clin. Endocr. Metab.* **17**, 238.

Bonne, C. and Raynaud, J. P. (1974). *Mol. Cell. Endocr.* **2**, 59.

Boyar, R. M., Rosenfeld, R. S., Knapen, S., Finkelstein, J. W., Roffwarg, M. P., Weizman, E. D. and Hellman, L. (1974). *J. clin. Invest.* **54**, 609.

Breuer, J., Schneider, H. T. and Breuer, H. (1970). *Z. klin. Chem. klin. Biochem.* **8**, 626.

Brown, D. M., Markland, C. and Dehner, L. P. (1978). *J. clin. Endocr. Metab.* **46**, 1.

Brownie, A. C., Van der Molen, H. S., Nishizawa, E. E. and Eik-Nes, K. B. (1964). *J. clin. Endocr. Metab.* **24**, 1091.

Bruchovsky, N. and Wilson, G. D. (1968a). *J. biol. Chem.* **243**, 5953.

Bruchovsky, N. and Wilson, G. D. (1968b). *Clin. Res.* **14**, 72.

Bundschu, H. D., Rager, K., Heller, S., Hayduk, D., Pfeiffer, E. H., Lüders, G. and Liebau, G. (1976). *Klin. Wschr.* **54**, 1039.

Burger, H. G., Ken, S. R. and Kellie, A. E. (1964). *J. clin. Endocr. Metab.* **24**, 432.

Buster, J. E. and Abraham, G. E. (1972). *Anal. Lett.* **5**, 543.

Calvin, H. I., Van de Wiele, R. and Lieberman, S. (1964a). *Biochemistry,* **2**, 648.

Calvin, H. I., Van de Wiele, R. and Lieberman, S. (1964b). *Biochemistry,* **3**, 259.

Catt, K. J. and Dufau, M. L. (1973). *Nature New Biol.* **244**, 219.

Catt, K. J., Dufau, M. L. and Tsuruhara, T. (1972). *J. clin. Endocr. Metab.* **34**, 123.

Chapdelaine, A. and Lanthier, A. (1966). Int. Cong. Ser. No. 111, Abst. 523. Excerpta Medica Foundation, Amsterdam.

Chapdelaine, A., MacDonald, P. C., Gonzalez, O., Gurpide, E., Van de Wiele, R. and Lieberman, S. (1965). *J. clin. Endocr. Metab.* **25**, 1569.

Chen, J. C., Vidt, D. G., Zorn, E. M., Hallberg, M. C. and Wieland, R. G. (1970).

J. clin. Endocr. Metab. **31**, 14.

Childs, B., Grumbach, M. V. and Van Wyck, J. J. (1956). *J. clin. Invest.* **35**, 213.

Chopra, I. J., Tulchinsky, D. and Greenway, F. L. (1973). *Ann. int. Med.* **79**, 198.

Chopra, I. J. and Tulchinsky, D. (1974). *J. clin. Endocr. Metab.* **38**, 269.

Christensen, A. K. and Mason, N. R. (1965). *Endocrinology,* **76**, 646.

Clark, A. F. and Bird, C. E. (1973). *J. Endocr.* **57**, 289.

Clark, A. F., Carson, G. D., DeLory, B., Clemow, M. E. and Bird, C. E. (1973). *Clin. Endocr.* **2**, 361.

Cohn, G. L. and Hume, M. (1960). *J. clin. Invest.* **39**, 1584.

Colas, A., Heinrichs, W. L. and Tatum, H. S. (1964). *Steroids,* **3**, 417.

Collu, R. and Ducharme, J. R. (1975). *J. ster. Biochem.* **6**, 869.

Condom, R. and Desfosses, B. (1977). *J. ster. Biochem.* **8**, 1085.

Conney, A. H., Kuntzman, R. and Jacobson (1966). Proc. 2nd Int. Cong. Horm. Steroids., Int. Cong. Ser. No. 111, Abst. 232. Excerpta Medica Foundation, Amsterdam.

Coppage, W. S. and Cooner, A. E. (1965). *New Engl. J. Med.* **273**, 903.

Corvol, P., Bertagna, L. and Bedrossian, J. (1974). *Acta endocr., Copenh.* **75**, 756.

Corvol, P., Michaud, A., Menard, J., Freifeld, M. and Mahoudeau, J. (1975). *Endocrinology,* **97**, 52.

Cox, P. A. and Kellie, A. E. (1965). *In* "Hormonal Steroids" (L. Martini and A. Pecile, eds), Vol. 2, pp. 575. Academic Press, New York and London.

Coyotupa, J., Parlow, A. F. and Abraham, G. E. (1972). *Anal. Lett.* **5**, 329.

Cunningham, G. R., Goldzieher, J. W., de la Pena, A. and Oliver, M. (1978). *J. clin. Metab.* **46**, 8.

Cushman, P. (1973). *Am. J. Med.* **55**, 452.

Davies, P. and Griffith, K. (1973). *Biochem. J.* **136**, 611.

Davis, T. E., Lipsett, M. B. and Korenman, S. G. (1965). *J. clin. Endocr. Metab.* **25**, 476.

Degenhart, H. S., Visser, H. K. A., Wilmink, R. and Exley, D. (1966). *In* "Androgens in Normal and Pathological Conditions" (A. Vermeulen and D. Exley, eds), Int. Cong. Ser. 101. Excerpta Medica Foundation, Amsterdam.

Dehennin, L., Reiffsteck, A. and Scholler, R. (1974). *J. ster. Biochem.* **5**, 81.

Demisch, K., Magnet, W., Neubauer, M. and Schöffling, K. (1973). *J. clin. Endocr. Metab.* **37**, 129.

De Neve, L. and Vermeulen, A. (1965). *J. Endocr.* **32**, 295.

De Peretti, E. and Forest, M. G., (1976). *J. clin. Endocr. Metab.* **43**, 982.

Dessypris, A. G. (1975). *J. ster. Biochem.* **6**, 1287.

Dessypris, A., Kuoppasalmi, K. and Adlercreutz, H. (1961). *J. ster. Biochem.* **7**, 33.

Dessypris, A., Drosdowsky, M. A., McNiven, N. L. and Dorfman, R. I. (1966). *Proc. Soc. exp. Biol. Med.* **121**, 1128.

Diez D'Aux, D. C. and Murphy, B. E. P. (1974). *J. ster. Biochem.* **5**, 207.

Dignam, W. J., Pion, R. I., Lamb, E. J. and Simmer, H. H. (1964). *Acta endocr. Copenh.* **45**, 254.

Doerr, P. and Pirke, K. M. (1976). *J. clin. Endocr. Metab.* **43**, 622.

Dorfman, R. I. and Ungar, F. (1965). *In* "Metabolism of Steroid Hormones", 2nd edition, p. 125. Academic Press, London and New York.

Dray, F. (1966). *C. r. Acad. Sc. Paris,* **262**, 679.

Dray, R., Reinberg, A. and Sebaoun, J. (1965). *C. r. Acad. Sci. Paris,* **261**, 573.

Dray, F., Sebaoun, J., Delzan, G., Ledru, M. J. and Mowszowicz, I. (1968). *Rev. fr. Etud. clin. biol.* **19**, 622.

Dray, F. Sebaoun, J., Mowszowicz, I., Delzan, G., Dergez, P. and Dreyfus, G. (1967). *C. r. Acad. Sci. Paris*, **264**, 2578.

Drucker, W. D., Blumberg, J. M., Gandy, H. M., David, R. R. and Verde, A. L. (1972). *J. clin. Endocr. Metab.* **35**, 78.

Dufau, M. L., de Kretser, D. M. and Hudson, B. (1971). *Endocrinology*, **88**, 825.

Dymling, J. F., Nilsson, K. O. and Hökfelt, B. (1972). *Acta endocr., Copenh.* **70**, 104.

Eik-Nes, K. (1964). *Can. J. Physiol. Pharmacol.* **42**, 671.

Eik-Nes, K. (1970). "The Androgens of the Testis." Dekker, New York.

Ettinger, B., Van Werder, K., Thenaers, G. C. and Forsham, P. H. (1971). *Am. J. Med.* **51**, 170.

Fang, S., Anderson, K. M. and Liao, S. (1969). *J. biol. Chem.* **244**, 6584.

Finkelstein, M., Forchielli, E. and Dorfman, R. I. (1961). *J. clin. Endocr. Metab.* **21**, 98.

Fiorelli, G., Borrelli, D., Forti, G., Gonnelli, P., Pazzagli, M. and Serio, M. (1976). *J. ster. Biochem.* **7**, 113.

Fleetwood, J. A., Leigh, R. J., Hall, R. and Smith, P. A. (1974). *Clin. Endocr.* **3**, 457.

Fogh, M., Corker, C. S., McLean, A., Bruunshuus-Petersen, I., Philip, S. and Skakkebaek, N. E. (1978). *Acta endocr., Copenh.* **87**, 643.

Forchielli, E., Dorfman, R. I., Ichii, S. and Menon, K. (1965). *Cancer Res.* **25**, 1076.

Forest, M. G. (1975). *Clin. Endocr.* **4**, 569.

Forest, M. G. and Bertrand, J. (1975). *J. ster. Biochem.* **6**, XXIV.

Forest, M. G. and Cathiard, A. M. (1975). *J. clin. Endocr. Metab.* **41**, 977.

Forest, M. G., Cathiard, A. M. and Bertrand, J. A. (1973). *J. clin. Endocr. Metab.* **37**, 148.

Forest, M. G., Cathiard, A. M., Bourgeois, J. and Genoud, J. (1974a). Int. Symp. Sex. Endocr. Perinat. Period. *INSERM*, **32**, 315.

Forest, M. G., Sizonenko, P. C., Cathiard, A. M. and Bertrand, J. (1974b). *J. clin. Invest.* **53**, 819.

Furuyama, S., Mayes, D. and Nugent, C. A. (1970). *Steroids*, **16**, 415.

Galvao Teles, A., Anderson, D. C., Burke, C. W. and Marshall, J. C. (1973). *Lancet*, **i**, 173.

Gandy, H. M. (1970). In "Endocrinology of Pregnancy" (F. Fuchs and A. Klopper, eds), p. 130. Harper and Row, New York.

Gandy, H. M. and Peterson, R. E. (1968). *J. clin. Endocr. Metab.* **28**, 949.

Gant, M. F., Hutchinson, H. T., Siiteri, P. and MacDonald, P. (1971). *Am. J. Obstet. Gynec.* **111**, 555.

Girard, J. and Baumann, J. B. (1975). *Pediat. Res.* **9**, 669.

Givens, J. R., Andersen, R. M., Umstot, E. S. and Wiser, W. L. (1976a). *Obstet. Gynec.* **47**, 388.

Givens, J. R., Andersen, R. M., Ragland, J. B., Wiser, W. L. and Umstot, E. S. (1975). *J. clin. Endocr. Metab.* **40**, 988.

Givens, J. R., Andersen, R. M., Wiser, W. L., Coleman, S. A. and Fish, S. A. (1974). *J. clin. Endocr. Metab.* **38**, 126.

Givens, J. R., Andersen, R. M., Wiser, W. L., Umstot, E. S. and Fish, S. A. (1976b). *Am. J. Obstet. Gynec.* **124**, 333.

Gordon, G. G., Olivo, J., Rafii, F. and Southren, L. (1975). *J. clin. Endocr. Metab.* **40**, 1018.

Gordon, G. G., Altman, K., Southren, A. L., Rubin, E. and Lieber, C. S. (1976). *New Engl. J. Med.* **295**, 793.

Gordon, G. G., Southren, A. L., Tochimoto, G., Rand, J. and Olivo, J. (1969). *J.*

clin. Endocr. Metab. **29**, 164.

Gordon, G. G., Southren, A. L., Tochimoto, G., Olivo, J., Altman, K., Rand, J. and Lemberger, L. (1970). *J. clin. Endocr. Metab.* **30**, 449.

Greenblatt, R. B. and Mahesh, V. B. (1976). *Am. J. Obstet. Gynec.* **125**, 712.

Grodin, J. M., Siiteri, P. K. and MacDonald, P. C. (1973). *J. clin. Endocr. Metab.* **47**, 383.

Grumbach, M. M. and Kaplan, S. L. (1973) *In* "Advances in Foetal and Neonatal Physiology" (K. S. Comline, K. W. Cross, G. S. Dawes and P. W. Nathanielz, eds), p. 462. Cambridge University Press, Cambridge.

Gupta, D., McCafferty, E. and Rager, K. (1972). *Steroids,* **19**, 411.

Hall, P. F. (1964). *Endocrinology,* **74**, 201.

Hall, P. F., Irby, D. C. and De Kretser, D. M. (1969). *Endocrinology,* **84**, 488.

Hall, R., Smith, P. A. and Harkness, S. A. (1970). *Proc. R. Soc. Med.* **63**, 140.

Hammond, G. L., Ruokonen, A., Kontturi, M., Koskela, E. and Vihko, R. (1977). *J. clin. Endocr. Metab.* **45**, 16.

Hemsell, D. L., Grodin, J. M., Brenner, P. F., Siiteri, P. K. and MacDonald, P. C. (1974). *J. clin. Endocr. Metab.* **38**, 476.

Hopper, B. R. and Yen, S. S. C. (1975). *J. clin. Endocr. Metab.* **40**, 458.

Horton, R. and Frasier, S. D. (1967). *J. clin. Invest.* **46**, 1003.

Horton, R. and Neisler, J. (1968). *J. clin. Endocr. Metab.* **28**, 479.

Horton, R. and Tait, J. F. (1966). *J. clin. Invest.* **45**, 301.

Horton, R. and Tait, J. F. (1967). *J. clin. Endocr. Metab.* **27**, 79.

Horton, R. Kato, T. and Sherins, R. J. (1967). *Steroids,* **10**, 245.

Horton, R., Romanoff, E. and Walker, J. (1966). *J. clin. Endocr. Metab.* **26**, 1267.

Hudson, B., Coghlan, J. P., Dulmanis, A., Wintour, M. and Ekkel, L. (1963). *Aust. J. exp. Biol. Med. Sci.* **41**, 235.

Huttunen, M. O., Härkönen, M., Niskanen, P., Leino, T. and Ylikahri, R. (1976). *J. Stud. alcohol,* **37**, 1165.

Imperato McGinley, J. and Peterson, R. E. (1976). *Am. J. Med.* **61**, 251.

Imperato McGinley, J., Guerrero, L., Gauthier, T. and Peterson, R. E. (1974). *Science,* **186**, 1213.

Irvine, W. J., Toft, A. D., Wilson, K. S., Fraser, R., Wilson, A., Young J., Hunter, W. M., Ismail, A. A. A. and Burger, P. E. (1974). *J. clin. Endocr. Metab.* **39**, 522.

Ismail, A. A., Niswender, G. D. and Midgley, E. R. (1972). *J. clin. Endocr. Metab.* **34**, 177.

Ishimaru, T., Pages, L. and Horton, R. (1977). *J. clin. Endocr. Metab.* **45**, 695.

Ishimaru, T., Edmiston, W. A., Pages, L. and Horton, R. (1978). *J. clin. Endocr. Metab.* **46**, 528.

Ito, T. and Horton, R. (1971). *J. clin. Invest.* **50**, 1261.

Jänne, O., Perheentupa, J., Viinikka, L. and Vihko, R. (1974). *J. clin. Endocr. Metab.* **39**, 206.

Jänne, O., Perheentupa, J., Viinikka, L. and Vihko, R. (1975). *Clin. Endocr.* **4**, 39.

Jayle, M. F., Scholler, R., Mauvais Jarvis, P. and Szper, E. M. (1962). *Clin. chim. Acta,* **7**, 322.

Jeanloz, R. W., Levy, H., Jacobson, R. P., Hechter, O., Schenker, V. and Pincus, G. (1953). *J. biol. Chem.* **203**, 453.

Jaffee, W., Russell, V., Longcope C. K. and Vaitukaitis J (1978). Abst. 60th Ann. Meet. p. 110.

Jeffcoate, S. L., Brooks, R. V., London, D. R., Smith, P. M., Spathis, G. S. and Prunty, F. F. G. (1968). *J. Endocr.* **42**, 213.

Johnsen, S. G., Bennett, E. P. and Jensen, V. G. (1974). *Lancet,* **ii**, 1473.

Johnsen, S. G., Kampmann, J. P., Bennett, E. P. and Schønau-Jørgensen (1976). *Clin. Pharm. Ther.* **20**, 233.

Johnson, B. H. and Ewing, L. (1971). *Science,* **173**, 635.

Joyce, B. G., Fahmy, D. and Hillier, S. G. (1975). *Clin. chim. Acta,* **62**, 231.

Judd, H. L. and Yen, S. S. C. (1973). *J. clin. Endocr. Metab.* **36**, 475.

Judd, H. L., Rigg, L. A., Anderson, D. C. and Yen, S. S. C. (1976). *J. clin. Endocr. Metab.* **43**, 347.

Kellie, A. E. and Smith, E. R. (1957). *Biochem. J.* **66**, 490.

Kent, J. R. and Acone, A. B. (1966). *In* "Androgens in Normal and Pathological Conditions" E. M. F., ICS 101, p. 31.

Kim, M. H., Hosseinian, A. H. and Dupon, C. (1974). *J. clin. Endocr. Metab.* **39**, 706.

Kim, M. H., Rosenfield, R. L. and Dupon, C. (1976). *Am. J. Obstet. Gynec.* **126**, 982.

King, R. J. B. and Mainwaring, W. P. (1974). "Steroid Cell Interactions." Butterworth, London.

Kinouchi, T. and Horton, R. (1974a). *J. clin. Endocr. Metab.* **38**, 261.

Kinouchi, T. and Horton, R. (1974b). *J. clin. Invest.* **54**, 646.

Kinouchi, T., Pages, L. and Horton, R. (1973). *J. Lab. clin. Med.* **82**, 309.

Kirkay, J. and Westphal, U. (1968). *Bioch. biophys. Acta,* **170**, 324.

Kirschner, M. A. and Bardin, C. W. (1972). *Metabolism,* **21**, 667.

Kirschner, M. A. and Jacobs, S. M. (1971). *J. clin. Endocr. Metab.* **33**, 199.

Kirschner, M. A., Lipsett, M. B. and Collins, D. R. (1965). *J. clin. Invest.* **44**, 657.

Kirschner, M. A., Zucker, I. R. and Jespersen, D. (1976). *New Engl. J. Med.* **294**, 637.

Kirschner, M. A., Bardin, C. W., Hembree, W. C. and Ross, G. T. (1970). *J. clin. Endocr. Metab.* **30**, 727.

Kirschner, M. A., Sinhamahapatra, S., Zucker, I. R., Loriaux, L. and Nieschlag, E. (1973). *J. clin. Endocr. Metab.* **37**, 183.

Klemm, W., Liebich, H. M. and Gupta, D. (1976). *J. clin. Endocr. Metab.* **42**, 514.

Kley, H. K., Nieschlag, E. and Krüskemper, H. L. (1975). *Horm. Metab. Res.* **7**, 99.

Kley, H. K., Nieschlag, E., Wiegelman, W., Solbach, H. G. and Krüskemper, H. L. (1975). *Acta endocr., Copenh.* **79**, 275.

Kley, H. K., Wiegelmann, W., Nieschlag, E., Solbach, H. G., Zimmermann, H. and Krüskemper, H. L. (1974). *Acta endocr., Copenh.* **75**, 417.

Korenman, S. G. and Lipsett, M. B. (1964). *J. clin. Invest.* **43**, 2125.

Korenman, S. G., Wilson, H. and Lipsett, M. D. (1964). *J. biol. Chem.* **239**, 1004.

Korth-Schutz, S., Levine, L. S. and New, M. I. (1976). *J. clin. Endocr. Metab.* **42**, 117.

Kowarski, A., Thompson, R. C., Migeon, C. J. and Blizzard, R. M. (1971). *J. clin. Endocr. Metab.* **32**, 356.

Kreuz, L. E., Rose, R. M. and Jennings, J. (1972). *Arch. Psychiat.* **26**, 479.

Kuttenn, F. and Mauvais Jarvis, P. (1975). *Acta endocr., Copenh.* **79**, 1644.

Laatikainen, T. and Peltonen, J. (1975). *Acta endocr., Copenh.* **79**, 577.

Laatikainen, T., Laitinen, E. A. and Vihko, R. (1969). *J. clin. Endocr. Metab.* **29**, 219.

Laatikainen, T., Laitinen, A. and Vihko, R. (1971). *J. clin. Endocr. Metab.* **32**, 59.

Lacy, D. (1973). *In* "The Endocrine Function of the Human Testes" (V. H. T. James, M. Serio and L. Martini, eds), Vol. I, p. 493. Academic Press, London and New York.

Larson, B. A., Vanderlaan, W. P., Judd, H. L. and McCullough, D. L. (1976). *J. clin. Endocr. Metab.* **42**, 882.

Lasnitski, I. and Franklin, A. R. (1972). *J. Endocr.* **54**, 333.

Leichter, S. B. and Daughaday, W. H. (1974). *Ann. int. Med.* **81**, 638.

Levin, J., Lloyd, C. W., Lobotsky, S. and Friedreich, E. H. (1967). *Acta endocr., Copenh.* **55**, 184.

Liang, T., Tymoczko, J. L., Chan, K. M. B., Hung, S. C. and Liao, S. (1977). *In* "Androgens and Antiandrogens" (L. Martini and M. Molta, eds). Raven Press, New York.

Liao, S. and Fang, S. (1969). *Vit. Horm.* **27**, 17.

Lim, V. S. and Fang, V. S. (1975). *Am. J. Med.* **58**, 655.

Lipsett, M. B. (1973). *New Engl. J. Med.* **289**, 802.

Lipsett, M. B., Davis, T. E., Wilson, II. and Canfield, C. J. (1965). *J. clin. Endocr. Metab.* **25**, 1027.

Lipsett, M. B., Wilson, H., Kirschner, M. A., Korenman, S. G., Fishman, L. M., Sarfaty, G. A. and Bardin, C. W. (1966). *Rec. Prog. Horm. Res.* **22**, 245.

Little, M., Szendro, P., Teran, C., Hughes, A. and Jungblut, P. W. (1975). *J. ster. Biochem.* **6**, 493.

Loeb, P. M. and Wilson, J. D. (1965). *Clin. Res.* **13**, 45.

Longcope, C. (1973). *Steroids,* **21**, 583.

Longcope, C., Kato, T. and Horton, R. (1969). *J. clin. Invest.* **48**, 2191.

Longcope, C., Pratt, J. H., Schneider, S. H. and Fineberg (1978). *J. clin. Endocr. Metab.* **46**, 146.

Lopez, J. M., Migeon, C. J. and Jones, G. E. S. (1967). *Am. J. Obstet. Gynec.* **198**, 749.

Loriaux, D. L. and Lipsett, M. B. (1972). *Steroids,* **19**, 681.

MacDonald, P. C., Chapdelaine, A., Gonzales, O., Gurpide, E., Van de Wiele, R. L. and Lieberman, S. (1965). *J. clin. Endocr. Metab.* **25**, 1557.

MacDonald, P. C. and Siiteri, P. K. (1965). *J. clin. Invest.* **44**, 465.

Mahesh, V. B. and Greenblatt, R. B. (1962). *J. clin. Endocr. Metab.* **22**, 441.

Mahoudeau, J. A., Bardin, C. W. and Lipsett, M. B., (1971). *J. clin. Invest.* **50**, 1338.

Mahoudeau, J. A., Valcke, J. C. and Bricaire, H. (1975). *J. clin. Endocr. Metab.* **41**, 13.

Mainwaring, W. I. B. (1975). *Vit. Horm.* **33**, 223.

Mangan, F. R., Neal, G. E. and Williams, D. C. (1968). *Arch. biochim. Biophys.* **124**, 27.

Maroulis, G. B., Mamlimos, F. S., Garza, R. and Abraham G. E. (1976). *Obstet. Gynec.* **48**, 388.

Maroulis, G. B., Mamlimos, F. S. and Abraham, G. (1977). *Obstet. Gynec.* **49**, 454.

Marsh, J. M., Savard, K. and Lemaire, W. J. (1976) *In* "The Endocrine Function of the Ovary" (V. H. T. James, M. Serio and G. Giusti, eds), p. 37. Academic Press, London and New York.

Martin, R. P., Loriaux, D. L. and Farnham, G. S. (1965). *Steroids,* **5** (suppl. 2), 149.

Marynick, S. P., Sherins, R. J., Pita, J. C. and Lipsett, M. B. (1975). Abst. 148, 59th Ann. Meet. Endocr. Soc.

Mauvais Jarvis, P. and Baulieu, E. E. (1965). *J. clin. Endocr. Metab.* **25**, 1167.

Mauvais Jarvis, P., Bercovici, J. P. and Floch, H. H. (1969). *Rev. fr. Etud. clin. biol.* **14**, 159.

Mauvais Jarvis, P., Charransol, G. and Bobas-Masson, F. (1973). *J. clin. Endocr. Metab.* **36**, 452.

McKenna, T. S., Jennings, A. S., Liddle, C. W. and Burr, I. M. (1976). *J. clin. Endocr. Metab.* **42**, 918.

Menard, R. H., Stripp, B. and Gillette, J. R. (1974). *Endocrinology,* **94**, 1628.

Mendelson, J. H. and Mello, N. R. (1975). *Clin. Pharm. Ther.* **17**, 529.

Mendelson, J. H., Mendelson, J. E. and Patel, V. D. (1975). *J. Pharmacol. Exp. Ther.* **192**, 211.

Mendelson, J. H., Kuehnle, J., Ellingboe, J. and Babor, T. F. (1974). *New Engl. J. Med.* **291**, 1051.

Menon, K. M. J., Dorfman, R. I. and Forchielli, E. (1965). *Steroids*, **2**, 165.

Mercier, C., Alfsen, A. and Baulieu, E. E. (1966). *In* "Androgens in Normal and Pathological Conditions" (A. Vermeulen and D. Exley, eds), p. 212. Int. Cong. Ser. No. 101, Excerpta Medica Foundation, Amsterdam.

Meyer, R. (1931). *Am. J. Obstet. Gynec.* **22**, 697.

Mikhail, G. (1970). *Gynaec. Invest.* **1**, 5.

Mills, I. H. (1968). *In* "The Investigation of Hypothalamic Pituitary Adrenal Function" (V. H. T. James and J. Landon, eds). Cambridge University Press, Cambridge.

Mizuno, M., Lobotsky, J., Lloyd, C. W., Kobayashi, T. and Murasawa, Y. (1968). *J. clin. Endocr. Metab.* **28**, 1133.

Morris, M. D. and Chaikoff, T. L. (1959). *J. biol. Chem.* **234**, 1095

Mowszowicz, I., Kahn, D. and Dray, F. (1970). *J. clin. Endocr. Metab.* **31**, 584.

Mulder, E., van Beurden-Lamers, W. M. O., Brinkmann, A. O., Mechielsen, M. J. and van der Molen, H. S. (1974). *J. ster. Biochem.* **5**, 955.

Murphy, B. E. P. (1970). *In* "Steroid Assay by Protein Binding" (E. Diczfalusy, ed.). *Acta endocr., Copenh.* (Suppl. 147), p. 37.

Naftolin, E. and Judd, J. H., and Yen, S. S. C. (1973). *J. clin. Endocr. Metab.* **36**, 285.

Neher, R. and Wettstein, A. (1960). *Acta endocr., Copenh.* **35**, 1.

Newmark, S., Dluhy, R. G., Williams, G. H., Pochi, P. and Rose, L. I. (1977). *Am. J. Gynec. Obstet.* **127**, 594.

Nieschlag, E. and Loriaux, D. (1972). *Z. Klin. Chem. Klin. Biochem.* **10**, 164.

Nieschlag, E., Cüppers, J. H. and Wickings, E. S. (1977). *Eur. J. Clin. Invest.* **7**, 145.

Nieschlag, E., Loriaux, D. L. and Lipsett, M. B. (1972). *Steroids*, **19**, 669.

Nieschlag, E., Walk, T. and Schindler, A. E. (1974). *Horm. Metab. Res.* **6**, 170.

Nilsson, K. and Hökfelt, B. (1971). *Acta endocr., Copenh.* **68**, 576.

Odell, W. D. and Swerdloff, R. S. (1974). *In* "The Control of the Onset of Puberty", p. 313. John Wiley, New York.

Oertel, G. W. and Eik-Nes, K. (1961). *Arch. biochem. Biophys.* **92**, 150.

Oertel, G. W. and Kaiser, E. (1962). *Clin. chim. Acta*, **7**, 221.

Oseko, F., Yoshimi, T., Fukase, M. and Kono, T. (1974). *Acta endocr., Copenh.* **76**, 332.

Panicucci, F. (1966). *In* "Androgens in Normal and Pathological Conditions" (A. Vermeulen and D. Exley, eds), p. 25. Int. Cong. Ser. No. 101.

Patton, W. C., Berger, M. S., Thompson, E. E., Chong, A. P., Grimes, E. M. and Taymor, M. L. (1975). *Am. J. Obstet. Gynec.* **121**, 383.

Parks, G. A., Bermudez, S. A., Anast, C. S., Bongiovanni, A. M. and New, M. I. (1971). *J. clin. Endocr. Metab.* **33**, 269.

Pazzagli, M., Borrelli, D., Forti, G. and Serio, M. (1974). *Acta endocr., Copenh.* **76**, 388.

Pearlman, W. H. and Crepy, (1967). *J. biol. Chem.* **242**, 182.

Pearlman, W. H., Pearlman, M. R. S. and Rakoff, A. E. (1954). *J. biol. Chem.* **209**, 803.

Petry, R., Mauss, J., Rausch-Strooman, J. G. and Vermeulen, A. (1972). *Horm. Metab. Res.* **4**, 381.

Pincus, G. and Romanoff, E. B. (1955). *Ciba Found. Colloq. Endocr.* **8**, 97.

Pirke, K. M. (1977). *Steroids*, **30**, 53.

Pirke, K. M., Doerr, P., Sintermann, R. and Vogt, H. J. (1977). *Acta endocr., Copenh.*

86, 415.

Poortman, S., Andriesse, R., Agema, A., Donker, G., Mulder, G. and Thyssen, J. H. H. (1977). *J. ster. Biochem.* **9**, I.

Rager, K., Bundschu, H. and Gupta, D. (1975). *J. reprod. Fert.* **42**, 113.

Rees, L. H. (1977). *Clin. Endocr.* **6**, 137.

Reinberg, A., Lagoguey, M., Chauffournier, M. and Cesselin, F. (1975). *Ann. Endocr.* **36**, 44.

Reyes, F. I., Winter, J. S. D. and Faiman, C. (1973). *J. clin. Endocr. Metab.* **37**, 74.

Reyes, F. I., Boroditsky, M. S., Winter, J. S. D. and Faiman, C. (1974). *J. clin. Endocr. Metab.* **38**, 612.

Riondel, A., Tait, J. F., Gut, M., Tait, S. A. S., Joachim, E. and Little, B. (1963). *J. clin. Endocr. Metab.* **23**, 620.

Rivarola, M. A., Singleton, R. T. and Migeon, C. J. (1967). *J. clin. Invest.* **46**, 2095.

Rivarola, M. A., Saez, J. M., Jones, H. W., Jones, S. G. and Migeon, C. J. (1967). *Johns Hopkins Med. J.* **121**, 82.

Rivarola, M. A., Saez, J. M., Meyer, W. J., Jenkins, M. E. and Migeon, C. J. (1966). *J. clin. Endocr. Metab.* **26**, 1203.

Robel, P., Emiliozzi, R. and Baulieu, E. E. (1966). *J. biol. Chem.* **241**, 20.

Robinson, J. D., Judd, H. L., Young, P. E., Jones, O. W. and Yen, S. S. C. (1977). *J. clin. Endocr. Metab.* **45**, 755.

Raboch, J., Neuwirth, J. and Starka, L. (1975). *Andrologia,* **7**, 77.

Rosenbaum, W., Christy, M. P. and Kelly, W. G. (1966). *J. clin. Endocr. Metab.* **26**, 1399.

Rosenfeld, R. S., Rosenberg, B. S. and Hellman, L. (1975a). *Steroids,* **25**, 799.

Rosenfeld, R. S., Rosenberg, B. S., Fukushima, D. K. and Hellman, L. (1975b). *J. clin. Endocr. Metab.* **40**, 850.

Rosenfeld, R. S., Hellman, L., Roffwarg, H., Weitzmann, E. D., Fukushima, D. K. and Gallagher, T. F. (1971). *J. clin. Endocr. Metab.* **33**, 87.

Rosenfield, R. L. (1971). *J. clin. Endocr. Metab.* **32**, 717.

Rosenfield, R. L. and Otto, P. (1972). *J. clin. Endocr. Metab.* **35**, 818.

Rosenfield, R. L., Ehrlich, E. M. and Cleary, R. A. (1972). *J. clin. Endocr. Metab.* **34**, 92.

Rosenfield, R. L., Barmach de Niepomniszsze, A., Kenny, F. M. and Genel, M. (1974). *J. clin. Endocr. Metab.* **39**, 370.

Rosner, W. (1972). *J. clin. Endocr. Metab.* **34**, 983.

Rubens, R., Dhont, M. and Vermeulen, A. (1974). *J. clin. Endocr. Metab.* **39**, 40.

Rubin, R. T., Poland, R. E. and Tower, B. B. (1976). *J. clin. Endocr. Metab.* **42**, 112.

Saez, J. M., Bertrand, J. and Migeon, C. J. (1971). *Steroids,* **17**, 435.

Saez, J. M., Rivarola, M. A. and Migeon, C. J. (1967). *J. clin. Endocr. Metab.* **27**, 615.

Saez, J. M., Saez, S. and Migeon, C. J. (1967). *Steroids,* **9**, 1.

Saez, J. M., Forest, M. G., Morera, A. M. and Bertrand, J. (1972). *J. clin. Invest.* **51**, 1226.

Saez, J. M., De Peretti, E., Morera, A. M., David, M. and Bertrand, J. (1971). *J. clin. Endocr. Metab.* **32**, 604.

Sanchez, R. S., Murthy, G. G., Mehta, J., Shreeve, W. W. and Singh, F. (1976). *Fert. Steril.* **27**, 667.

Sandberg, A. A. and Slaunwhite, W. R. (1956). *J. clin. Invest.* **35**, 1331.

Sandberg, D. H., Ahmed, M., Zachmann, M. and Cleveland, W. W. (1965). *Steroids,* **6**, 777.

Sandberg, E., Gurpide and Lieberman, S. (1964). *Biochemistry,* **3**, 1256.

Savard, K., Marsh, J. M. and Rice, B. F. (1965). *Rec. Prog. Horm. Res.* **21**, 294.

Scaglia, H. E., Medina, M., Gual, C., Cabeza, M. and Perez-Palacios, G. (1976). *Fert. Steril.* **27**, 243.

Schneider, H. P. G., Bohnet, G. A. and Mühlenstedt, D. (1977), *Acta endocr., Copenh.* **85** (Suppl. 212), 17.

Schneider, G., Genel, M., Bongiovanni, A. M., Goldman, A. S. and Rosenfield, R. L. (1975). *J. clin. Invest.* **55**, 681.

Schubert, R., Weinberger, K. and Frankenberg, G. (1964). *Steroids,* **3**, 579.

Sekihara, H., Ohsawa, N. and Ibayashi, H. (1972). *Steroids,* **20**, 813.

Serio, M., Cattaneo, S., Borrelli, D., Gonnelli, P., Pazzagli, M., Forti, G., Fiorelli, G., Giannotti, P. and Giusti, G. (1977) *In* "Androgens and Antiandrogens" (L. Martini and D. L. Motta, eds). Raven Press, New York.

Sheard, M. H., Marini, J. L. and Giddings, S. S. (1977). *Dis. Nerv. Syst.* **38**, 765.

Sherins, R. J. and Loriaux, D. L. (1973). *J. clin. Endocr. Metab.* **36**, 886.

Shimizu, K. (1965). *J. bioch. Chem.* **6**, 301.

Shimizu, K. and Gut, K. (1965). *Steroids,* **6**, 301.

Sholiton, L. I., Srïvastava, L. and Taylor, B. B. (1976). *Steroids,* **26**, 809.

Siiteri, P. K. and MacDonald, P. C. (1973). *In* "Handbook of Physiology" (S. R. Geiger, E. B. Astwood and R. O. Greep, eds), Vol. II, Part I, p. 615. American Physiological Society.

Silman, R. E., Chard, T., Lowry, P. J., Mullen, P. E., Smith, I. and Young, I. M. (1977). *J. Ster. Biochem.* **8**, 553.

Simmer, H. H., Easterling, W. E., Pion, R. J. and Dignam, W. J. (1965). *Steroids,* **4**, 125.

Sizonenko, P. C. and Paunier, L. (1975). *J. clin. Endocr. Metab.* **41**, 894.

Sizonenko, P. C., Schindler, A. M., Kohlberg, I. S. and Paunier, L. (1972). *Acta endocr., Copenh.* **71**, 539.

Slaunwhite, W. R. and Samuels, L. T. (1956). *J. biol. Chem.* **220**, 341.

Smals, A. G. H., Kloppenborg, P. W. C. and Benraad, Th. J. (1974). *Acta endocr., Copenh.* **77**, 753.

Smals, A. G. H., Kloppenborg, P. W. C. and Benraad, Th. J. (1975). *Acta endocr., Copenh.* **78**, 604.

Smals, A. G. H., Kloppenborg, P. W. C. and Benraad, Th. J. (1977). *J. clin. Endocr. Metab.* **45**, 240.

Smith, K. D., Chetri, M. K., Johanson, A. M., Radfar, N. and Migeon, C. J. (1975). *J. clin. Endocr. Metab.* **41**, 60.

Southren, A. L., Gordon, G. G. and Tochimoto, S. (1968). *J. clin. Endocr. Metab.* **28**, 1105.

Southren, A. L., Tochimoto, S., Carmody, N. C. and Isurugi, K. (1965). *J. clin. Endocr. Metab.* **25**, 1441.

Southren, A. L., Gordon, G. G., Olivo, J., Rafii, F. and Rosenthal, W. S. (1973). *Metabolism,* **22**, 695.

Southren, A. L., Gordon, G. G., Tochimoto, S., Krikun, E. and Krieger, D. (1969). *J. clin. Endocr. Metab.* **29**, 251.

Southren, A. L., Gordon, G. G., Tochimoto, S., Olivo, J., Sherman, D. H. and Pinzon, G. (1969). *J. clin. Endocr. Metab.* **29**, 1356.

Southren, A. L., Gordon, G. G., Tochimoto, S., Pinzon, G., Lane, D. R. and Stypulkowski, W. (1967). *J. clin. Endocr. Metab.* **27**, 686.

Southren, A. L., Olivo, J., Gordon, G. G., Vittek, J., Brener, J. and Rafii, F. (1974). *J. clin. Endocr. Metab.* **38**, 207.

Stein, T. F. and Leventhal, M. L. (1935). *Am. J. Obstet. Gynec.* **219**, 181.

Stewart-Bentley, M. and Horton, R. (1973). *Metabolism,* **22**, 875.

Stewart-Bentley, M., Gans, D. and Horton, R. (1974a). *Metabolism,* **23**, 1065.

Stewart-Bentley, M., Odell, W. and Horton, R. (1974b). *J. clin. Endocr. Metab.* **38**, 545.

Tait, J. F. (1963). *J. clin. Endocr. Metab.* **23**, 1285.

Tait, J. F. and Burstein, J. (1964). *In* "The Hormones" (G. Pincus, K. V. Thimann and E. B. Astwood, eds) Vol. V, p. 441. Academic Press, London and New York.

Tait, J. F. and Horton, R. (1966). *In* "Steroid Dynamics" (G. Pincus, T. Nakao and J. F. Tait, eds), p. 393. Academic Press, New York and London.

Tait, J. F., Little, B., Tait, S. A. S. and Flood, C. (1962). *J. clin. Invest.* **41**, 2093.

Tourniaire, J., Audi-Parera, L., Loras, B., Blum, J., Castelnovo, P. and Forest, M. G. (1976). *Clin. Endocr.* **5**, 53.

Turnipseed, M. R., Bentley, R. and Reynolds, J. W. (1976). *J. clin. Endocr. Metab.* **43**, 1219.

Tyler, J. P. P., Newton, J. R. and Collins, W. P. (1975). *Acta endocr., Copenh.* **80**, 542.

Valladares, L. and Mingnell, J. (1975). *Steroids,* **25**, 13.

Van Look, P. T. A., Hunter, W. M., Corker, C. S. and Baird, T. (1977). *Clin. Endocr.* **7**, 353.

Van Thiel, D. H., Lester, R. and Sherins, R. J. (1974). *Gastroenterology,* **67**, 1188.

Van Thiel, D. H., Gavaler, J. S., Lester, R. and Goodman, M. D. (1975). *Gastroenterology,* **69**, 326.

Vermeulen, A. (1967). *In* "C. R. Table Ronde—Paris 1967. Chromatographie en Phase Gazeuse des Steroides Hormonaux" (R. Scholler and M. F. Jayle, eds). Dunod, Paris.

Vermeulen, A. (1968). *In* "Testosterone" (J. Tamm, ed.), p. 171. G. Thieme Verlag, Stuttgart.

Vermeulen, A. (1973). *Verh. Kon. VI. Acad. Gen. Belgïe,* **35**, 95.

Vermeulen, A. (1974). *In* "The Endocrine Function of the Human Testis" (V. H. T. James and M. Serio, eds), Vol. II. Academic Press, London and New York.

Vermeulen, A. (1976a). Proc. 5th Int. Cong. Endocr., Hamburg (V. H. T. James, ed.), Vol. 2, p. 41. Excerpta Medica Foundation.

Vermeulen, A. (1976b). *J. clin. Endocr. Metab.* **42**, 247.

Vermeulen, A. (1976c). *Acta endocr., Copenh.* **83**, 651.

Vermeulen, A. (1977). *In* "Androgens and Antiandrogens" (L. Martini and M. Motta, eds). Raven Press, New York.

Vermeulen, A., and Ando, S. (1978). *Clin. Endocr.* **8**, 295.

Vermeulen, A. and Comhaire, F. (1978). *Fert. Steril.* **29**, 320;

Vermeulen, A. and Verdonck, L. (1967). *Res. Ster.* **III**, 55.

Vermeulen, A. and Verdonck, L. (1968). *Steroids,* **11**, 609.

Vermeulen, A. and Verdonck, L. (1976a). *J. Ster. Biochem.* **7**, 1.

Vermeulen, A. and Verdonck, L. (1976b). *Am. J. Obstet. Gynec.* **125**, 491.

Vermeulen, A. and Verdonck, L. (1978). *Clin. Endocr.* **9**, 59.

Vermeulen, A., Mussche, M. and Verdonck, L. (1972a). Abst. 2nd Int. Cong. Endocr. Int. Cong. Ser. No. 256, p. 123. Excerpta Medica Foundation.

Vermeulen, A., Rubens, R. and Verdonck, L. (1972b). *J. clin. Endocr. Metab.* **34**, 370.

Vermeulen, A., Stoica, T. and Verdonck, L. (1971). *J. clin. Endocr. Metab.* **33**, 709.

Vermeulen, A., Suy, E. and Rubens, R. (1977). *J. clin. Endocr. Metab.* **44**, 1222.

Vermeulen, A., Dhondt, M., Thiery, M. and Vandekerckhove, D. (1976). *Fert. Steril.* **27**, 773.

Vermeulen, A., Verdonck, L., Van der Straeten and M. Orie (1969). *J. clin. Endocr. Metab.* **29**, 1470.

Vermeulen, A., Vandeweghe, M., Rubens, R., Comhaire, R. and Verdonck, L. (1974). *In* "Recent Progress in Reproductive Endocrinology" (P. S. Crosignani and V. H. T. James, eds), p. 633. Academic Press, London and New York.

Vihko, R. (1966). *Acta endocr., Copenh.* (Suppl. 109).

Vihko, R. and Ruokonen, A. (1974). *J. ster. Biochem.* **5**, 843.

Villee, D. B., Engib, L. L., Loring, J. M. and Villee, C. M. (1961). *Endocrinology,* **69**, 354.

Wang, C., Baker, H. W. G., Burger, H. G., de Kretser, D. M. and Hudson, B. (1975). *Clin. Endocr.* **4**, 399.

Wang, D. Y., Bulbrook, R. D., Sneddon, A. and Hamilton, T. (1967). *J. Endocr.* **38**, 307.

Weinstein, R. L., Kelch, R. P., Jenner, M. S., Kaplan, S. L. and Grumbach, M. M. (1974). *J. clin. Invest.* **53**, 1.

Werk, E. E., Sholiton, L. J. and Kaleis, L. (1973). *New Engl. J. Med.* **289**, 767.

Wieland, R. G., de Courcy, C., Levy, R. P., Zala, A. P. and Hirschman, H. (1965). *J. clin. Invest.* **44**, 159.

Wilson, J. D., Harrod, M. J., Goldstein, J. L., Hemsell, D. L. and MacDonald, P. C. (1971). *New Engl. J. Med.* **290**, 1097.

Winter, J. S. D., Hughes, I. A., Reyes, F. I. and Faiman, C. (1976). *J. clin. Endocr. Metab.* **42**, 679.

Yanaihara, T. and Troen, P. (1972). *J. clin. Endocr. Metab.* **34**, 783.

Yen, S. S. C., Vela, P. and Rankin, J. (1970). *J. clin. Endocr. Metab.* **39**, 435.

Younglai, E. V. (1972). *J. Endocr.* **54**, 513.

Youssefnejadian, E., Collins, W. P. and Sommerville, I. F. (1970). *Steroids,* **22**, 63.

Zachman, M., Völlmin, J. A., Hamilton, W. and Prader, A. (1972). *Clin. Endocr.* **1**, 369.

Zanisi, M., Motta, M. and Martini, L. (1974). *In* "The Endocrine Function of the Human Testes", Vol. I, p. 533. Academic Press, London and New York.

Zondek, T., Mansfield, M. D. and Zondek, H. L. (1977). *Br. J. Obstet. Gynaec.* **84**, 714.

VIII. Progesterone. I. Physico-chemical and Biochemical Aspects

H. J. VAN DER MOLEN

INTRODUCTION

The existence of progesterone was suggested by early observations (Prenant, 1898; Fraenkel, 1903; Loeb, 1907; Bouin and Ancel, 1910; Corner, 1928) that the corpora lutea of the ovary of several animals produces a substance responsible for the secretory response of the endometrium and also necessary for the implantation of the fertilised ovum. This resulted in the preparation of extracts from sow corpora lutea that would maintain pregnancy in castrated rabbits (Allen and Corner, 1929, 1930; Corner and Allen, 1929). Initially the name "progestin" was coined for this active principle of the corpus luteum (Allen, 1930). Subsequently, several groups (Allen and Wintersteiner, 1934; Butenandt, Westphal and Cobler, 1934; Slotta, Ruschig and Fels, 1934; Hartmann and Wettstein, 1934) isolated the biologically active pure crystalline compound, the structure of which was also elucidated by Butenandt and Schmidt (1934). The name "progesterone" was adopted by a conference on the standardisation of sex hormones in 1935 (League of Nations, 1935; Allen, Butenandt, Corner and Slotta, 1935; Allen, 1974). Accounts of several historical aspects of early research on progesterone have recently been published (Allen, 1974; Butenandt and Westphal, 1974; Greep, 1977).

Endometrial changes during the menstrual cycle resembling the endometrial changes in women under influence of administered progesterone and the isolation from urine of pregnanediol (Pearlman, 1948), which was known to be a metabolite of progesterone, were considered evidence for the occurrence of progesterone in the human. Moreover, using biological assays, the presence of progestationally active material in serum of pregnant women was detected by Haskins (1941), whereas Forbes (1950) demonstrated progestational activity in plasma of women before ovulation. Not until 1952 was progesterone isolated from human material (placenta) and identified by chemical criteria (Diczfalusy, 1952; Pearlman and Cerceo, 1952; Salhanick, Noall, Zarrow and Samuels, 1952). Zander (1954) isolated progesterone from human pregnancy plasma and confirmed the structure of the isolated compound by a variety of physico-chemical techniques, including ultraviolet and infrared spectrometry. Finally, Woolever and Goldfien (1963), using a double isotope dilution derivative procedure, obtained the first meaningful estimate of progesterone in blood from normal non-pregnant women. Thereafter, other workers (Riondel, Tait, Tait, Gut and Little, 1965; van der Molen and Groen, 1965), with a variety of sensitive physico-chemical detection techniques, were able to obtain quantitative estimates of progesterone in blood from normal men and women; in other studies (Rünnebaum, van der Molen and Zander, 1965; van der Molen et al., 1965) progesterone was rigorously identified in such plasma samples.

Several authoritative reviews concerning progesterone have been published. These reviews have discussed the occurrence and estimation in blood (Pearlman, 1960; Short, 1961; Zander, 1962; Hendeles, 1965; van der Molen and Aakvaag, 1967; Cooke, 1976), biosynthesis and metabolism (Fotherby, 1964; Dorfman and Unger, 1965; Langecker and Damrosch, 1968), the interrelationship between progesterone and gonadotrophins in the regulation of ovulation and cyclical ovarian and pituitary function (Fotherby, 1964; Rothschild, 1965; Greep, 1973), biological assays (Miyake, 1962), protein binding (Slaunwhite, 1960; Sandberg, Rosenthal, Schneider and Slaunwhite, 1966), secretion and production (Eik-Nes and Hall, 1965) and biochemical actions of progesterone (Gurpide, 1977). The chemistry, including chemical synthesis of progesterone, has been treated extensively by Fieser and Fieser (1959).

A. SOME PHYSICO-CHEMICAL AND CHEMICAL CHARACTERISTICS OF PROGESTERONE

Progesterone (pregn-4-ene-3,20-dione) has the empirical formula $C_{21}H_{30}O_2$ and a molecular weight of 314·4. Progesterone may occur in two interconvertible polymorphic crystalline modifications. Slow crystallisation from ethanol–water mixture results in prisms with a melting point of 129°, whereas rapid crystallisation from ligroin or light petroleum results in needles having a melting point of 121°.

The solubility of progesterone in water, as for most of the naturally occurring steroids, is low, and has been estimated in the order of 5–10 μmol/l (1–3 μg/ml) (Haskins, 1949; Haskins and Taubert, 1963). Progesterone dissolves easily, however, in many organic solvents. Due to its low polarity, its solubility in most of the non-polar solvents that are commonly used in steroid chemistry, such as hexane, heptane, ligroin and light petroleum, is excellent. This has advantageously been used for extraction and chromatography under conditions which will separate progesterone from other, more polar, steroids.

The presence of the Δ^4-3 oxo structure in the progesterone molecule results in a maximal absorption at approximately 240 mμ. This property is widely used for localisation of the compound when present in sufficiently large quantity during chromatography and for quantitative estimations. Other physico-chemical characteristics of progesterone may be demonstrated by infrared spectrometry, mass spectrometry, nuclear magnetic resonance, optical rotation and rotatory dispersion. The optical rotation of progesterone in acetone solution is $(\alpha)_D = +175°$, but in ethanol solution $(\alpha)_D = +192°$. Such techniques, however, have mainly been used when problems of identification and characterisation are involved, whereas they find little application for problems involving routine analysis of progesterone in blood.

Formation of derivatives of progesterone has frequently been used during estimation and characterisation of progesterone to modify or improve the sensitivity of detection in spectrophotometry, gas chromatography, or to introduce a radioactive isotope. Moreover, derivative formation modifies the chromatographic properties of progesterone to permit separation from contaminating compounds during column, paper, thin layer or gas chromatography.

By virtue of the presence of oxo groups at C-3 and C-20, progesterone will generally react with reagents such as thiosemicarbazide, dinitrophenyl-hydrazine and isonicotinic acid hydrazide. More specifically applied to separations involving gas chromatography, derivatives involving ketonic reagents, such as the dimethylhydrazones (Gardiner and Horning, 1966), methoximes (Van den Heuvel and Horning, 1963) and ethylenethioketals (Zmigrod and Lindner, 1966) have been used. It is relatively easy to reduce the oxo groups in the progesterone molecule. Reductions performed with specific enzymes, such as 20α-hydroxysteroid dehydrogenase (Wiest, 1959; Wiest and Wilcox, 1961) or 20β-hydroxysteroid dehydrogenase (Hübener, Sahrholz, Schmidt-Thomé, Nesemann and Junk, 1959; Henning and Zander, 1962; Purdue, Halla and Little, 1964) will, under proper conditions, result in almost quantitative conversion to a single well defined substance, 20α-hydroxypregn-4-en-3-one or 20β-hydroxypregn-4-en-3-one respectively. Chemical reduction of progesterone using sodium or potassium borohydride (Norymberski and Woods, 1955) or lithium aluminium hydride may under controlled conditions (e.g. low borohydride concentrations in the cold) yield a mixture of the 20-hydroxy epimers, containing mainly 20β-hydroxypregn-4-en-3-one. With excess reagents, or at higher temperature, progesterone will be converted to a mixture of pregn-4-ene-3,20-diols.

After reduction of progesterone, it is possible to perform further chemical transformations involving the resulting hydroxyl groups. In this respect acetylation has frequently been used, although, especially in combination with gas chromatography, other derivatives such as the chloroacetates, heptafluorobutyrates, trimethylsilylethers, trifluoroacetates, and chloro-difluoroacetates have been used after reduction of progesterone isolated from biological sources. Methods for progesterone measurements involving its conversion to 20-hydroxypregn-4-en-3-ones may equally well be applied to the measurement of the 20-hydroxypregn-4-en-3-ones present in blood and tissues, if these compounds are separated from progesterone and from one another before reduction.

The occurrence of progesterone in urine was doubtful for a long time. Small amounts of biologically active progesterone-like material were found in urine of pregnant and non-pregnant women as early as 1931 (De Fremery, Luchs and Tausk, 1931; Loewe and Voss, 1934; Fels, 1937). Progesterone lacks free hydroxyl groups and can thus not be conjugated with sulphuric or glucuronic acid. Ismail and Harkness (1966) obtained physico-chemical evidence for the presence of about 5 µg progesterone/l in urine obtained from pregnant women. Also with sensitive gas chromatographic techniques the occurrence of about 1 µg progesterone/24 hr in urine of non-pregnant women during the menstrual cycle has been demonstrated (van der Molen and Corpéchot, 1968) and urinary progesterone has been used as an index of ovulation and corpus luteum function (Chattoraj, Rankin, Turner and Lowe, 1976).

B. SITES OF PRODUCTION AND MODE OF BIOSYNTHESIS

Progesterone has been considered a key intermediate in the biosynthesis of steroid hormones. Recently, however, it has become evident that progesterone is not an obligatory intermediate in the production of corticosteroids in the adrenal (Weliky and Engel, 1962), or of androgens in the testis (Neher and Wettstein, 1960; Eik-Nes and Hall, 1962), while the results of Ryan and Smith (1961) indicate that androgens and oestrogens might be formed in the ovary by a biosynthetic pathway not involving progesterone. In this other pathway the Δ^5-3β-hydroxy configuration of pregnenolone is maintained while other parts of the molecule are changed, for example, by introduction of a hydroxyl group in 17α-position or by removal of the side chain at C-17. This pathway may be the more important one in the canine ovary *in vivo* (Aakvaag and Eik-Nes, 1964, 1965).

Cholesterol sulphate as well as steroid sulphates can serve as substrates for the various enzymes involved in the biosynthesis of steroid hormones (Calvin and Lieberman, 1966), and Pion, Conrad and Wolf (1966) have demonstrated the conversion of pregnenolone sulphate to progesterone by human placentae.

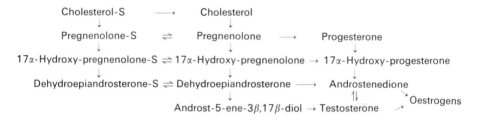

Fig. 1. Pathways for steroid biosynthesis originating from cholesterol (S = sulphate).

1. Ovary

Progesterone has been measured in the ovarian vein blood of several animal species (Table 1), thus supporting the evidence for synthesis and secretion of progesterone by the ovary. The steroid biosynthetic capacity of the different compartments of the human ovary has been studied by incubations of tissue slices or minces *in vitro* (Savard *et al.*, 1965; Ryan and Smith, 1965) and by cultures of separated cell types (Channing, 1969). It has been shown that the Graafian follicle may produce progesterone, but the corpus luteum secretes much more progesterone into the ovarian effluent. Little or no progesterone production has been found in ovarian stroma (Rice and Savard, 1966).

Table 1

Progesterone in the ovarian venous effluent from various animal species.

Species	Physiological condition	Progesterone (μg/100 ml plasma)[c]	References
Rabbit[a]	Pre-ovulatory	n.d.	Hilliard et al. (1963)
Rabbit[a]	Post-ovulatory	12 ± 4.5^b	Hilliard et al. (1963)
Rabbit[a]	Pregnant	70–130	Hafez et al. (1965)
Rat	Early di-oestrus	50 (n.d.–125)	Eto et al. (1962)
Rat	Late pro-oestrus	125 (80–180)	Eto et al. (1962)
Rat	Pregnant (day 15)	280	Eto et al. (1962)
Ewe	Follicular phase	n.d.	Short et al. (1963)
Ewe	Mid-luteal phase	95.3 ± 46.1	Short et al. (1963)
Ewe	Late-luteal phase	104.3 ± 37.4	Short et al. (1963)
Dog	Anoestrus	n.d.	Telegdy and Endröczi (1961)
Dog	Luteal phase	61.2 (5.5–228)	Telegdy and Endröczi (1961)
Human	Follicular phase	n.d.	Mikhail et al. (1963)
Human	Follicular phase	n.d.–8.1	Aakvaag and Fylling (1966)
Human	Follicular phase	0.393–1.550	Mikhail (1967); De Jong et al. (1974)
Human	Luteal phase	14.8–110.0	Mikhail and Allen (1966); Mikhail et al. (1963); De Jong et al. (1974)
Human	Pregnant	6.4–58.1	Lurie et al. (1966)
Human	Pregnant	152	Aakvaag and Fylling (1966)

[a] Produces mainly pregn-4-en-20α-ol-3-one.
[b] Secretion rate (μg/hr).
[c] n.d. = not detectable.

(a) Graafian follicle

During the follicular phase of the cycle very little progesterone is found in the ovarian vein blood, although substantial concentrations have been demonstrated in follicular fluid (Zander, Forbes, von Münstermann and Neher, 1958; De Jong, Baird and van der Molen, 1974). It may thus be concluded that the Graafian follicle produces progesterone *in vivo*, but apparently does not secrete it significantly (Aakvaag and Fylling, 1966). Ryan and Smith (1961) demonstrated the formation of progesterone from acetate by follicular tissue *in vitro* and showed that the formation of progesterone in follicular tissue follows the same pathways as steroid production in other organs. It is debatable whether both the granulosa cells and the theca cells have the ability to carry out the complete biosynthesis from acetate to progesterone separately, or that products formed by one kind of tissue cells need to be further transformed by the other cells (Short, 1964).

Ryan and Short (1966) separated the granulosa cells from the theca cells in the follicle of the mare, and showed that both cell types form cholesterol from acetate *in vitro*. They failed, however, in demonstrating any formation of steroid hormones. Granulosa cells as well as theca cells from human follicles can transform pregnenolone to progesterone *in vitro* (Ryan and Petro, 1966).

It has been suggested that the granulosa cells are primarily responsible for the progesterone production in the follicle. Ryan and Petro (1966) and Channing (1969) have substantiated this, demonstrating that the metabolism of the human granulosa, cells closely resembles that of the corpus luteum (Ryan, 1963).

(b) Corpus luteum

Granulosa cells of the Graafian follicle are not close to blood vessels, and their secretory products do not readily enter the blood-stream. When ovulation occurs, blood vessels and fibroblasts grow into the collapsed follicle, and the granulosa cells are converted into lutein cells; the progesterone produced by these cells can readily pass into the vascular system (Short, 1962).

This sequence of events is considered to be the physiological background for the cyclic variation observed in the urinary pregnanediol excretion and in the plasma concentration of progesterone throughout the menstrual cycle. Progesterone has been isolated from human corpora lutea (Zander *et al.*, 1958) as well as from corpora lutea of other animals (Rowlands and Short, 1959).

During the life span of the corpus luteum in women, Mikhail, Zander and Allen (1963) found the concentration of progesterone in ovarian vein blood to decrease from day 5 after ovulation onwards. This pattern is also found for the concentration of progesterone in peripheral blood plasma (see Ch. IX). Moreover, it appears that the corpus luteum *in vitro* produces maximum amounts of progesterone about day 5 after ovulation (Savard, Marsh and Rice, 1965).

2. Testis

Progesterone is produced by testicular tissue as an intermediate in the production of androgens. There are indications that the pathway through progesterone to C_{19} steroids is not the main one for production of testosterone (Eik-Nes and Kekre, 1963; Hagen and Eik-Nes, 1964; van der Molen and Eik-Nes, 1971). The presence of progesterone in testicular venous blood of the dog has been demonstrated (van der Molen and Eik-Nes, 1971), but there is no convincing evidence that progesterone is a secretory product of the testis in man (Strott *et al.*, 1969).

3. Adrenal Cortex

Progesterone has been isolated from the adrenal gland (Beall and Reichstein, 1938), but although adrenal contribution to plasma progesterone is assumed to be of little physiological significance the amount secreted by the adrenal gland is not known. Progesterone has been isolated in the adrenal venous effluent in women (Short, 1960a) and in domestic animals (Balfour, Comline and Short, 1957; Heap, Holzbauer and Newport, 1966). ACTH administration did not increase the plasma progesterone (Wolever, 1963). Several workers have observed that the excretion of pregnanediol in human urine may increase after ACTH administration. As pointed out by Arcos *et al.* (1964), the specific activity of pregnanediol in the urine after injection of labelled progesterone cannot be used to calculate secretion rate of progesterone since compounds other than progesterone contributed to urinary pregnanediol, especially in non-pregnant individuals. The increment in urinary pregnanediol excretion observed after ACTH may therefore be due to an increased adrenal output of pregnenolone or pregnenolone sulphate (Arcos, Gurpide, van der Wiele and Lieberman, 1964).

4. Placenta

The placental production of steroid hormones has been the subject of several reviews (Cassmer, 1959; Diczfalusy, 1964; Solomon, 1966) and many important contributions to the understanding of this parameter of placental function have appeared. The placenta is unique among endocrine organs in that its existence is temporary, and during this limited life span the output of steroid hormones, at least in the human, exceeds that of any other steroid-producing organ.

The placenta seems to differ from other steroid-producing organs with regard to the mode of biosynthesis of steroids. The pathway for steroid production from acetate through squalene, lanosterol and cholesterol, prevailing in other endocrine organs (Fig. 2) (Samuels, 1960), does not play the same role in the placenta. Zalewski and Villee (1966) obtained results which might indicate that the pathway for placental biosynthesis of cholesterol from acetate via squalence and lanosterol might differ from the pathway used for this conversion through mevalonate. Placental perfusions, as well as incubations with placental tissue, have failed to demonstrate the formation of progesterone from acetate (Levitz, Emerman and Dancis, 1962; van Leusden and Villee, 1965).

Acetyl-CoA → ... → Mevalonic acid → ... →

→ Squalene → Lanosterol → ... → Cholesterol →

→ 20α-Hydroxycholesterol → 20α,22-Dihydroxycholesterol →

→ Pregnenolone → Progesterone

Fig. 2. The biosynthesis of progesterone from "acetate". For a detailed discussion of steps in this biosynthetic sequence and the importance of separate pools of a single compound see Savard *et al.* (1965).

Cholesterol is probably an obligatory precursor for placental progesterone production. This compound is present in ample amounts in the maternal blood. By perfusing the placenta with blood containing [4-^{14}C]-cholesterol Solomon (1960) isolated radioactive progesterone in the perfusate. The radioactive precursor yielded 0·1% progesterone. The rate of conversion observed *in vitro* is large enough to account for the progesterone production *in vivo* in late pregnancy.

Placental conversion of pregnenolone or pregnenolone sulphate of adrenal origin in the maternal circulation may also be taken into consideration. The nearly normal pregnanediol excretion observed by Harkness, Menini, Charles, Kenny and Rombaut (1966) in a pregnant adrenalectomised woman, however, points to a limited role of the maternal adrenal in progesterone production during pregnancy.

The midterm foetus lacks the ability to convert Δ^5-3β-hydroxy steroids into the corresponding Δ^4-3-oxo steroids (Mancuso, Dell'acqua, Eriksson, Wiqvist and Diczfalusy, 1966; Bolté, Wiqvist and Diczfalusy, 1966), and all progesterone formed by the foetal–placental unit is probably synthesised in the placenta.

Although the foetus may contribute to the cholesterol or pregnenolone (or its sulphate) that is converted to progesterone in the placenta (Pion, Jaffe, Eriksson, Wiqvist and Diczfalusy, 1965; Palmer, Wiqvist, Eriksson and Diczfalusy, 1966a), the results of Cassmer (1959) indicate that the foetal contribution of precursors for placental progesterone production is small as compared with that of the mother. It has been shown that progesterone transported from the placenta to the foetus may be partly converted by the foetus to other steroids. Among the steroids formed is 20α-hydroxy-pregn-4-en-3-one, which may be reoxidised to progesterone upon recirculation through the placenta (Palmer, Blair, Eriksson and Diczfalusy, 1966b). However small or large the foetal contribution to placental progesterone production may be, this progesterone production is ultimately dependent upon the amount of sterol and steroid precursors transported to the foetus via the placenta.

C. DETECTION TECHNIQUES FOR ESTIMATION OF PROGESTERONE IN BLOOD

Several techniques that potentially could be applied for detection of progesterone have found limited application for estimation of progesterone in biological samples. Such techniques include polarographic detection of Girard derivatives (Butt, Morris, Morris and Williams, 1951), infrared spectrophotometry (Zander, 1955; van der Molen *et al.*, 1965) spectrophotometry and fluorimetry in sulphuric acid (Zaffaroni, 1950), the Zimmermann reaction and sodium hydroxide fluorescence (Bush, 1952) and potassium *t*-butoxide fluorescence (Abelson and Bondy, 1955). Due to the (relative) lack of specificity and sensitivity these techniques have been used merely for qualitative purposes.

Levels of progesterone in peripheral plasma of human subjects range between 20 and 50 ng/100 ml plasma for men, between 20 and 400 ng/100 ml plasma for women in the follicular phase of the cycle and between 140 and 2000 ng/100 ml plasma in the luteal phase of the cycle. Only methods that are sensitive enough to measure progesterone at the nanogram level can, therefore, be used for the detection of progesterone in 10 ml plasma samples from normal men and women.

Although several attempts were made to apply the ultra-violet absorption of progesterone for its quantitative measurement in biological extracts (Reynolds and Ginsberg, 1942; Haskins, 1950; Butt *et al.*, 1951), it was only in 1953, that Edgar (1953) succeeded in measuring progesterone isolated from biological material. The first physico-chemical method for the reliable determination of progesterone in human blood was introduced by Zander (1954). The sensitivity of this and other spectrophotometric methods (300–500 ng) limited the application of this method for reasonable blood volumes to analysis of human blood during the second half of pregnancy. The rapid development of more sensitive saturation analyses for progesterone estimation since 1960, notably competitive protein binding and radioimmunoassay methods, have offered several possibilities for the large scale application of progesterone assays in human blood.

1. Bioassays

Numerous bioassay methods using different endpoints have been suggested for the estimation of progesterone (Miyake, 1962). Such methods have generally employed the effect of progesterone on the uterine endometrium and the ovary, or the capacity to maintain pregnancy in a variety of animals. Cytological or biological changes in the test animals have most frequently been used as parameter for the biological activity of progesterone. Pincus, Miyake, Merril and Longo (1957) and Miyake and Pincus (1958) have used the increase in endometrial carbonic anhydrase of immature female rabbits as an index of "progestational" activity.

Although the sensitivity of early bioassay methods for progesterone was poor, the sensitivity of the methods of McGinty, Anderson and McCullough (1939) ($0 \cdot 1$–$0 \cdot 05$ µg) or Hooker and Forbes (1947) ($0 \cdot 0002$ µg) was as good as, or better than, the sensitivity of many of the physico-chemical techniques that have been used for progesterone detection. In the technique developed by McGinty *et al.* (1939) proliferation of the endometrium after injection of the unknown extracts into an isolated segment of the uterine horns of immature female rabbits, is employed as parameter. The Hooker-Forbes test depends on the hypertrophy of stromal nuclei in the endometrium of ovariectomised mice after intra-uterine injection of progesterone-containing extracts.

Most or all of the bioassay techniques lack specificity in that several compounds, other than progesterone, may exert similar effects. It has for example been shown that 16α- or 17α-hydroxyprogesterone, 20α- or 20β-hydroxypregn-4-en-3-one or oestrogens, may exert synergistic or antagonistic actions on the effect of progesterone in the Hooker-Forbes test, depending upon the amounts of these compounds present in progesterone-containing extracts (Forbes, 1959; 1964).

A more serious disadvantage, which renders such bioassay techniques less valuable for the reliable quantitation of progesterone, is the variation of the relative responses to similar compounds in different tests. This is clearly demonstrated when comparing the responses to progesterone and 20-dihydroprogesterone observed in different techniques (Table 2). It appears

Table 2

Comparison of biological activities of progesterone, 20α-hydroxypregn-4-en-3-one (20α-OH-pregn.) and 20β-hydroxypregn-4-en-3-one (20β-OH-pregn.) in different assay methods. The activity of progesterone in each test is arbitrarily designated 100%.

Assay method	Progesterone	20α-OH-pregn.	20β-OH-pregn.	References
Hooker-Forbes	100	40	200	Zander *et al.* (1958)
Clauberg	100	30–50	10–50	Zander *et al.* (1958)
Maintenance of pregnancy in spayed rats or mice	100	5	5	Talwalker *et al.* (1966); Wiest and Forbes (1964)
Implantation in ovariectomised rabbits	100	10	10	Rennie and Davies (1965)

that the effect of 20α- and 20β-dihydroprogesterone on the maintenance of pregnancy is much lower than the effect on the uterine mucosa.

Variations in specificity and reactivity of different strains of the same animal species may influence the results of bioassay as demonstrated by the effect of 17α-hydroxyprogesterone in the Hooker-Forbes test. Zarrow, Neher, Lasowasem and Salhanick (1957) found an activity of 17α-hydroxyprogesterone 60 times as large as that of progesterone, whereas Zander, Forbes, Neher and Desaulles (1957), using the same test with a different strain of mice, found 17α-hydroxyprogesterone to be inactive.

Lack of specificity, however, applies equally well to most of the physico-chemical detection techniques for progesterone estimation. The isolation of fractions containing progesterone, without contaminating substances, might be expected to overcome this. Although with bioassay methods reliable quantitative estimates might be obtained under strictly standardised conditions, the risk that unexpected contaminating impurities may influence the biological response seems larger than with a physico-chemical technique. This, in addition to the possibility of spontaneous variations between test animals, and the cost and time required for biological testing, renders physico-chemical techniques or saturation analyses for mass estimation to be recommended.

Biological assays, by virtue of the progestational effects that can be studied, may be expected to remain important in the evaluation and characterisation of biological activities of substances relative to the biological activity of progesterone, especially on account of the numerous "progestins" that are being synthesised industrially. Since the quantitation by chemical means of these synthetic compounds is often difficult and because such synthetic compounds derive their importance from their biological activities, initial testing or screening by biological techniques is indispensable.

2. Spectrophotometry

The absorption of the ultraviolet radiation at 240 mμ resulting from the presence of the Δ^4-3-oxo structure in the progesterone molecule, has been widely used for quantitative estimation (Reynolds and Ginsberg, 1942; Haskins, 1950, 1954; Diczfalusy, 1952; Pearlman and Cerceo, 1952; Edgar, 1953; Zander and Simmer, 1954; Short, 1956, 1958; Marti and Schindler, 1961) (Table 3).

The presence of the oxo-groups in the progesterone molecule has frequently been used to prepare coloured derivatives that can be measured spectrophotometrically. Thus, Hinsberg, Pelzer and Seuken (1956), Hilliard, Endröczi and Sawyer (1961), and Telegdy and Endröczi (1961) have employed the absorption of progesterone-bis-dinitrophenylhydrazone in acid

Table 3

Sensitivity of detection of some physico-chemical techniques that have been used for the quantitative estimation of progesterone isolated from biological sources.

Principle of detection	Sensitivity (ng)	References
UV absorption of progesterone ($\varepsilon_{240} = ca$ 17,000)	300–500	Zander and Simmer (1954); Short (1958)
Absorption of dinitrophenylhydrazone derivative ($\varepsilon_{380} = ca$ 40,000)	100–200	Hinsberg et al. (1956)
Absorption of isonicotinic acid hydrazide derivative ($\varepsilon_{380} = ca$ 12,000)	500–1000	Sommerville and Deshpande (1958)
Absorption of sulphuric acid–ethanol chromogen ($\varepsilon_{290} = ca$ 20,000)	300–500	Oertel et al. (1959)
Absorption of thiosemicarbazide derivative ($\varepsilon_{300} = ca$ 40,000)	100–200	Pearlman and Cerceo (1953); Simmer and Simmer (1959)
KOH-sulphuric acid fluorescence	50–100	Touchstone and Murawec (1960); Short and Levett (1962)
Sulphuric acid fluorescence after conversion to 20β-dihydroprogesterone	3–5	Heap (1964)
Double isotope derivative (^{3}H and ^{14}C) measuring 20-^{3}H-20β-dihydroprogesterone	100	Woolever and Goldfien (1963)
Double isotope derivative (^{3}H and ^{35}S) measuring progesterone-^{35}S-thiosemicarbazide-2′,4′-diacetate	2	Riondel et al. (1965)
Double isotope derivative (^{3}H and ^{14}C) measuring 20β-dihydroprogesterone-^{3}H-acetate	10–20	Wiest et al. (1966)
Argon ionisation detection after gas–liquid chromatography	10–100	Collins and Sommerville (1964)
Flame ionisation detection after gas–liquid chromatography	5–100	Yannone et al. (1964); Lurie et al. (1966a)
Electron capture detection of the chloroacetate derivative of 20β-dihydroprogesterone	1	van der Molen and Groen (1965)
Competitive protein binding	0·5–1·0	Reeves et al. (1970)
Radioimmunoassay	0·01–0·02	Abraham et al. (1971)
Enzyme immunoassay	0·01–0·02	Dray et al. (1975)

or neutral solution at 380 mμ, whereas Rombauts and Piton (1963) used the absorption of the same derivative in alkaline solution at 445 mμ. Although the molar extinction coefficients for the dinitrophenylhydrazone of progesterone in acid solution (ε_{380} = about 36,600) and in alkaline solution

(ε_{445} = about 31,000) appear to be comparable, the main advantage of Rombauts and Piton's procedure appears to be removal of excess reagent by a simple solvent extraction without chromatographic purification.

Application of the spectral absorption of the thiosemicarbazone derivative of progesterone for quantitative measurement has been attempted by several workers (Pearlman and Cerceo, 1953; Simmer and Simmer, 1959; Sommerville, Pickett, Collins and Denyer, 1963). Despite the high molecular absorption coefficient of this derivative (Table 3), impurities from glassware and reagents frequently interfere with specific measurement of progesterone. Thus corrections have to be applied, and the sensitivity of measurement for this derivative is little better than that for other progesterone derivatives when measured by spectrophotometric techniques.

The isonicotinic acid hydrazone derivative has been applied for measurement of plasma progesterone by Sommerville and Deshpande (1958). Although Oertel, Weiss and Eik-Nes (1959) have claimed the absorption at 290 mμ of the chromogen formed from progesterone after treatment with a sulphuric acid–ethanol reagent to be more sensitive for progesterone detection than ultraviolet absorption at 240 mμ, later work (Short, 1961; van der Molen, 1963) has shown these techniques to be of comparable sensitivity.

The application of nearly all of these spectrophotometric procedures to the analysis of progesterone in biological samples has required the use of Allen's (1950) procedure to correct for the interference of unspecific absorption of contaminating impurities. The actual sensitivity of detection may therefore be less than might be expected from the molecular extinction coefficients at the wavelengths of maximal absorption. Using appropriate microcells (total capacity 0·2–0·3 ml), the smallest amounts of progesterone that can be measured spectrophotometrically fall in the range of 0·1–0·5 µg (Table 3).

3. Fluorescence

Short and Levett (1962), using the KOH-sulphuric acid fluorescence described by Touchstone and Murawec (1960) for progesterone measurement, could estimate as little as 0·05 µg progesterone and have applied this to detection of progesterone isolated from human peripheral blood. Heap (1964) described a method for progesterone assay in which the hormone is converted enzymically to 20β-hydroxy-pregn-4-en-3-one. The latter compound could be measured by fluorescence in a sulphuric acid–ethanol reagent with a sensitivity of detection of 3–5 ng.

4. Detection after Gas Chromatography

The application of gas chromatography to the isolation and quantitative estimation of progesterone has been reviewed by Wotiz and Clark (1966) and van der Molen (1967). In combination with gas–liquid chromatography, a number of physical methods for detection of compounds have become available. Detection by flame ionisation, argon ionisation and electron capture has proved to be sensitive enough for estimation of the small amounts of progesterone (or derivatives) isolated from biological sources. Argon ionisation (Futterweit, McNiven and Dorfman, 1963; Collins and Sommerville, 1964) and flame ionisation detectors (Yannone, McGomas and Goldfien, 1964; Lurie *et al.*, 1966a; van der Molen and Groen, 1967) will permit estimation of amounts of progesterone of the order of 0·1–0·01 µg.

Although progesterone does not capture electrons to an extent that will permit sensitive detection, electron capture of appropriate derivatives of progesterone may permit estimation of amounts in the nanogram range. Van der Molen and Groen (1965) have used the chloroacetate derivative of 20β-dihydroprogesterone in a method for the estimation of progesterone in peripheral plasma; they were able to detect as little as 1 ng of the chloroacetate derivative. Moreover, Raisinghani, Dorfman and Forchielli (1966) have reported detection and estimation of nanogram quantities of progesterone as the chlorodifluoro acetate derivative of 20β-dihydroprogesterone. The application of heptafluorobutyrate derivatives in combination with electron capture detection (van der Molen and Groen, 1967) has permitted detection of amounts of the order of 0·1–0·2 ng for 20β-dihydroprogesterone heptafluorobutyrate. Combination of gas–liquid chromatography with detection of radioactivity in the effluent gas, has been used by Collins and Sommerville (1964) for detection of radioactively labelled progesterone.

Although the detection systems as applied in gas chromatography may show a specificity for some compounds, they are in general relatively non-specific. Thus, the specificity of estimations using detection in combination with gas chromatography will generally depend upon separation of progesterone (or a derivative) from other compounds before reaching the detector. See Ch. 3 for determination of progesterone and its metabolites by GLC–MS.

5. Isotope Labelling

The use of radioactively labelled reagents that will react with progesterone has permitted the preparation of labelled progesterone derivatives. After purification of such derivatives, the amount of radioactivity in the final residue will be proportional to the amount of progesterone or its derivative.

Isotope derivative techniques for estimation of progesterone have involved preparation of derivatives such as 20β-dihydroprogesterone using sodium [3H]-borohydride (Woolever and Goldfien, 1963), progesterone-thiosemicarbazide-diacetate using [35S]-thiosemicarbazide (Riondel *et al.*, 1965) and 20β-dihydroprogesterone acetate after reduction and acetylation with [3H]-acetic anhydride (Wiest, Kerengi and Csapo, 1966). The sensitivity of such techniques depends on the sensitivity of estimation of radioactivity and the specific activity of the labelling reagents. To ensure accuracy and precision, the isotope derivative procedure has been applied predominantly in combination with the isotope dilution procedure to correct for losses during the purification of the sample.

This approach has been applied using combinations of [14C]-progesterone and [3H]-acetic anhydride (van der Molen *et al.*, 1965; Wiest *et al.*, 1966), [14C]-progesterone and sodium [3H]-borohydride (Woolever and Goldfien, 1963), [14C]-progesterone and [35S]-thiosemicarbazide (Riondel *et al.*, 1965).

The sensitivity and precision of such techniques depend upon the measurement of the two isotopes in the derivatives and appropriate standards, and is mainly limited by the specific activity of the radioactive compounds and the efficiency for simultaneous counting of isotopes with different energy spectra. Depending on the combinations used, the sensitivity of double isotope dilution derivative techniques has been reported to be from 0·1 (Woolever and Goldfien, 1963; Wiest *et al.*, 1966) to 0·002 µg (Riondel *et al.*, 1965) (Table 3).

The specificity of these techniques depends upon the rigorous purification of the labelled derivative and removal of all radioactive contaminants before the final counting. Precision of estimation is mainly dependent on the ratio of the mass of labelled steroid added as indicator and the mass of steroid present in the sample.

6. Saturation Analyses

(a) Competitive protein binding

Since the suggestion of Murphy (1967) that the method of competitive protein binding might be used for the estimation of progesterone, several methods have used this principle (Neill, Johansson and Knobil, 1967); Yoshimi and Lipsett, 1968; Reeves, de Souza, Thompson and Diczfalusy, 1970; Martin, Cooke and Black, 1970). Amounts as small as 0·1–0·2 ng of progesterone have been estimated (Reeves *et al.*, 1970). Corticosteroid binding globulin (CBG) is normally used as the binding protein, the source of CBG being diluted whole plasma obtained from dogs, from pregnant women (after removal of endogenous steroids) or from oestrogen-treated ovariectomised women. [^{3}H]-Progesterone as well as [^{3}H]-corticosterone (compound B) have been used as indicator steroids for competitive binding of progesterone. Competitive binding methods are rapid to perform, but due to the great sensitivity of these techniques and a relatively low specificity, particular care must be taken in estimating low amounts (< 1 ng) of progesterone.

(b) Radioimmunoassay

Since the introduction of the radioimmunoassay technique to progesterone estimation (Furuyama and Nugent, 1971; Abraham, Swerdloff, Tulchinsky and Odell, 1971) this technique undoubtedly has become the most widely used detection technique in progesterone assays. This development has resulted from the high specificity of antisera, the high sensitivity (10–20 pg) of detection and the relative ease of application of this technique in methods for routine applications in clinical situations. Details of this methodology have been discussed by Abraham (1974) and it is considered further, together with competitive protein-binding in Ch. IX.

(c) Enzyme immunoassay

In order to avoid the use of radiolabels required in radioimmunoassays, several attempts have been made to develop immunoassays of steroid-haptens using other kinds of labelling. A sensitive enzyme immunoassay for progesterone has been described (Dray, Andrieu and Renaud, 1975) using β-galactosidase coupled to progesterone as label. The progesterone-β-galactosidase conjugate will compete with progesterone for binding to progesterone antisera and the enzyme activity of the conjugate can be determined spectrophotometrically with O-nitrophenyl-β-D-galactoside as substrate. The specificity and sensitivity (10–20 pg) of this enzyme immunoassay (Dray et al., 1975) makes it an attractive alternative to radioimmunoassay for progesterone.

REFERENCES

Aakvaag, A. and Eik-Nes, K. B. (1964). *Biochim. biophys. Acta*, **86**, 380.
Aakvaag, A. and Eik-Nes, K. B. (1965). *Biochim. biophys. Acta*, **111**, 273.
Aakvaag, A. and Fylling, P. (1966). *Acta obstet. gynec. Scand.* (Suppl. 9), 158.
Abelson, D. and Bondy, P. K. (1955). *Arch. biochem. Biophys.* **57**, 208.
Abraham, G. E. (1974). *Acta endocr., Copenh.* **75** (Suppl. 183).
Abraham, G. E., Swerdloff, R., Tulchinsky, D. and Odell, W. D. (1971). *J. clin. Endocr. Metab.* **32**, 619.
Allen, W. M. (1930). *J. Physiol., Lond.* **92**, 174.
Allen, W. M. (1974). *Gynec. Invest.* **5**, 142.

434 H. J. VAN DER MOLEN

Allen, W. M. and Corner, G. W. (1929). *Am. J. Physiol.* **88**, 340.
Allen, W. M. and Corner, G. W. (1930). *Proc. Soc. exp. Biol. Med.* **27**, 403.
Allen, W. M. and Wintersteiner, O. (1934). *Science, N.Y.* **80**, 190.
Allen, W. M., Butenandt, A., Corner, G. W. and Slotta, K. H. (1935). *Science, N.Y.* **82**, 153.
Arcos, M., Gurpide, E., Vande Wiele, R. L. and Lieberman, S. (1964). *J. clin. Endocr. Metab.* **24**, 237.
Balfour, W. E., Comline, R. S. and Short, R. V. (1957). *Nature, Lond.* **180**, 1480.
Beall, D. and Reichstein, T. (1938). *Nature, Lond.* **142**, 479.
Bolté, E., Wiqvist, N. and Diczfalusy, E. (1966). *Acta endocr., Copenh.* **52**, 583.
Bouin, P. and Ancel, P. (1910). *J. Physiol. Path. gén.* **12**, 1.
Bush, I. E. (1952). *Biochem. J.* **50**, 370.
Butenandt, A. and Schmidt, J. (1934). *Ber. dt. Chem. Ges.* **67**, 2068.
Butenandt, A. and Westphal, U. (1974). *Am. J. Obstet. Gynec.* **120**, 138.
Butenandt, A., Westphal, U. and Cobler, H. (1934). *Ber. dt. Chem. Ges.* **67**, 1611.
Butt, W. R., Morris, P., Morris, C. J. O. R. and Williams, D. C. (1951). *Biochem. J.* **49**, 434.
Calvin, H. J. and Lieberman, S. (1966). *J. clin. Endocr.* **26**, 402.
Cassmer, O. (1959). *Acta endocr., Copenh.* (Suppl. 45), 33.
Channing, C. P. (1969). *J. Endocr.* **45**, 297.
Chattoraj, S. C., Rankin, J. S., Turner, A. K. and Lowe, E. W. (1976). *J. clin. Endocr. Metab.* **43** 1402.
Collins, W. P. and Sommerville, I. F. (1964). *Nature, Lond.* **203**, 836.
Cooke, I. D. (1976). *In* "Hormone Assays and their Clinical Applications", Ch. 14. Churchill Livingstone, Edinburgh.
Corner, G. W. (1928). *Am. J. Physiol.* **86**, 74.
Corner, G. W. and Allen, W. M. (1929). *Am. J. Physiol.* **88**, 326.
De Jong, F. H., Baird, D. T. and van der Molen, H. J. (1974). *Acta endocr., Copenh.* **77**, 575.
Diczfalusy, E. (1952). *Acta endocr., Copenh.* **10**, 373.
Diczfalusy, E. (1964). *Fed. Proc.* **23**, 791.
Dorfman, R. I. and Ungar, F. (1965). "Metabolism of Steroid Hormones." Academic Press, New York and London.
Dray, F., Andrieu, J. M. and Renaud, F. (1975). *Biochim. biophys. Acta,* **403**, 131.
Edgar, D. G. (1953). *Biochem. J.* **54**, 50.
Eik-Nes, K. B. and Hall, P. F. (1962). *Proc. Soc. exp. Biol. Med.* **111**, 280.
Eik-Nes, K. B. and Hall, P. F. (1965). *Vit. Horm.* **23**, 153.
Eik-Nes, K. B. and Kehre, M. (1963). *Biochim. biophys. Acta,* **78**, 449.
Eto, T., Masuda, M., Suzuki, Y. and Hosi, T. (1962). *Jap. J. anim. Reprod.* **8**, 34.
Fels, E. (1937). "Das Hormon des Corpus Luteum" (Biologie, Chemie und Klinik), p. 95. Franz Deuticke, Leipzig and Vienna.
Fieser, L. F. and Fieser, M. (1959). "Steroids." Reinhold, New York.
Forbes, T. R. (1950). *Am. J. Obstet. Gynec.* **60**, 180.
Forbes, T. R. (1959). *In* "Recent Progress in the Endocrinology of Reproduction" (C. W. Lloyd, ed.), p. 279. Academic Press, New York and London.
Forbes, T. R. (1964). *Endocrinology,* **75**, 799.
Fotherby, K. (1964). *Vit. Horm.* **22**, 153.
Fraenkel, L. (1903). *Arch. Gynak.* **68**, 438.
Fremery, P. de, Luchs, A. and Tausk, M. (1931). *Arch. ges. Physiol.* **231**, 341.
Furuyama, S. and Nugent, C. A. (1971). *Steroids,* **17**, 663.

Futterweit, W., McNiven, N. L. and Dorfman, R. I. (1963). *Biochim. biophys. Acta*, **71**, 474.

Gardiner, W. L. and Horning, E. C. (1966). *Biochim. biophys. Acta*, **115**, 524.

Greep, R. O. (Ed.) (1973). *In* "Handbook of Physiology, Sect. 7; Endocrinology, Vol. II, Female Reproductive System, Part 1." American Physiology Society, Washington.

Greep, R. O. (1977). *Ann. N.Y. Acad. Sci.* **286**, 1.

Gurpide, E. (1977). *Ann. N.Y. Acad. Sci.* **286**, 1.

Hafez, E. S., Tsutsumi, Y. and Khan, M. A. (1965). *Proc. Soc. exp. Biol. Med.* **120**, 75.

Hagen, A. A. and Eik-Nes, K. B. (1964). *Biochim. biophys. Acta*, **90**, 593.

Harkness, R. A., Menini, E., Charles, D., Kenny, F. M. and Rombaut, R. (1966). *Acta endocr. Copenh.* **52**, 409.

Hartmann, M. and Wettstein, A. (1934). *Helv. chim. Acta*, **17**, 878.

Haskins, A. L. (1941). *J. clin. Endocr. Metab.* **1**, 65.

Haskins, A. L. (1949). *Proc. Soc. exp. Biol. Med.* **70**, 228.

Haskins, A. L. (1950). *Proc. Soc. exp. Biol. Med.* **73**, 439.

Haskins, A. L. (1954). *Am. J. Obstet. Gynec.* **67**, 330.

Haskins, A. L. and Taubert, H. D. (1963). *Obstet. Gynec.* **21**, 395.

Heap, R. B. (1964). *J. Endocr.* **30**, 293.

Heap, R. B., Holzbauer, M. and Newport, H. M. (1966). *J. Endocr.* **36**, 159.

Hendeles, S. M. (1965). *Bull. Soc. R. Belge. Gynec. Obstet.* **35**, 355.

Henning, H. D. and Zander, J. (1962). *Hoppe-Seyler's Z. physiol. Chem.* **330**, 31.

Hilliard, J., Endröczi, J. and Sawyer, C. H. (1961). *Proc. Soc. exp. Biol. Med.* **108**, 154.

Hilliard, J., Archibald, A. and Sawyer, C. H. (1963). *Endocrinology*, **72**, 59.

Hinsberg, K., Pelzer, H. and Seuken, A. (1956). *Biochem. Z.* **328**, 117.

Hooker, C. W. and Forbes, T. R. (1949). *Endocrinology*, **45**, 71.

Hübener, H. J., Sahrholz, F. G., Schmidt-Thomé, J., Nesemann, G. and Junk, R. (1959). *Biochim. biophys. Acta*, **35**, 270.

Ismail, A. A. A. and Harkness, R. A. (1966). *Biochem. J.* **98**, 15 P.

Langecker, H. and Damrosch, L. (1968). "Handbook of Experimental Pharmacology", Vol. XXII/1. Springer, Berlin.

League of Nations (1935). *Q. Bull. Hlth. Org.* **4**, 618.

Leusden, H. van, and Villee, C. A. (1965). *Steroids*, **6**, 31.

Levitz, M., Emerman, S. and Dancis, J. (1962). Excerpta Med. Int. Cong. Ser. No. 51, 266.

Loeb, L. (1907). *Zentbl. allg. Path.* **18**, 563.

Loewe, J. and Voss, H. E. (1934). *Schweiz. med. Wschr.* **64**, 1049.

Lurie, A. O., Villee, C. A. and Reid, D. E. (1966a). *J. clin. Endocr. Metab.* **26**, 742.

Lurie, A. O., Reid, D. E. and Villee, C. A. (1966b). *Am. J. Obstet. Gynec.* **96**, 670.

Mancuso, S., Dell'acqua, S., Eriksson, G., Wiqvist, N. and Diczfalusy, E. (1966). *Steroids*, **5**, 183.

Marti, M. and Schindler, O. (1961). *Gynaecologia*, **151**, 67.

Martin, B. T., Cooke, B. A. and Black, W. P. (1970). *J. Endocr.* **46**, 369.

McGinty, D. A., Anderson, L. P. and McCullough, N. B. (1939). *Endocrinology*, **24**, 829.

Mikhail, G. (1967). *Clin. Obstet. Gynaec.* **10**, 29.

Mikhail, G. and Allen, W. M. (1966). Excerpta Med. Int. Cong. Ser. No. 111, 150.

Mikhail, G., Zander, J. and Allen, W. M. (1963). *J. clin. Endocr. Metab.* **23**, 1267.

Miyake, T. (1962). *In* "Methods in Hormone Research" (R. I. Dorfman, ed.), Vol. II. Academic Press, New York and London.

Miyake, T. and Pincus, G. (1958). *Endocrinology*, **63**, 816.

Murphy, B. E. P. (1967). *J. clin. Endocr.* **27**, 973.

Neher, R. and Wettstein, A. (1960). *Acta endocr., Copenh.* **35**, 1.

Neill, J. D., Johansson, E. D. B. and Knobil, E. (1967). *J. clin. Endocr.* **27**, 1167.

Norymberski, J. K. and Woods, G. F. (1955). *J. chem. Soc.* **4**, 3426.

Oertel, G. W., Weiss, S. P. and Eik-Nes, K. B. (1959). *J. clin. Endocr. Metab.* **19**, 213.

Palmer, R., Eriksson, G., Wiqvist, N. and Diczfalusy, E. (1966a). *Acta endocr., Copenh.* **52**, 598.

Palmer, R. A., Blair, J. A., Eriksson, G. and Diczfalusy, E. (1966b). *Acta endocr., Copenh.* **53**, 407.

Pearlman, W. H. (1948). *In* "The Hormones" (G. Pincus and K. V. Thimann, eds), Vol. 1, Ch. II. Academic Press, New York and London.

Pearlman, W. H. (1960). *In* "Hormones in Human Plasma" (N. H. Antoniades, ed.), Ch. 14. Churchill, London.

Pearlman, W. H. and Cerceo, E. (1952). *J. biol. Chem.* **198**, 79.

Pearlman, W. H. and Cerceo, E. (1953). *J. biol. Chem.* **203**, 127.

Pincus, G., Miyake, T., Merril, A. P. and Longo, P. R. (1957). *Endocrinology*, **61**, 528.

Pion, R., Jaffe, R., Eriksson, G., Wiqvist, N. and Diczfalusy, E. (1965). *Acta endocr., Copenh.* **48**, 234.

Pion, R. J., Conrad, S. H. and Wolf, B. J. (1966). *J. clin. Endocr. Metab.* **26**, 225.

Prenant, A. (1898). *Rev. gén. Sci.* **9**, 646.

Purdue, R. H., Halla, M. and Little, B. (1964). *Steroids*, **4**, 625.

Raisinghani, K. H., Dorfman, R. I. and Forchielli, E. (1966). Abst. Meet. Gas Chromat. Determ. Horm. Steroids, Rome.

Reeves, B. D., de Souza, M. L. A., Thompson, I. E. and Diczfalusy, E. (1970). *Acta endocr., Copenh.* **63**, 225.

Rennie, P. and Davies, J. (1965). *Endocrinology*, **76**, 535.

Reynolds, S. R. M. and Ginsberg, N. (1942). *Endocrinology*, **31**, 147.

Rice, B. F. and Savard, K. (1966). *J. clin. Endocr. Metab.* **26**, 593.

Riondel, A., Tait, J. F., Tait, S. A. S., Gut, M. and Little, B. (1965). *J. clin. Endocr. Metab.* **25**, 229.

Rombauts, P. and Piton, C. (1963). *Ann. Biol. anim. Biochem. Biophys.* **3**, 437.

Rothchild, I. (1965). *Vit. Horm.* **23**, 210.

Rowlands, J. W. and Short, R. V. (1959). *J. Endocr.* **19**, 81.

Rünnebaum, B., van der Molen, H. and Zander, J. (1965). *Steroids*, (Suppl. II), 189.

Ryan, K. J. (1963). *Acta endocr., Copenh.* **44**, 81.

Ryan, K. J. and Petro, Z. (1966). *J. clin. Endocr. Metab.* **26**, 46.

Ryan, K. J. and Short, R. V. (1966). *Endocrinology*, **78**, 214.

Ryan, K. J. and Smith, O. W. (1961). *J. biol. Chem.* **236**, 2207.

Ryan, K. J. and Smith, O. W. (1965). *Rec. Prog. Horm. Res.* **21**, 367.

Salhanick, H. A., Noall, M. W., Zarrow, M. X. and Samuels, L. T. (1952). *Science, N.Y.* **115**, 708.

Samuels, L. T. (1960). *In* "Metabolic Pathways" (D. M. Greenberg, ed.). Academic Press, New York and London.

Sandberg, A. A., Rosenthal, H., Schneider, S. L. and Slaunwhite, W. R. (1966). *In* "Steroid Dynamics" (G. Pincus, T. Nakao and J. F. Tait, eds), p. 1. Academic Press, New York and London.

Savard, K., Marsh, J. and Rice, B. F. (1965). *Rec. Prog. Horm. Res.* **21**, 285.

Short, R. V. (1956). *Nature, Lond.* **178**, 743.

Short, R. V. (1958). *J. Endocr.* **16**, 415.

Short, R. V. (1960a). *Biochem. Soc. Symp.* **18**, 59.
Short, R. V. (1961). *In* "Hormones in Blood" (C. H. Gray and A. L. Bacharach, eds.), p. 397, 1st edition. Academic Press, New York and London.
Short, R. V. (1962). *J. Endocr.* **24**, 59.
Short, R. V. (1964). *Rec. Prog. Horm. Res.* **20**, 303.
Short, R. V. and Levett, I. (1962). *J. Endocr.* **25**, 239.
Short, R. V., McDonald, M. F. and Rowson, L. E. A. (1963). *J. Endocr.* **26**, 169.
Simmer, H. and Simmer, I. (1959). *Klin. Wschr.* **37**, 971.
Slaunwhite, W. R. (1960). *In* "Hormones in Human Plasma" (H. N. Antoniades, ed.), p. 478. Little, Brown, Boston.
Slotta, K. H., Ruschig, H. and Fels, E. (1934). *Ber. dt. Chem. Ges.* **67**, 1624.
Solomon, S. (1960). *In* "The Placenta and Fetal Membranes" (C. A. Villee, ed.), p. 200. Williams and Wilkins Co., New York.
Solomon, S. (1966). *J. clin. Endocr. Metab.* **26**, 762.
Sommerville, I. F. and Deshpande, G. N. (1958). *J. clin. Endocr. Metab.* **18**, 1223.
Sommerville, I. F., Pickett, M. T., Collins, W. P. and Denyer, D. C. (1963). *Acta endocr., Copenh.* **43**, 101.
Strott, C. A., Yoshimi, T. and Lipsett, M. B. (1969). *J. clin. Invest.* **48**, 930.
Talwalker, P. K., Krähenbühl, C. and Desaulles, P. A. (1966). *Nature, Lond.* **209**, 5018.
Telegdy, G. and Endröczi, E. (1961). *Acta physiol. hung.* **20**, 277.
Touchstone, J. C. and Murawec, T. (1960). *Anal. Chem.* **7**, 822.
Van den Heuvel, W. J. A. and Horning, E. C. (1963). *Biochem. biophys. Acta,* **74**, 560.
van der Molen, H. J. (1963). *Clin. chim. Acta,* **8**, 943.
van der Molen, H. J. (1967). *In* "Gas Phase Chromatography of Steroids" (K. B. Eik-Nes and E. C. Horning, eds). Springer Verlag, Heidelberg.
van der Molen, H. J. and Aakvaag, A. (1967). *In* "Hormones in Blood" (C. H. Gray and A. L. Bacharach, eds), p. 221, 2nd edition. Academic Press, London and New York.
van der Molen, H. J. and Groen, D. (1965). *J. clin. Endocr. Metab.* **25**, 1625.
van der Molen, H. J. and Groen, D. (1967). *In* "Steroid Gas Chromatography", Endocr. Memoir No. 16 (J. K. Grant, ed.). Cambridge University Press, Cambridge.
van der Molen, H. J. and Corpêchot, C. (1968). *J. clin. Endocr. Metab.* **28**, 1361.
van der Molen, H. J. and Eik-Nes, K. B. (1971). *Biochim. biophys. Acta,* **248**, 343.
van der Molen, H. J., Rünnebaum, B., Nishizawa, E. E., Kristensen, E., Kirschbaum, T., Wiest, W. G. and Eik-Nes, K. B. (1965). *J. clin. Endocr. Metab.* **25**, 170.
Weliky, I. and Engel, L. L. (1962). *Fed. Proc.* **20**, 179.
Wiest, W. G. (1959). *J. biol. Chem.* **234**, 3115.
Wiest, W. G. and Wilcox, R. B. (1961). *J. biol. Chem.* **236**, 2425.
Wiest, W. G. and Forbes, T. R. (1964). *Endocrinology,* **74**, 149.
Wiest, W. G., Kerenyi, T. and Csapo, A. I. (1966). Excerpta Med. Int. Cong. Ser., No. 111, p. 114.
Woolever, C. A. (1963). *Am. J. Obstet. Gynec.* **85**, 981.
Woolever, C. A. and Goldfien, A. (1962). Excerpta Med. Int. Cong. Ser. No. 51, p. 81.
Woolever, C. A. and Goldfien, A. (1963). *Int. J. appl. Radiat. Isotopes,* **14**, 163.
Wotiz, H. H. and Clark, S. J. (1966). "Gas Chromatography in the Analysis of Steroid Hormones." Plenum Press, New York.
Yannone, M. E., McComas, D. B. and Goldfien, A. (1964). *J. Gas Chromat.* **2**, 30.
Yoshimi, T. and Lipsett, M. B. (1968). *Steroids,* **11**, 527.
Zaffaroni, A. (1950). *J. Am. chem. Soc.* **72**, 3828.

Zander, J. (1954). *Nature, Lond.* **174**, 406.

Zander, J. (1955). *Klin. Wschr.* **33**, 697.

Zander, J. (1962). *In* "Methods in Hormone Research" (R. I. Dorfman, ed.), Vol. I, p. 91. Academic Press, New York and London.

Zander, J. and Simmer, H. (1954). *Klin. Wschr.* **32**, 529.

Zander, J., Forbes, T. R., Neher, R. and Desaulles, P. (1957). *Klin. Wschr.* **35**, 143.

Zander, J., Forbes, T. R., von Münstermann, A. M. and Neher, R. (1958). *J. clin. Endocr. Metab.* **18**, 377.

Zarrow, M. X., Neher, G. M., Lasowasem, E. A. and Salhanick, H. A. (1957). *J. clin. Endocr. Metab.* **17**, 658.

Zelewski, L. and Villee, C. A. (1966). *Biochemistry,* **5**, 1805.

Zmigrod, A. and Lindner, H. R. (1966). *Steroids,* **8**, 119.

IX. Progesterone. II. Clinical Aspects

K. FOTHERBY

INTRODUCTION

This review will be concerned only with progesterone and its metabolites in human blood and will deal almost entirely with information accumulated during the past decade. The major developments of the clinical aspects of progesterone since the survey by van der Molen and Aakvaag (1967) have been due to improved methods of estimation of progesterone and its metabolites. The earlier tedious methods have been superseded by techniques depending upon saturation analysis, either by competitive protein-binding or by radioimmunoassay. The simplicity, sensitivity and accuracy of these methods have permitted acquisition of much new information concerning progesterone, much of which has resulted from a reinvestigation of topics previously studied by earlier less satisfactory methods of estimating progesterone in blood and of pregnandiol in urine.

Compared with other steroid hormones, the clinical usefulness of progesterone measurements is limited (MacNaughton, 1976). However, the application of the improved methods based on saturation analysis has been useful in two particular areas: the study of the relationship between ovarian and pituitary hormones during the menstrual cycle, and the use of blood progesterone measurements as an indicator of a functional corpus luteum and hence to provide evidence for ovulation. This last area has been particularly useful in the assessment of the mode of action of steroidal contraceptives and in the development of newer forms of contraceptives as well as in monitoring the effect of agents used clinically for stimulating ovarian function.

Some important reviews of progesterone are by Junkmann (1968), Tausk (1971), Scholler, Tea and Castanier (1973), Aufrere and Benson (1976) and Cooke (1976).

A. SOME ASPECTS OF PROGESTERONE METABOLISM

The level of progesterone in blood will be determined by the rate at which it is being produced and entering the circulation and by the rate at which it is leaving the circulation due to excretion or tissue metabolism.

The blood production rates of progesterone in non-pregnant subjects, calculated from the metabolic clearance rate (MCR), were summarised by van der Molen and Aakvaag (1967). In men and ovariectomised women values of 0·6–0·8 mg/day (1·9–2·5 µmol/day) were obtained. Higher values were found in women during the follicular phase (2·9 mg/day; 9·2 µmol/day) and greatly increased values during the luteal phase (22 mg/day; 70 µmol/day). In pregnant women, with large amounts of progesterone being secreted by the placenta, there was no significant discrepancy between values for the production rate calculated from the MCR and that calculated by measuring the specific activity of a urinary metabolite after administration of labelled progesterone. In the last trimester of pregnancy, reported values range from 132–563 mg/day (420–1790 µmol/day) (Zander and Munstermann, 1956; Pearlman, 1957; Bengtsson and Ejarque, 1964; Solomon, Watanabe, Dominguez, Gray, Meeker and Sims, 1964; Lin, Lin, Erlenmeyer, Kline, Underwood, Billiar and Little, 1972). Solomon *et al.* (1964) quote a mean of 92 mg/day (292 µmol/day) for subjects in the 15th week of pregnancy and Bengtsson and Ejarque (1964) 76 mg/day (237 µmol/day) for mid-pregnancy.

Maternal plasma cholesterol appears to be the precursor of these large amounts of progesterone produced during pregnancy (Hellig, Gattereau, Lefebvre and Bolte, 1970). Weiner and Allen (1967) suggest that 20α-dihydro-progesterone may be involved in the control of progesterone synthesis in the placenta since this steroid inhibits the conversion of pregnenolone to pro-gesterone. The peripheral contribution of pregnenolone to the progesterone production rate in pregnancy is small. Little, Billiar, Halla, Heinsons, Jassani, Kline and Purdy (1971) found the conversion in the last trimester of pregnancy to be from 18–32%. The plasma concentration and production rate of pregnenolone were 7·3 ng/ml (23·1 nmol/l) and 23·4 ± 3·9 mg/day (73·9 ± 9·1 μmol/day) compared with values for progesterone of 100·9 ng/ml (321 nmol/l) and 212 mg/day (674 μmol/day) on the same samples. Thus in the last trimester of pregnancy the peripheral contribution of pregnenolone to the progesterone production rate was only about 6 mg/day (19 μmol/day). Scommegna, Burd and Bieniarz (1972) have shown that pregnenolone sulphate from the maternal adrenal is not a major contributor to pro-gesterone synthesis since increasing the maternal plasma pregnenolone sulphate concentration by intravenous infusion of the compound or de-creasing its plasma concentration by giving dexamethasone did not affect the maternal plasma progesterone level.

The dynamics of progesterone metabolism in humans and some other species have been studied in detail (Little, Billiar, Rahman, Johnson, Takaoka and White, 1975). The plasma MCR in humans varied from 1800–2500 l/day with values in women slightly higher than in men. The MCR of progesterone does not appear to change during the menstrual cycle. These values correspond to a blood MCR of about 60–70 l/day/kg in agreement with the findings of Lin et al. (1972). A major site of metabolism of pro-gesterone is the liver and Little, Billiar, Bougas and Tait (1973) calculated the splanchnic clearance to be 704 l/day and the extra-splanchnic to be 1091 l/day so that 60% of the total MCR was extra-splanchnic. The incomplete hepatic extraction may be due to the binding of progesterone to plasma proteins. Little et al. (1973) suggest that there is an inverse correlation between the splanchnic extraction and the levels of cortisol-binding globulin in plasma. However, administration of oestrogens to women (Billiar, Jassani and Little, 1975a) increased the plasma concentration of cortisol-binding globulin leading to a decrease in the MCR of cortisol but was without effect on that of progesterone, although there was a decrease in the conversion rate of progesterone to 20α-dihydroprogesterone.

Other organs in the body are involved in the metabolism of progesterone. In rhesus monkeys the brain extraction of progesterone was 25% and the calculated brain clearance (Billiar, Little, Kline, Reier, Takaoka and White, 1975b) was 20 l/day (6% of total MCR). Part of this clearance was due to the metabolism of progesterone to 20α-dihydroprogesterone and 5α-pregnane-

3,20-dione. Backstrom, Carstensen and Sodergard (1976) have shown the transfer of about 10% of plasma progesterone to cerebrospinal fluid.

Both proliferative and secretory endometria from human uteri (Pollow, Lubbert, Boquoi and Pollow, 1975; Garzon, Aznar, Olivera, Gallegos, 1977) as well as human myometrium (Mickan, 1976) convert progesterone into a number of metabolites. The rate of metabolism of progesterone by endometrium is higher than that of myometrium (Sweat and Bryson, 1970). In pregnancy, progesterone in myometrium varies from 40–630 µg/100 g (130–2000 nmol/100 g) tissue with no difference in the first trimester or at term (see Aufrere and Benson, 1976).

Similar values were also obtained in the human endometrium in pregnancy (Nilsson, 1972). The concentration of progesterone in samples of myometrium from 33 women at delivery was 92.2 ± 6.8 ng/g (293 ± 22 pmol/g) tissue and the plasma level was 175.3 ± 11.3 ng/ml (557 ± 36 nmol/l); these values were higher than those obtained (Batra and Bengtsson, 1978) in five samples of tissue taken between the 17th and 20th week of pregnancy (myometrial progesterone 54.7 ± 16.9 ng/g (174 ± 54 pmol/g) tissue) and plasma progesterone 27.2 ± 8.4 ng/ml (86 ± 27 nmol/l) suggesting a possible decrease during pregnancy in the ratio of myometrial to plasma progesterone. There was no significant difference of progesterone concentration in myometrium near to from that distal to the placental site. These findings confirmed those of Runnebaum and Zander (1971) that in spite of the great increase in plasma levels of progesterone with advancing pregnancy, there was a smaller increase in the levels in the myometrium.

Batra, Grundsell and Sjoberg (1977) found a mean endometrial progesterone of 7.2 ± 1.8 ng/g (23 ± 6 pmol/g) tissue during the proliferative phase of the menstrual cycle when the mean plasma level was 0.26 ng/ml (0.83 nmol/l) whereas during the secretory phase the plasma level increased to 10.5 ng/ml (33.4 nmol/l) but the endometrial level only to 27.1 ± 2.35 ng/g (86 ± 7 pmol/g) tissue. If the latter findings are correct, the tissue:plasma ratio was less in the secretory phase (M. 4.2) than in the proliferative phase (M. 38.7). Similar values were obtained by Hagenfeldt and Landgren (1975) although higher values were found by Nilsson (1972) and Grundsell, Nilsson and Nordqvist (1973). During the menstrual cycle Bayard, Louvet, Monrozies, Boulard and Pontonnier (1975) found a good correlation between endometrial and plasma progesterone levels but this was not confirmed by Guerrero, Landgren, Montiel, Cekan and Diczfalusy (1975) or by Batra et al. (1977). If these latter findings are correct, plasma progesterone levels need to be interpreted with caution if used to assess tissue responses to the hormone.

The half-life of progesterone in blood is short, but the reported values vary widely (Thijssen and Zander, 1966). The controversy regarding the half-life of progesterone discussed by van der Molen and Aakvaag (1967) has been resolved to some extent by Fylling (1970) who removed both the corpus luteum and the foetoplacental unit from women in the first trimester of pregnancy who were undergoing legal abortion and sterilisation. During the first 6 min after operation progesterone disappeared rapidly from the circulation with a half-life of about 6 min (Fig. 1). The disappearance rate then decreased and the half-life was about 95 min. Similar values were obtained when labelled progesterone was given by intravenous infusion. When the labelled steroid was given by intravenous injection the disappearance rate was greater, the half-life of the second phase being about 45 min. Thus differences in the way in which progesterone is administered and the sensitivity or specificity of the methods used in its estimation probably account for many of the differences in the disappearance rate reported by various investigators. However, Lin *et al.* (1972) found after administration of the hormone by injection the half-life of the second phase of progesterone to be 19 min. Since progesterone is not stored in the corpus luteum, and since the half-life is short, the plasma concentration of the hormone is a reliable indicator of its production by the corpus luteum.

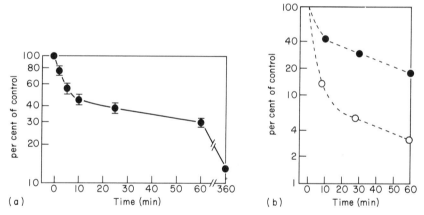

Fig. 1. Disappearance of progesterone from blood. (a) M. ± S.D. percentage change of plasma progesterone after simultaneous removal of both corpus luteum and foetoplacental unit. (b) Disappearance of tritiated progesterone in two post-menopausal women after a single i.v. injection of 10 μCi (open circles) and i.v. infusion of 1 μCi/min for 15 min (closed circles) (from Fylling, 1970).

1. Protein Binding

Progesterone does not bind to erythrocytes or to platelets as shown by Lin *et al.* (1972), who found, after i.v. administration of [³H]-progesterone to women, a plasma-blood ratio of radioactivity of 1·55 compared with the calculated value of 1·59. In human plasma or serum, small amounts of progesterone exist in the unbound state, the remainder is bound to serum albumin, corticosteroid-binding globulin (CBG) and to the α-acid glyco-protein, orosomucoid. With serum from pregnant women, Westphal, Stroupe and Cheng (1977) found that 43–48% of progesterone was bound to CBG, 50–54% to albumin, 1–2% was unbound and only a small amount to orosomucoid. The concentration of the progesterone bound to CBG was about half of that of the cortisol bound to CBG. The association constant of CBG for progesterone at 37° was about 500 times higher than that of albumin but albumin binding was important because of the high plasma albumin concentration. Rosenthal, Slaunwhite and Sandberg (1969) agree was Westphal et al. (1977) that only about 2% of progesterone circulates in the free state but, in normal non-pregnant women only 37% and 18% of the plasma progesterone was bound to CBG and albumin respectively with 36% to unassigned binding proteins. There was little change in these values in pregnancy, although the CBG-bound fraction increased slightly at the expense of the albumin-bound fraction. In molar terms, however, due to the increase in plasma progesterone concentration during pregnancy, the amount bound to CBG changed from 0·067 to 0·167 μmol/l (21·1 to 52·5 ng/ml), for albumin from 0·035 to 0·066 μmol/l (10·1 to 20·1 ng/ml), to unassigned binding pro-teins 0·07 to 0·151 μmol/l (22·0 to 47·5 ng/ml) and the free fraction increased from 0·003 to 0·007 μmol/l (0·9 to 2·2 ng/ml).

However, Yannone, Mueller and Osborn (1969) also using equilibrium dialysis found the unbound progesterone to be much greater (8–10%), as did Tulchinsky and Okada (1975) who found about 5% of plasma progesterone to be unbound (Table 1).

Table 1

Total and unbound plasma progesterone concentrations (M. ± S.E.) in maternal and foetal plasma (1 ng/ml = 3·18 nmol/l) (from Tulchinsky and Okada, 1975).

Source of plasma samples	Total (ng/ml)	%	Unbound ng/ml
Luteal phase	17 ± 3	4·83 ± 0·1	0·82 ± 0·14
End of first trimester	41 ± 5	4·93 ± 0·1	2·03 ± 0·24
Term pregnancy	160 ± 10	5·02 ± 0·1	8·03 ± 0·50
Umbilical vein at term	788 ± 30	7·01 ± 0·2	55·20 ± 2·10

Both groups of workers agree with Rosenthal et al. (1969) that the percentage of unbound progesterone does not change during the menstrual cycle or pregnancy. However, Batra, Bengtsson, Grundsell and Sjoberg (1976) using a microfiltration method found 5–6% unbound progesterone at week 24 of pregnancy and this increased to about 13% at the end of pregnancy. If the percentage of unbound progesterone in plasma is constant during the menstrual cycle and in pregnancy, the concentration of unbound progesterone in plasma will vary directly with the total plasma concentration of the hormone. The amount of unbound progesterone in umbilical vein blood is significantly higher than in peripheral blood probably due to the lower CBG content of cord blood compared with that of maternal blood (Table 1).

As with other steroid hormones, probably only the unbound progesterone in blood is biologically active. The binding of progesterone to orosomucoid (Westphal and Forbes, 1963), or to CBG or albumin (Hoffman, Forbes and Westphal, 1969) causes a loss of biological activity.

2. Circadian Rhythm

The possibility that progesterone levels in blood may undergo a diurnal variation has been widely investigated. Johansson (1969a) reported progesterone levels in non-pregnant women were higher in the morning compared with the remainder of the day. Florensa, Sommerville, Harrison, Johnson and Youssefnejadian (1976) collected samples four-hourly during the follicular phase of the cycle, and also found the progesterone levels to be higher in the morning with a decrease towards evening, the lowest concentration being found at 08.00 hr. In contrast 20α-dihydroprogesterone showed a peak at 20.00 hr with low values in the morning. Runnebaum and Zander (1971) found no significant circadian variation in ten women during the luteal phase of the cycle. West, Mahajan, Chavre, Nabors and Tyler (1973) collected samples every 20 min over a 24-hr-period from one female and one male subject. Although the results suggested that progesterone was secreted episodically, the plasma levels did not correlate with those of cortisol, testosterone or 17α-hydroxyprogesterone. In contrast, Younglai, Smith, Cleghorn and Streiner (1975), who measured the plasma levels of oestradiol and progesterone in samples taken every 20 min during the day found a good correlation ($r = 0.9$) between the levels of the two hormones but no evidence for the episodic release of either steroid, although values were significantly lower in the afternoon than in the morning.

No significant circadian variation was found in ten women during the first trimester of pregnancy (Runnebaum, Holzman, Bierworth-v, Munstermann and Zander, 1972) although in the latter half of pregnancy the progesterone concentration increased from 08.00 hr until the evening. Similar findings were made by Craft, Carriere and Youssefnejadian (1974), who found a variation in women near the end of pregnancy with the 16.00 hr and 04.00 hr samples higher than the 08.00 hr ones, and by Coats, Walker, Youssef-nedjadian and Craft (1977) and by Teoh, Dawood, Ratnam, Ambrose and Das (1973). The last workers found no consistent pattern in the levels of plasma progesterone in five pregnant women from whom samples were taken every 6 hr although in four of the women the value tended to be highest in the late evening; however, the difference between samples could be ±22% of the mean. Lindberg, Nilsson and Johansson (1974) measured the plasma level of progesterone every 2 hr during a 24 hr period in seven subjects. There was no consistent pattern in relation to the time of the day but there were large variations over the 24 hr period, the difference between samples on occasions being more than 100 ng/ml (318 nmol/l). Large variations between samples were also found in five women from whom blood samples were taken every 5 min over a 1 hr period. Luisi, Levanti and Franchi (1971) found no consistent pattern in the plasma levels of progesterone in three patients studied in the second trimester of pregnancy. Thus firm evidence for a circadian variation of progesterone levels in blood is lacking.

3. Progesterone Metabolites

Two metabolites of progesterone of potential biological importance also occur in blood, 5α-pregnane-3,20-dione and 20α-dihydroprogesterone.

(a) 5α-Pregnane-3,20-dione

The pattern of concentration of 5α-pregnanedione in blood is similar to that of progesterone. Stoa and Bessesen (1975) found the concentration to be about 19·6 ng/ml (61·9 nmol/l) at 27–29 weeks of pregnancy and 57 ng/ml (180 nmol/l) at the end of pregnancy. The ratio of progesterone to 5α-pregnanedione was about three. Milewich, Gomez-Sanchez, Madden and MacDonald (1975) found a ratio of 3·6 ± 1·5. In four women the concentration of pregnanedione during the follicular phase was 0·01–0·44 ng/ml (0·03–1·39 nmol/l), similar to that of progesterone, and at the peak of the luteal phase the concentration varied from 1·4–2·8 ng/ml (4·4–8·8 nmol/l) (Milewich, Gomez-Sanchez, Crowley, Porter, Madden and MacDonald, 1977). It seems likely therefore that 5α-pregnanedione in plasma arises directly from progesterone as a result of the action of 5α-reductase.

(b) 20α-Dihydroprogesterone

Small amounts of 20α-dihydroprogesterone, a weakly progestational steroid, are found in peripheral plasma and the steroid appears to be a secretory product of the ovary. Mikhail (1967) detected this steroid in ovarian vein plasma both in the follicular phase (active ovary 1·1 ng/ml (3·5 nmol/l), inactive 0·4 ng/ml (1·3 nmol/l)) and in the luteal phase (ovary with corpus luteum 1·4 ng/ml (4·4 nmol/l); ovary without corpus luteum 0·5 ng/ml (1·6 nmol/l)).

Florensa and Somerville (1973) found by radioimmunoassay the levels in men and in women during the early follicular phase (0·1–0·3 ng/ml (0·3–0·9 nmol/l) and 0·12–0·48 ng/ml (0·38–1·52 nmol/l) respectively) to be similar to those of progesterone itself. In women during the luteal phase, levels were only about half those of progesterone (0·24–3·8 ng/ml; 0·8–12·0 nmol/l) whereas in the third trimester of pregnancy the ratio of 20α-dihydro-progesterone to progesterone was much lower (approximately 0·25). Levels of 20α-dihydroprogesterone in the last trimester of pregnancy varied from 8·4–40·9 ng/ml (26·5–129 nmol/l). Similar values were found by Little et al. (1971). The decrease in the ratio of 20α-dihydroprogesterone to progesterone in late pregnancy may be due to the large amounts of oestrogens being secreted at this time since Billiar et al. (1975a) have shown that administration of oestrogen will decrease the conversion rate of progesterone to 20α-dihydro-progesterone. Wu, Prazak, Flickinger and Mikhail (1974) found the mean level during the follicular phase to be 0·4 ± 0·05 ng/ml (1·26 ± 0·16 nmol/l) with a slow rise after ovulation to a peak of 3·4 ± 0·5 ng/ml (10·7 ± 1·6 nmol/l) in the mid-luteal phase. They found the ratio of the 20α-dihydro-progesterone to progesterone (0·15–0·22) to be fairly constant throughout the luteal phase. Similar results have been reported by Aedo, Landgren, Cekan and Diczfalusy (1976) who studied the levels during 15 normal menstrual cycles. There was a significant correlation between the levels of progesterone and 20α-dihydroprogesterone. Levels of the latter during the proliferative phase were about 0·24 ng/ml (0·75 nmol/l). The first significant increase was observed between days LH − 1 and LH 0. Peak levels on day LH + 8 were similar to those reported by Wu et al. (1974).

Billiar et al. (1974) found the metabolic clearance rate of 20α-dihydropro-gesterone to be 1700 l/day. Florensa et al. (1976) suggested that there was a circadian variation in the plasma levels of 20α-dihydroprogesterone with a peak at 08.00 hr and lower values at 16.00 hr and 24.00 hr. 20α-Dihydro-progesterone may be important in the control of progesterone synthesis in the placenta since Wiener and Allen (1967) have shown that dihydro-progesterone will inhibit the conversion of pregnenolone to progesterone.

Levels of 20β-dihydroprogesterone in both peripheral and ovarian vein plasma are much lower than those of 20α-dihydroprogesterone (Mikhail, 1967).

B. ESTIMATION OF PROGESTERONE IN BLOOD

The methods described by van der Molen and Aakvaag (1967) were either non-specific or technically complex and were subsequently replaced by methods depending upon saturation analysis. In 1971 competitive protein binding was the method of choice (Solomon and Fuchs, 1971; Reeves and Diczfalusy, 1971) but, as shown below, radioimmunoassay of progesterone would now be considered a superior technique.

It is impossible to discuss in detail all the methods for the assay of progesterone which have been published. Only two methods will be outlined as being basic methods. The first is the "quick" competitive protein-binding assay described by Johansson (1969a), modified from the method of Neill, Johansson, Datta and Knobil (1967); the chromatographic stage is omitted and specificity is dependent upon the ability of certain grades of light petroleum to extract progesterone from plasma unaccompanied by significant quantities of interfering steroids. This method is described since it is simple to perform, has been widely used and, although not as sensitive as radioimmunoassay, is adequate for levels of progesterone greater than 1 ng/ml (3 nmol/l). Thus it is satisfactory for routine clinical use in that it can readily distinguish ovulatory from non-ovulatory menstrual cycles and for studies in pregnancy. Although the method first described by Neill et al. (1967) and subsequent modifications of this method, involve a chromatographic separation with an improvement in specificity and sensitivity, radioimmunoassay is preferred for accurate estimation of low levels of progesterone.

1. Competitive Protein Binding

The method (Johansson, 1969a) involves the following stages:

(i) extraction of plasma (0·25 ml) to be assayed with light petroleum ([^{3}H]-progesterone is usually added to correct for losses);

(ii) evaporation of the light petroleum in suitably small tubes;

(iii) incubation of the extract with [^{3}H]-corticosterone (or [^{3}H]-progesterone) and cortisol-binding globulin (CBG);

(iv) separation of the free and bound corticosterone by absorption of free steroid with Florisil;

(v) estimation of bound radioactivity in the supernatant.

Accurate timing in many of the stages is essential. The method is sensitive to 50 pg (0·16 pmol) per tube, but because of variable blank values the overall sensitivity is probably not less than 500 pg/ml (1·6 nmol/l) plasma. The recovery of progesterone was 85·5 ± 3·4%. The accuracy and precision of the method seemed satisfactory and the coefficient of variation for amounts of progesterone above 0·2 ng (0·6 pmol) was about 5%.

(a) Extraction

Since no chromatographic separation is involved, the specificity of the method depends on the light petroleum used for extraction. Light petroleum is an ill-defined entity, and various batches do not always fulfil the requirements of the assay. Under defined conditions, this solvent (i) should extract more than 80% of progesterone in one extraction; (ii) should extract less than 0·25% of cortisol, corticosterone or 11-deoxycortisol and less than 25% 17α-hydroxyprogesterone; and (iii) give no interference in the assay. Exclusion of cortisol and corticosterone is necessary since the large amounts of these steroids in plasma would seriously interfere in the estimation of progesterone. During the normal menstrual cycle only 17α-hydroxyprogesterone and 20α-dihydroprogesterone are likely to interfere significantly, but the contribution from 17α-hydroxyprogesterone is limited by its low extractability (14%) and that of 20α-dihydroprogesterone by its lower affinity for CBG. Interference from other steroids appears to be minimal since there is no significant difference in the values obtained using this "quick" method and those given in the original method of Neill et al. (1967) involving a thin-layer chromatographic separation. If a chromatographic separation is included in the assay, ether can be used instead of light petroleum for extracting the plasma (Yoshimi and Lipsett, 1968).

(b) Purification of the plasma extract

Various investigators have used column chromatography on Celite (Stone, Nakamura, Mishell and Thorneycroft, 1971) or Sephadex (Holmdahl and Johansson, 1972a), thin-layer chromatography on silica gel (Reeves, de Souza, Thompson and Diczfalusy, 1970; Yoshimi and Lipsett, 1968) and paper chromatography (Martin, Cooke and Black, 1970).

(c) Binding protein

As a source of binding protein, Neill et al. (1967) and many subsequent workers used dog plasma (Hagerman and Williams, 1969; Luisi et al., 1971). However, Reeves et al. (1970) showed that such plasma gave a less sensitive assay than human plasma. Reeves et al. (1970) and Yoshimi and Lipsett (1970) and other workers have used plasma from ovariectomised women treated with oestrogens to increase the plasma content of CBG and dexamethasone to suppress endogenous cortisol production. Johansson (1969a) used diluted plasma from healthy young women treated for two weeks with 100 µg ethynyloestradiol daily. Other sources include women taking oral contraceptives and treated with dexamethasone (Stone et al., 1971), post-menopausal women treated with dexamethasone (Shaaban and Klopper, 1973), late pregnancy plasma (Demetriou and Austin, 1971; Fylling, 1970), chick plasma (Morgan and Cooke, 1972) and plasma from pregnant guinea-pigs (Swain, 1972; Pichon and Milgrom, 1973; Stoa and Bessesen, 1975; Wajchenberg, Sugawara, Mesquita, Lerario, Wachslicht, Pieroni and Mattar, 1976). Each sample of plasma must be tested before use to ensure that its binding characteristics are satisfactory.

(d) Separation of free from the bound ligand

Most investigators have used Florisil although Yoshimi and Lipsett (1968) employed Sephadex columns for this purpose.

2. Radioimmunoassay

The steps involved in this assay are similar to those for competitive protein binding and involve the following:
(i) extraction of sample after addition of a small amount (about 500 dpm) of [^{3}H]-progesterone to act as internal standard;
(ii) purification of progesterone by chromatography;
(iii) incubation of extract with [^{3}H]-progesterone and antiserum;
(iv) separation of free radioactivity from that bound to the antibody;
(v) estimation of either free or bound radioactivity.
Variations on this basic procedure depend upon the source of the antiserum and its specificity, purification of the plasma extract by chromatography and the method used for the separation of the free radioactivity from that bound to the antibody protein.
Abraham et al. (1971) and Furuyama and Nugent (1971) were the first to describe radioimmunoassays for progesterone. Abraham et al. (1971) used an antiserum raised in sheep against the 21-hemisuccinate of 11-deoxy-cortisol coupled to bovine serum albumin. Chromatography on Celite columns was necessary to separate progesterone from 17α-hydroxypro-gesterone and oestradiol. Furuyama and Nugent (1971) conjugated pro-gesterone to bovine serum albumin via the 3-carboxymethyloxime and raised an antibody in rabbits. Plasma extracts were purified by chromato-graphy on alumina columns and saturated ammonium sulphate was used to separate the free from the bound progesterone. The sensitivity of both these methods was about 25 pg (0·08 pmol) per tube.

Thorneycroft and Stone (1972) described a radioimmunoassay in which chromatographic purification of the plasma extract could be omitted. They used a specific antiserum raised in rabbits against 11α-hydroxyprogesterone hemisuccinate-bovine serum albumin conjugate. Only 11α-hydroxyprogesterone had a cross-reaction higher than that of progesterone. Of the other steroids tested, the only ones showing a significant cross-reaction compared with progesterone were 5β-pregnane-3,20-dione (11–18%); deoxycorticosterone (3·8–9·7%) and pregnenolone (2·5–3·3%). They used dextran-charcoal for the separation of free and bound progesterone and this adsorbent has been widely used in radioimmunoassays. They reported that the blank values were always less than 10 pg (0·03 pmol) per tube, the intra-assay and the inter-assay coefficients of variation were about 8% and 13% respectively. The sensitivity of the assay was about 20 pg/ml (64 pmol/l) and similar values were obtained when plasma samples were assayed after direct extraction and after a chromatographic purification. Assays based upon the use of antibodies to the 11α-hydroxyprogesterone antigen are now widely used and methods utilising them have been published by Furr (1973), West et al. (1973), de Jong, Baird and van der Molen (1974), Laborde, Carril, Cheviakoff, Croxatto, Pedroza and Rosner (1976), Spieler, Webb, Saldarini and Coppola (1972), de Villa, Roberts, Wiest, Mikhail and Flickinger (1972) and Tea, Castanier, Roger and Scholler (1975). The last investigators showed that there was a good correlation between the values obtained by radioimmunoassay and those obtained by a method based upon gas chromatography-mass spectrometry.

One advantage of using a chromatographic separation is that it enables a number of other steroids present in the extract to be assayed (see, for example, Abraham, Odell, Swerdloff and Hopper (1972); Dupon, Hosseinion and Kim (1973); Powell and Stevens (1973); West et al. (1973); Parker, Ellergood and Mahesh (1975); Tea et al. (1975) and Aedo et al. (1976).

Bodley, Chapdelaine, Flickinger, Mikhail, Yauerbaum and Roberts (1973) have described a solid phase assay for progesterone, and Hammond, Viinikka and Vihko (1977) have described an automated technique.

Niswender (1973) found good agreement between the values obtained on plasma samples analysed by a double isotope derivative method, by competitive protein-binding and by radioimmunoassay using the 11α-hydroxyprogesterone antiserum but all samples tested had a concentration greater than 3 ng/ml (10 nmol/l). Morgan and Cooke (1972) compared values obtained by competitive protein-binding using chick plasma as the binding reagent with those obtained by radioimmunoassay. They found a good correlation between the two sets of values ($r = 0.95$) but the radioimmunoassay was less prone to interference, less dependent upon the type of petroleum ether used for extraction and had better reproducibility. Wajchenberg et al.

(1976) compared competitive protein-binding using guinea pig plasma with radioimmunoassay using the 11α-hydroxyprogesterone antiserum. They found no difference between the two sets of values if a chromatographic separation was used but without chromatography, values obtained by competitive protein-binding were greater than those obtained by radioimmunoassay in samples taken during the follicular phase but not in the luteal phase. Thus for most purposes competitive protein-binding assays and radioimmunoassay give comparable results but the greater sensitivity and specificity of radioimmunoassay together with its convenience make it the method of choice.

In order to find a specific antibody for progesterone, comparisons have been made between antisera raised to antigens formed by linkages to different positions of the progesterone molecule. Niswender (1973) compared antibodies formed in rabbits from progesterone linked through the C-3 and C-20-oxo group via the carboxymethyloxime, through the 11α-hydroxy group via the chloroformate and through the 6α- and 6β-hydroxy groups via the hemisuccinate. He used an iodinated tyrosine methylether derivative of progesterone as labelled ligand and the double antibody procedure for the separation of bound and free radioactivity. The specificity of the antisera was assessed by testing the ability of twenty-four different steroids to displace labelled progesterone. Specificity is determined not only by the nature of the antiserum but also by the nature of the labelled ligand (Warren and Fotherby, 1975), Niswender (1973) suggested that conjugation of progesterone via the B and C rings gave rise to antisera with greater specificity. The antiserum raised from the C-20 conjugate was relatively non-specific in that it reacted with a number of other 4-en-3-oxosteroids. The antiserum raised to the C-3 antigen was more specific and those from the C-6 and C-11 antigens were very specific. There was little difference between the antisera from the C-6α and C-6β antigens but both were slightly less specific than the antiserum to the 11α-hydroxy antigen in that the last showed less cross-reaction with 5α-pregnanedione and pregnenolone. A similar finding in respect of the C-6 and C-11 linked antigens was made by Jones and Mason (1974) and by Lindner, Perel, Friedlander and Zeitlin (1972) who used a progesterone-6-(carboxymethylene)thioether-bovine serum albumin conjugate. The findings in respect of the C-3 and the C-11α-hydroxy antigens were confirmed by Scarisbrick and Cameron (1975). Bauminger, Lindner and Weinstein (1973) raised an antiserum in rabbits to progesterone-7α-carboxyethylthio-ether-BSA conjugate and found that its specificity was superior to that obtained using C-3, C-6 and C-20 conjugates of progesterone but less specific than the C-11α-hydroxyprogesterone conjugate. Milewich et al. (1975) raised an antiserum also in rabbits to progesterone-11-carboxyethylthio-ether coupled to thyroglobulin but this antiserum showed a large cross-reaction with 5α-pregnanedione (137%), 5β-pregnanedione (53%) and 11β-hydroxyprogesterone (28%). It was therefore much less specific than antisera raised to the 11α-hydroxyprogesterone conjugate.

C. PROGESTERONE IN BLOOD DURING THE MENSTRUAL CYCLE

1. The Normal Cycle and its Disorders

The application of the newer methods of analysis has allowed the plasma levels of progesterone during the menstrual cycle to be more accurately defined. In spite of this, many problems, for example the role of plasma progesterone in the regulation of gonadotrophin secretion, the factors responsible for formation and regression of the corpus luteum, the origin and function of the periovulatory secretion of progesterone and other aspects of the role of progesterone remain to be elucidated.

Plasma progesterone levels during the menstrual cycle have been measured by the following: Faiman and Ryan (1967), Burger, Catt and Brown (1968), Midgley and Jaffe (1968), Cargille, Ross and Yoshimi (1969), Johansson (1969a), Ross, Cargille, Lipsett, Rayford, Marshall, Strott and Rodbard (1970), Strott, Cargille, Ross and Lipsett (1970), van de Wiele, Bogumil, Dyrenfurth, Ferin, Jewelewics, Warren, Rizkallah and Mikhail (1970), Yen, Vela, Rankin and Littell (1970), Yussman and Taymor (1970), Johansson (1969a), Mishell, Nakamura, Crosignani, Stone, Kharma, Nagata and Thorneycroft (1971), Newton, Joyce, Pearce, Revell and Tyler (1971), Somerville (1971), Speroff and van de Wiele (1971), Thorneycroft, Mischell, Stone, Kharma and Nakamura (1971), Abraham et al. (1972), Fogel, Rubin and Ossowski (1972), Holmdahl and Johansson (1972a), Moghissi, Syner and Evans (1972), Taymor, Berger, Thompson and Karam (1972), Dupon, Hosseinian and Kim (1973), Korenman and Sherman (1973), Shaaban and Klopper (1973), Kim, Hosseinian and Dupon (1974), Lundy, Lee, Levy, Woodruff, Wu and Abdalla (1974), Thorneycroft, Scribyatta, Tom, Nakamura and Mishell (1974), Saxena, Dusitsin, Poshyachinda and Smith (1974), Akande (1975), Dodson, Coutts and Macnaughton (1975), Kletzky, Nakamura, Thorneycroft and Mishell (1975), Sherman and Korenman (1975), Tea et al. (1975), Younglai et al. (1975), Aedo et al. (1976), Guerrero, Aso, Brenner, Cekan, Landgren, Hagenfeldt and Diczfalusy (1976), Laborde et al. (1976), Feng, Rodbard, Rebar and Ross (1977), Landgren, Aedo, Nunez, Cekan and Diczfalusy (1977) and Pauerstein, Eddy, Croxatto, Hess, Silerkhodr and Croxatto (1978).

The pattern of progesterone secretion during the menstrual cycle in relation to that of oestradiol, LH and FSH is shown in Fig. 2. Both Kletzky *et al.* (1975) and Guerrero *et al.* (1976) have shown that the range of plasma levels of the ovarian steroids and gonadotrophins in groups of women at the same stage of the menstrual cycle follow a log-normal rather than a normal distribution.

As far as progesterone is concerned, there are now several areas of agreement:

(i) During the follicular phase of the cycle plasma progesterone levels are usually less than 1 ng/ml (3 nmol/l) depending on the method employed. Guerrero *et al.* (1976) found a mean value of 0·3 ng/ml (1 nmol/l) using radioimmunoassay. Johansson (1969a) had also quoted a mean value of 0·3 ng/ml (1 nmol/l) using competitive protein binding.

(ii) During the luteal phase, plasma progesterone levels rise to reach a peak between days 5 and 8 after the LH peak. The mean peak level is about 15 ng/ml (48 nmol/l) but there is a wide range from about 5–35 ng/ml (16–112 nmol/l) (see Fig. 2).

(iii) If fertilisation of the ovum does not occur, the corpus luteum begins to regress and secretion of progesterone decreases. Plasma levels of the hormone have usually decreased below 1 ng/ml (3 nmol/l) at the onset of menstruation (see Fig. 3).

During both the follicular and luteal phase of the cycle the concentration of progesterone in plasma in a bilaterally adrenalectomised woman was within the range of those found in normal women suggesting that even during the follicular phase of the cycle the adrenocortical contribution of progesterone was negligible (Abraham and Chakmajian, 1973). Kim *et al.* (1974) showed that the plasma levels of oestradiol and progesterone during cycles in which women were treated with dexamethasone to suppress adrenocortical function were similar to those during normal untreated cycles again suggesting that the source of the steroids was primarily the ovary.

Johansson (1969a) found the variation in plasma progesterone levels to be larger between menstrual cycles of different women than between menstrual cycles of the same woman. In one subject the pattern of plasma progesterone was consistent when measured during four cycles during one year. Marked changes in the hormonal pattern of the menstrual cycle occur in the different phases of reproductive life from the menarché to the menopause (Sherman and Korenman, 1975). Reyes, Winter and Faiman (1977) who studied 58 cycles from women of different ages observed lower luteal phase plasma progesterone levels in older menstruating women than in younger ones.

There is controversy regarding changes in progesterone levels at midcycle. Early studies (see van der Molen and Aakvaag, 1967) suggested that

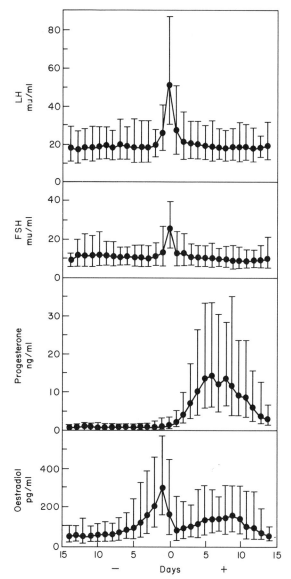

Fig. 2. Plasma levels of progesterone, oestradiol and gonadotrophins during normal menstrual cycles (from Kletzky *et al.*, 1975).

in some cycles there may be a slight increase in plasma progesterone at about the time of ovulation. Yussman and Taymor (1970) who took samples

every eight hours during a five day period at mid-cycle and Abraham *et al.*
(1972) noted at the time of the LH peak in many of the cycles a small rise
with levels reaching about 1·5 ng/ml (4·8 nmol/l) on the day of the LH
peak. This level persisted for one to two days when there was a more marked
increase. Johansson (1969a) had also found a rise in progesterone levels
on the day of the LH peak, but Thorneycroft and Stone (1972) detected a

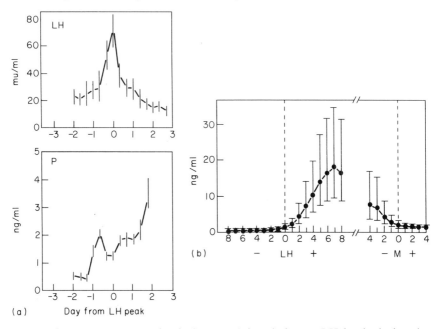

Fig. 3. Plasma progesterone levels (M. ± S.E.) in relation to LH levels during the
menstrual cycle—from Laborde *et al.*, 1976; (b) from Guerrero *et al.*, 1976.

marked increase in progesterone levels 24–36 hr after the LH peak in
menstrual cycles of three of four subjects they studied. Laborde *et al.* (1976)
obtained samples at eight-hourly intervals during days 11–16 of the
menstrual cycle from 13 women with normal ovulatory cycles confirmed by
corpus luteum biopsy. Plasma progesterone in all subjects began to increase
22 hr before the LH peak, reaching a peak of about 2 ng/ml (6 nmol/l) 12 hr
later, and then fell slightly during the LH peak and subsequently rose to
luteal phase levels (Fig. 3a).

    The periovulatory rise has also been studied in detail (Fig. 3b) by Guerrero
et al. (1976). In 15 of 17 subjects the difference between plasma progesterone
concentrations on days LH − 2 and LH − 1 of the pre-ovulatory period
was less than 0·35 ng/ml (1·1 nmol/l), whereas the difference between
LH − 1 and LH 0 was greater than 0·35 ng/ml (1·1 nmol/l) in 13 of the

subjects. A difference greater than 0·35 ng/ml (1·1 nmol/l) in plasma progesterone concentration between two consecutive days of the cycle occurred for the first time on the day of the LH peak for 13 of the 17 subjects. They therefore suggest that due to the association of the first marked elevation of progesterone with the LH peak daily measurements of progesterone can be used to predict ovulation. They found no decrease in the rate of progesterone secretion after the LH peak, as observed by Laborde et al. (1976). These findings have been extended by Landgren et al. (1977) by continuously withdrawing blood from ten normally menstruating women during the periovulatory period. The first significant increase in progesterone level occurred 6–9 hr after LH began to increase to its peak.

Although a rise in plasma progesterone before ovulation now seems well-founded, its role in still conjectural. Whether it is due to the final maturation of the follicle or to changes in its vascularisation remains to be elucidated as does its possible role in the regulation of LH secretion. It may be relevant that progesterone injected into women will release LH by a positive feedback effect (Leyendecker, Wardlaw and Nocke, 1972) and may also affect the pituitary response to LHRH (Shaw, Butt and London, 1975).

The source of the periovulatory progesterone is probably the ovarian follicle. Ryan and Petro (1966) showed that both the granulosa cells of the follicle and, to a lesser extent, the theca interna synthesise progesterone from pregnenolone in vitro. The structural relationship between these two cell types has been described by Baird (1972). Any steroid formed in the granulosa cells would readily pass into the follicular fluid but would probably have to cross to the theca interna in order to enter the circulation since the granulosa cell layer is relatively avascular. Thus part of the increase in the plasma levels of progesterone at mid-cycle may result from the release of progesterone when the follicle ruptures at ovulation. Although this contribution would probably be relatively small, the increase of plasma levels of progesterone before ovulation occurs would suggest that some progesterone is secreted by the theca interna cells or is formed in the granulosa cells and finds its way into the circulation.

Early work, reviewed in Ch. VIII showed the presence of progesterone in ovarian vein blood even during the follicular phase of the cycle. More detailed investigations have since shown concentrations of up to 15 ng/ml (48 nmol/l) during the follicular phase (Mikhail, 1967, 1970; Lloyd, Lobotsky, Baird, McCracken, Weisz, Pupkin, Zanartu and Puga, 1971; de Jong et al., 1974). The last workers found that the ovary containing a Graafian follicle in one woman in the late proliferative phase was secreting almost 50 µg (159 nmol) of progesterone per day. The concentration of progesterone in ovarian venous plasma from the ovary containing the Graafian follicle was always higher than that from the contralateral ovary suggesting that progesterone was synthesised by the theca or granulosa cells and that some was secreted from the stroma of ovaries not containing a developing follicle or corpus luteum. During the luteal phase the concentration of progesterone in ovarian venous blood increased dramatically, sometimes to about 2000 ng/ml (6·4 µmol/l), from the ovary bearing the corpus luteum but even the contralateral ovary appeared to secrete an increased amount of progesterone. De Jong et al. (1974) calculated the secretion rate of progesterone during the luteal phase in two women to be 17·3 (55) and 24·5 mg/day (78 µmol/day).

Progesterone is secreted during in vitro perfusion of human ovaries, even though they may not contain an active corpus luteum (Fukunishi, Mickan and Zander, 1975).

Although little progesterone is secreted by the ovary during the follicular phase and only small amounts are found in ovarian vein blood the follicle is capable of producing large amounts of progesterone as shown by the high content in follicular fluid. The progesterone concentration varied from 65–18,000 ng/ml (0·2–57 µmol/l) in follicular fluid from human ovaries primed with gonadotrophins, the concentration increasing with increasing size of the follicle (Edwards, Steptoe, Abraham, Walters, Purdy and Fotherby, 1972). In follicular fluid aspirated from normally menstruating women undergoing surgery, Sanyal, Berger, Thompson, Taymor and Horne (1974) reported progesterone levels to rise from a mean of 154 ng/ml (0·5 µmol/l) on days 4 and 5 of the cycle to 366 ng/ml (1·2 µmol/l) on days 8 and 9 and to a mean value of 1042 ng/ml (3·3 µmol/l) on days 10 and 11. Friederich, Breitenecker, Salzer and Holzner (1974) found that in tertiary follicles at different stages of the menstrual cycle the progesterone content estimated by gas-liquid chromatography varied from 9–1900 ng/ml (0·03–6·0 µmol/l) (м. 290 ng/ml (0·9 µmol/l)) with no change during the cycle whereas in Graafian follicles the progesterone content was 2290–14,000 ng/ml (7·3–45 µmol/l).

Since the large Graafian follicles of the later proliferative phase contain such a high concentration of progesterone, they are possibly the source of the pre-ovulatory progesterone in the circulation. The high concentration of progesterone in follicular fluid suggests that the progesterone produced in the follicle must be poorly secreted into the circulation. This is supported by Younglai and Short (1970) who detected only small amounts of radioactivity in ovarian venous plasma after injection of labelled progesterone into the follicle.

From the studies of hormone secretion during the menstrual cycle, Johansson, Wide and Gemzell (1971) found nine of 51 cycles that did not fulfil their criteria for normality. Seven of these nine cycles were shorter than 25 days, with a progesterone level below 5 ng/ml (16 nmol/l) and were classified as the short luteal phase type. Strott *et al.* (1970) had described seven similar cases characterised by plasma progesterone levels below the normal range and a peak three to four days after the initial LH surge rather than at six to eight days. Although the subjects had a biphasic temperature chart, the luteal phase defect was postulated as due to a low secretion of FSH at the beginning of the cycle with abnormal follicular development giving rise to inadequate luteinisation. Sherman and Korenman (1974a) described 11 similar cycles and further found that in two women this type of hormonal pattern occurred regularly in cycles analysed for up to one year.

These studies provide a hormonal background to the defect first described on the basis of clinical findings or on an endometrial biopsy (Jones, 1976; Aksel, Wiebe, Tyson and Jones, 1976). Jones (1976) has defined the "luteal phase defect" as:

> a deficiency of corpus luteum progesterone steroidogenesis either in amount or duration or both. The clinical manifestations include either primary infertility or repeated first trimester abortions. The diagnosis can only be made clinically on the basis of a well-timed endometrial biopsy that is read histologically as two or more days out of phase with the next period in at least two cycles. The deficiency is not due to a single etiology.

This defect would include those disorders of the menstrual cycle which have been termed the short luteal phase as well as those described by Sherman and Korenman (1974b) where the luteal phase is a normal length but the amount of progesterone secreted appears to be inadequate. This latter type of cycle with an inadequate luteal phase may be characteristic of oligomenorrheic obese infertile women. Sommerville (1971) has described another type of abnormal cycle in which the oestradiol peak did not occur until the seventeenth day of the cycle and was followed by menstruation about six days later. Plasma progesterone levels remained low throughout the cycle. This pattern is similar to that described by Fotherby and Brown (1964) on the basis of urinary steroid analyses.

Premenstrual tension has long been said to be associated with an imbalance between progesterone and oestrogen production during the luteal phase of the cycle. Backstrom, Wide, Sodergard and Carstensen (1976) compared hormone levels in a group of 15 women with premenstrual tension to those in a control group of 17 women and found that progesterone levels were consistently lower and oestrogen levels significantly higher in the group with premenstrual tension.

2. As an Index of Luteal Function

The studies described above have shown that measurements of plasma progesterone can be used to provide information about the occurrence of ovulation and the formation of a functional corpus luteum. Measurements of blood progesterone are likely to be a more precise indicator of luteal function than endometrial biopsies or recordings of the basal body temperature. However, daily sampling for plasma progesterone measurements is inconvenient so that it is necessary to know the minimum number of samples that need to be analysed to provide a reliable indicator of the presence of a functional corpus luteum.

Steele and Robertson (1972) showed that by determining progesterone in blood samples taken weekly, clear evidence of ovulation was obtained in 139 out of 147 cycles (94%). Sobotka and Kirton (1970) measured plasma progesterone levels on both day 8 and day 22 of the cycle and considered that ovulation had occurred if there was a change of more than 0·75 ng/ml (2·4 nmol/l) between the values on the two days, or if the plasma progesterone on day 22 was greater than 3 ng/ml (10 nmol/l). Israel, Mischell, Stone, Thorneycroft and Moyer (1972) suggested that only a single plasma progesterone measurement was necessary. Eighty-six women were studied using a competitive protein binding technique; a serum progesterone greater than 3 ng/ml (10 nmol/l) during the mid-luteal phase was always accompanied by a secretory endometrium. Saxena et al. (1974) found a serum progesterone level greater than 3 ng/ml (10 nmol/l) in 70–80% of samples taken in the mid-luteal phase.

Nadji, Reyniak, Sedlis, Szarowski and Bartosik (1975) put the lower limit of progesterone concentration at 2 ng/ml (6 nmol/l) on the basis of a study on day 20 or later of 24 women in whom plasma progesterone measurements and endometrial biopsies were assessed. In seven the endometrium was in a proliferative state and in these women the plasma progesterone concentration was less than 1 ng/ml (3 nmol/l). In the remaining 17 a secretory endometrium was observed and only two women had progesterone values less than 1 ng/ml (3 nmol/l). Askalani, Smuk, Sugar, Delvoye, Robyn and Schwers (1974a) studied 54 women and found the serum progesterone levels in the proliferative phase to range from 0·15–1·3 (M. 0·44) ng/ml (0·5–4·1 (M. 1·4) nmol/l) and in the secretory phase from 1·8–17·6 (M. 5·6) ng/ml (5·7–1·3 (M. 18) nmol/l). This discrimination between the two phases of the cycle was better than that obtained by measurements of urinary pregnanediol (proliferative phase range, 0·15–1·2 mg/24 hr (0·47–3·7 μmol/24 hr); secretory phase range, 1·2–10·1 mg/24 hr (3·7–31·5 μmol/24 hr)). They suggested therefore that a single measurement of plasma progesterone after day 20 of the cycle indicated the presence of a corpus luteum if a value greater than 1·8 ng/ml (5·7 nmol/l) was obtained.

However, other investigators have suggested that the lower limit of a single estimate of plasma progesterone which is consistent with the presence of a functional corpus luteum should be 5 ng/ml (16 nmol/l). Ross et al.

(1970) suggested that a level of 5 ng/ml (16 nmol/l), 5–8 days after the LH peak represented the lower limits of normal. This is supported by Shaaban and Klopper (1973), Lundy *et al.* (1974) and by Guerrero *et al.* (1976) who found the lowest individual progesterone value between days LH + 5 to LH + 8 was 6·7 ng/ml (21 nmol/l). Shepard and Senturia (1977) found a progesterone level greater than 3 ng/ml (10 nmol/l) in the mid-luteal phase (days 19–23 of the cycle) of 91% of cycles examined in 55 infertile women and 81% of endometrial biopsies taken at the same time showed a secretory pattern.

Black *et al.* (1972) compared plasma progesterone levels and endometrial biopsies in 103 patients and suggested that whereas a plasma progesterone level greater than 5 ng/ml (16 nmol/l) indicated the presence of a functional corpus luteum, repeated sampling or a single value of 10 ng/ml (32 nmol/l) increased the predictive value. Abraham *et al.* (1974) found that several of their anovulatory patients had plasma progesterone values greater than 3 ng/ml (10 nmol/l) and preferred to rely on measurements obtained from three samples taken from 4–11 days before the next menstrual period. Their criterion for normality was that the summed concentrations of progesterone in these three samples should be equal to or greater than 15 ng/ml (48 nmol/l). Such an approach is cumbersome and inconvenient compared with collection of a single blood sample. Although there is no consensus regarding the lower level of plasma progesterone consistent with the presence of a functional corpus luteum, review of the levels obtained from the various studies of plasma progesterone concentrations during the menstrual cycle would suggest that a value greater than 3 ng/ml (10 nmol/l), obtained by a reliable radioimmunoassay, would give few false positive results and a limit of 5 ng/ml (16 nmol/l) probably none.

Askalani, Wilkin and Schwers (1974b) also investigated other indices of luteal function. Vaginal cytology had only a poor correlation with the serum progesterone level. Of 26 women in whom the progesterone values were in the proliferative range, 20 showed oestrogenic vaginal smears and six showed a mixed pattern. In 16 women where the progesterone levels were in the secretory range, 14 showed a mixed pattern and only two showed an oestrogenic smear. Whereas a biphasic body temperature curve was associated with elevated levels of progesterone showing the presence of a corpus luteum, a monophasic temperature chart did not necessarily indicate anovulation. Endometrial biopsies were obtained from 21 women with low levels of serum progesterone and in 19 of these the endometrium was in a proliferative state whereas of 17 women with luteal phase levels of progesterone, 16 showed a secretory endometrium.

Radwanska, Hughesdon and Swyer (1976a) from an analysis of plasma progesterone estimations and endometrial biopsies on 140 infertile women, concluded that the plasma progesterone measurement was more precise in the diagnosis of corpus luteum insufficiency than an endometrial biopsy. Rosenfeld and Garcia (1976) carried out a retrospective analysis of endometrial biopsies with simultaneous plasma progesterone estimations from 230 women attending an infertility clinic and found a high degree of correlation between the two measurements.

The conclusion from the above studies is that estimation of plasma progesterone is a more precise indicator of the presence of a functional corpus luteum than other parameters such as an endometrial biopsy. The simplicity of taking a blood sample compared to the inconvenience of taking a biopsy is in favour of the blood measurement. However, the type of information given by the two evaluations is different. Jones and Wentz (1974) claimed that a properly taken, accurately dated endometrial biopsy serves as a bioassay measuring the hormonal effect at the tissue level and is the best clinical method for diagnosing a luteal phase defect.

Although there is a good correlation between an elevated plasma progesterone value and a secretory endometrium there appears to be a poorer correlation between plasma progesterone levels and histological dating of the endometrium. Cooke, Morgan and Parry (1972) studied 59 women attending an infertility clinic. In 34, the histological dating of the endometrium showed a good correlation with the chronological dating of the day of the cycle and in these women the plasma progesterone levels were within the normal range for the time of the cycle. In a further 16 women the histological dating was at least three days less than the chronological assessment and in only five of these was the progesterone level within the normal range for the time of the cycle. In the remaining nine subjects the histological dating was at least three days later than the chronological assessment showing a more mature endometrium than anticipated and five of these had plasma progesterone levels within the normal range. Overall therefore there was a poor correlation between the endometrial dating and plasma progesterone levels. A similar finding was reported by Shepard and Senturia (1977), who found that in only 11 of 33 cycles were the endometrial pattern and progesterone levels consistent with each other and with the presumed time of ovulation. Whereas the progesterone level was inconsistent with the time of ovulation in only two cycles, the endometrial pattern was inconsistent in twenty.

The concentration of progesterone in blood required for a successful pregnancy if fertilisation occurs in not known. Inadequate corpus luteal function is known clinically to be related either to primary infertility or to recurrent early abortion (Jones and Wentz, 1974; Yip and Sung, 1977). Jones and Wentz found that the progesterone levels in ten patients with infertility were significantly lower than those of eight subjects with normal luteal function. Dodson *et al.* (1975) found that, compared to a group of normal women, a group of infertile patients produced "poor" corpora lutea in that the normal increase in plasma progesterone was delayed and the number of days of peak hormone production was less, although the progesterone levels in the two groups were not significantly different. Radwanska, McGarrigle and Swyer (1976b) have suggested that a mid-luteal phase level of progesterone less than 10 ng/ml (32 nmol/l) indicated deficient secretion of progesterone and may be a cause of infertility. They studied 299 menstruating women attending an infertility clinic. In 145 with a non-hormonal cause for the infertility such as tubal occlusion, endometriosis, infertile husband, the mid-luteal plasma progesterone level was 14·5 ± 4·4 ng/ml (46·1 ± 1·4 nmol/l) and values lower than 10 ng/ml (32 nmol/l) were found in 21 women (14%). In the remaining 154 women with no obvious non-hormonal cause for the infertility the mean mid-luteal plasma progesterone level (11·9 ± 5·3 ng/ml; 38·1 ± 16·8 nmol/l) was significantly lower than that in the first group. Values lower than 10 ng/ml (32 nmol/l) were found in 61 women (40%) of this group. The authors suggest therefore that a large number of women with unexplained infertility have luteal insufficiency. Similar findings have been reported by Karow and Gentry (1976) and by Shepard and Senturia (1977). However, Cooke *et al.* (1972) in their study of endometrial biopsies and plasma progesterone levels in infertile women found no difference in the incidence of successful pregnancy between those women in which the dating of the biopsy correlated with the plasma progesterone levels and in those in whom there was no correlation.

3. Factors Affecting Progesterone Secretion in Humans

Although neither the factors governing the life-span of the human corpus luteum nor the nature of the control of its synthesis of progesterone is known, the secretion of progesterone is affected by a number of administered substances. In many species the uterus appears to produce a luteolysin which induces regression of the corpus luteum so that hysterectomy leads to prolongation of the life-span of the corpus luteum. The comparative aspects of uterine–luteal relationships have been reviewed by Anderson, Bland and Melampy (1969). In humans no such activity has been detected in the uterus and hysterectomy does not prolong the activity of the corpus luteum (Beling, Stewart and Markham, 1970). Doyle, Barclay, Duncan and Kirton (1971) have also shown that normal cyclicity continued in five women after hysterectomy between days 18 and 22 of the menstrual cycle and in whom measurements of plasma progesterone and LH were made at weekly intervals for 13 weeks.

(a) Effect of oestrogens

In many species oestrogens have been shown to be luteolytic and to cause a decrease in progesterone synthesis in the corpus luteum. Some studies have suggested that a similar effect may occur in humans. Post-coital administration of oestrogens soon after ovulation has long been known to prevent pregnancy (see reviews by Blye, 1973, and Haspels, 1976). Blye (1973) showed a luteolytic effect of diethylstilboestrol in doses of 50 mg daily for five days starting three days after the rise in basal body temperature. The length of the luteal phase was decreased by two to four days, and there was a marked decrease in the plasma progesterone concentration on the third day after starting treatment. Similar findings were obtained by Gore, Caldwell and Speroff (1973) and also by Board, Bhatnagar and Bush (1973) using a dose of 25 mg diethylstilboestrol daily. Lehmann, Just-Nastansky, Behrendt, Czygan and Bettendorf (1975) compared the effect of 60 mg diethylstilboestrol daily with the very high dose of 30 mg mestranol (ethynyloestradiol-3-methyl ether). Compared with control cycles in the same women they found no decrease in the length of the luteal phase, but there was a suppression of corpus luteal function.

Oestrogens administered in the first half of the cycle may also affect luteal function. Dhont, Vandekerckhove and Vermeulen (1974) treated two groups of regularly menstruating women with 100 µg ethynyloestradiol daily either on days 7 and 8 or on days 10 and 11 of the cycle. Administration on days 7 and 8 appeared to have little effect on hormone secretion, but on days 10 and 11 it increased the plasma levels of LH and also oestrogen and progesterone during the luteal phase.

(b) Effect of synthetic gestagens

The effect of synthetic gestagens on corpus luteum function has been studied in detail (Johansson, 1971, 1973; Nygren and Johansson, 1975). The gestagens were administered daily starting three days after the presumed day of ovulation. A depression in the plasma progesterone level was observed and the lowest total dose of the gestagens required to produce this effect was 30 mg norethisterone, 12 mg d-norgestrel, 300 mg chlormadinone acetate or 360 mg medroxyprogesterone acetate. Menstruation was delayed in spite of the plasma levels of progesterone decreasing to below 1 ng/ml (3 nmol/l) due to the administered gestagen maintaining the uterine endometrium. The gestagen appeared to inhibit progesterone synthesis in the corpus luteum. Since the corpus luteum in such circumstances is able to respond to injections of human chorionic gonadotrophin, the gestagens are without a luteolytic effect. Administration of the same gestagens in high doses (Nygren and

Johansson, 1975) to women in the early stages of pregnancy when plasma levels of progesterone were elevated (from 20–80 ng/ml; 64–254 nmol/l) produced no consistent effect on the plasma progesterone levels. Neither Johansson (1973) nor Aksel and Jones (1974) found intramuscular injection of 17α-hydroxyprogesterone caproate in doses up to 500 mg caused no decrease in progesterone production as judged by plasma levels.

Much lower doses of the gestagens administered daily from the beginning of the cycle, for example 50–75 μg norgestrel or 450 μg norethisterone will depress corpus luteum function and the plasma progesterone level in many women (see Fotherby, 1977) without inhibiting ovulation. This effect also seems to be brought about by inhibiting progesterone synthesis in the corpus luteum (Mukherjee, Wright, Davidson and Fotherby, 1972) since a histologically normal corpus luteum is observed at laparotomy (Wright, Fotherby and Fairweather, 1970).

(c) Effect of human chorionic gonadotrophin (hCG)

Earlier findings regarding the effect of hCG in extending the life-span of the corpus luteum and its ability to increase progesterone secretion as determined by urinary pregnanediol excretion have been confirmed by measurements of plasma progesterone levels. Strott, Yoshimi, Ross and Lipsett (1969) showed that intramuscular administration of 2000 u hCG for 10 days during the luteal phase of the cycle caused a two-fold increase in plasma progesterone concentration and an increase in the length of the menstrual cycle. Similar results were obtained by Hanson, Powell and Stevens (1971). Runnebaum, Holzmann, Munstermann and Zander (1972b) administered 5000 u hCG by intravenous infusion over a 2-hr period during the luteal phase of the cycle and found that the stimulatory effect upon the corpus luteum may last for up to 15 hr. With larger doses (20,000 u) there was a greater increase in the progesterone levels and in some women the levels were still elevated 20 hr after starting the infusion (Fig. 4).

With intramuscular injection the increased levels of progesterone could be maintained for a much longer period of time. When these same doses of hCG were administered to women in early pregnancy, little effect on the plasma progesterone concentration was observed. Kaiser and Geiger (1971) showed that during early pregnancy very high doses of hCG (up to 80,000 u daily) may be necessary to stimulate the corpus luteum.

(d) Effect of other compounds

The role of prostaglandins in the physiology and biochemistry of the corpus luteum has been reviewed by Pharriss, Tillson and Erickson (1972). In many species prostaglandins are luteolytic and cause regression of the corpus luteum, but in humans they appear not to have this effect. Jones and Wentz (1972) infused 25 mg of prostaglandin $PGF_{2\alpha}$ over an 8-hr-period into 21 women during the luteal phase of the cycle. Thirteen of the 21 women showed a slight shortening of the luteal phase, but there was no consistent change in the serum progesterone levels. A similar lack of effect was found by Okamura, Aso, Yoshida and Mishimura (1974) who administered 75 mg of the same prostaglandin intravaginally to three women during the mid-luteal phase and found no significant effect on the plasma progesterone levels or on the corpus luteum examined either histochemically or by electron microscopy.

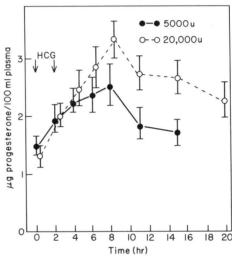

Fig. 4. Plasma progesterone concentrations (M. ± S.D.) before, during and after a 2 hr infusion of 5000 u (six women) and of 20,000 u HCG (four women) on day 5 in the hyperthermic phase of the cycle (from Runnebaum *et al.*, 1972b).

The steroid oxymethylone (2-hydroxymethylene-17α-methyl-5α-dihydro-testosterone) is an inhibitor of 3β-hydroxysteroid dehydrogenase steroid isomerase and appears to affect corpus luteum function. Klaiber, Henzl, Lloyd and Segre (1973) administered 100 mg of the compound daily for seven days to 12 women and found that the menstrual cycles decreased in length by about six days. When treatment was started before day LH + 4, plasma progesterone decreased by 28–74%. This compound appears to exert a specific effect upon progesterone synthesis since it had no effect upon oestrogen production from the corpus luteum and the effect could be reversed by the simultaneous administration of hCG.

Infusion of αMSH during the luteal phase of the cycle produced no significant change in progesterone levels (Runnebaum, Heep, Geiger, Vecsei and Andor, 1976).

Insertion of an intrauterine device may shorten the luteal phase of the cycle by up to two days (Brenner and Mishell, 1975) but does not decrease the secretion of ovarian steroids. The action appears to be by a local effect on the endometrium which results in menstruation occurring about two days earlier than usual and at a time when plasma progesterone and oestradiol levels are higher than they usually are at the time of menstruation.

Continuous cervical dilatation will increase plasma progesterone levels during the first trimester of human pregnancy (Fylling and Norman, 1970) as will the intravenous infusion of vasopressin and theophyllamine (Fylling, 1973). The increases produced by cervical dilatation, and by vasopressin, but not that produced by theophyllamine can be prevented by administration of the β-receptor blocking agent propranolol. Similarly, administration of dexamethasone (2·5 mg four times daily orally or a single intramuscular injection of 24 mg) did not affect plasma progesterone levels, but abolished the increase produced by cervical dilatation and vasopressin (Fylling, 1972).

D. PROGESTERONE IN BLOOD DURING PREGNANCY

1. Early Pregnancy

Some aspects of progesterone metabolism in women during early pregnancy were reported by James, Fotherby and MacNaughton (1969) and hormone production during early pregnancy was reviewed by Fotherby (1971). During the menstrual cycle, regression of the corpus luteum, as shown by the decrease in plasma progesterone, begins about seven to eight days after ovulation. If fertilisation occurs, some signal, the nature of which is at present unknown (Short, 1969), from the fertilised ovum must reach the corpus luteum by this time to maintain it in a functional state and to prevent regression. One of the factors presumably responsible for maintaining the function of the corpus luteum is hCG, which begins to be secreted about nine days after ovulation and is thereafter secreted in rapidly increasing amounts, reaching a peak 50–65 days after ovulation. Milwidsky, Adoni, Segal and Palti (1977) have suggested that another factor may also be involved since in 11 out of 17 patients with ectopic pregnancy, plasma progesterone levels were lower than those in normal pregnancies, and in eight cases proliferative phase levels were found in spite of hCG levels within the normal range. In spite of the rapid rise in hCG production, there is no corresponding marked increase in progesterone production and the corpus luteum becomes increasingly refractory to the stimulatory effects of hCG (see p. 465). In fact, progesterone production as estimated on the basis of pregnanediol excretion or plasma progesterone levels exceeds that of the luteal peak only at the eighth or ninth week of pregnancy.

These findings have been confirmed in more recent investigations (Johansson, 1969a; Yoshimi, Strott, Marshall and Lipsett, 1969; Holmdahl and Johansson, 1972; Mishell, Thorneycroft, Nagata, Murata and Naka-mura, 1973; Tulchinsky and Hobel, 1973 and Corker, Michie, Hobson and Parboosingh, 1976). In most of these studies there was a slight decrease in plasma progesterone levels up to the seventh to ninth week of pregnancy

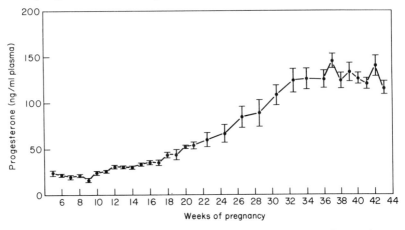

Fig. 5. Levels of plasma progesterone (M. ± S.E.) during pregnancy (from Johansson, 1969b).

and after this time progesterone levels again begin to increase (Fig. 5). This time appears to correspond with the end of the corpus luteum as the source of progesterone and the beginning of secretion of progesterone from the trophoblast.

Holmdahl, Johansson and Wide (1971) measured the disappearance of progesterone from the plasma of 17 women undergoing therapeutic abortion between the seventh and sixteenth week of pregnancy. Plasma progesterone levels remained elevated for a much longer time when vacuum aspiration of uterine contents was performed in weeks 7 and 8 of pregnancy in contrast to those obtained when aspiration was carried out between weeks 12 and 16, suggesting that in the latter group the placenta was the main source of progesterone production, whereas in the former group it was the corpus luteum.

2. Mid and Late Pregnancy

Although the above studies suggest that the corpus luteum is not essential after about the ninth week of pregnancy, it remains active throughout pregnancy. LeMaire, Rice and Savard (1968) showed that the corpus luteum during pregnancy and up to four days post-partum retained the ability to synthesise progesterone from acetate *in vitro* and was also capable of responding to hCG. It seems likely that the hCG secreted during pregnancy is responsible for the maintenance of the corpus luteum of pregnancy since, with the disappearance of the source of hCG at delivery, corpus luteum function decreases. The activity of the corpus luteum, however, could be maintained by daily administration of hCG in large doses post-partum (LeMaire, Conley, Moffet, Spellacy, Cleveland and Savard, 1971).

In vivo investigations also suggest that the corpus luteum of pregnancy secretes progesterone. Mikhail and Allen (1967) found the concentration of progesterone in venous blood from corpus luteum-bearing ovaries in pregnant women to be 480–800 ng/ml (1·5–2·5 μmol/l) at mid-pregnancy and 50–150 ng/ml (160–480 nmol/l) at the end of pregnancy. LeMaire, Conly, Moffet and Cleveland (1970) found that at the end of pregnancy the concentration of progesterone in venous plasma from the ovary without a corpus luteum varied from 80–160 ng/ml (254–510 nmol/l), м. 110 ng/ml (350 nmol/l), whereas that in plasma from the ovary with a corpus luteum was significantly higher, 100–310 ng/ml (318–986 nmol/l) м. 200 ng/ml (700 nmol/l). Similar results were reported by Weiss and Rifken (1975) who measured plasma progesterone levels in peripheral and ovarian venous blood 20–30 min after delivery of the placenta from nine women undergoing Caesarean section. The mean concentration of progesterone in peripheral blood was 44·9 ± 9·7 ng/ml (143 ± 31 nmol/l); in blood from the ovary not containing a corpus luteum the value was 56·2 ± 5·1 ng/ml (179 ± 16 nmol/l) and in blood from the ovary containing the corpus luteum the concentration was significantly higher (116·9 ± 25·8 ng/ml; 372 ± 82 nmol/l).

Guraya (1972) has reviewed the histochemical, biochemical and morphological evidence showing that the corpus luteum is a functioning endocrine organ throughout pregnancy, and Crisp, Dessouky and Denys (1973) have also made a detailed histological examination of the corpus luteum of pregnancy and suggested that such corpora are functional.

Thus, although the corpus luteum retains the ability to synthesise and secrete progesterone throughout pregnancy, quantitatively the amounts are small compared to placental secretion.

The pattern of plasma progesterone levels during pregnancy described by van der Molen and Aakvaag (1967) has since been confirmed in a number of subsequent studies. The levels found by Johansson (1969b) using a competitive protein binding assay increased from the ninth to the thirty-second week of gestation with the most marked increase occurring between the eighteenth and thirtieth weeks (Fig. 5). The mean levels at weeks 9 and 32 were 16·7 ± 7·4 ng/ml (53 ± 23 nmol/l) and 125 ± 37·9 ng/ml (397 ± 120 nmol/l) respectively. Measurements of urinary pregnanediol have shown that the amount excreted did not change during the last 8 to 10 weeks of pregnancy and, similarly, there was no increase in the plasma progesterone levels during this time. The levels of progesterone in plasma reported by Johansson (1969b) show a close correlation with urinary pregnanediol estimations (Fotherby, 1975). Similar values have been found by Luisi et al. (1971), Lindberg et al. (1974) and Christensen, Froyshov and Fylling (1974) who studied 32 women serially throughout pregnancy using competitive protein binding assay and by Coats et al. (1977) and Tulchinsky, Hobel, Yeager and Marshall (1972a) using radioimmunoassay. The last workers found the ratio of plasma progesterone to unconjugated oestradiol and to unconjugated oestriol to remain fairly constant during the second half of pregnancy. Levels in Asian women (Teoh et al., 1973; Dawood, 1976) are similar to the above values. Spellacy, Conly, Cleveland and Buhi (1975) measured the serum progesterone and hCG concentrations in 268 normal pregnant women within the last four days of pregnancy. Although there was a weak correlation of the serum progesterone level with the placental weight ($r = 0.24$), there was no correlation with the hCG level, foetal weight or sex. These findings are confirmed by the results of a similar study carried out by Boroditzky, Reyes, Winter and Faiman (1975). Contrary to these results, Conly, Spellacy and Cleveland (1972) found plasma progesterone levels in the last month of gestation to be significantly higher in women bearing female foetuses (93.4 ± 6.7 ng/ml; 297 ± 21 nmol/l) than in those bearing male foetuses (75.5 ± 5.2 ng/ml; 240 ± 16 nmol/l) although women with female foetuses had similar placentae (408 ± 14.9) than women carrying male foetuses (471 ± 19.7). There was no difference in the gestational ages or birth weights. Antonipillai and Murphy (1977) found higher levels of progesterone in primiparous women compared with multiparous ones, but found no correlation with foetal sex.

Most investigators agree that variations in the levels of progesterone in blood during pregnancy are considerable and detract from the usefulness of its measurement as an index of placental function. Klopper and Shaaban (1974) found the day-to-day variation during the last four weeks of pregnancy in the same subject to be 22% and a subject-to-subject variation of 27%. Christensen et al. (1974) reported individual variations of up to 100 ng/ml (318 nmol/l) from one day to another. Of 32 women from whom samples were taken weekly, 25 showed a variation between samples of more than 50 ng/ml (159 nmol/l) and five a variation of more than 100 ng/ml (318 nmol/l) (Lindberg et al., 1974).

Tulchinsky and Okada (1975) claimed that cortisol or ACTH produced no significant change in the maternal or foetal plasma progesterone levels, suggesting that neither the maternal nor foetal adrenals were producing significant amounts of progesterone at this time.

Winkel, Gaede and Lyngbye (1976) devised a mathematical model, based upon the assumption that the plasma progesterone concentration is correlated with the growth rate of the placenta, which can be used for monitoring placental growth from the plasma progesterone levels.

3. Parturition and Abortion

The increased production of oestrogens and progesterone throughout pregnancy and the marked decrease in plasma levels after parturition have long suggested that these steroid hormones may play a key role in the process of parturition. Parturition, however, is a complex physiological process involving many interrelated factors and it is unlikely that changes in any one of these components alone will be sufficient to explain the process. This section will deal only with changes in blood progesterone levels during parturition. The endocrine factors involved in labour have been discussed in detail (Klopper and Gardner, 1973; Pierrepoint, 1973; Liggins, Forester, Grieves and Schwartz, 1977; Turnbull and Anderson, 1978; Ryan, 1971).

The emphasis on the role of progesterone in labour stems partly from the suggestion of Csapo and Wood (1968) that the increasing levels of progesterone in blood during pregnancy have a sedating effect on uterine myometrial activity until, at parturition, a decrease in the progesterone level in blood and in the myometrium removes the block to myometrial activity. In most studies no significant decrease in progesterone levels has been observed before parturition, although in all studies a marked fall in progesterone levels has been shown to occur after expulsion of the placenta (van der Molen and Aakvaag, 1967).

Bengtsson (1973) and Fuchs (1972) conclude that the evidence that the onset of human labour is due to a withdrawal of progesterone is meagre. Llauro et al. (1968) performed serial determinations of progesterone before, during and after labour in a group of 13 pregnant women. The mean values obtained are shown in Fig. 6. There was no significant change in the plasma progesterone concentrations between the thirty-fourth week of pregnancy, the onset of labour and the stage when the cervix was fully dilated, although 10 subjects showed a fall between the onset of labour and the stage of full dilatation of the cervix. The most marked fall occurred after removal of the placenta. The progesterone concentration continued to decrease and was in the range of luteal phase levels 24 hr after delivery. Yannone, McCurdy and Goldfien (1968) also found no relationship between plasma progesterone levels and the progress of labour, and in some cases the levels of progesterone rose during labour.

Craft, Wyman and Sommerville (1969) took several blood samples daily from four women before spontaneous delivery and during labour and found

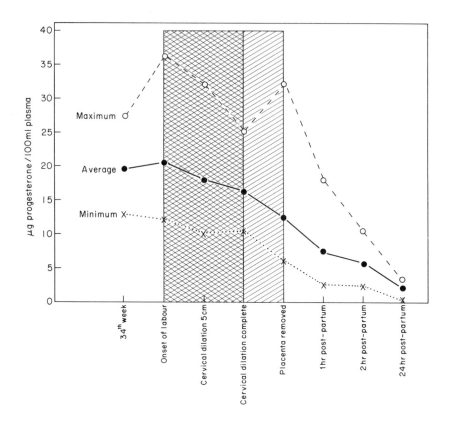

Fig. 6. Levels of progesterone (1 nmol/l = μg/dl × 3180) in plasma during labour. Values are means for 13 women (from Llauro *et al.*, 1968).

no consistent change in the plasma progesterone levels. Ances, Hisley and Haskins (1971), using a competitive protein-binding assay, studied 14 women in whom labour was induced by oxytocin infusions. There was a consistent fall in progesterone levels at the beginning of labour when the cervix was dilated 4–6 cm and the values returned to the pre-labour levels during the phase when the cervix was dilated 8–9 cm. Shaaban and Klopper (1973) found a wide variation in progesterone levels but without any consistent change over the last three weeks of pregnancy. The progesterone concentration during labour was not different from that found before labour. Okada, Tulchinsky, Ross and Hobel (1974) studied six nulliparous women admitted to hospital for induction of labour by amniotomy. Spontaneous labour occurred within 1 hr of amniotomy, but there was no significant change in the mean values for plasma progesterone in samples taken hourly for 9 hr from the beginning of the induction. They found wide fluctuations in the plasma progesterone concentration from hour-to-hour without any consistent pattern.

No decrease occurred in the concentration of free (ultrafiltrable) progesterone in plasma before labour (Batra et al., 1976) and neither these investigators nor Cousins, Hobel, Chang, Okada and Marshall (1977) found any significant change in the progesterone or oestradiol levels before normal term labour. Haning, Barrett, Alberino, Lynskey, Donabedian and Speroff (1978) measured several hormones and a prostaglandin $PGF_{2\alpha}$ metabolite in samples of maternal and umbilical cord venous blood at delivery. They studied four groups of women, one undergoing Caesarian section before the onset of labour, one undergoing Caesarian section once labour had begun spontaneously, a third group of women having spontaneous onset of labour and a fourth group in whom labour was induced with oxytocin. There was no significant difference in the progesterone levels between these four groups and in all cases progesterone levels in venous cord blood were two- to tenfold higher than in maternal venous blood. Similar results were found by Pokoly and Jordan (1975).

Antonipillai and Murphy (1977) measured progesterone levels in maternal blood and in the umbilical vein and artery in women immediately after delivery of the infant but before delivery of the placenta. Both umbilical artery and vein levels were significantly lower in women undergoing elective Caesarian section than after spontaneous delivery or induced delivery with oxytocin, but there were no differences in the maternal levels of progesterone. Values measured in umbilical artery and venous blood at end of labour induced by oxytocin were significantly higher than those obtained at elective Caesarian section. Arai and Yanaihara (1977) found no change in the foetal plasma progesterone between the first and second stages of labour.

Two studies have shown a decrease in plasma progesterone concentrations in women during labour. Csapo, Knobil, van der Molen and Wiest (1971) took plasma samples from 12 nulliparous women with normal pregnancies during the last seven weeks of pregnancy and during labour. The samples were analysed by different methods in three separate laboratories. Although there were differences in the time at which plasma progesterone levels reached a peak during the last four weeks of pregnancy, all subjects showed a decrease at the onset of labour. Two to three weeks before the onset of labour in 11 nulliparous women with normal pregnancies, the mean plasma progesterone level was 173 ± 6 ng/ml (550 ± 19 nmol/l) and was significantly higher than that found at the onset of labour (146 ± 11 ng/ml; 464 ± 35 nmol/l). Furthermore, there appeared to be a correlation between the progesterone level and the duration of labour. Six of the 11 women had a mean progesterone concentration of 169 ± 7 ng/ml (540 ± 22 nmol/l) and were in active labour for 8·0 ± 1·3 hr, while the remaining five had a lower progesterone concentration (116 ± 6 ng/ml; 369 ± 19 nmol/l) and were in labour for only 2·8 ± 0·4 hr. The authors interpreted these results as showing a fall in circulating progesterone at the beginning of labour, but because large variations occur in the plasma progesterone level, this work needs repeating with a larger series of patients. It receives some support from the work of Turnbull, Flint, Jeremy, Patten, Keirse and Anderson (1974) who measured the plasma progesterone levels in 33 primigravidae with uncomplicated pregnancies and in whom labour began spontaneously within 12 days of the expected date. They found a three-fold increase in the plasma progesterone levels between the twentieth and thirty-sixth weeks of pregnancy, followed by a marked fall from a mean value of about 150 ng/ml (477 nmol/l) at week 36 to a value of 105 ng/ml (334 nmol/l) at the fortieth week. Levels observed during the second stage of labour were not significantly different from those found in the week before labour. The decrease in plasma progesterone levels at the end of pregnancy seemed unlikely to be due to placental insufficiency since plasma oestradiol values continued to increase during this time.

Even small decreases in the blood progesterone level at the end of pregnancy may be important and Csapo, Sauvage and Wiest (1970) extended the hypothesis to suggest that the contractile activity of the myometrium is governed by the ratio of the uterine volume to the plasma progesterone level. During pregnancy the uterine volume and the ratio increases and a further increase would be produced if the plasma progesterone level decreased at the end of pregnancy. An increased uterine volume stimulates the synthesis of prostaglandins which would further stimulate myometrial activity unless this activity were inhibited by an increased concentration of progesterone. Thus, in order to maintain pregnancy there must be a proper balance between the levels of prostaglandin and progesterone in the myometrium and an increase in the ratio would tend to induce labour. The relationship between uterine volume, plasma progesterone levels and intrauterine pressure has also been studied by Pulkkinen, Liukko, Rauramo and Willman (1974) whose results support the findings of Csapo et al. (1970). However, in non-pregnant women Gibor, Pandya, Bieniarz and Scommegna (1971) failed to find any relationship between uterine contractility and the plasma progesterone level. Recordings of uterine contractility were made in four non-pregnant subjects during the course of 60 menstrual cycles. During some cycles progesterone was administered locally into the uterus but without effect on uterine contractility.

Moreover the level of progesterone in myometrial tissue shows little change during pregnancy (Runnebaum and Zander, 1971; Batra and

Bengtsson, 1978). Csapo (1969) has suggested that the binding of progesterone may not be uniform throughout the myometrium and that local changes, for example at the site of attachment of the placenta, may occur which would not be reflected throughout the myometrium as a whole. However, this is negated by the results of the studies cited above (see p. 442).

(a) Premature labour

Csapo, Pohanka and Kaihola (1974) have extended their studies to include premature labour. The mean values for plasma progesterone in 11 women admitted to hospital for threatened premature labour were 100 ± 8 ng/ml (318 ± 25 nmol/l) at week 35 of pregnancy and 71 ± 6 ng/ml (226 ± 19 nmol/l) during premature labour. These values were significantly lower than those found in a control group (173 ± 6 ng/ml (550 ± 19 nmol/l) at week 37 and 141 ± 6 ng/ml (448 ± 19 nmol/l) during labour). They also found a correlation between the birth weight of the baby and the progesterone concentration. Six of the mothers had babies weighing less than 2 kg and during labour the plasma progesterone concentration was 52 ± 9 ng/ml (165 ± 19 nmol/l). In the remaining five pregnancies the birth weights were more than 2 kg and the progesterone level was significantly higher (90 ± 12 ng/ml; 286 ± 38 nmol/l). Csapo et al. (1974) suggest that in the group with the larger babies the uterine volume would be larger so that progesterone production would have to increase to maintain the ratio of uterine volume to plasma progesterone levels similar to the two groups.

Although there was a marked increase in plasma oestradiol levels preceding the onset of premature labour in a group of women studied by Tambyraja, Anderson and Turnbull (1974), there was no consistent change in progesterone levels. Cousins et al. (1977) found that women in premature labour had significantly lower levels of both progesterone and oestradiol than control subjects. They further suggest that the extent to which the plasma levels were depressed depended upon the type of premature labour. Women with idiopathic premature labour had significantly lower levels than those where labour was induced by premature rupture of the membranes.

(b) Therapeutic abortion

No significant decrease in the plasma progesterone levels in women undergoing therapeutic abortion has been observed by most investigators irrespective of the agents used to produce abortion. No significant changes were observed with the use of intra-amniotic hypertonic saline (Osborn, Goplerud and Yannone, 1968), hypertonic urea (Raud, Balsdon and Collins, 1972) or prostaglandin-$PGF_{2\alpha}$ (Cantor, Jewelewicz, Warren,

Dyrenfurth, Patner and Van de Wiele, 1972; Symonds, Fahmy, Morgan, Roberts, Gomershall and Turnbull, 1972) although the findings of Craft et al. (1974) are at variance with those of the two last groups of investigators, and Koren, Schulman, Lev-Gur, Gatz, Thysen and Bloch (1976) found a decrease in progesterone levels during the first 3 hr after intra-amniotic administration of prostaglandin-$PGF_{2\alpha}$ but no subsequent further decrease. Csapo et al. (1969) have also reported changes in the plasma progesterone levels during abortion induced with hypertonic saline. Plasma samples were obtained from six patients in the sixteenth week of normal pregnancy and analysed with good agreement in four separate laboratories. Plasma progesterone levels decreased from a pre-induction value of 38 ± 4 ng/ml (121 ± 13 nmol/l) to 26 ± 2 ng/ml (83 ± 6 nmol/l) 10 hr later and to 23 ± 3 ng/ml (73 ± 10 nmol/l) at the onset of clinical abortion 14 hr later. During the next 3 hr the values decreased to 17 ± 3 ng/ml (54 ± 10 nmol/l). The fall was seen in all six patients and uterine contractility commenced during the first 10 hr. Ruttner (1969) has obtained evidence in support of Csapo's hypothesis by showing that administration of progesterone to women undergoing hypertonic saline-induced abortions more than doubled the time until abortion began.

4. Disorders of Pregnancy

The measurement of urinary pregnanediol excretion in disorders of pregnancy has been of little clinical value (Klopper, 1969). From the few studies of pregnancy disorders, blood progesterone levels are little more informative than measurements of urinary pregnanediol excretion, mainly because of the wide day-to-day variations of plasma progesterone values.

(a) Threatened abortion

Plasma progesterone levels are reported to be lower than normal in spontaneous abortion (Johansson, 1969b; Luisi et al., 1971). Kunz and Keller (1976) reported that 89% of 65 women with threatened abortion had serum progesterone values below the normal range and that normal values predicted continuation of the pregnancy with an accuracy of 60%. They concluded therefore that measurements of progesterone were as reliable as the measurement of oestradiol, hCG and hPL. The results of other investigators do not support these findings. Nygren, Johansson and Wide (1973) found no correlation between the progesterone level and threatened abortion, and McNaughton (1976) observed levels within the normal range in women who had recurrent abortions in the first trimester. More recently Jovanovic, Dawood, Landesman and Saxena (1978) measured the serum levels of several hormones in 12 women who were identified as potential aborters on the basis of a low serum hCG, but whether the pregnancies went to term or ended in abortion serum progesterone values remained within the normal range.

(b) Toxaemia of pregnancy and foetal death

Johansson (1969b) and Luisi et al. (1971) reported low progesterone levels in each of two patients with intrauterine foetal death due to toxaemia. However, Tulchinsky and Okada (1975) found levels below normal in only two of 11 patients with pre-eclampsia which led to intrauterine death. Even after death of the foetus the plasma progesterone levels remained unchanged in seven of the patients. Christensen et al. (1974) found no changes in the progesterone concentration in either mild or severe pre-eclampsia although the levels of the other hormones were reduced. Lindberg et al. (1974) and Dawood (1976) also found levels to be normal in most cases of intrauterine foetal death. Normal progesterone values in pregnancies with an anencephalic foetus have been reported by Tulchinsky and Okada (1975) and Dawood (1976). There was no consistent change in the serum progesterone levels in nine patients with severe hypertensive disorders of pregnancy (Dawood, 1976) or in pregnant women with essential hypertension (Christensen et al., 1974).

(c) Rh-isoimmunisation

Tulchinsky, Hobel, Yeager and Marshall (1972b) suggested that the progesterone : oestriol ratio was of use in predicting foetal well-being in patients with Rh-isoimmunisation disease. Lindberg et al. (1974) found values within the normal range in cases of Rh-immunisation except in severely affected groups when the values tended to increase.

(d) Diabetic pregnancy

An increased incidence of complications occurs during pregnancies of diabetic women with an increased perinatal mortality. Lin et al. (1972) detected no significant difference in the plasma progesterone concentrations, the metabolic clearance rates and production rates in the third trimester of pregnancy in 10 women with an abnormal intravenous glucose tolerance curve and seven insulin-dependent diabetics compared with 30 normal pregnant women.

(e) Hydatidiform mole and choriocarcinoma

The serum progesterone concentration in 26 women with intact molar pregnancies without theca lutein cysts ranged from 18–289 ng/ml (57–919 nmol/l) with a mean value of 65·9 ng/ml (210 nmol/l), whereas in 16 subjects with cysts the range of values was similar (34–288 ng/ml; 108–916 nmol/l) but the mean value was significantly higher (134 ng/ml; 426 nmol/l). Low concentrations of progesterone were found after abortion of the moles (Teoh, Das, Dawood and Ratnam, 1972a; Dawood and Med, 1974; Dawood, 1975a; Dawood and Teoh, 1975). In subjects with choriocarcinoma the serum progesterone ranged from 1–61 ng/ml (3–194 nmol/l) with a mean value of 16·9 ng/ml (54 nmol/l), suggesting that progesterone synthesis was not greatly increased in spite of the high hCG secretion (Teoh, Das, Dawood and Ratnam, 1972b). In a subsequent paper (Dawood, 1975b) much higher serum progesterone values were obtained in choriocarcinoma (1·3–183 ng/ml (4·1–582 nmol/l) with a mean value of 36 ng/ml (114 nmol/l)). Values for the concentration of progesterone in molar tissue and in molar vesicle fluid and changes produced after removal of the mole have also been reported (Dawood and Teoh, 1975; Dawood and Das, 1975; Dawood, 1975c).

(f) Ectopic pregnancy

In 17 women with ectopic pregnancies hCG levels were within normal range, but in eight progesterone levels were less than 1 ng/ml (3 nmol/l) and in a further eight they were between 2·3 (7·3) and 6·9 ng/ml (21·9 nmol/l), i.e. within the normal range (Milwidsky et al., 1977).

5. Umbilical Cord Blood

More recent measurements of the progesterone concentration in umbilical venous and arterial plasma confirm the values recorded by van der Molen and Aakvaag (1967). The values reported since (Table 2) show that the foetus is exposed to very high levels of progesterone, particularly since the concentration of unbound progesterone in cord blood is higher than that in maternal peripheral blood.

Levels in the arterial blood are much lower than those in the venous blood, suggesting that the foetus is active in the metabolism of progesterone. Effer, Gupta and Younglai (1973) calculated that only about 44% of progesterone returned unchanged from the foetus to the placenta. Tulchinsky and Okada (1975) suggest that the secretion rate of progesterone into the foetal circulation is about 23 mg/day (73 µmol/day) but Dawood and Helmkamp (1977) found a much higher value (84 mg/day; 267 µmol/day). Runnebaum and Zander (1962) showed that levels of progesterone and its metabolites (20α-dihydro-, 20β-dihydro- and 17α-hydroxy-progesterone) were inversely related in

Table 2

Concentration of progesterone (M. ± S.E.) in umbilical artery and vein
(1 ng/ml = 3·18 nmol/l).

Umbilical artery (ng/ml)	Umbilical vein (ng/ml)	References
436 ± 58	724 ± 42	Harbert et al. (1964)
339	496	Craft et al. (1969)
536 ± 55	966 ± 88	Scommegna et al. (1972)
378 ± 54	677 ± 94	Effer et al. (1973)
390 ± 1600	960 ± 2320	Hagemenas and Kittinger (1973)
134 ± 5	767 ± 73	Dawood (1974)
318 ± 39	440 ± 69	Tulchinsky and Okada (1975)
260 ± 20	340 ± 20	Arai and Yanaihara (1977)
520 ± 38	1295 ± 73	Dawood and Helmkamp (1977)
425 ± 48	718 ± 75	Male foetus ⎫ Antonipillai and
372 ± 46	620 ± 74	Female foetus ⎭ Murphy (1977)

umbilical arterial and venous blood. The foetus is probably also able to hydroxylate progesterone at C-6 (James, Fotherby and Klopper, 1972).

Hagemenas and Kittinger (1973) found that whereas the concentrations of progesterone in the umbilical venous blood of male and female foetuses were not significantly different, the arterio-venous difference was significantly greater in female than in male foetuses. This difference was not, however, confirmed by Tulchinsky and Okada (1975) who studied 13 male and 15 female foetuses, by Dawood and Helmkamp (1977) or by Warne, Faiman, Reyes and Winter (1977). Tulchinsky and Okada (1975) found no change in the umbilical venous and arterial levels when the mothers were treated with 150 mg (414 μmol) cortisol or with ACTH. There was no correlation of the levels with the weight of the foetus, method of delivery, Apgar score or duration of labour (Dawood and Helmkamp, 1977). In contrast with progesterone the concentration of pregnenolone sulphate (Scommegna et al., 1972) was higher in the umbilical artery (1700 ± 265 ng/ml; 4·3 ± 0·7 μmol/l) than in the umbilical vein (1240 ± 177 ng/ml; 3·1 ± 0·4 μmol/l).

6. Amniotic Fluid

Zander and von Munstermann (1956) measured progesterone in amniotic fluid from the second month to the end of pregnancy and found a mean value of 140 ng/ml (445 nmol/l) with a range from 10–500 ng/ml (32–1590 nmol/l). Low concentrations (59–75 ng/ml; 188–238 nmol/l) were detected by Harbert, McGaughey, Scoggin and Thorton (1964) in amniotic fluid obtained at delivery and similar values were found in late pregnancy by Schindler and Siiteri (1968). Lower values were obtained by competitive binding (Younglai, Effer and Pelletier, 1971) and by radioimmunoassay (Warne *et al.*, 1977).

Johansson and Jonasson (1971) showed the levels in amniotic fluid early in pregnancy were higher than in plasma but that as pregnancy advances the concentration decreases (Fig. 7). There was a correlation ($r = 0.5$) between amniotic fluid progesterone concentration and placental weight. The low concentration of progesterone in amniotic fluid and its decrease with advancing pregnancy, when increasing amounts of progesterone were being transferred to the foetus, suggests that urinary excretion by the foetus is not a major metabolic pathway.

Jonasson and Johansson (1971) extended their studies to include samples from women with pregnancies complicated by Rh-immunisation or cholestasis of pregnancy. There was no difference from values observed in

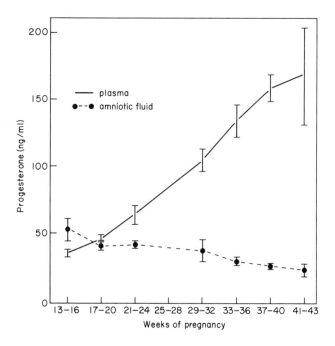

Fig. 7. Levels (M. ± S.E.) of progesterone (1 nmol/l = ng/ml × 318) in plasma and amniotic fluid during pregnancy (from Johansson and Jonasson, 1971).

normal pregnancies except for a significant increase at 37 weeks of pregnancy in amniotic fluid concentration of progesterone in pregnancies with severe foetal erythroblastosis or with cholestasis. The authors conclude that the estimation of amniotic fluid progesterone has little value in the evaluation of foetal well-being in pregnancies complicated by Rh-disease.

Koren et al. (1976) measured progesterone in amniotic fluid from 11 women undergoing induced abortion by intra-amniotic administration of prostaglandin-$PGF_{2\alpha}$ in the mid-trimester of pregnancy. In plasma the progesterone concentrations declined from a value of about 48 ng/ml (153 nmol/l) at the beginning of the infusion to about 30 ng/ml (95 nmol/l) 3 hr later with no further decrease to 12 hr, whereas in amniotic fluid the progesterone concentration increased from a mean value of about 50 ng/ml (159 nmol/l) at the beginning of the infusion to more than 200 ng/ml (636 nmol/l) 12 hr later.

E. PROGESTERONE IN BLOOD OF CHILDREN

Harbert et al. (1964) found measurable amounts of progesterone in blood from neonates for up to 24 hr after expulsion of the placenta. In premature and full-term infants progesterone levels ranged from 4–34 (M. 15) ng/ml (13–108 (M. 48) nmol/l) at 12 hr of life, decreasing to 2–6 (M. 3) ng/ml (6–19 (M. 10) nmol/l) at 24 hr, and these low concentrations persisted for the next two to three days (Conly et al., 1970). In infants aged from 2–11 months Tea et al. (1975) found a mean value of 0·2 ng/ml (0·6 nmol/l) (range 0·1–0·4 ng/ml; 0·3–1·3 nmol/l) and in pre-pubertal children aged from 2–12 years, the mean value (0·25 ng/ml; 0·79 nmol/l) was not significantly different. Widholm, Kantero, Axelson, Johansson and Wide (1974) studied 148 healthy female subjects ranging from a bone age of eight years up to young adults from whom samples were obtained between days seven and 10 of the menstrual cycle. Before menarché plasma levels of progesterone were often undetectable and did not exceed 0·2 ng/ml (0·6 nmol/l). Similar low values also occurred during the second year of menstruation but after the second post-menarchal year and after stage four of puberty, mean values increased markedly.

Strott et al. (1969) found plasma progesterone levels ranging from 2–11 ng/ml (6–35 nmol/l) in two children with congenital adrenal hyperplasia. Blood production rates were 3·3 (10·5) and 6·5 mg/day (20·7 μmol/day) in these two children and metabolic clearance rates were 1590 and 1090 l/day. In a more detailed study plasma progesterone levels in a control group of children were 0·17–0·68 ng/ml (0·54–2·2 nmol/l), whereas in children with the 21-hydroxylase deficiency there was a marked increase with a range of

1·4–17·5 ng/ml (4·5–5·6 nmol/l) (Janne, Perheentupa, Viinikka and Wihko, 1975).

F. PROGESTERONE IN BLOOD OF MAN

Levels of plasma progesterone in men less than 50 years of age ranged from 0·08–0·37 (м. 0·18) ng/ml (0·25–1·18 (м. 0·57) nmol/l) and were not significantly different from those of men more than 50 years of age (Vermeulen and Verdonck, 1976). Most of the progesterone in blood of males appeared to arise from the adrenal cortex since progesterone levels were markedly increased after administration of ACTH and markedly decreased after administration of dexamethasone. Bermudez and Lipsett (1972) also reported that levels of progesterone in men could be increased by administration of ACTH. Administration of hCG significantly increased plasma levels of testosterone and androstenedione but not those of progesterone and levels of progesterone in eight orchidectomised males were not significantly different from those of intact males.

However, Scholler, Nahoul, Grenier, Charles and Netter (1975) showed that progesterone was a secretory product of the testes and more recently Hammond, Ruokonen, Kontturi, Koskela and Vihko (1977) found the concentration of progesterone in human spermatic venous blood to be 1·5–33·2 (м. 10·2) ng/ml (4·8–105 (м. 32·4) nmol/l) compared with a mean level of 0·3 ng/ml (1·0 nmol/l) in peripheral venous blood. Strott, Yoshimi and Lipsett (1969) found the levels of progesterone in men to range from 0·1–0·4 (м. 0·2) ng/ml (0·3–1·3 (м. 0·6) nmol/l). They calculated that the blood production rate was about 0·3 mg/day (1·0 μmol/day) and the metabolic clearance rate about 2000 l/day.

Using radioimmunoassay, Tea et al. (1975) reported the range of plasma levels of progesterone in men to be from 0·5–1·2 (м. 0·27) ng/ml (0·2–3·8 (м. 0·86) nmol/l) and Thorneycroft and Stone (1972) found 0·15–0·28 (м. 0·19) ng/ml (0·48–0·89 (м. 0·60) nmol/l). The mean values for males obtained by both groups of investigators agree with those reported by others using gas-chromatography, double isotope dilution, competitive protein binding or radioimmunoassay. Gutai, Meyer, Kowarski and Migeon (1976) collected blood continuously over 24 hr from five normal males and obtained a mean value (±s.d.) of 0·25 ± 0·05 ng/ml (0·79 ± 0·16 nmol/l).

5α-Pregnane 3,20-dione is also present in male blood in similar concentrations to that of progesterone (Milevich et al., 1975).

REFERENCES

Abraham, G. E. and Chakmakjian, Z. H. (1973). *J. clin. Endocr. Metab.* **37**, 581.

Abraham, G. E., Maroulis, G. B. and Marshall, J. R. (1974). *Obstet. Gynec.* **44**, 522.

Abraham, G. E., Odell, W. D., Swerdloff, R. S. and Hopper, K. (1972). *J. clin. Endocr. Metab.* **34**, 312.

Abraham, G. E., Swerdloff, R., Tulchinsky, D. and Odell, W. D. (1971). *J. clin. Endocr. Metab.* **32**, 619.

Aedo, A. R., Landgren, B. M., Cekan, Z. and Diczfalusy, E. (1976). *Acta endocr., Copenh.* **82**, 600.

Akande, E. O. (1975). *Am. J. Obstet. Gynec.* **122**, 887.

Aksel, S. and Jones, G. S. (1974). *Am. J. Obstet. Gynec.* **118**, 466.

Aksel, S., Wiebe, R. H., Tyson, J. E. and Jones, G. S. (1976). *Obstet. Gynec.* **48**, 598.

Ances, I. G., Hisley, J. C. and Haskins, A. L. (1971). *Am. J. Obstet. Gynec.* **109**, 36.

Anderson, L. L., Bland, K. P. and Melampy, R. M. (1969). *Rec. Prog. Horm. Res.* **25**, 57.

Antonipillai, I. and Murphy, B. E. P. (1977). *J. Obstet. Gynec. Br. Commonw.* **84**, 179.

Askalani, H., Smuk, M., Sugar, J., Delvoye, P., Robyn, C. and Schwers, J. (1974a). *Am. J. Obstet. Gynec.* **118**, 1054.

Askalani, H., Wilkin, P. and Schwers, J. (1974b). *Am. J. Obstet. Gynec.* **118**, 1064.

Arai, K. and Yanaihara, T. (1977). *Am. J. Obstet. Gynec.* **127**, 879.

Aufrere, M. B. and Benson, H. (1976). *J. pharm. Sci.* **65**, 783.

Backstrom, T., Carstensen, H. and Sodergard, R. (1976). *J. ster. Biochem.* **7**, 469.

Backstrom, T., Wide, L., Sodergard, R. and Carstensen, H. (1976). *J. ster. Biochem.* **7**, 473.

Baird, D. T. (1972). *In* "Hormones in Reproduction" (C. R. Austin and R. V. Short, eds), Vol. 3, p. 1. Cambridge University Press, Cambridge.

Batra, S. and Bengtsson, L. P. (1978). *J. clin. Endocr. Metab.* **46**, 622.

Batra, S., Bengtsson, L. P., Grundsell, H. and Sjoberg, N.-O. (1976). *J. clin. Endocr. Metab.* **42**, 1041.

Batra, S., Grundsell, H. and Sjoberg, N.-O. (1977). *Contraception,* **16**, 217.

Bauminger, S., Lindner, H. R. and Weinstein, A. (1973). *Steroids,* **21**, 847.

Bayard, F., Louvet, J. P., Monrozies, M., Boulard, A. and Pontonnier, G. (1975). *J. clin. Endocr. Metab.* **41**, 412.

Bengtsson, L. P. (1973). *In* "Endocrine Factors in Labour" (A. Klopper and J. Gardner, eds), Vol. 20, p. 37. Mem. Soc. Endocrinol., Cambridge University Press, Cambridge.

Bengtsson, L. P. and Ejarque, P. M. (1964). *Acta obstet. gynec. scand.* **43**, 49.

Beling, C. G., Stewart, L. M. and Markham, S. M. (1970). *J. clin. Endocr. Metab.* **30**, 30.

Bermudez, J. A. and Lipsett, M. B. (1972). *J. clin. Endocr. Metab.* **34**, 241.

Billiar, R. B., Jassani, M. and Little, B. (1975a). *Am. J. Obstet. Gynec.* **121**, 877.

Billiar, R. B., Little, B., Kline, I., Reier, P., Takaoka, Y. and White, R. J. (1975b). *Brain Res.* **94**, 99.

Black, W. P., Martin, B. T. and Whyte, W. G. (1972). *J. Obstet. Gynaec. Br. Commonw.* **79**, 363.

Blye, R. P. (1973). *Am. J. Obstet. Gynec.* **116**, 1044.

484 K. FOTHERBY

Board, J. A., Bhatnager, A. S. and Bush, C. W. (1973). *Fert. Steril.* **24**, 95.

Bodley, F. H., Chapdelaine, A., Flickinger, G., Mikhail, G., Yauerbaum, S. and Roberts, K. D. (1973). *Steroids*, **21**, 1.

Boroditsky, R. S., Reyes, F. I., Winter, J. S. D. and Faiman, C. (1975). *Am. J. Obstet. Gynec.* **121**, 238.

Brenner, P. F. and Mishell, D. R. (1975). *Obstet. Gynec.* **46**, 456.

Burger, H. G., Catt, K. J. and Brown, J. B. (1968). *J. clin. Endocr. Metab.* **28**, 1508.

Cantor, B., Jewelewicz, R., Warren, M., Dyrenfurth, I., Patner, A. and Van de Wiele, R. L. (1972). *Am. J. Obstet. Gynec.* **113**, 607.

Cargille, C. M., Ross, G. T. and Yoshimi, T. (1969). *J. clin. Endocr. Metab.* **29**, 12.

Christensen, A., Froyshov, D. and Fylling, P. (1974). *Acta endocr., Copenh.* **76**, 201.

Coats, P., Walker, E., Youssefnejadian, E. and Craft, I. L. (1977). *Acta obstet. gynec. scand.* **56**, 453.

Cooke, I. D. (1976). *In* "Hormone Assays and their Clinical Application" (J. A. Loraine and E. T. Bell, eds), 4th edition, p. 447. Churchill, Livingstone, Edinburgh.

Cooke, I. D., Morgan, C. A. and Parry, T. E. (1972). *J. Obstet. Gynaec. Br. Commonw.* **79**, 647.

Corker, C. S., Michie, E., Hobson, B. and Parboosingh, J. (1976). *J. Obstet. Gynaec. Br. Commonw.* **83**, 489.

Corker, C. S., Naftolin, F. and Exley, D. (1969). *Nature, Lond.* **222**, 1063.

Conly, P. W., Morrison, T., Sandberg, D. H. and Cleveland, W. W. (1970). *Pediat. Res.* **4**, 76.

Conly, P. W., Spellacy, W. M. and Cleveland, W. W. (1972). *Clin. Res.* **20**, 94.

Cousins, L. M., Hobel, C. J., Chang, R. J., Okada, D. M. and Marshall, J. R. (1977). *Am. J. Obstet. Gynec.* **127**, 612.

Craft, I., Carriere, E. and Youssefnejadian, E. (1974). *Obstet. Gynec.* **44**, 135.

Craft, I., Wyman, H. and Sommerville, I. F. (1969). *J. Obstet. Gynaec. Br. Commonw.* **76**, 1080.

Crisp, T. M., Dessouky, D. A. and Denys, F. R. (1973). *Am. J. Obstet. Gynec.* **115**, 901.

Csapo, A. I. (1961). *In* "Progesterone and the Defense Mechanism of Pregnancy", Ciba Foundation Study Group No. 9 (G. E. W. Wolstenholme and H. P. Cameron, eds), p. 3. J. and A. Churchill, London.

Csapo, A. I. (1969). *In* "The Regulatory Effect of Progesterone on the Myometrium", Ciba Foundation Study Group No. 34. J. and A. Churchill, London.

Csapo, A. I., Knobil, E., Pulkkinen, M., van der Molen, H. J., Sommerville, I. F. and Wiest, W. G. (1969). *Am. J. Obstet. Gynec.* **105**, 1132.

Csapo, A. I., Knobil, E., van der Molen, H. J. and Wiest, W. G. (1971). *Am. J. Obstet. Gynec.* **110**, 630.

Csapo, A. I., Pohanka, O. and Kaihola, H. L. (1974). *Br. med. J.* **1**, 137.

Csapo, A. I., Sauvage, J. P. and Wiest, W. G. (1970). *Am. J. Obstet. Gynec.* **108**, 950.

Csapo, A. I. and Wood, C. (1968). *In* "Recent Advances in Endocrinology" (V. H. T. James, ed.), Ch. 7, p. 207. J. and A. Churchill, London.

Dawood, M. Y. (1975a). *Acta endocr., Copenh.* **79**, 729.

Dawood, M. Y. (1975b). *Am. J. Obstet. Gynec.* **123**, 762.

Dawood, M. Y. (1975c). *Obstet. Gynec.* **45**, 531.

Dawood, M. Y. (1976). *Am. J. Obstet. Gynec.* **125**, 832.

Dawood, M. Y. and Das, N. P. (1975). *Obstet. Gynec.* **45**, 171.

Dawood, M. Y. and Helmkamp, F. (1977). *Obstet. Gynec.* **50**, 450.

Dawood, M. Y. and Med, M. (1974). *Am. J. Obstet. Gynec.* **119**, 911.

Dawood, M. Y. and Teoh, E. S. (1975). *Obstet. Gynec.* **45**, 9.

Demetriou, J. A. and Austin, F. G. (1971). *Clin. chim. Acta*, **33**, 21.

Dhont, M., Vandekerckhove, D. and Vermeulen, A. (1974). *J. clin. Endocr. Metab.* **39**, 465.

Dignam, W. J., Parlow, A. E. and Daane, T. A. (1969). *Am. J. Obstet. Gynec.* **104**, 679.

Dodson, K. S., Coutts, J. R. T. and Macnaughton, M. C. (1975). *J. Obstet. Gynaec. Br. Commonw.* **82**, 602.

Doyle, L. L., Barclay, D. L., Duncan, G. W. and Kirton, K. T. (1971). *Am. J. Obstet. Gynec.* **110**, 92.

Dupon, C., Hosseinian, A. and Kim, M. H. (1973). *Steroids,* **22**, 47.

Edwards, R. G., Steptoe, P. C., Abraham, G. E., Walters, E., Purdy, J. M. and Fotherby, K. (1972). *Lancet,* **ii**, 611.

Effer, S. B., Gupta, K. and Younglai, E. V. (1973). *Am. J. Obstet. Gynec.* **116**, 643.

Faiman, C. and Ryan, R. J. (1967). *J. clin. Endocr. Metab.* **27**, 1711.

Feng, L.-J., Rodbard, D., Rebar, R. and Ross, G. T. (1977). *J. clin. Endocr. Metab.* **45**, 775.

Florensa, E. and Sommerville, I. F. (1973). *Steroids,* **22**, 451.

Florensa, E., Sommerville, I. F., Harrison, R. F., Johnson, M. W. and Youssefne-jadian, E. (1976). *J. ster. Biochem.* **7**, 769.

Fogel, M., Rubin, B. L. and Ossowski, R. (1972). *Am. J. Obstet. Gynec.* **112**, 629.

Fotherby, K. (1971). *Biblphy Reprod.* **17**, 589 and 703.

Fotherby, K. (1975). *In* "Biochemistry of Steroid Hormones" (H. L. J. Makin, ed.), p. 249. Blackwell Scientific Publications, Oxford.

Fotherby, K. (1977). *In* "Regulation of Human Fertility" WHO Symposium Moscow (E. Diczfalusy, ed.), p. 283. Scriptor, Copenhagen.

Fotherby, K. and Brown, J. B. (1964). *J. Endocr.* **29**, 55.

Friedrich, F., Breitenecker, G., Salzer, H. and Holzner, J. H. (1974). *Acta endocr.,* Copenh. **76**, 343.

Fuchs, F. (1972). *In* "Endocrine Factors in Labour" (A. Klopper and J. Gardner, eds), Vol. 20, p. 1. Mem. Soc. Endocrinol. Cambridge University Press, Cambridge.

Fukunishi, H., Mickan, H. and Zander, J. (1975). *Acta endocr., Copenh.* **79**, 111.

Furr, B. J. A. (1973). *Acta endocr., Copenh.* **72**, 89.

Furuyama, S. and Nugent, C. A. (1971). *Steroids,* **17**, 663.

Fylling, P. (1970a). *Acta endocr., Copenh.* **65**, 273.

Fylling, P. (1970b). *Acta endocr., Copenh.* **65**, 284.

Fylling, P. (1972). *Acta endocr., Copenh.* **69**, 602.

Fylling, P. (1973). *Acta endocr., Copenh.* **72**, 569.

Fylling, P. and Norman, N. (1970). *Acta endocr., Copenh.* **65**, 293.

Garzon, P., Aznar, R., Olivera, E. and Gallegos, A. J. (1977). *Contraception,* **16**, 79.

Gibor, Y., Pandya, G. N., Bieniarz, J. and Scommegna, A. (1971). *Am. J. Obstet. Gynec.* **109**, 542.

Gore, B. Z., Caldwell, B. V. and Speroff, L. (1973). *J. clin. Endocr. Metab.* **36**, 615.

Grundsell, H., Nilsson, I. and Nordqvist, S. (1973). *Lancet,* **i**, 888.

Guerrero, R., Aso, T., Brenner, P. F., Cekan, Z., Landgren, B. M., Hagenfeldt, K. and Diczfalusy, E. (1976). *Acta endocr., Copenh.* **81**, 133.

Guerrero, R., Landgren, B.-M., Montiel, R., Cekan, Z. and Diczfalusy, E. (1975). *Contraception,* **11**, 169.

Guraya, S. S. (1972). *Acta endocr., Copenh.* **69**, 107.

Gutai, J. P., Meyer, W. J., Kowarski, A. A. and Migeon, C. J. (1976). *J. clin. Endocr. Metab.* **43**, 116.

Hagemenas, F. C. and Kittinger, G. W. (1973). *J. clin. Endocr. Metab.* **36**, 389.

Hagenfeldt, K. and Landgren, B.-M. (1975). *J. ster. Biochem.* **6**, 895.

Hagerman, D. D. and Williams, K. L. (1969). *Am. J. Obstet. Gynec.* **104**, 114.

Hammond, G. L., Ruokonen, A., Kontturi, M., Koskela, E. and Vihko, R. (1977b). *J. clin. Endocr. Metab.* **45**, 16.

Hammond, G. L., Viinikka, L. and Vihko, R. (1977a). *Clin. Chem.* **23**, 1250.

Hanson, F. W., Powell, J. E. and Stevens, V. C. (1971). *J. clin. Endocr. Metab.* **32**, 211.

Haning, R. V., Barrett, D. A., Alberino, S. P., Lynskey, M. T., Donabedian, R. and Speroff, L. (1978). *Am. J. Obstet. Gynec.* **130**, 204.

Harbert, G. M., McGaughey, H. S., Scoggin, W. A. and Thorton, W. N. (1964). *Obstet. Gynec.* **23**, 413.

Haspels, A. A. (1976). *Contraception,* **14**, 375.

Hellig, H., Gattereau, D., Lefebvre, Y. and Bolte, E. (1970). *J. clin. Endocr. Metab.* **30**, 624.

Hoffmann, W., Forbes, T. R. and Westphal, U. (1969). *Endocrinology,* **85**, 778.

Holmdahl, T. H. and Johansson, E. D. B. (1972a). *Acta endocr., Copenh.* **71**, 743.

Holmdahl, T. H. and Johansson, E. D. B. (1972b). *Acta endocr., Copenh.* **71**, 765.

Holmdahl, T. H., Johansson, E. D. B. and Wide, L. (1971). *Acta endocr., Copenh.* **67**, 353.

Hooker, C. W. and Forbes, T. R. (1949). *Endocrinology,* **44**, 61.

Israel, R., Mishell, D. R., Stone, S. C., Thorneycroft, I. H. and Moyer, D. L. (1972). *Am. J. Obstet. Gynec.* **112**, 1043.

James, F., Fotherby, K. and Klopper, A. (1972). *Clin. Endocr.* **1**, 73.

James, F., Fotherby, K. and MacNaughton, M. C. (1969). *Endokrinologie,* **55**, 34.

Janne, O., Perheentupa, J., Viinikka, L. and Vihko, R. (1975). *Clin. Endocr.* **4**, 39.

Johansson, E. D. B. (1969a). *Acta endocr., Copenh.* **61**, 592.

Johansson, E. D. B. (1969b). *Acta endocr., Copenh.* **61**, 607.

Johansson, E. D. B. (1971). *Acta endocr., Copenh.* **68**, 779.

Johansson, E. D. B. (1973). *Acta obstet. gynec. scand.* **52**, 37.

Johansson, E. D. B. and Gemzell, C. (1971). *Acta endocr., Copenh.* **68**, 551.

Johansson, E. D. B. and Jonasson, L.-E. (1971). *Acta obstet. gynec. scand.* **50**, 339.

Johansson, E. D. B., Wide, L. and Gemzell, C. (1971). *Acta endocr., Copenh.* **68**, 502.

Jonasson, L.-E. and Johansson, E. D. B. (1971). *Acta obstet. gynec. scand.* **50**, 345.

Jones, C. D. and Mason, N. R. (1974). *Steroids,* **23**, 323.

Jones, G. S. (1976). *Fert. Steril.* **27**, 351.

Jones, G. S. and Wentz, A. C. (1972). *Obstet. Gynec.* **44**, 26.

de Jong, F. H., Baird, D. T. and van der Molen, H. J. (1974). *Acta endocr. Copenh.* **77**, 575.

Jovanovic, L., Dawood, M. Y., Landesman, R. and Saxena, B. B. (1978). *Am. J. Obstet. Gynec.* **130**, 274.

Junkmann, K. (1968). *In* "The Gestagens" Handbook of Experimental Pharmacology (K. Junkmann, ed.), Vol. XXII/I. Springer-Verlag, Berlin and New York.

Kaiser, R. and Geiger, W. (1971). *Acta endocr., Copenh.* **67**, 331.

Karow, W. G. and Gentry, W. C. (1976). *Obstet. Gynec.* **48**, 603.

Kim, M. H., Hosseinian, A. H. and Dupon, C. (1974). *J. clin. Endocr. Metab.* **39**, 706.

Klaiber, E. L., Henzl, M. R., Lloyd, C. W. and Segre, E. J. (1973). *J. clin. Endocr. Metab.* **36**, 142.

Kletzky, O. A., Nakamura, R. M., Thorneycroft, I. H. and Mishell, D. R. (1975). *Am. J. Obstet. Gynec.* **121**, 688.

Klopper, A. (1969). *In* "Foetus and Placenta" (A. Klopper and E. Diczfalusy, eds), p. 471. Blackwell Scientific Publications, Oxford.

Klopper, A. and Gardner, J. (1972). *In* "Endocrine Factors in Labour", Mem. Soc. Endocrinol., Vol. 20. Cambridge University Press, Cambridge.

Klopper, A. and Shaaban, M. M. (1974). *Obstet. Gynec.* **44**, 187.

Koren, Z., Schulman, H., Lev-Gur, M., Gatz, M., Thysen, B. and Bloch, E. (1976). *Obstet. Gynec.* **48**, 472.

Korenman, S. G. and Sherman, B. M. (1973). *J. clin. Endocr. Metab.* **36**, 1205.

Kunz, J. and Keller, P. J. (1976). *J. Obstet. Gynaec. Br. Commonw.* **83**, 640.

Laborde, N., Carril, M., Cheviakoff, S., Croxatto, H. D., Pedroza, E. and Rosner, J. M. (1976). *J. clin. Endocr. Metab.* **43**, 1157.

Landgren, B.-M., Aedo, A.-R., Nunez, M., Cekan, S. Z. and Diczfalusy, E. (1977). *Acta endocr., Copenh.* **84**, 620.

Lee, P. A., Xenakis, T., Winer, J. and Matsenbaugh, S. (1976). *J. clin. Endocr. Metab.* **43**, 775.

Lehmann, F., Just-Nastansky, I., Behrendt, B., Czygan, P.-J. and Bettendorf, G. (1975). *Acta endocr., Copenh.* **79**, 329.

LeMaire, W. J., Conly, P. W., Moffett, A. and Cleveland, W. W. (1970). *Am. J. Obstet. Gynec.* **108**, 132.

LeMaire, W. J., Conly, P. W., Moffett, A., Spellacy, W. N., Cleveland, W. W. and Savard, K. (1971). *Am. J. Obstet. Gynec.* **110**, 612.

LeMaire, W. J., Rice, B. F. and Savard, K. (1968). *J. clin. Endocr. Metab.* **28**, 1249.

Leyendecker, G., Wardlaw, S. and Nocke, W. (1972). *Acta endocr., Copenh.* **71**, 160.

Lindner, H. R., Perel, E., Friedlander, A. and Zeitlin, A. (1972). *Steroids,* **19**, 357.

Liggins, G. C., Forester, C. S., Grieves, S. A. and Schwartz, A. L. (1977). *Biol. Reprod.* **16**, 39.

Lin, T. J., Lin, S. C., Erlenmeyer, F., Kline, I. T., Underwood, R., Billiear, R. B. and Little, B. (1972). *J. clin. Endocr. Metab.* **34**, 287.

Lindberg, B. S., Nilsson, B. A. and Johansson, E. D. B. (1974). *Acta obstet. gynec. scand.* **53**, 329.

Little, B., Billiar, R. B., Bougas, J. and Tait, J. F. (1973). *J. clin. Endocr. Metab.* **36**, 1222.

Little, B., Billiar, R. B., Halla, M., Heinsons, A., Jassani, M., Kline, I. T. and Purdy, R. H. (1971). *Am. J. Obstet. Gynec.* **111**, 505.

Little, B., Billiar, R. B., Rahman, S. S., Johnson, W. A., Takaoka, Y. and White, R. J. (1975). *Am. J. Obstet. Gynec.* **123**, 527.

Llauro, J. L., Runnebaum, B. and Zander, J. (1968). *Am. J. Obstet. Gynec.* **101**, 867.

Lloyd, C. W., Lobotsky, J., Baird, D. T., McCracken, J. A., Weisz, J., Pupkin, M., Zanartu, J. and Puga, J. (1971). *J. clin. Endocr. Metab.* **32**, 155.

Lomax, C. W., May, H. V., Panko, W. B. and Thornton, W. N. (1977). *Obstet. Gynec.* **50**, 39s.

Lundy, L. E., Lee, S. G., Levy, W., Woodruff, J. D., Wu, C.-H. and Abdalla, M. (1974). *Obstet. Gynec.* **44**, 14.

Luisi, M., Levanti, S. and Franchi, F. (1971). *Fert. Steril.* **22**, 435.

MacNaughton, M. C. (1976). *In* "Plasma Hormone Assay in Evaluation of Fetal Well Being" (A. Klopper, ed.), Ch. 3. Churchill, Livingstone, Edinburgh.

Martin, B. T., Cooke, B. A. and Black, W. P. (1970). *J. Endocr.* **46**, 369.

Mickan, H. (1976). *Steroids,* **27**, 65.

Midgley, A. R. and Jaffe, R. B. (1968). *J. clin. Endocr. Metab.* **28**, 1699.

Mikhail, G. (1967). *Clin. Obstet. Gynec.* **10**, 29.

Mikhail, G. (1970). *Gynec. Invest.* **1**, 5.

Mikhail, G. and Allen, W. M. (1967). *Am. J. Obstet. Gynec.* **99**, 308.

Milewich, L., Gomez-Sanchez, C., Crowley, G., Porter, J. C., Madden, J. D. and MacDonald, P. C. (1977). *J. clin. Endocr. Metab.* **45**, 617.

Milewich, L., Gomez-Sanchez, C., Madden, J. D. and MacDonald, P. C. (1975). *Gynec. Invest.* **6**, 291.

Milwidsky, A., Adoni, A., Segal, S. and Palti, Z. (1977). *Obstet. Gynec.* **50**, 145.

Mishell, D. R., Thorneycroft, I. H., Nagata, Y., Murata, T. and Nakamura, R. M. (1973). *Am. J. Obstet. Gynec.* **117**, 631.

Mishell, D. R., Nakamura, R. M., Crosignani, P. G., Stone, S., Kharma, K., Nagata, Y. and Thorneycroft, I. H. (1971). *Am. J. Obstet. Gynec.* **111**, 60.

Moghissi, K. S., Syner, F. N. and Evans, T. N. (1972). *Am. J. Obstet. Gynec.* **114**, 405.

van der Molen, H. J. and Aakvaag, A. (1967). *In* "Hormones in Blood" (C. H. Gray and A. L. Bacharach, eds), Vol. 2, p. 221, 2nd edition. Academic Press, London and New York.

Morgan, C. A. and Cooke, I. D. (1972). *J. Endocr.* **54**, 445.

Mukherjee, T. K., Wright, S. W., Davidson, N. J. H. and Fotherby, K. (1972). *J. Obstet. Gynaec. Br. Commonw.* **79**, 175.

Nadji, P., Reyniak, J. V., Sedlis, A., Szarowski, D. H. and Bartosik, D. (1975). *Obstet. Gynec.* **45**, 193.

Neill, J. D., Johansson, E. D. B., Datta, J. K. and Knobil, E. (1967). *J. clin. Endocr. Metab.* **27**, 1167.

Newton, J., Joyce, D., Pearce, B., Revell, C. and Tyler, J. (1971). *J. Reprod. Fert.* **27**, 481.

Nilsson, I. (1972). *Acta obstet. gynec. scand.* **51**, 117.

Niswender, G. D. (1973). *Steroids,* **22**, 413.

Nygren, K.-G. and Johansson, E. D. B. (1975). *Acta obstet. gynec. scand.* **54**, 54.

Nygren, K.-G., Johansson, E. D. B. and Wide, L. (1973). *Am. J. Obstet. Gynec.* **116**, 916.

Okada, D. M., Tulchinsky, D., Ross, J. W. and Hobel, C. J. (1974). *Am. J. Obstet. Gynec.* **119**, 502.

Okamura, H., Aso, T., Yoshida, Y. and Mishimura, T. (1974). *Obstet. Gynec.* **44**, 127.

Osborn, R. H., Goplerud, C. P. and Yannone, M. E. (1968). *Am. J. Obstet. Gynec.* **101**, 1073.

Parker, C. R., Ellergood, J. O. and Mahesh, V. B. (1975). *J. ster. Biochem.* **6**, 1.

Pauerstein, C. J., Eddy, C. A., Croxatto, H. D., Hess, R., Siler-Khedr, T. M. and Croxatto, H. B. (1978). *Am. J. Obstet. Gynec.* **130**, 876.

Pearlman, W. H. (1957). *Biochem. J.* **67**, 1.

Pharriss, B. B., Tillson, S. A. and Erikson, R. R. (1972). *Rec. Prog. Horm. Res.* **28**, 51.

Pichon, M.-F. and Milgrom, E. (1973). *Steroids,* **21**, 335.

Pokoly, T. B. and Jordan, V. C. (1975). *Obstet. Gynec.* **46**, 577.

Pollow, K., Lubbert, H., Boquoi, E. and Pollow, B. (1975). *J. clin. Endocr. Metab.* **41**, 729.

Powell, J. E. and Stevens, V. C. (1973). *Clin. Chem.* **19**, 210.

Pulkkinen, M. O., Liukko, P., Rauramo, L. and Willman, K. (1974). *Acta obstet. gynec. scand.* **53**, 287.

Radwanska, E., Hughesdon, P. E. and Swyer, G. I. M. (1976a). *Mat. Med. Pol.* **1**, 1.

Radwanska, E., McGarrigle, H. H. G. and Swyer, G. I. M. (1976b). *Acta eur. fertil.* **7**, 39.

Raud, H. R., Balsdon, J. J. and Collins, J. A. (1972). *Am. J. Obstet. Gynec.* **113**, 887.

Reeves, B. D. and Diczfalusy, E. (1971). *Am. J. Obstet. Gynec.* **109**, 775.

Reeves, B. D., de Souza, M. L. A., Thompson, I. E. and Diczfalusy, E. (1970). *Acta endocr., Copenh.* **63**, 225.

Reyes, F. I., Winter, J. S. D. and Faiman, C. (1977). *Am. J. Obstet. Gynec.* **129**, 557.

Rosenfeld, D. L. and Garcia, C.-R. (1976). *Fert. Steril.* **27**, 1256.
Rosenthal, H. E., Slaunwhite, W. R. and Sandberg, A. A. (1969). *J. clin. Endocr. Metab.* **29**, 352.
Ross, G. T., Cargille, C. M., Lipsett, M. B., Rayford, P. L., Marshall, J. R., Strott, C. A. and Rodbard, D. (1970). *Rec. Prog. Horm. Res.* **26**, 1.
Runnebaum, B., Heep, J., Geiger, W., Vecsei, P. and Andor, J. (1976). *Acta endocr., Copenh.* **81**, 243.
Runnebaum, B., Holzmann, K., Bierwirth-v. Munstermann, A.-M. and Zander, J. (1972b). *Acta endocr., Copenh.* **69**, 739.
Runnebaum, B., Rieben, W., Munstermann, A.-M. and Zander, J. (1972a). *Acta endocr., Copenh.* **69**, 731.
Runnebaum, B. and Zander, J. (1971). *Acta endocr., Copenh.* (Suppl. 150), 5.
Runnebaum, B. and Zander, J. (1962). *Klin. Wschr.* **40**, 453.
Ruttner, B. (1969). *Am. J. Obstet. Gynec.* **105**, 547.
Ryan, K. J. (1971). *Am. J. Obstet. Gynec.* **109**, 299.
Ryan, K. J. and Petro, Z. (1966). *J. clin. Endocr. Metab.* **26**, 46.
Sanyal, M. K., Berger, M. J., Thompson, I. E., Taymor, M. L. and Horne, H. W. (1974). *J. clin. Endocr. Metab.* **38**, 828.
Saxena, B. N., Dusitsin, N., Poshyachinda, V. and Smith, I. (1974). *J. Obstet. Gynaec. Br. Commonw.* **81**, 113.
Scarisbrick, J. and Cameron, E. H. D. (1975). *J. ster. Biochem.* **6**, 51.
Schindler, A. E. and Siiteri, P. K. (1968). *J. clin. Endocr. Metab.* **28**, 1189.
Scholler, R., Nahoul, K., Grenier, J., Charles, J. F. and Netter, A. (1975). *Ann. Endocr.* **36**, 353.
Scholler, R., Tea, N. T. and Castanier, M. (1973). In "Le Corps Jaune" (R. Denamur and A. Netter, eds), p. 95. Masson et Cie, Paris.
Scommegna, A., Burd, L., Bieniarz, J. (1972). *Am. J. Obstet. Gynec.* **113**, 60.
Shaaban, M. M. and Klopper, A. (1973). *J. Obstet. Gynaec. Br. Commonw.* **80**, 210.
Shaw, R. W., Butt, W. R. and London, D. R. (1975). *Clin. Endocr.* **4**, 543.
Shepard, M. K. and Senturia, Y. D. (1977). *Fert. Steril.* **28**, 541.
Sherman, B. M. and Korenman, S. G. (1974). *J. clin. Endocr. Metab.* **38**, 89.
Sherman, B. M. and Korenman, S. G. (1975). *J. clin. Invest.* **55**, 699.
Short, R. V. (1969). In "Foetal Autonomy" (G. E. W. Wolstenholme and M. O'Connor, eds), p. 2. Churchill, London.
Sobota, J. T. and Kirton, K. T. (1970). *Obstet. Gynec.* **35**, 752.
Solomon, S. and Fuchs, F. (1971). In "Endocrinology of Pregnancy" (A. Klopper and F. Fuchs, eds), Ch. 4, p. 66. Harper and Row, New York and London.
Solomon, S., Watanabe, M., Dominguez, O. V., Gray, M. J., Meeker, C. I. and Sims, E. A. H. (1964). Int. Cong. Series, No. 51, 267. Excerpta Medica, Amsterdam.
Somerville, B. W. (1971). *Am. J. Obstet. Gynec.* **111**, 419.
Spellacy, W. N., Conly, P. W., Cleveland, W. W. and Buhi, W. C. (1975). *Am. J. Obstet. Gynec.* **122**, 278.
Speroff, L. and van de Wiele, R. L. (1971). *Am. J. Obstet. Gynec.* **109**, 234.
Spieler, J. M., Webb, R. L., Saldarini, R. J., Coppola, J. A. (1972). *Steroids,* **19**, 751.
Steele, S. J. and Robertson, D. M. (1972). *Obstet. Gynec.* **40**, 152.
Stoa, K. F. and Bessesen, A. (1975). *J. ster. Biochem.* **6**, 21.
Stone, S., Nakamura, P. M., Mishell, D. R. and Thorneycroft, I. H. (1971). *Steroids,* **17**, 411.
Strott, C. A., Cargille, C. M., Ross, G. T. and Lipsett, M. B. (1970). *J. clin. Endocr. Metab.* **30**, 246.

Strott, C. A., Yoshimi, T. and Lipsett, M. B. (1969). *J. clin. Invest.* **48**, 930.

Strott, C. A., Yoshimi, T., Ross, G. T. and Lipsett, M. B. (1969). *J. clin. Endocr. Metab.* **29**, 1157.

Swain, M. C. (1972). *Clin. chim. Acta,* **39**, 455.

Sweat, M. L. and Bryson, M. J. (1970). *Am. J. Obstet. Gynec.* **106**, 193.

Symonds, E. M., Fahmy, D., Morgan, C., Roberts, G., Gomershall, C. R. and Turnbull, A. C. (1972). *J. Obstet. Gynaec. Br. Commonw.* **79**, 976.

Tambyraja, R. L., Anderson, A. B. M. and Turnbull, A. C. (1974). *Br. med. J.* **4**, 67.

Tausk, M. (1971). "International Encyclopedia of Pharmacology and Therapeutics", Sect. 48. Pergamon Press, New York and London.

Taymor, M. L., Berger, M. J., Thompson, I. E. and Karam, K. S. (1972). *Am. J. Obstet. Gynec.* **114**, 445.

Tea, N. T., Castanier, M., Roger, M. and Scholler, R. (1975). *J. ster. Biochem.* **6**, 1509.

Teoh, E. S., Das, N. P., Dawood, M. Y. and Ratnam, S. S. (1972a). *Acta endocr., Copenh.* **70**, 791.

Teoh, E. S., Das, N. P., Dawood, M. Y. and Ratnam, S. S. (1972b). *Acta endocr., Copenh.* **71**, 773.

Teoh, E. S., Dawood, M. Y., Ratnam, S. S., Ambrose, A. and Das, N. P. (1973). *Aust. N.Z. J. Obstet. Gynec.* **13**, 198.

Thijssen, J. H. H. and Zander, J. (1966). *Acta endocr., Copenh.* **51**, 563.

Thorneycroft, I. H., Mishell, D. R., Stone, S. C., Kharma, K. M., Nakamura, R. M. (1971). *Am. J. Obstet. Gynec.* **111**, 947.

Thorneycroft, I. H., Scribyatta, B., Tom, W. K., Nakamura, R. M. and Mishell, D. R. (1974). *J. clin. Endocr. Metab.* **39**, 754.

Thorneycroft, I. H. and Stone, S. C. (1972). *Contraception,* **5**, 129.

Tulchinsky, D. and Hobel, C. J. (1973). *Am. J. Obstet. Gynec.* **117**, 884.

Tulchinsky, D., Hobel, C. J., Yeager, E. and Marshall, J. R. (1972a). *Am. J. Obstet. Gynec.* **113**, 766.

Tulchinsky, D., Hobel, C. J., Yeager, E. and Marshall, J. R. (1972b). *Am. J. Obstet. Gynec.* **112**, 1095.

Tulchinsky, D. and Okada, D. M. (1975). *Am. J. Obstet. Gynec.* **121**, 293.

Turnbull, A. C. and Anderson, A. B. M. (1978). *In* "Scientific Basis of Obstetrics and Gynaecology" (R. R. McDonald, ed.), p. 79, 2nd edition. Churchill, Livingstone, London.

Turnbull, A. C., Flint, A. P. F., Jeremy, J. Y., Patten, P. T., Keirse, M. J. N. C. and Anderson, A. B. M. (1974). *Lancet,* **i**, 101.

Vermeulen, A. and Verdonck, L. (1976). *J. ster. Biochem.* **7**, 1.

de Villa, G. O., Roberts, K., Wiest, W. G., Mikhail, G. and Flickinger, G. (1972). *J. clin. Endocr. Metab.* **35**, 458.

Wajchenberg, B. L., Sugawara, S. H., Mesquita, C. H., Lerario, A. C., Wachslicht, H., Pieroni, R. R. and Mattar, E. (1976). *Clin. chim. Acta,* **68**, 67.

Warne, G. L., Faiman, C., Reyes, F. I. and Winter, J. D. (1977). *J. clin. Endocr. Metab.* **44**, 934.

Warren, R. J. and Fotherby, K. (1975). *J. ster. Biochem.* **6**, 1151.

Weiss, G. and Rifkin, I. (1975). *Obstet. Gynec.* **46**, 557.

West, C. D., Mahajan, D. K., Chavre, V. J., Nabors, C. J. and Tyler, F. H. (1973). *J. clin. Endocr. Metab.* **36**, 1230.

Westphal, U. and Forbes, T. R. (1963). *Endocrinology,* **73**, 504.

Westphal, C. D., Mahajan, D. K., Chavre, V. J., Nabors, C. J. and Tyler, F. H. (1973). *J. clin. Endocr. Metab.* **36**, 1230.

Westphal, U., Stroupe, S. D. and Cheng, S.-L. (1977). *Ann. N.Y. Acad. Sci.* **286**, 10.

Widholm, O., Kantero, R.-L., Axelson, E., Johansson, E. D. B. and Wide, L. (1974). *Acta obstet. gynec. scand.* **53**, 197.

Wu, C.-H., Prazak, L., Flickinger, G. L. and Mikhail, G. (1974). *J. clin. Endocr. Metab.* **39**, 536.

van de Wiele, R. L., Bogumil, F., Dyrenfurth, I., Ferin, M., Jewelewicz, F., Warren, M., Rizkallah, T. and Mikhail, G. (1970). *Rec. Prog. Horm. Res.* **26**, 63.

Wiener, M. and Allen, S. H. G. (1967). *Steroids,* **9**, 567.

Winkel, P., Gaede, P. and Lyngbye, J. (1976). *Clin. Chem.* **22**, 422.

Wright, S. W., Fotherby, K. and Fairweather, F. (1970). *J. Obstet. Gynaec. Br. Commonw.* **77**, 65.

Yannone, M. E., McCurdy, J. R. and Goldfien, A. (1968). *Am. J. Obstet. Gynec.* **101**, 1058.

Yannone, M. E., Mueller, J. R. and Osborn, R. H. (1969). *Steroids,* **13**, 773.

Yen, S. S. C., Vela, P., Rankin, J. and Littell, A. S. (1970). *J. Am. med. Assoc.* **211**, 1513.

Yip, S. R. and Sung, M. L. (1977). *Fert. Steril.* **28**, 151.

Younglai, E. V., Effer, S. B. and Pelletier, C. (1971). *Am. J. Obstet. Gynec.* **111**, 833.

Younglai, E. V. and Short, R. V. (1970). *J. Endocr.* **47**, 321.

Younglai, E. V., Smith, S. L., Cleghorn, J. M. and Streiner, D. L. (1975). *Clin. Biochem.* **8**, 234.

Yoshimi, T. and Lipsett, M. B. (1968). *Steroids,* **11**, 527.

Yoshimi, T., Strott, C. A., Marshall, J. R. and Lipsett, M. B. (1969). *J. clin. Endocr. Metab.* **29**, 225.

Yussman, M. A. and Taymor, M. L. (1970). *J. clin. Endocr. Metab.* **30**, 396.

Zander, J. and von Munstermann, A. M. (1956). *Klin. Wschr.* **34**, 944.

X. Aldosterone

J. P. COGHLAN, B. A. SCOGGINS and E. M. WINTOUR

R

A. PROPERTIES OF ALDOSTERONE

1. Physico-chemical Properties

The structure of aldosterone, $11\beta,21$-dihydroxy-18-oxo-pregn-4-ene-3,20-dione, is set out in Fig. 1. Aldosterone is unique amongst the corticosteroids secreted by the adrenal gland in that it has an aldehyde grouping on C-18. In solution it exists as a hemi-acetal (Fig. 1.2) (Simpson, Tait, Wettstein, Neher, Von Euw, Schindler and Reichstein, 1954a). Recent studies of molecular configuration have demonstrated only two tautomeric forms in solution, the 11-18 hemi-acetal and the 11-18 hemi-acetal, 18-20 hemi ketal (Genard, Palem-Vliers, Denoel, Van Cauwenberge and Erchaute, 1975).

The aldosterone isolated originally was dextrorotatory, $\alpha D + 152 \cdot 2°$, with a molecular weight of 360·4. The original crystalline hydrated form had a melting point of 108–112° while the value for the anhydrous form was 164° (Simpson et al., 1954b). Because aldosterone contains a Δ^4-3-oxo group it absorbs ultraviolet light ($\gamma_{max} = 240$ mμ, $\Sigma_{mol} = 16,000$).

17-iso-Aldosterone (Fig. 1.3) can be formed from aldosterone under alkaline conditions (Schmidlin, Anner, Billeter, Hensler, Ueberwasser, Wieland and Wettstein, 1957). This isomerisation can occur on storage to a significant extent, particularly if soda glass ampoules are used (Tait and Tait, 1962; Coghlan, Wintour and Scoggins, unpublished observations). Neher and Wettstein (1960) isolated this material from hog adrenals, but recently Flood, Pincus, Tait, Tait and Willoughby (1967) have shown the secretion rate of this isomer to be insignificant in normal subjects and that aldosterone is not significantly converted to the 17-iso isomer in vivo. Before infusion of aldosterone, or its use as an internal indicator, the presence of this isomer must be excluded carefully (Coghlan and Scoggins, 1967; Flood et al., 1967b).

Various combinations of the di- or monoacetate forms of aldosterone and the 11,18-lactone-21-monoacetate (Fig. 1) were used with double labelling procedures based on the use of radioactive acetate (see Section C.1). Other radioactive derivatives have been formed after esterification of the 21-hydroxyl, e.g. pipsyl (p-iodo benzene sulphonate) Bojesen and Degn, 1961), tosyl (toluene sulphonate) (Bojesen and Thuneberg, 1967). Bojesen has also used methylation of the 18 position (Bojesen and Degn, 1961). Reduction of the 20-oxo to the 20-alcohol has been used during purification (Coghlan *et al.*, 1966).

At present the interest in forming derivatives of aldosterone is generally to introduce a chemical grouping to allow coupling to a suitable hapten as a preliminary to raising antibodies against aldosterone for use in radioimmunoassay. Many minor modifications have been made by various authors for forming these special derivatives. The formation of the 21-hemisuccinate and 18,21 di-hemisuccinate has been described by Haning, McCracken, St. Cyr, Underwood, Williams and Abraham (1972). The procedures of Erlanger, Borek, Beiser and Lieberman (1957) have been used to form the 3-oxime and 3-carboxymethyl oxime. One consideration frequently overlooked is that these oxime derivatives are a mixture of syn and anti forms.

The formation of a derivative into which ^{125}I can be introduced before or after derivative formation is an important adjunct to radioimmunoassay. Gomez-Sanchez, Milevid and Holland (1977) have described the use of [^{125}I]-aldosterone-3-(p-hydroxybenzoyl)hydrazone. Aldosterone-3-oxime-^{125}I histamine has been described by Al-Dugaili and Edwards (1978) and Ogihara, Innuma, Nishi, Arakawa, Takagi, Kubata, Miyia and Kunahara (1977) have employed aldosterone-3-oxime coupled to an ^{125}I iodinated phenolic ring.

Although suitable derivatives, e.g. Horning and Mauna (1969) for gas-liquid chromatography have been described, this has not proved to be acceptable for routine assay. High pressure liquid chromatography (de Vries, Popp Snijders, de Kreviet and Ackerman Faber, 1977; Ch. II) is unlikely in the near future to supersede radioimmunoassay (Section C.1).

2. Biological Properties

The role of aldosterone as a salt-retaining steroid is well established. This feature of the biological properties of aldosterone has formed the basis of various bioassays. One of the earliest (Simpson and Tait, 1952) was critical for following the "specific" activity during initial isolation procedures. A method still used in our own laboratory for monitoring and screening experimental procedures is based on changes in the parotid salivary sodium to potassium ratio in the sheep (Blair-West, Coghlan, Denton, Goding, Wintour and Wright, 1963a; Blair-West, Coghlan, Denton, Goding and Wright, 1963b; Blair-West, Coghlan, Denton, Nelson, Wright and Yamauchi, 1969). The action of mineralocorticoids on salivary glands in man and animals has been reviewed by Blair-West, Coghlan, Denton and Wright (1967b).

Several questions were raised at one time as to whether aldosterone had a causal or permissive role in renal conservation of sodium (O'Connor, 1962). Blair-West, Coghlan, Denton, Scott and Wright (1967c) concluded that, in the sheep, renal conservation of sodium during sodium deficiency is

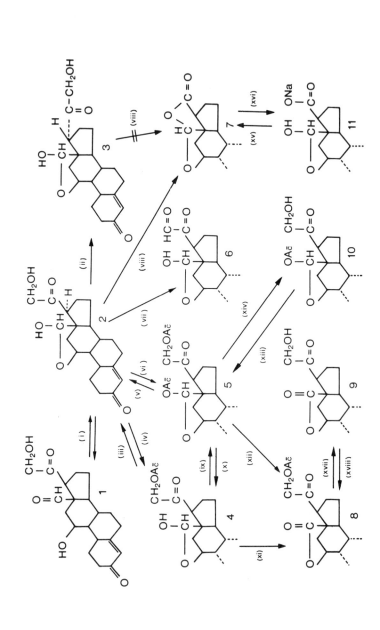

Compound (trivial name)	Reactions		
	Detail		References
1 Aldosterone	(i)	Solution	Simpson et al. (1954a)
2 Aldosterone hemiacetal	(ii)	Alkaline conditions	Schmidlin et al. (1957)
3 17-iso-aldosterone	(iii) (v)	Enzyme hydrolysis	Coghlan et al. (1966)
4 Aldosterone-21-mono-acetate	(iv)	Dilute acetic anhydride	Brodie et al. (1967)
5 Aldosterone-18,21-di-acetate	(vi) (xiii)	Acetic anhydride	Kliman and Peterson (1960)
6 Aldosterone-21-aldehyde(glyoxal)	(vii)	Methanolic cupric acetate	Lewbart and Mattox (1961)
7 Aldosterone-γ-lactone	(viii)	Periodic oxidation	Simpson et al. (1954)
8 Aldosterone-11,18-lactone-21-mono-acetate	(ix)	Acetic anhydride	Brodie et al. (1967)
9 Aldosterone-11,18-lactone	(x)	Dilute acid hydrolysis	Peterson (1964)
10 Aldosterone-18-mono-acetate	(xi) (xii)	Chromic acid oxidation	Kliman and Peterson (1960)
11 Aldosterone-γ-lactone (saponified)	(xiv)	Enzyme hydrolysis	Mattox and Mason (1956)
	(xv) (xvi)	Saponification, relactonisation	Ulick and Vetter (1965)

Fig. 1. Aldosterone and various derivatives which can be formed. These derivatives are oriented toward double isotope methods. The compounds and reactions leading to their formation are tabulated in the accompanying key.

proportional to the effective level of aldosterone. In normal subjects given aldosterone there is eventually "renal escape" (August, Nelson and Thorn, 1958). This may explain the lack of oedema and the rapid excretion of a sodium load in primary aldosteronism (Biglieri and Forsham, 1961). Oedema in secondary hyperaldosteronism may be due to operation of a sensitising factor preventing "escape" (Blair-West et al., 1963b; Urquhart, Davis and Higgins, 1964; Blair-West et al., 1967c).

The phenomenon of increased sensitivity of the target organs of aldosterone may be of importance in clinical situations where excess sodium is retained seemingly without evident cause. The sensitivity does not result from a large increase in receptor affinity or number (Butkus, Coghlan, Paterson, Scoggins, Robinson and Funder, 1976) but an increased response to aldosterone induced by sodium deficiency by a small number of strategically placed cells could not be excluded. Adam and Funder (1977) have also examined the increased renal sensitivity to aldosterone in the rat, induced by a high K diet.

Cox, Platts, Horn, Adams and Miller (1966), using a cumulative dose of 2000 µg/day for 6–8 days in humans, found an increase in total exchangeable sodium but estimated there was no change in exchangeable intracellular sodium. Streeten, Rapoport and Conn (1963) found patients with primary aldosteronism had a normal exchangeable sodium/kg body weight but the presence of a slowly exchangeable pool of body sodium could not be demonstrated after 24 hr. Libel, Schalekamp, Beevers, Brown, Davies, Fraser, Kremer, Lever, Morton, Robertson, Tree and Wilson (1974) have recently shown exchangeable sodium to be elevated in untreated primary aldosteronism. In studies of this type, as in those concerning fluid volume, age–weight matched controls are an essential requirement for any valid comparisons. Because plasma sodium is elevated, it may have been predicted that plasma volume would not be elevated (Tarazi, Dustan, Frohlich, Gifford and Hoffman, 1970).

The 60–90 min delay in electrolyte transfer in aldosterone-responsive tissues does not seem to be due to delay in the steroid reaching the nucleus. Aldosterone induces DNA-dependent RNA and protein synthesis but energy-producing substrate is also required (for review see Sharp and Leaf, 1966).

A vast literature exists on recent studies of aldosterone action. These will be outlined only, as others have reviewed them (Pelletier, Lirdens and Fanestil, 1972; Feldman, Funder and Edelman, 1972; Morris and Davis, 1974; Edelman, 1975). It has been possible to inhibit an aldosterone-induced antinatriuresis without altering the kaliuresis, thus leading to the important implication that steroidal regulation of Na excretion may be independent of the steroidal regulation of K (Lipshitz, Schrier and Edelman, 1973). In the rat, sex differences in physiological response have been demonstrated — there being a significantly larger kaliuretic response in the male (Morris and Davis, 1974).

The nature and role of the aldosterone-induced protein(s) is still a matter of controversy. The debate centres around three propositions: (i) the permease theory—more sodium enters the cell from the mucosal or tubular side, (ii) the energy theory—more ATP is synthesised, and (iii) the pump theory—that the aldosterone-induced protein has a specific action on the Na pump (Na + K activated ATPase). This raises an immediate possible association between aldosterone and the Na pump. Some time ago it was noted that cooling changes intracellular electrolyte composition of red cells and the return to normal composition on warming can be blocked with digitoxin. This digitoxin effect can be overcome by mineralocorticoids (Wilbrandt, 1959). Whilst it does not seem that this particular aspect has received much attention a great deal of effort has focused on the relationship between aldosterone and Na pump. The direct evidence is not persuasive, but ouabain abolished the increase in sodium transport produced by aldosterone (Sharp and Leaf, 1966; Edelman and Fanestil, 1970). Notwithstanding, a most interesting recent paper has implicated phospholipase A and prostaglandins in a crucial role in the action of aldosterone (Yoroi and Bentley, 1978).

There was a suggestion that colonic potential difference may be used as indication of aldosterone concentration in man (Efstratopoulos, Peart and Wilson, 1974). This was disputed by Nicholls, Arcus and Espiner (1975). However, a modification of the original procedure, whereby random fluctuation in potential difference, probably due to the activity of the autonomic nerves, can be corrected, has established that the procedure may be of value as an estimate of *in vivo* mineralocorticoid activity (Skrabal, Auböck, Edwards and Braunsteiner, 1978).

B. BIOCHEMISTRY

1. Biosynthesis

Aldosterone is secreted by the adrenal cortex only, and from data on adrenalectomised humans there would appear to be no other site of synthesis in man (Kowarski, Finkelstein, Loras and Migeon, 1964; Brodie and Tait, 1967; Coghlan and Scoggins, 1967) even during pregnancy (Baulieu, de Vigan, Bricaire and Jayle, 1957; Laidlaw, Cohen and Gornall, 1958). Pasqualini, Wiqvist and Diczfalusy (1966) were able to demonstrate that the adrenals of previable foetuses contained labelled aldosterone after perfusion with [^{3}H]-corticosterone. In earlier similar studies aldosterone was not isolated from the perfusate (Solomon, Bird, Wilson, Wiqvist and Diczfalusy, 1964). Studies in the sheep have established that aldosterone is secreted by the sheep foetal adrenal at the earliest time it is possible to make the measurements (Wintour, Brown, Denton, Hardy, McDougall, Oddie and Whipp,

1975). There is an early report of aldosterone production from an ovarian androblastoma (Ehrlich, Dominguez, Samuels, Lynch, Oberhelman and Warner, 1963), though reversal of the symptoms of hyperaldosteronism also involved removal of one adrenal, said to be microscopically normal. Two other cases support the proposition of extra adrenal aldosterone production (Flanagan and McDonald, 1967; Todesco, Mantero, Terribile, Guarnieri and Borsatti, 1973).

Earliest identifications in adrenal vein blood were by Simpson, Tait and Bush (1952) in the monkey and dog, and by Farrell and Richards (1953) in the dog. It was also shown that aldosterone is specifically elaborated by the zona glomerulosa (Ayres, Gould, Simpson and Tait, 1956; Giroud, Stachenko and Venning, 1956). This so-called functional zonation originally formulated by Swann (1940) has presented difficulties because several important precursors can arise in both zones. Their specific activities in radioactive tracer studies become of little use as indicators of pathways in a single zone. Manual separation of the zones has been used to divide the function of the two zones. In regard to functional zonation in the rat, 18-OH corticosterone and aldosterone are produced by the zona glomerulosa (Giroud et al., 1956; Stachenko and Giroud, 1959; Lucis, Dyrenfurth and Venning, 1961; Sandor and Lanthier, 1963; Sheppard, Mowles, Chart, Renzi and Howie, 1964) and 18-hydroxydeoxycorticosterone despite its 18-oxygen function is produced mainly by the fasciculata and reticularis. 18-OH-DOC, however, would appear to be under the control of ACTH as judged from responses *in vitro* (Birmingham and Kurlents, 1958; Peron, 1961) and *in vivo* (Cortes, Peron and Dorfman, 1963; Williams, Braley and Underwood, 1976). A small amount of 18-OH-DOC is also produced by the zona glomerulosa (Sheppard, Swenson and Mowles, 1963; Lucis, Carballeira and Venning, 1965; Baniukiewicz et al., 1967). Corticosterone has been shown to arise from both zones in the rat and ox (Ayres et al., 1956; Stachenko and Giroud, 1959). Functionally complete separation may only be true for aldosterone and cortisol in those glands capable of producing it. Baniukiewicz et al. (1967) report that small but significant amounts of 18-OH-corticosterone are produced by the fasciculata-reticularis complex in the rat. Marusic and Mulrow (1967) have shown that 18-OH-corticosterone can also be produced by the beef fascicular zone.

These several aspects of functional zonation have in the main been confirmed by recent experience with isolated adrenal cell suspensions for investigating aldosterone secretion (Swallow and Sayers, 1969; Haning, Tait and Tait, 1970; Tait, Tait, Gould and Mee, 1973; Fredland, Saltman and Catt, 1975; Peach and Chiu, 1974). The function of the reticularis zone is not well defined. Hyatt, Bill, Gould, Tait and Tait (1976) in a preliminary publication showed that reticularis cells were capable of producing DOC. The impact of this particular finding upon the current concept concerning the control of mineralocorticoid secretion needs to be urgently explored further.

Figure 2 shows a schematic diagram of adrenal biosynthesis. The accepted route of synthesis to aldosterone is cholesterol, pregnenolone, progesterone, deoxycorticosterone, corticosterone, 18-OH-corticosterone and aldosterone. It is assumed that the conversion to 18-aldehyde can only proceed via the 18-hydroxyl. Obviously many alternative pathways are possible. The precursor materials known to be converted to aldosterone, regardless of yield, are included in Table 1.

Table 1

Precursors converted to aldosterone.

Precursor	References
Acetate	Lommer and Wolff (1966)
Cholesterol	Muller (1966) Kaplan and Bartter (1962) Ayers et al. (1960)
Pregnenolone	Muller (1966)
Progesterone	Muller (1965) Davis et al. (1966) Sandor and Lanthier (1963)
11-OH-Progesterone	Giroud, Stachenko and Piletta (1958) Stachenko and Giroud (1964)
18-OH-Progesterone	Nicolis and Ulick (1965)
Deoxycorticosterone	Muller (1966) Kaplan and Bartter (1962) Stachenko and Giroud (1964)
18-OH-Deoxycorticosterone	Nicolis and Ulick (1965)
11-Dehydro-corticosterone	Stachenko and Giroud (1964)
Corticosterone	Muller (1966) Baniukiewicz et al. (1967) Davis et al. (1966)
18-OH-Corticosterone	Nicolis and Ulick (1965) Pasqualini (1964a) Sandor and Lanthier (1963) Grekin, Dale and Melby (1973)

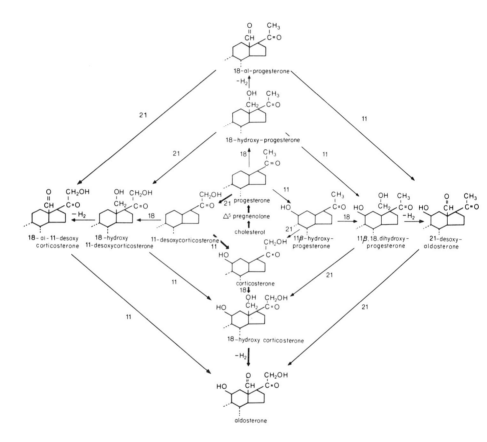

Fig. 2. Schematic representation of the biosynthesis of aldosterone from cholesterol (redrawn from Wettstein, 1961). The accepted pathway is shown by arrows. Many of the compounds are theoretical intermediates only. The numbers associated with arrows indicate the positions at which hydroxylations occur.

Figure 3 is a scheme for aldosterone biosynthesis showing the major sites of action of the known proximate stimuli (from Muller, 1971). Aldosterone biosynthesis has been reviewed by Muller (1971) and Blair-West, Coghlan, Denton and Scoggins (1973). Even now there are several unresolved questions

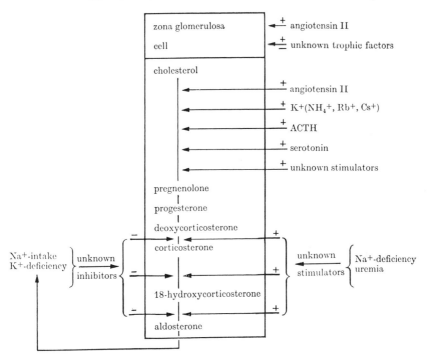

Fig. 3. Scheme of regulation of aldosterone biosynthesis in the rat (Muller, 1971).

concerning aldosterone regulation. This is a composite scheme based on data for several species. Experimental evidence to support the known action at various biosynthetic steps is often based on quite complex studies. The major recognised proximate stimuli at an "early" biosynthetic site. Na deficiency or deprivation seems to act at an "early" and "late" site, thus immediately the question whether or not these stimuli are sufficient alone or together to explain the control of aldosterone biosynthesis. K^+ does have a complex influence over these "late" steps. If Na deficiency cannot be explained by the known facts then the model or the experimental results must be suspect in some way. There are two obvious possibilities. First, most biosynthetic studies using stimuli are completed over a few hours whereas sodium deficient states or chronic sodium deprivation takes days. The design of the experimental protocols thus has limitations of times of exposure. Catt's group have recently completed ingenious studies examining this particular question and would assign to angiotensin II in the rat a trophic action, inducer of angiotensin II receptors and stimulation of aldosterone secretion (Hauger, Aguilera and Catt, 1978; Aguilera, Hauger and Catt, 1978; Aguilera and Catt, 1978). Second, the single path model or concept used by most investigators may not be correct. Figure 2 illustrates the vast number of alternative possibilities. A hypothesis based on an alternative route through 180H DOC could explain some of the difficulties in interpretation, and was proposed by Blair-West, Cain, Catt, Coghlan, Denton, Funder, Scoggins, Stockigt and Wright (1972). This has not been substantiated but difficulties with the availability and purity of 18-hydroxylated steroids until quite recently have hampered studies along that particular line (Coghlan and Blair-West, 1967). Difficulties inherent in the use of these 18-hydroxylated steroids have not been fully appreciated until the recent clarification of many real and potential problems, including the formation of dimers (Roy, Ramirez and Ulick, 1976; Genard et al., 1975; Arazones, Aros, Lantos and Luciano, 1976; Kondo, Mitsuzi and Tori, 1965).

The biosynthetic events leading to increased aldosterone secretion are not fully understood. In the conjectural scheme for the biosynthesis of aldosterone with special emphasis on angiotensin II put together by Blair-West et al. (1972), all the major data which were used to construct this model were from in vivo experiments.

Over the past few years many experiments examining biochemical processes leading to aldosterone production have been concerned with the role of intracellular potassium as a factor common to all stimuli, and the role of cAMP. An exhaustive consideration of these problems is not possible here, but changed intracellular K^+ is clearly not associated with all proximate stimuli and cAMP does not appear to be the second messenger for all stimuli, except that with small numbers of cells in some experiments it may not have been possible to measure relevant changes. Pertinent references are Mendelsohn and Mackie (1975); Tait and Tait (1976); Tait, Tait, Albano, Brown and Mendelsohn (1975).

2. Distribution

There are only a few studies concerned with distribution in the human. If a single injection of $[^3H]$-aldosterone is given into the antecubital vein the disappearance curve indicates that aldosterone is distributed into two apparent anatomical compartments if sampling starts between 8–10 min. Generally, venous blood samples are taken to demonstrate these features. Formally it is important in this type of experiment to be sure that there is no metabolic removal of the steroid in the vascular bed drained by the sampling vein. If this should occur then the compartments would be artificially large. Studies of the whole body distribution of aldosterone were carried out initially by Tait, Tait, Little and Laumus (1961), Tait, Little, Tait and Flood (1962). The earliest sampling time in these studies was 7·5 min after injection. Theoretical aspects of interpretation of disappearance curves have been presented by Tait (1963) and Tait and Burstein (1964). Figure 4 is a typical disappearance curve taken from Tait and Burstein (1964) with the postulated model. The mean initial volume of distribution is 27 l and at zero time 3·7% of the dose remained per litre of plasma (Tait et al., 1961).

During the initial mixing a compartment in rapid equilibrium with blood is established with an apparent volume of 27 l, the inner compartment. The rate of disappearance from plasma is artifactually high, as steroid is leaving the blood and entering the outer compartment as well as being irreversibly metabolised. At the point of inflection, the outer and inner compartments are in equilibrium with respect to specific activity. The rate of disappearance from this point becomes a function of return from the outer compartment and metabolism from the inner. Sampling from the outer compartment is not possible since precise definition of a sampling site cannot be arrived at and it is merely convenient to refer to this dimensionally as a volume. It represents the integrated handling at intracellular sites of concentration, or other localisation not in rapid equilibrium with the plasma. The mean value for this outer compartment expressed as a volume was 14 l. It is more likely that the inner compartment dimensionally is a volume but this cannot be taken for granted. George, Lazarus, Hickie, Freeman and Kinnane (1964) suggested that there was an additional compartment revealed only by earlier sampling. Certainly in sheep where there are two aldosterone compartments the first would be missed by sampling as late as 7·5 min (Scoggins, Coghlan and Blair-West, 1966). In the human, however, there is other evidence set out below to indicate that, except in congestive cardiac failure, the question of a small third compartment is not a serious problem. Cheville, Luetscher, Hancock, Dowdy and Nokes (1966) also commented upon this question. Indeed, Cheville et al. (1966) reported that in congestive heart failure the volume of distribution of the first compartment was reduced from 27 l, quoted above, to the blood volume. The physiological implication suggested was that this smaller initial volume of distribution would render the peripheral blood concentration more labile when secretion rate changed. This might occur for example during postural change which is a potent stimulus to aldosterone secretion. It was difficult for us to accept that in congestive cardiac failure there was a significant alteration in the distribution of aldosterone which was not simply a consequence of the lengthened circulation time in these subjects. This question was re-examined in normal subjects and those with congestive heart failure. Provided samples are taken

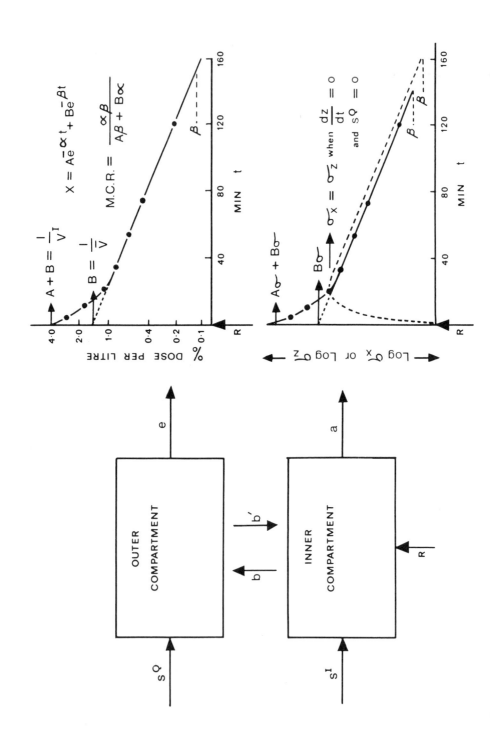

after 1–2 min the disappearance curves are resolvable into three components, the first compartment approximating the blood volume (Coghlan, Scoggins, Stockigt, Meerkin and Hudson, 1971). This third exponential component was discernable in the older studies, e.g. Cheville *et al.*, of patients with congestive cardiac failure because of the increased circulation time and therefore mixing time in this early compartment. These findings are very important in terms of current concepts of how steroid hormones are handled by the body. The significance of the "third" compartment on metabolic clearance rate will be discussed in Section B.3.

Two papers have drawn attention to what appears to be specific ^{3}H aldosterone binding in brain (Anderson and Fanestil, 1976; Ermesch and Rühte, 1978).

In the human, Bojesen (1962, 1964) found that aldosterone was distributed at the same concentration in the plasma and red cells. However, a more recent study (Chavarri, Luetscher, Dowdy and Ganguly, 1977) suggests that the red cell concentration is lower, about 70% at 37°, but is dependent upon the temperature and prevailing cortisol concentration. Aldosterone is distributed equally in red cells and plasma in the sheep and dog (Blair-West *et al.*, 1963a; Davis, Kliman, Yankopoulos and Peterson, 1958). Aldosterone is protein bound in blood both to albumin and transcortin (Meyer, Layne, Tait and Pincus, 1961; Zager, Burlis, Luetscher, Dowdy and Sood, 1976; Pratt, Dale and Melby, 1976; Messerli, Nowaczynski, Honda, Genest and Kuchel, 1976; Zipser, Speckart, Zia, Edmeston, Lau and Horton, 1976).

Fig. 4. The theoretical two-compartmental model suitable for the description of the behaviour and distribution of aldosterone (redrawn from Tait and Burstein, 1964). The upper right-hand panel shows a typical two-compartment disappearance curve. The lower right-hand panel shows the theoretical changes in specific activity within the two compartments. The broken line represents the specific activity of aldosterone in the outer compartment. The following abbreviations have been used: S^I = secretion into the inner compartment, S^Q = secretion into the outer compartment, R = Radioactivity injected into the inner compartment, z = total radioactivity in the outer pool as a fraction of the dose injected, b = rate of transfer of steroid from inner to outer compartment, b' = rate of transfer of steroid from outer to inner compartment, a = rate of metabolism from the inner compartment, e = rate of metabolism from the outer compartment, V^I = distribution in the inner compartment as volume, $\bar{V}$ = volume of distribution obtained by extrapolating the later part of the radioactive disappearance curve to the ordinate, X = concentration of radioactive steroid as a fraction of injected dose per unit volume, σ_x = specific activity of hormone in inner pool, σ_z = specific activity of the hormone in outer pool, α = fractional rate constant describing the disappearance of plasma radioactive concentration, β = fractional rate constant describing the disappearance of plasma radioactive concentration-in fact gradient of later curve, A and B = parameters used in describing the disappearance of radioactivity as aldosterone from the inner compartment.

The binding to transcortin affects the metabolic clearance rate depending on the saturation of transcortin sites with cortisol.

3. Metabolism

There have been very few important papers on metabolism since the last edition of this book, to which the reader is referred for details of earlier extensive studies. Figure 5 (from Pasqualini *et al.*, 1966) shows the major metabolites and their approximate proportions.

C. METHODS OF DETERMINATION IN PERIPHERAL BLOOD AND PLASMA

Most of the information concerning the concentration of aldosterone in blood which is now available has been derived from radioimmunoassay procedures of one type or another. The isotopic methods originally used were all complex, though once established they were time-consuming rather than technically demanding. For some special situations especially where specificity is absolutely crucial, they still have their place.

1. Direct Methods

(a) Radioimmunoassay

Antibodies to aldosterone were first produced in 1964 (Neri, Tolksdorf, Beiser, Erlanger, Agate and Lieberman, 1964). However, the first radioimmunoassays for aldosterone were not described until 1970 (Bayard, Beitins, Kowarski and Migeon, 1970; Mayes, Furuyama, Kem and Nugent, 1970; Wahlen, Tyler and West, 1970). Since that time over 140 papers have reported a variety of methodological approaches to the measurement of aldosterone in plasma and urine.

(*1*) *Preparation of antisera.* Structural modifications of the A ring to produce the 3-oxime (Coghlan and Scoggins, 1967; McKenzie and Clements, 1974), the 3-carboxymethoxime (Erlanger, Borek, Beiser and Lieberman, 1957; Vetter, Armbruster, Tschudi and Vetter, 1974), the 3-carboxymethoxime of 18-21 diacetate (Pham-Huu-Trung and Corvol, 1974) and the 3-hydrazone (Vetter, Freedlender and Haber, 1974), or of the C-21 side chain to produce the 18,21-dihemisuccinate (Haning, McCracken, St. Cyr, Underwood, Williams and Abraham, 1972), the 21-hemisuccinate (Haning *et al.*, 1972), the γ-lactone (Wettstein, 1954) and the 3-carboxymethoxime of the γ-lactone (Farmer, Roup, Pellizzari and Fabre, 1972) have been used to

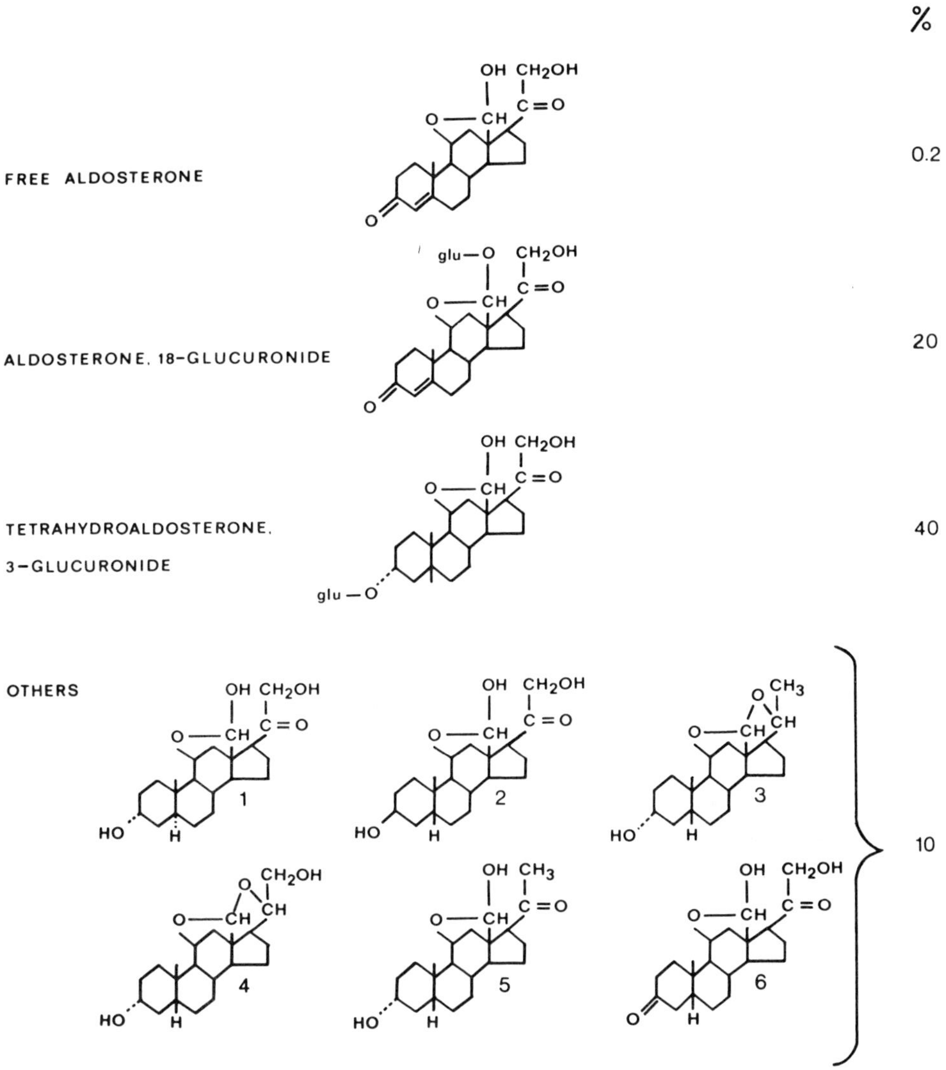

%

FREE ALDOSTERONE

0.2

ALDOSTERONE, 18-GLUCURONIDE

20

TETRAHYDROALDOSTERONE,

3-GLUCURONIDE

40

OTHERS

1

2

3

4

5

6

10

Fig. 5. The most abundant urinary metabolites of aldosterone that have been isolated. The approximate percentages they represent of the daily production are also shown (redrawn from Pasqualini, 1966). 1—3α,11β,21-trihydroxy-5α-pregnan-20-one-18al; 2—3β,11β,21-trihydroxy-5β-pregnan-20-one-18al; 3—3α-hydroxy-5β-pregnane(11β, 18S) (18S, 20α) dioxide; 4—3α,21-dihydroxy-5β-pregnane (11β, 18S) (18S, 20α) dioxide; 5—21-deoxytetrahydroaldosterone; 6—dihydroaldosterone.

enable the steroid to be coupled to an antigenic hapten such as bovine or rabbit serum albumin or bovine gamma globulin.

Methods of coupling the aldosterone derivatives to protein are generally those first described by Erlanger, Borek, Beiser and Lieberman (1957) using isobutylchlorocarbonate. Others (Bayard, Beitins, Kowarski and Migeon, 1970) have used the carbodiimide method (Goodfriend and Levine, 1964) as modified by Gocke, Gerten, Sherwood and Laragh (1969). The molar incorporation ratios are of the order 15–20 mol of aldosterone per mol of bovine serum albumin (Haning et al., 1972; McKenzie and Clements, 1974; Pham-Huu-Trung and Corvol, 1974). Although Vetter, Armbruster, Tschudi and Vetter (1974) failed to show any effect of the hapten-steroid ratio in an experimental study using aldosterone-carbomethoxime, the most specific antisera (Al-Dujaili and Edwards, 1978) have a high molar incorporation ratio. Immunisation programmes producing useful antibodies have been described for sheep (Haning et al., 1972) and rabbits (Vetter and Vetter, 1974; McKenzie and Clements, 1974). The most specific antisera (those permitting assay of aldosterone without purification) have been produced by conjugation of aldosterone-3-oxime to albumin by the carbodiimide reaction (McKenzie and Clements, 1974; Ogihara, Iinuma, Nishi, Arakawa, Tagaki, Kurata, Miyai and Kumahara, 1977; Al-Dujaili and Edwards, 1978)

Evaluation of the specificity related to site of coupling has been examined by Vetter et al. (1974) with rabbit antisera. However, their results showing a less specific antisera using the 3-hydrazone compared with the 3,20 dioxime have not been confirmed by Vetter and Vetter (1974); McKenzie and Clements (1974); Ogihara et al. (1977) and Al-Dujaili and Edwards (1978). An increase in specificity would have been predicted if coupling between steroid and protein is remote from the functional groups of the molecule (Beisér, Erlanger, Agate and Lieberman, 1959).

(2) *Tracer.* 1-2,^{3}H-aldosterone (s.a. 50 Ci/mmol) has been most often used (McKenzie and Clements, 1974) but 1,2,6,7^{3}H-aldosterone (s.a. 90 Ci/mmol) was used by Varsano-Aharon and Ulick (1973). More recently the preparation and use of ^{125}I-aldosterone (s.a. 360–800 Ci/mmol) has been described by Gomez-Sanchez et al. (1977), Ogihara et al. (1977) and Al-Dujaili and Edwards (1978).

(3) *Analytical procedures.* It is not possible to describe in detail all published radioimmunoassays for aldosterone. Seven different types of assay— a classification based primarily on the method of sample purification—have been published. An example of each type together with the relevant details of the procedure are shown on Table 2. The majority of publications have described methods in which purification of the sample before radioimmuno-

assay is essential due to the poor specificity of the antisera and the need to exclude cross-reacting steroids such as cortisol. More recently highly specific antisera have been produced and enabled the direct assay of aldosterone in small volumes of plasma (0·1 ml) with great sensitivity, accuracy and precision (Ogihara *et al.*, 1977; Al-Dujaili and Edwards, 1978). Overall plasma levels determined by radioimmunoassay are similar to those determined by double isotope derivative dilution procedures (Coghlan and Scoggins, 1967; Brodie *et al.*, 1967). Although the immunoassay procedures provide great sensitivity and very rapid assay, rigorous establishment of specificity is difficult to achieve. The requirement to measure assay blanks in plasma from adrenalectomised patients should not be forgotten as has often been the case in published radioimmunoassay procedures.

(b) Isotopic assays

These were dealt with *in extenso* in the previous edition (Coghlan and Blair-West, 1967), although not all the procedures had been published in full at that time. The three most commonly used procedures based on the use of ^3H acetic anhydride were Brodie, Shimiyu, Tait and Tait (1967), Coghlan and Scoggins (1967) and James and Fraser (1966). One modification of the Bojesen and Thuneberg (1967) ^{35}S-*p*-toluene sulphonic anhydride method has been described (Scholer, Riondel and Manning, 1972).

2. Indirect Methods

Target organ responses to aldosterone during both physiological and pathological variations are most directly correlated with peripheral concentration of this hormone. Before the availability of effective methods for measuring the peripheral level the best estimates available were by inference from a knowledge of secretion rate, or even earlier, from a knowledge of renal excretion of the hormone. This approach involves a series of extrapolations which are to some extent overcome by the utilisation of methods which measure the rate of clearance of aldosterone.

These indirect estimates, therefore, fall into three groups, those where the aldosterone concentration can be calculated from other measurements; and those where after estimation of secretion rate, or excretion rate, a relation with peripheral level is assumed. Both these latter methods have had wide usage, particularly for clinical studies. As opposed to the direct estimation in blood, a wide variety of measurements are available for determination of aldosterone or its metabolites from urine (Tait and Tait, 1962; Brodie and Tait, 1967).

Tabl

Summary of seven different types of radioimmunoas
used to measure levels of aldosterone in plasma (1 pg/ml = 2·775 pmo

Type of assay	Paper chromatography purification	Column chromato- graphy purification	TL chromatography purification
References	Mayes *et al.* (1970)	Ito *et al.* (1972)	Kurtz and Bartter, (1976)
Plasma (ml)	1–5	1–2	2–3
[^{3}H]–Aldo	Yes	Yes	Yes
% Recovery	77 ± 5%	57 ± 14%	75%
Extraction	Dichloromethane	Dichloromethane	Dichloromethane
Purification	Paper chromatography Be: MeOH: W	LH 20	TLC Chl: MeOH: W: tB
Antibody	3–Oxime	3–c Methox	18–21 DiSucc
Protein	BSA	BSA	BSA
Species	Rabbit	Rabbit	Sheep (NIH)
Separation (B/f)	$(NH_4)_2 SO_4$	Florisil	$(NH_4)_2 SO_4$
Sensitivity (pg)	20	6	2·6
Intra-assay CV% (n)	6	11	4·4
Interassay CV% (n)	—	—	12·2
Specificity	X-reacting steroids + other chromato- graphy	*cf.* with paper chroma- tography and DIDDA	No details
Blank		<6 pg	20 pg/ml
Normal values			
Recumbent	74 ± 42 (13)	—	89 (45–180) (?)
Upright	132 ± 89 (8)	—	200 (110–400) (?)
Comment	One of first published RIA for aldosterone	—	$(NH_4)_2 SO_4$ partitio free Aldo into toluer scintillant

(a) Calculation of peripheral level

This can be carried out if both the secretion rate based on specific activity of a urinary metabolite and the clearance rate are known.

Peripheral concentration (ng/l) = SR(ng/day)/MCR(l/day).

Some estimates of peripheral concentration have been made in this way, notably by Tait *et al.* (1961), Camargo, Dowdy, Hancock and Luetscher (1965), Hickie and Lazarus (1966) and Kono, Yoshimi and Miyake (1966).

e 2—*continued*

ctone ation	Immunological purification	Direct assay with extraction	Direct assay
nes *et al.* (1976)	Gomez-Sanchez *et al.* (1973)	McKenzie and Clements (1974)	Al-Dujaili and Edwards (1978)
	0·5–2·0	2	0·1
	Yes	No	No
6%	64 ± 12%		
loromethane	Dichloromethane	Dichloromethane	No
γ–lactone	Ab + $(NH_4)_2SO_4$ + dextran charcoal	No	No
Methox	18, 21 DiSucc	3–Oxime	3–Oxime
	BSA	RSA	BSA
o	Sheep (NIH)	Rabbit	Rabbit
ran–charcoal	$(NH_4)_2 SO_4$	Dextran–charcoal	Dextran–charcoal
	4	10	1·0
	12·8	9·2% between dupl.	7·6 (n = 12)
	16·3	6·2	9·3 (n = 15)
uate except DOC	*cf.* with paper chromatography	Excellent	Excellent *cf.* paper chromatography
g/ml	2 pg	0	0
10 (10)	—	—	78 ± 26 (20)
	—	105 ± 59 (10)	170 ± 61 (20)
lactone formation clude competing ds	Uses Ab purification but requires charcoal extraction to lower blank	Standard curve thru assay so no need for intern. recovery	Uses ^{125}I as tracer

Requirements for determination of plasma metabolic clearance rate have been detailed above. Some of these are identical with those for determination of secretion rate by isotope dilution. The determination of secretion rate is detailed in Section C.2.b. In the situation where secretion rate estimations are to be made, it is worth considering whether the isotope should be administered in such a way that clearance rate can be determined. It involves very little more technical work, especially if a continuous infusion is used, and it offers advantages especially if any change in aldosterone degradation is suspected or expected.

(b) *Secretion rate*

The basic assumptions underlining the determination of aldosterone secretion rate have been described fully elsewhere (Coghlan and Blair-West, 1967). Because a secretion rate estimation is the integrated output over a fixed time period it is sometimes more useful than random sampling of peripheral blood concentration. Direct sampling of adrenal vein blood for secretion rate estimation is a common experimental procedure. Various procedures have been introduced so that adrenal vein blood may be obtained in experimental animals (Hume and Nelson, 1954; Weaver and Eik-Nes, 1959). Other procedures suitable for long term access for sampling in conscious sheep have been introduced from this laboratory (McDonald, Goding and Wright, 1958; Blair-West, Coghlan, Denton, Goding, Munro, Wintour and Wright, 1962b; Goding and Wright, 1964). This approach has even been used in the human (Hume, 1962).

(c) *Urinary excretion rate*

This requires only that the urine be collected for a known time. It must be considered as only a rough indicator of peripheral level, and serves chiefly to demonstrate large variations from normal. Generally, the free aldosterone, and the aldosterone released at pH 1 from the 18-glucuronide, are measured together, or the latter alone. Any change in steady state excretory or metabolic pattern will have serious consequences in this determination.

D. PHYSIOLOGICAL VARIATIONS

1. Normal Regulatory Mechanisms

The control of the secretion rate of aldosterone in the several species which have been studied is recognised as being multifactorial (see Table 3). A concensus view can easily be gathered about some issues over which there would be no interspecies variation. For example, increased plasma K is a potent stimulus to aldosterone whilst hypokalaemia is often associated with blunted aldosterone responses and, if severe enough, with very low aldosterone secretion rates.

ACTH is an important vector for episodic increases in aldosterone secretion rate although it may be more potent in man than in other species. Continued stimulation of the adrenal with ACTH leads ultimately to a severe reduction in aldosterone secretion rate even during sodium deficiency (Newton and Laragh, 1968; Scoggins, Coghlan, Denton, Fan, McDougall,

Table 3

Aldosterone normal values (1pg/ml = 2·775 pmol/l).

Na/K intake (mmol)	Posture	Plasma aldosterone (pg/ml)	References
Na 100	Supine	60 ± 27	Best *et al.* (1971)
	Upright	107 ± 27	
Na 10	Supine	179 ± 94	
	Upright	261 ± 109	
Na 150 K80	Supine	98 ± 27	Michelakis and Horton (1970)
Na 10 K80	Supine	241 ± 81	
Na 100	Supine	116 ± 21	Chinn *et al.* (1970)
Na 10	Supine	277 ± 32	
Na 100	Supine	65 ± 10	Oddie *et al.* (1972)
Na 100	Supine	58 ± 6	McCaa *et al.* (1972)
	Upright	229 ± 22	
Na 10	Supine	183 ± 17	
	Upright	371 ± 24	
Na 200	Supine	19 ± 3	
	Upright	37 ± 3	
Na 200 K100	Supine	58 ± 13	Mendelsohn *et al.* (1972)
Na 20 K100	Supine	153 ± 24	
Na 170	Supine	66 ± 18	Mason *et al.* (1977)
Na 15	Supine	180 ± 64	

Oddie and Shulkes, 1974). Once this "refractory stage" is attained the other known proximate stimuli also fail to cause an increase in aldosterone secretion. Studies of our own using morphological indices indicate that at this time there is an enormous reduction in the number of subcapsular cells. This finding would also explain the totally "refractory" behaviour of the zona glomerulosa and the slow return to normal of the response. Thus under a variety of circumstances changes in ACTH or plasma K concentrations can influence the prevailing secretion rate of aldosterone in normal subjects.

In addition it is clearly established that angiotensin II is a potent direct stimulus to increased secretion. Whilst again in a variety of physiological situations angiotensin II may act concurrently with increased plasma K or

ACTH concentration, the major thrust of most of the research in many species has been to analyse the individual roles of those proximate stimuli during sodium restriction or deprivation. The control of sodium economy through aldosterone has of course, a central role in homeostasis. Is the increased aldosterone secretion of sodium restriction of deprivation caused solely by increased angiotensin II concentration? Some controversy has surrounded this debate, species variations being difficult to reconcile. Other unknown factors appear to be more important from quite early studies in sheep and the rat continually has presented interpretative difficulties (Blair-West et al., 1973).

Since it was first shown that the des[1] analogue (heptapeptide) (AIII) of angiotensin II was equipotent in vivo on the zona glomerulosa with regard to aldosterone secretion (Blair-West, Coghlan, Denton, Funder, Scoggins and Wright, 1971) there has been a great preoccupation with the question as to whether AII or AIII is the most important. Studies in many species have utilised the new generation of potent antagonist analogues of AII and AIII or inhibition of converting enzyme. Whilst this is an important question, the role of angiotensin be it AII or AIII in aldosterone regulation has not been resolved in full. In biosynthetic terms their action appears to be the same but related potency may vary from species to species and from in vivo to in vitro and depends on sodium status.

One point needs re-emphasis. In the sheep graded sodium deficiency ranging from 100 mmol to 800 mmol has been used as a stimulus to aldosterone secretion. This has been contrived by progressive loss of parotid saliva. In other species, including man, a sodium restricted diet is generally employed sometimes together with some short term challenge with a diuretic. These various manipulations of sodium balance are not necessarily equatable in physiological terms (Blair-West et al., 1976). Aguilera and Catt (1978) have also commented on this type of dichotomy in their studies in the rat. It is unlikely that sodium restriction does cause a really negative sodium status although the homeostatic mechanisms respond to this challenge and conserve sodium (Ford et al., 1968). A frequent complication is that changes in potassium intake accompany the sodium restriction (see below). However, very early sodium depletion can probably be compared with dietary sodium restriction but moderate to severe deficiency in the sheep probably represents a much greater physiological stimulus than can be contrived in man. In fact this is one of the important reasons that this model system has been used (Blair-West et al., 1963). Indeed, it could be argued that certain features of the control of aldosterone secretion may be best observed when the system is severely stressed.

There is no doubt that in most instances of sodium depletion or restriction if plasma [K] is not increased then angiotensin is a crucial vector. There is common concensus that the kidney is essential for the normal increased secretion rate.

Is the prevailing angiotensin II concentration causal, contributory causal, or permissive? The increasing angiotensin II concentration shows an excellent correlation with increasing aldosterone secretion during the onset of sodium restriction or depletion. Correlation does not, however, establish cause and effect. Studies in sheep have been carried out over 20 years seeking answers to these questions. Recent methodological developments have resulted in a plethora of publications in man and animals but many have recovered old ground.

In sheep, considerations concerning altered sensitivity of the adrenal gland during sodium deficiency were put forward as early as 1962 (Blair-West et al., 1963). Infusion of angiotensin II to moderately sodium deficient sheep did not cause an increase in aldosterone secretion whereas increased sodium deficiency did. That increasing sensitivity of the gland was a likely explanation of this finding was put forward by Blair-West, Coghlan, Denton, Goding, Orchard, Scoggins, Wintour and Wright (1967) and Blair-West, Coghlan, Denton, Scoggins, Wintour and Wright (1970). Likewise progressively increased sensitivity of the zona glomerulosa was a cogent explanation of the normal aldosterone secretion increases during sodium deficiency when the angiotensin II concentration was held in the normal sodium replete range (Blair-West, Coghlan, Cran, Denton, Funder and Scoggins, 1973) or was held outside the normal range by systemic infusion of angiotensin II (Blair-West, Cain, Catt, Coghlan, Denton, Funder, Scoggins, Wintour and Wright, 1970; Coghlan et al., 1971). Since in the experiments cited above the full gamut of response could occur in aldosterone secretion without increase in angiotensin II, a "fourth" factor in aldosterone regulation was proposed and this could be adrenal sensitivity, at least in part. Also, these results indicated that the role of angiotensin II in the increased aldosterone secretion was permissive (Blair-West et al., 1970; Blair-West, Coghlan, Denton, Funder, Oddie and Scoggins, 1973). The role of angiotensin II may appear to be permissive because the sensitivity of the zona glomerulosa is increased to such a great extent that angiotensin II concentration in the normal range can now elicit a maximal response. This maximal response at any point in time seems to be determined by sodium status.

Studies in man have concluded that increased adrenal sensitivity to angiotensin II is a crucial feature of the response to sodium restriction (Oelkers et al., 1974; Hollenberg et al., 1974). Although these papers are frequently cited in support of each other the differences are very substantial. Oelkers et al. (1974) can demonstrate increased sensitivity by log linearisation of their dose response curves: however, the linear regression used by Hollenberg et al. (1974) does not give persuasive results with data from Oelkers et al.

(1974). In the Hollenberg paper aldosterone responses are still found in sodium replete subjects at higher concentrations of angiotensin II in sharp contrast to findings of Oelkers et al., who state: "In sodium repletion the biggest increments in aldosterone were observed at angiotensin infusion rates of 2 vs. 4 ng/kg/min with little or no additional rise in aldosterone at the highest dose (8 ng/kg/min) in any subject". Thus while the same conclusion is drawn the results between the two studies are not easily compatible. Further studies (Oelkers et al., 1975) also report increased sensitivity of the zona glomerulosa to angiotensin II during sodium deficiency. Oelkers et al. (1978) have addressed themselves to two further questions. Will angiotensin II sustain increased aldosterone secretion and is angiotension II a trophic hormone for the adrenal glomerulosa zone. The answer to the question of sustained secretion reported is in the affirmative but the studies are difficult to interpret. This is because the angiotensin II infusion caused sodium retention and dietary restriction was used to control balance. Dietary restriction alone would have increased the aldosterone. A definitive conclusion from these results is therefore compromised. This logical fallacy does have enduring qualities as the earlier results of Ames et al. (1965) were compromised in the same way over the same issue. Because sodium intake has been altered the question of the trophic action is not completely persuasive. As well, a further consideration has been added by the findings of Carey, Vaughan, Peach and Ayers (1978). While in general terms increased adrenal sensitivity to AII has been confirmed, it appears that this increase in sensitivity is more marked for AIII than AII. In anephric man poor responses to angiotensin II have been reported (McCaa et al., 1973) and quoted in support of the trophic action proposition. In another series of anephric patients (Deheneffe et al., 1976) it would appear that the adrenal sensitivity can be implicated. In this series, however, the angiotensin concentrations are reported as near normal and this would support the idea of a permissive trophic action.

In terms of aldosterone control, studies in the rat over several years have resulted in seemingly paradoxical findings compared to other species. In more recent studies in conscious and even trained animals many of the enigmas have been swept away. This has highlighted, if nothing else, the need for the use of conscious, preferably trained animals and patients experienced in the procedures if the physiology of aldosterone is to be really understood. In this regard, the studies of Catt will suffice to illustrate the present position. Angiotensin II does appear to be a crucial vector in increased aldosterone secretion following sodium restriction (Aguilera and Catt, 1978; Aguilera, Hauger and Catt, 1978; Hauger, Aguilera and Catt, 1978). Furthermore, it is claimed that angiotensin II did sustain aldosterone secretion without change in sodium status. The whole issue hangs upon this fact. Angiotensin II does appear to have a trophic role as far as number of receptors are concerned and to fulfil the critical requirements of stimulus of the late biosynthetic pathway. Though Aguilera and Catt (1978) interpreted their studies as illustrating a cause and effect relationship rather than a permissive role, this could only really be concluded from extensive studies where the angiotensin II level was kept constant while the degree of sodium restriction was varied. In all species the increasing sensitivity may be a continuum increasing progressively with increasing sodium deficit until angiotensin II concentration in the normal range will suffice to give a full response. If the change in sensitivity could be induced progressively by serial increases in angiotensin II without changed sodium status this would be cause and effect. This is yet to be proven. Oelkers et al. (1978) found room for other factors in the increased sensitivity. In experiments cited above in the sheep, sensitivity would appear to be more related to the prevailing level of sodium deficit than the prevailing concentration of angiotensin II.

In sodium deficient sheep, when sodium status is restored, the prompt fall in aldosterone secretion can be divorced from a concurrent fall in angiotensin II concentration. This strongly implicates additional factors in aldosterone control (Blair-West et al., 1971; Coghlan et al., 1971; Blair-West et al., 1973). The concept of further factors being involved in "turn off" is strongly supported by the fact that during sodium deficiency, perfusion of the brain ventricles with high sodium CSF reduces aldosterone secretion into the normal range—albeit slowly (Abraham, Blair-West, Coghlan, Denton, Mouw and Scoggins, 1976).

In man there are an increasing number of studies where the nexus between angiotensin and aldosterone can be broken, e.g. during hypoxia, during ascent to higher altitudes, during postural changes, in congestive cardiac failure, in essential hypertension, during fasting, following treatment with β blockers, in inappropriate ADH secretion and in familial dysautonomia (see below).

In summary it may be said that angiotensin II is essential for a normal increase in aldosterone secretion following sodium restriction or deficiency. It has a trophic role in that it induces an increased number of receptors for itself in the zona glomerulosa, thereby contributing to the increased sensitivity of the adrenal in sodium deficiency. It seems highly probable that additional factors are required to fully explain the increased sensitivity during "turn on" of aldosterone secretion. It cannot be said at this time whether reduced sensitivity has a role in "turn off" but aldosterone secretion can certainly be reduced to the normal range independent of a concurrent change in angiotensin II. Again unrecognised factors are implicated. Clinical situations where the correlation between angiotensin and aldosterone is poor without evident change in other recognised stimuli are worthy of further investigation.

2. Renin–Angiotensis System

(a) Angiotensin II

Angiotensin II (AII) is a potent stimulus to aldosterone production in man (see Table 4) (Laragh, Angers, Kelley and Lieberman, 1960; Fraser, James, Brown, Isaac, Lever and Robertson, 1965; Mendelsohn, Johnson, Doyle, Scoggins, Denton and Coghlan, 1972; Speckart, Zia, Zipser and Horton, 1977). It increases aldosterone at physiological concentrations and at rates of infusions which are sub-pressor (Michelakis and Horton, 1970; Mendelsohn *et al.*, 1972; Hollenberg, Chenitz, Adams and Williams, 1974). The effects on plasma aldosterone are rapid (10 min) (Scholer, Birkhauser, Peytremann, Riondel, Vallotton and Muller, 1973) and similar responses are produced by equimolar infusions of either valine 5 or isoleucine 5 AII (Boyd, Adamson, Arnold, James and Peart, 1972; Oelkers, Schoneshofer, Schultze, Brown, Fraser, Morton, Lever and Robertson, 1975). During infusion of AII endogenous levels of renin and angiotensin II are suppressed (Genest, de Chamberlain, Veyrat, Boucher, Tremblay, Strong, Koiw, Marc-Aurele, 1965). At sub-pressor doses aldosterone increases are not associated with change in plasma cortisol but pressor doses may interact with ACTH and produce suppression of cortisol (Rayyis and Horton, 1971).

Although it is clear that AII is involved in producing hypersecretion of aldosterone under a variety of physiological situations, the area of greatest significance has been the role of the peptide in the aldosterone response to Na depletion. This is discussed in detail below.

(b) Angiotensin III

After the demonstration that the 2-8 heptapeptide of angiotensin II (AII), [des-Asparty[1]]–angiotensin II (angiotensin III, AIII) had similar *in vivo* potency to angiotensin II on aldosterone secretion in the sheep (Blair-West, Coghlan, Denton, Funder and Scoggins, 1971) the role of this peptide has been investigated in man (Table 5). Kono, Oseko, Shimpo, Nanno and Endo (1975) showed that equimolar infusions of AII and AIII (20 ng/kg/min) both increased plasma aldosterone from 85 ± 16 to 221 ± 45 pg/ml (236 ± 44 to 613 ± 125 pmol/l) (AII) and from 83 ± 23 to 172 ± 29 pg/ml (230 ± 64 to 477 ± 80 pmol/l) AIII. AIII had only 20% of the pressor activity. Contrary to this report, a more detailed study on two levels of Na intake (Carey, Vaughan, Peach and Ayers, 1978) has shown AIII to have only 15–30% of the effect of AII on aldosterone on a normal Na intake. The dose-response curves were not parallel and the authors postulated the existence of different receptor sites within the adrenal. During Na deprivation

Table 4

The effect of angiotensin II on plasma aldosterone concentration in man.

	Na/K intake (mmol)	Posture	Infusion	BP	Plasma aldosterone (pg/ml)[a]		References
					Basal	Maximum	
Angiotensin II	Na 150 K 80	Supine	2 ng/kg/min	=	78 ± 13	152 ± 61	Michelakis and Horton (1970)
	Na 150 K 80	Supine	9 ng/kg/min	↑	104 ± 35	438 ± 164	
	Na 200 K 100	Supine	100 ng/min	=	58 ± 13	104 ± 21	Mendelsohn et al. (1972)
	Na 20 K 100	Supine	100 ng/min	=	153 ± 24	196 ± 36	
	Ad lib	Supine	10 ng/kg/min	↑	73 ± 30	285 ± 5	Rayyis and Horton (1971)
	Na 10 K 100	Supine	0·1 ng/kg/min	=	150 ± 20	180 ± 30	Williams et al. (1977)
			0·3 ng/kg/min	=	—	180 ± 30	
			1·0 ng/kg/min	=	—	260 ± 40	
			3·0 ng/kg/min		—	400 ± 50	
	Na 200 K 100	Supine	0·1 ng/kg/m	=	70 ± 10	70 ± 10	
			0·3 ng/kg/m	=	—	90 ± 20	
			1·0 ng/kg/m	↑	—	110 ± 20	
			3·0 ng/kg/m	↑	—	190 ± 40	
	Ad lib	Supine	20 ng/kg/min		53 ± 3	118 ± 22	Kono et al. (1977)
	Na 200	Supine	10 ng/kg/min		31 ± 7	122 ± 19	Speckart et al. (1977)
	Na 10	Supine	10 ng/kg/min		153 ± 34	390 ± 43	
	Ad lib	Supine	7 ng/kg/min		75 ±	225 ±	Birkhauser et al. (1973)

[a] 1 pg/ml = 2·775 pmol/l.

Table 5

The effect of angiotensin III and angiotensin analogues on plasma aldosterone concentration in man.

	Na/K intake (mmol)	Posture	Infusion	BP	Plasma aldosterone (pg/ml)[a] Basal	Maximum	References
Angiotensin III	Ad lib	Supine	20 ng/kg/min		46 ± 2	100 ± 10	Kono et al. (1978)
Sar[1], Ala[8]–AII	Ad lib	Supine	1–20µg/kg/min		98 ± 21	165 ± 48	Kono et al. (1978)
	Na 10 K 75	Supine	1–20µg/kg/min		300 ± 61	224 ± 38	
des Asp[1], Ile[8] –AII	Ad lib	Supine	600 ng/kg/min		109 ± 7	114 ± 9	Kono et al. (1977)
	Ad lib	Supine	600 ng/kg/min		49 ± 9	61 ± 12	Kono et al. (1978)
	Ad lib	Supine	600 ng/kg/min		67 ± 9	82 ± 11	

[a] 1 pg/ml = 2·775 pmol/l.

the response to both AII and AIII was increased with a greater increase being observed in the AIII response. The effects on blood pressure were similar to those reported by Kono et al. (1975). A possible role for AIII in the renin–angiotensin system in man has been discussed by Goodfriend and Peach (1975) but clearly more clinical experimentation is required.

3. Sodium Depletion

A reduction in body Na status produced by either dietary Na restriction or by diuretic induced Na excretion is associated with an increase in aldosterone secretion (Luetscher and Axelrad, 1954; Ayres, Barlow, Garrod, Kellie, Tait, Tait and Walker, 1958; Espiner, Tucci, Jagger, Pauk and Lauler, 1967; Ford, Pieters and Bailey, 1968; Bull, Hillman, Cannon and Laragh, 1970), urinary excretion (Liddle, Duncan and Bartter, 1956; Johnson, Lieberman and Mulrow, 1957; Ford et al., 1968) and plasma concentration (Peterson, 1964; Coghlan and Scoggins, 1967; McCaa, McCaa, Reid, Bower and Guyton, 1972; Williams, Cain, Dluhy and Underwood, 1972; Walker, Moore, Horvath and Whelton, 1976). In two indigenous populations (Brazil/Venezuela and New Guinea) it has been possible to measure aldosterone excretion (Oliver, Cohen and Neel, 1975) and blood levels (Macfarlane, Coghlan, Scoggins and Skinner, unpublished observations) in people who have had no access to salt and who eat essentially a high K–low Na vegetarian diet. Aldosterone excretion and blood levels were elevated in these people and established that the hormonal adjustments to life-long low Na intake are similar to those found with acute Na restriction in civilised man. Over a wide range of Na intake a close relationship was found between urinary Na excretion and aldosterone production (Sealey, Buhler, Laragh, Manning and Brunner, 1972). There would appear to be no change in metabolic clearance rate of aldosterone in Na depletion (Ford et al., 1968). Although in diuretic-induced Na depletion a rise in both plasma renin concentration and angiotensin II is always observed (Gocke, Sherwood, Oppenhoff, Gerten and Laragh, 1968; Catt, Cain, Zimmet and Cran, 1969) this is not true for all studies involving dietary Na restriction. It has been shown by our group (Best, Bett, Coghlan, Cran and Scoggins, 1971) that restriction of dietary Na intake to less than 10 mmol/day for five days results in an increase in blood aldosterone concentration without change in arterial or venous angiotensin II levels. These observations were confirmed in a second independent study (Mendelsohn et al., 1972). This latter study used a different angiotensin II radioimmunoassay. It is also of interest to note that the observed increases in plasma renin activity were not paralleled by an increase in angiotensin II. An increase in the angiotensin II clearance rate has been observed in Na restriction and may have offset any increase in production (Johnston, Mendelsohn and Doyle, 1972). In both these studies the change to low salt diet involved an increase in K intake as well as a significant reduction in energy intake; both these factors may have influenced the ultimate outcome (see following sections).

Michelakis and Horton (1970) have also shown a lack of response of plasma renin to a low Na intake with an appropriate rise in aldosterone. However, in the majority of studies both plasma renin activity and concentration are increased (Brown, Davies, Lever, Robertson, 1963).

In contrast to the dissociation between angiotension II and aldosterone in our studies, others have reported a close correlation between the two parameters under similar conditions of experimentation (Brown, Fraser, Lever, Love, Morton and Robertson, 1972; Hollenberg *et al.*, 1974; Walker *et al.*, 1976).

The failure of plasma angiotensin II to rise with Na restriction led us to challenge the primacy of angiotensin II as the physiological stimulus to aldosterone secretion under these conditions. Our conclusions were supported by the studies of Boyd *et al.* (1972) which showed that while both angiotensin II and aldosterone levels were increased by diuretic-induced Na deficiency, the increase in aldosterone was greater in response to Na depletion than that produced by infused angiotensin II at comparable plasma angiotensin II levels. With ACTH, plasma $[Na^+]$ and $[K^+]$ unlikely to be involved, they suggested an additional unknown factor or factors to be necessary for the aldosterone response. This conclusion was supported by the considerable body of evidence in the sheep which suggested that angiotensin II may play a permissive rather than a direct contributory role in the aldosterone response to Na deficiency (Blair-West, Coghlan, Denton, Scoggins and Wright, 1974). Others working on the rabbit (Steele and Lowenstein, 1974) and dog (McCaa, McCaa and Guyton, 1975) have also produced evidence for a role for additional factors in aldosterone control.

The contrary position has been taken by a number of other groups (Brown *et al.*, 1972; Hollenberg *et al.*, 1974; Walker *et al.*, 1976). They propose a primary and regulatory role for angiotensin II in the control of aldosterone under conditions of Na depletion. Apart from the studies correlating angiotensin II levels with those of aldosterone (see above) a number of other investigations in favour of this position have been carried out in both normal and anephric man (see following section).

Although neither Mendelsohn *et al.* (1972) nor Boyd *et al.* (1974) could find evidence for changes in zona glomerulosa sensitivity to angiotensin II in Na depletion, it has been proposed that a significant increase in sensitivity does occur (Oelkers, Brown, Fraser, Lever, Morton and Robertson, 1974; Hollenberg *et al.*, 1974). There was no evidence for a change in angiotensin II clearance rate (Oelkers *et al.*, 1974). The mechanism of this increased responsiveness is unknown but is clearly not entirely dependent on increased levels of angiotensin II since it also occurs in anephric man (Deheneffe, Cuesta, Briggs, Brown, Fraser, Lever, Morton, Robertson and Tree, 1976).

In both the sheep (Blair-West, Coghlan, Denton, Funder and Scoggins, 1972) and dog (McCaa et al., 1975) AII fails to sustain elevated aldosterone secretion beyond 24 hr. This finding has thus been part of the case against a regulatory role for AII in the aldosterone response to Na depletion. The effect of prolonged pressor AII infusions (2–6 ng/kg/min) on plasma aldosterone has been investigated in both Na replete and depleted man and has been shown to sustain elevated levels of aldosterone (Oelkers et al., 1975; Oelkers, Schoneshofer, Schultze, Wenzler, Bauer, L'age and Fehm, 1978). The results of the latter study also confirmed previously published (Oelkers et al., 1974) short term studies showing that Na depletion sensitises the zona glomerulosa to AII. In an earlier study (Ames, Borkowski, Sicinski and Laragh, 1965) high doses of AII also sustained aldosterone secretion but there was no obvious increase in sensitivity in the Na depleted subjects. If this sensitisation does occur it is possible that unchanged levels of AII may be involved in the increased aldosterone of Na depletion.

The other approach used to examine the role of angiotensin in Na deficiency has been to examine the effect of angiotensin antagonists and angiotensin-converting enzyme inhibitor (Table 5).

The effect of the AII analogue saralasin (Sar[1]-Ala[8] AII) on plasma aldosterone levels has been examined in two normal supine individuals on a normal and Na restricted diet (Brown, Brown, Fraser, Lever, Morton, Robertson, Roser and Trust, 1976). After three hours of infusion of up to 10 µg/kg/min saralasin, plasma aldosterone had fallen to the upper limits of the normal range associated with a pronounced increase in AII levels. In a larger series of six subjects Noth, Tan and Mulrow (1977) found no significant fall in plasma aldosterone with saralasin infusions (1–20 µg/kg/min) over 60 min. On a normal Na intake no increase in aldosterone and only a slight rise in AII were observed (Brown et al., 1976). In contrast to this report a significant agonist action of saralasin on plasma aldosterone has been seen at much lower doses (1–3 µg/kg/min) by Hollenberg, Williams, Burger, Ishikawa and Adams (1976) and at infusions rates of 1–20 µg/kg/min (Noth et al., 1977). Similar findings have also been reported for a different analogue (Sar[1], Ile[8]-AII) in man (Yamamoto, Doi, Ogihara, Ichihara, Hatta and Kumahara, 1976). Since these subjects were on a high Na intake it is possible that under conditions of increased adrenal responsiveness such as Na restriction that saralasin will have an even greater agonist action. Thus although in man the analogues will block the aldosterone response to infused AII (Hollenberg et al., 1976; Kono, Oseko, Ikedo, Nanno and Endo, 1977) and AIII (Kono, Ikeda, Oseko, Nanno, Immura and Endo, 1978) its agonist action does not allow it to be used to decide between a permissive and direct contributory role for AII in the response to Na restriction.

An alternative approach has been to lower AII levels by blocking the angiotensin converting enzyme (CEI). The effect of CEI on the plasma aldosterone response to postural change ($\downarrow$ 70° tilt) and Na depletion has been evaluated in normal man (Sancho, Re, Burton, Barger and Haber, 1976). Their study showed that on both high and low Na diets aldosterone failed to respond to the tilt stimulus after CEI. CEI also lowered the supine plasma aldosterone on both levels of Na intake. Na replete levels fell from 211 ± 31 to 145 ± 26 pg/ml (586 ± 86 to 402 ± 72 pmol/l) and Na deplete from 271 ± 33 to 154 ± 18 pg/ml (752 ± 92 to 427 ± 50 pmol/l). Although the conclusions derived by the authors from this study regarding the role of angiotensin in aldosterone control appear straightforward, the Na replete plasma aldosterone concentration (156 ± 55 pg/ml; 433 ± 153 pmol/l) is much higher than that normally found in supine individuals (Coghlan and Scoggins, 1967). The aldosterone response to Na depletion was also poor with considerable intra-individual variation. In another study in normals on a low Na diet although CEI produced a significant fall in plasma aldosterone the mean level did not fall into the Na replete range (Mersey, Williams, Hollenberg and Dluhy, 1977). This study is difficult to interpret because there was only a small fall in AII.

Further evidence supporting a role for mechanisms other than the renin–angiotensin system has been derived from studies involving β-adrenergic blockade (Lowenstein and Steele, 1977). Administration of propranolol before and during Na depletion, despite unchanged or decreased plasma renin activity and AII concentration, produced a significant increase in plasma aldosterone after seven days of Na restriction. The increase in aldosterone was less than that normally seen in response to Na restriction but could not be attributed to changes in plasma [Na], [K] or ACTH. A role for change in adrenal responsiveness to AII can not be excluded. In subjects Na depleted before β-blockade a fall in plasma aldosterone from 157 ± 84 to 72 ± 29 pg/ml (436 ± 233 to 200 ± 80 pmol/l) associated with a parallel fall in plasma renin to control levels has been reported by Plouin, Corvol and Menard (1977).

In summary, dietary Na restriction in man results in an increase in plasma aldosterone. While this is often associated with increases in both plasma renin and AII it would appear that an increase in AII is not essential for the response. It is possible AII plays a permissive role which is amplified by a change in adrenal responsiveness rather than a primary regulatory role. Finally, irrespective of the type of role played by AII, evidence in both man and experimental animals suggests that additional and as yet unidentified factors may be involved.

4. Anephric Man

Over the past ten years there have been numerous clinical studies on aldosterone control in anephric man. It was hoped that study of the aldosterone secretion in the absence of the kidneys would enable the role of angiotensin II in aldosterone control in normal man to be resolved.

In normal man expansion of extracellular fluid volume by oral or intravenous saline suppresses aldosterone production and is usually associated with a decrease in the activity of the renin–angiotensin system. However, changes in plasma aldosterone in response to saline loading (Rossler and Gaiser, 1974) and Na depletion (Dalakos and Streeten, 1975) can be dissociated from volume changes. Studies in anephric man have been carried out in an attempt to clarify the role of the renin–angiotensin system in the response to volume and Na changes. Despite a number of studies the results are rather confused. In an early study, Mitra, Genuth, Berman and Vertes (1972) showed suppression of aldosterone from 178 to 67 pg/ml (494 to 186 pmol/l) with intravenous saline but their patients also changed from upright to supine. Others have examined the effect of volume expansion produced between dialyses and shown increases in plasma aldosterone (Bayard, Cooke, Tiller, Beitins, Kowarski, Walker and Migeon, 1971; Cooke, Ruiz-Maza, Kowarski, Migeon and Walker, 1973; Vetter, Zaruba, Armbruster, Beckerhoff, Reck and Siegenthaler, 1974). However, an increase in plasma [K] is also usually found and may well be responsible for the changes in aldosterone. Various studies in which volume depletion was produced by dialysis resulted in little effect on aldosterone in the majority of investigations (Mitra et al., 1972; Williams, Bailey, Hampers, Lauler, Merrill, Underwood, Blair-West, Coghlan, Denton, Scoggins and Wright, 1973; Weidman, Horton, Maxwell, Franklin and Fichmann, 1973; Birkhauser, Godard, Loirat and Vallotton, 1974; Goodwin, James and Peart, 1974; Deheneffe et al., 1976). The exceptions are those reported by McCaa, McCaa, Reid, Bower and Guyton, 1972; McCaa, Bower and McCaa, 1973; Reid, McCaa, Bower and McCaa, 1973. This group found an increase in aldosterone in response to ultrafiltration and dialysis but noted that with the latter method aldosterone only rose if plasma [Na] fell.

In an attempt to clarify the situation two other studies involving different approaches have been used. In the first, Epstein, Sancho, Perez, Haber, Re and Loutzenhiser (1978) have shown that immersion to the neck for three hours—resulting in central hypervolemia—had no effect on plasma aldosterone. This result is in contrast to that in normals where a fall of 60% was associated with a fall in plasma renin (Epstein, Pins, Sancho and Haber, 1975). The pre-immersion aldosterone levels for the normals was 374 (1038) compared with 70 pg/ml (194 pmol/l) for the anephric patients even though both groups had been equilibrated on a low Na diet. Additional evidence for an important role for the renin-angiotensin system has been provided by Olgaard, Madsen, Ladefoged and Regeur (1977) who found that plasma aldosterone was unchanged after extra cellular fluid volume (ECFV) expansion with 20% mannitol. This was in contrast to non-nephrectomised dialysis patients who exhibited a 35% fall. In both groups plasma [K] increased and cortisol fell. In similar experiments involving expansion of volume with glucose and reduction of K by insulin, Olgaard (1975) found an increase in plasma aldosterone in anephrics and the expected fall in renal failure patients. The results of this last study in anephric patients are in sharp contrast to those of Cooke, Horvath, Moore, Bledsoe and Walker (1973) who found a fall in plasma aldosterone from 144 to 66 pg/ml (400 to 183 pmol/l) associated with a fall in plasma [K] of 1.4 mmol/l on infusion of glucose and insulin.

In summary, the body of evidence would favour a role for the kidney and the renin–angiotensin system in the aldosterone response to changes in volume and Na status. This would be substantially in agreement with numerous studies in experimental animals. The difficulty with a simple interpretation of many of the studies detailed above is the failure to find normal responsiveness of the zona glomerulosa to the known agonists of aldosterone secretion—K, ACTH and angiotensin II.

Basal levels of plasma aldosterone are often low in anephric patients (Bayard et al., 1971; Weidmann et al., 1973; Williams et al., 1973) but have been reported to be within the normal range (McCaa et al., 1971, 1973). The metabolic clearance rate of aldosterone is significantly elevated in anephrics (2700 l/day) compared with normal (1600 l/day) and this will also tend to reduce plasma aldosterone levels (Corvol, Bertagna and Bedrossian, 1974).

The response to ACTH may be absent or blunted (Williams et al., 1973; Weidman et al., 1973; Goodwin et al., 1974; Olgaard and Madsen, 1977), although others have found an increase similar to that observed in normals (Mitra et al., 1972; McCaa, Read, Cowley, Bower, Smith and McCaa, 1973). Also for angiotensin II a variation in effect has been seen. Small but significant increases in plasma aldosterone were seen by Goodwin et al. (1974) and Deheneffe et al. (1976) while others have reported no effect (Weidmann et al., 1973; Williams et al., 1973; McCaa et al., 1973; Woods, McCaa, Bower and McCaa, 1974). It is of interest that Deheneffe et al. (1976) found that dialysis and Na restriction amplified the response to angiotensin II. This suggests that variations in Na status may play a role in modulating adrenal responsiveness in the anephric state as it does in normal man.

The aldosterone response to change in plasma [K] is clear cut in anephric patients and appears to be a major determinant of the secretion rate of the hormone in the absence of the renin–angiotensin system (Bayard *et al.*, 1971; Weidman *et al.*, 1973). Change in posture from supine to upright has also been used as a stimulus and since in normal man a large proportion of the effect on plasma aldosterone is due to increased secretion, which is dependent in part on angiotensin II, a blunted response might be expected in anephric man. This has been observed by Bayard *et al.* (1971), McCaa *et al.* (1973), Williams *et al.* (1973) and Weidmann *et al.* (1973). Only in one study was an increase observed but this was associated with an increase in cortisol (Mitra *et al.*, 1972).

Recent evidence utilising sensitive assays has shown that there are detectable levels of renin and angiotensin II in the anephric patient (Yu, Anderton, Skinner and Best, 1972; Deheneffe *et al.*, 1976). However, these basal levels do not respond to appropriate stimuli.

As in normal man, in the anephric state there are clearly subtle inter-relationships between all the factors involved in aldosterone regulation and the absence of one of these—angiotensin II—modifies zona glomerulosa responsiveness (Goodwin *et al.*, 1974). Changes in K and ACTH may well play a greater role in anephric man. It also appears that greater aldosterone responses are seen in those patients with the higher basal plasma aldosterone levels.

Although heparin has been shown to inhibit aldosterone secretion (Bailey and Ford, 1969) and was thought by Williams *et al.* (1972) to have played a role in their studies, others have shown that the amount of heparin routinely used in haemodialysis does not inhibit aldosterone (Weidmann *et al.*, 1973).

If these low basal levels of angiotensin II in the anephric play a per-missive role in aldosterone biosynthesis as has been proposed from experimental studies in the sheep (Blair-West *et al.*, 1974) then it is apparent that studies in nephrectomised subjects can not exclude such a role for the renin–angiotensin system in the response to volume and/or Na depletion in man. Under these circumstances additional factors may well be involved in aldosterone control as proposed in a number of studies in anephric man (Vetter *et al.*, 1974; Vetter *et al.*, 1975; Vetter, Zaruba, Armbruster, Beckerhoff, Uhlschmid, Furrer and Siegenthaler, 1976), and in studies involving changing Na status in the sheep (Blair-West *et al.*, 1974).

5. Potassium

That potassium loading increases aldosterone excretion was demonstrated by Falbriard, Muller, Neher and Mach (1955) and its effects were shown by Gann, Delea, Gill, Thomas and Bartter (1964) to be independent of changes in Na status. It was also established that while K loading increased aldosterone secretion (Cannon, Ames and Laragh, 1966), K depletion reduced it (Gann *et al.*, 1964; Cannon *et al.*, 1966). It was also shown that a low Na diet would amplify the effect of K loading while K depletion blunted the aldosterone response to Na depletion (Laragh, Cannon and Ames, 1966). Changes in plasma renin activity in response to changes in K status were the opposite to those observed for aldosterone (Brunner, Baer, Sealey, Ledingham and Laragh, 1970).

The plasma aldosterone response to changes in plasma [K] produced by KCl infusion have been examined in detail (Dluhy, Axelrod, Underwood and Williams, 1972; Birkhauser, Gaillard, Riondel, Scholer, Vallotton and Muller, 1973; Himathongkam, Dluhy and Williams, 1975; Hollenberg, Williams, Burger, Hooshmand, 1975; Moore-Ede, Meguid, Fitzpatrick, Boyden and Ball, 1978). Increases of 0·5 to 1·5 nmol/l of plasma [K] raised plasma aldosterone without change in plasma renin activity (Dluhy *et al.*, 1972). Prior dietary K loading produced an amplification of the aldosterone response to a similar change in plasma [K] produced by KCl infusion on both a restricted and a high Na diet (Dluhy *et al.*, 1972). Similarly, the aldosterone response to diuretic-induced Na depletion was increased by a high K intake (Dluhy, Cain and Williams, 1974). Previously, enhancement of the aldosterone response to ACTH had been shown by K loading (Williams *et al.*, 1970). The adrenal and renal vascular responses to infused angiotensin II are also modified by K intake on a high Na intake (Hollenberg *et al.*, 1975).

An important role for small changes in plasma [K] in regulating aldosterone in man was established by Himathongkam *et al.* (1975). Increases as small as 0·1 to 0·5 mmol/l produced by KCl infusion in subjects on a low Na diet were shown to produce significant increments in plasma aldosterone. This same group also examined plasma aldosterone levels following a fall in plasma [K] produced by glucose administration. Falls of 0·3 mmol/l of plasma [K] resulted in falls of aldosterone of up to 46% by 90 min. Subsequently aldosterone levels rose accompanied by an increase in plasma renin activity but without further change in plasma [K]. Similar falls after insulin and glucose have been seen in anephric man (Cooke, Horvath, Moore, Bledsoe and Walker, 1973).

The effect of KCl infusion on the pattern of urinary K excretion and on plasma [K] depends on the time of day (Moore-Ede *et al.*, 1978). However, although a greater increment in plasma [K] is obtained after infusion at midnight compared with midday, the increase in plasma aldosterone is similar.

In summary, changes in body potassium status produced by different levels of dietary K intake and fluctuations in urinary K excretion may produce changes in intracellular and extracellular [K] which plays an important regulatory role in aldosterone control. K also plays an important role in modulating the zona glomerulosa response to other factors known to stimulate aldosterone (ACTH, angiotensin II and Na depletion). Under most conditions the effects of K status on aldosterone are opposite to those on the renin–angiotensin system. The significance of this interaction has been evaluated and discussed by Laragh (1973).

6. Saline Loading

Intravenous infusion of 0·9% sodium chloride results in rapid suppression of aldosterone secretion (Table 6) (Espiner, Tucci, Jagger and Lauler, 1967; Bull, Hillman, Cannon and Laragh, 1970; Espiner, Christlieb, Amsterdam, Jagger, Dobrzinsky, Lauler and Hickler, 1971) and plasma concentrations (Kem, Weinberger, Mayes and Nugent, 1971; Williams, Tuck, Rose, Dluhy and Underwood, 1972; Birkhauser et al., 1973; Tuck, Dluhy and Williams, 1974; Wong, Talamo, Williams and Colman, 1975; Dluhy, Greenfield and Williams, 1977; Luft, Grim, Higgins and Weinberger, 1977). With the exception of two studies (Kem et al., 1971; Birkhauser et al., 1973) all infusions were carried out in subjects on a restricted Na intake. In the study by Bull et al. (1970) saline infusion resulted in a fall of aldosterone secretion even though blood volume was kept below control levels by haemorrhage. In all studies the fall in aldosterone has been associated with parallel changes in either plasma renin activity or angiotensin II. Infusion of 500 ml/hr of 0·9% sodium chloride for 6 hr reduced plasma aldosterone from 660 ± 70 to 360 ± 80 pg/ml (1832 ± 194 to 1000 ± 222 pmol/l) after 60 min and to 70 ± 10 pg/ml (194 ± 28 pmol/l) by the end of the infusion (Williams et al., 1972). There was no change in plasma Na or K and only a diurnal fall in plasma cortisol. A fall in angiotension II is seen with 10 min, and aldosterone is significantly reduced by 30 min (Tuck et al., 1974). Infusion of 5% glucose for 6 hr had no effect on angiotensin II or aldosterone and Dextran (250 ml/hr for 4 hr) produced a much delayed fall in aldosterone in association with a fall in angiotensin II and plasma [K] (Tuck et al., 1974). The role of plasma [K] during saline loading has been examined in normal subjects on a low Na diet by Dluhy et al. (1977). After 60 min of saline infusion they added KCl to raise the plasma [K] by 0·4 mmol/l. This resulted in a rise in plasma aldosterone with a continued fall in plasma renin. Conversely, addition of saline to a KCl infusion reduced plasma aldosterone. The changes in plasma aldosterone levels appeared to be the arithmetic sum of the changes produced in plasma renin activity and plasma [K]. Wong et al. (1975) have shown the changes in plasma aldosterone and renin activity during saline loading are also associated with a fall in plasma bradykinin. Although black subjects excrete less of the intravenous saline load and show a greater suppression of renin, they show a similar fall in plasma aldosterone to white subjects (Luft et al., 1977). Birkhauser et al. (1973) examined the mechanism of hyperosmotic

Table 6

The effect of saline loading and postural change on plasma aldosterone concentration in man.

	Na/K intake (mmol)	Posture	Method	Plasma aldosterone (pg/ml)[a]		References
Saline loading	Na 10 K 100	Supine	0·5 l/hr 4 hr	910 ± 70	130 ± 50	Williams et al. (1972)
	Na 10 K 100	Supine	0·5 l/hr 6 hr	360 ± 30	110 ± 20	Tuck et al. (1974)
	Na 10 K 100	Supine	0·5 l/hr 4 hr	420 ± 50	170 ± 20	Wong et al. (1975)
	Na 10 K 100	Supine	0·5 l/hr 6 hr	330 ± 30	60 ± 10	Tuck et al. (1976)
	Na 10 K 100	Supine	0·5 l/hr 1 hr	340 ± 70	190 ± 50	Dluhy et al. (1970)
	Ad lib	Upright→Supine	0·5 l/hr 4 hr	360 ± 40	46 ± 5	Luft et al. (1977)
Posture	Na 150 K 82	Supine→Upright	1 hr	79 ± 25	295 ± 106	Michelakis and Horton (1970)
	Na 10 K 82	Supine→Upright	1 hr	237 ± 57	778 ± 310	
	Na 10 K 100	Supine→Upright	3 hr	550 ± 70	1000 ± 170	Williams et al. (1972)
	Ad lib	Supine→Sitting	1·5 hr	11·2 ± 6	69 ± 21	Bajlikian et al. (1968)
		Supine→Upright	1·5 hr	26 ± 9	253 ± 61	
	Na 10 K 100	Supine→Upright	3 hr	330 ± 60	930 ± 160	Tuck et al. (1975)
	Na 200 K 100	Upright	3 hr	70 ± 20	330 ± 70	
	Na 10 K 100	Upright→Supine	4 hr	680 ± 70	120 ± 60	
	Na > 60	Supine→Upright	2 hr	139 ± 63	334 ± 68	Katz et al. (1972a)

Na <30	Upright	2 hr	471 ± 74	625 ± 160	Sassard et al. (1976)
Na 100	Supine→ Upright	2 hr	35 ± 7	262 ± 36	
	Upright→ Supine	1 hr	262 ± 36	211 ± 40	Peck et al. (1975)
Na 120	Supine→ Upright	3 hr	50 ± 20	124 ± 13	
Na 110 K 100	Supine→ Tilt	0·5 hr	156 ± 55	349 ± 92	Sancho et al. (1976)
Na 10 K 100	Tilt	0·5 hr	233 ± 90	402 ± 68	

[a] 1 pg/ml = 2·775 pmol/l.

and hyperoncotic plasma volume expansion on the suppression of aldosterone during angiotensin II infusion. From their experiments they proposed that both types of infusion are accompanied by shifts of intracellular K to the extracellular compartment. Further, since infusion of KCl will prevent the fall in plasma aldosterone and there is no simple correlation between plasma [K] and aldosterone, the intracellular [K] must be important. These conclusions need to be confirmed by further studies.

7. Deoxycorticosterone Acetate (DOCA)

Administration of DOCA on both high and low Na diets results in suppression of both plasma and urinary aldosterone in association with expansion of ECFV and a fall in plasma renin activity (Shade and Grim, 1975). In this study, in contrast to earlier studies (Rovner et al., 1965; Ehrlich and Lindheimer, 1972) but in agreement with a study involving administration of physiological doses of aldosterone (Adamson and Jamieson, 1972) no increase in K excretion was observed.

8. Corticotrophin (ACTH)

Administration of ACTH produces an increase in aldosterone secretion (Table 7) (Hume, 1962; Ulick, Nicolis and Vetter, 1963; Tucci, Espiner, Jagger, Pauk and Lauler, 1967; Benraad and Kloppenborg, 1970; Williams, Dluhy and Underwood, 1970; Rayfield, Rose, Dluhy and Williams, 1973; Pratt, Dale and Melby, 1976), excretion (Muller, Riondel, Manning and Mach, 1956; Venning, Dyrenfurth and Beck, 1957; Liddle, Duncan and Bartter, 1956; Lieberman and Luetscher, 1960; Biglieri, Schambelan and Slaton, 1969; Pratt et al., 1976) and plasma levels (Oddie, Coghlan and Scoggins, 1972; Dluhy, Himathongkam and Greenfield, 1974; Nicholls, Espiner and Donald, 1975; Kem, Gomez-Sanchez, Kramer, Holland and Higgins, 1975; Messerli, Nowaczynski, Honda, Genest and Kuchel, 1976). The effect of ACTH on aldosterone is not sustained and after three to four days aldosterone production (Liddle et al., 1956; Tucci et al., 1967; Newton and Laragh, 1968; Biglieri et al., 1969; Benraad and Kloppenborg, 1970) returns to basal levels. This transient stimulation of aldosterone is also seen in subjects on a low Na diet (Newton and Laragh, 1968; Biglieri et al., 1969; Benraad and Kloppenborg, 1970) with aldosterone levels on cessation of ACTH often being less than the pre-ACTH value. The mechanism of this inhibition of aldosterone production is not fully understood but it is not due to Na retention (Biglieri et al., 1969; Benraad and Kloppenborg, 1970) or suppression of plasma renin activity (Newton and Laragh, 1968; Biglieri et al., 1969). The inhibition can also be produced by glucocorticoids (Newton

Table 7

The effect of ACTH and potassium on plasma aldosterone concentration in man.

	Na/K intake (mmol)	Posture	Method	Plasma aldosterone (pg/ml)[a]		References
				Basal	Maximum	
ACTH	Ad lib	Supine	250 µg i.v.	82 ± 17	197 ± 41	Oddie et al. (1972)
	Ad lib	Supine	12·5 u/4 hr	55 ± 22	160 ± 48	Kem et al. (1975)
	Na 100	Supine and Dex	12·5 m u/0·5 hr	43	88	
	Na 100	Supine and Dex	100 m u/0·5 hr	43	212	
	Na 10	Supine and Dex	12·5 m u/0·5 hr	108	380	
	Na 10	Supine and Dex	100 m u/0·5 hr	108	750	
	Na 150 K 82	Supine	0·5 u/h	90 ± 35	553 ± 287	Michelakis and Horton (1970)
Potassium	Na 200 K 40	Supine	[K]p 4·2	52·2 ± 13		Hollengberg et al. (1975)
	Na 200 K 100	Supine	[K]p 4·4	52·2 ± 7		
	Na 200 K 200	Supine	[K]p 4·2	96·5 ± 14		
	Na 10 K 100	Supine	KCl i.v. Δ[K]p 0·2	280 ± 70	410 ± 60	Himathongkam et al. (1975)
	Na 10 K 100	Supine	KCl i.v. Δ[K]p 0·9	160 ± 40	330 ± 40	
	Na 10 K 40	Supine	KCl i.v. Δ[K]p 1·9	670 ± 160	980 ± 180	Dluhy et al. (1972)
	Na 10 K 200	Supine	KCl i.v. Δ[K]p 1·6	1060 ± 100	1940 ± 340	

[a] 1 pg/ml = 2·775 pmol/l.

and Laragh, 1968) and does not occur in patients with biosynthetic defects in cortisol production (Beitins, Bayard, Kowarski and Migeon, 1972). Morphological change and associated biosynthetic inhibition of aldosterone production within the zona glomerulosa rather than intra-adrenal modulation of aldosterone biosynthesis by ACTH would appear to be involved (McDougall, Coghlan, Robinson and Scoggins, 1978).

Dietary Na restriction enhances the aldosterone response to ACTH (Tucci et al., 1967; Williams et al., 1970; Rayfield et al., 1973; Kem et al., 1975). An increase in K intake (200 mmol/day on a normal Na intake (200 mmol/day) will also sensitise the response to ACTH (Williams et al., 1970). The enhanced aldosterone response in Na restriction may not be due to the rise in plasma renin activity since suppression of the renin by intravenous saline does not abolish the aldosterone increase (Kem et al., 1975). The human adrenal is very sensitive to ACTH and infusion of ACTH to raise the plasma ACTH level to within the physiological range (40–160 pg/ml) stimulates aldosterone in normal (Nicholls et al., 1975) and in dexamethasone-suppressed subjects (Kem et al., 1975). Studies examining the effects of ACTH on aldosterone metabolism have shown a significant increase in the plasma metabolic clearance rate after both long-term (after six days) (Pratt et al., 1975) and short-term ACTH administration (Messerli et al., 1976; Zipser, Speckart, Zia, Edmiston, Lau and Horton, 1976; Zager, Burtis, Luetscher, Dowdy and Sood, 1976; Chavarri, Luetscher, Dowdy and Ganguly, 1977). ACTH or cortisol treatment does not produce any consistent changes in hepatic blood flow (Zager et al., 1976; Messerli et al., 1976). Zager et al. (1976) have proposed that the increase in clearance is due to a fall in the plasma protein-bound (transcortin) fraction of aldosterone due to an increase in cortisol levels making a larger fraction available for metabolism. The plasma metabolic clearance rate increased by as much as 50% as cortisol levels were raised from 2 μg/100 ml to 50 μg/100 ml (55 nmol/l to 1379 nmol/l). Aldosterone has a lower affinity than cortisol for transcortin $2\cdot4$–$3\cdot0 \times 10^7 \text{M}^{-1}$ (Sandberg and Slaunwhite, 1971) cf. $6\cdot5 \times 10^6 \text{M}^{-1}$ (Doe and Seal, 1963) and 12–20% of aldosterone is bound to transcortin at normal physiological levels of cortisol (Zager et al., 1976). In contrast to the effect of ACTH on the plasma clearance rate described above, the blood metabolic clearance of aldosterone does not change (Zipser et al., 1976; Chavarri et al., 1977) with either ACTH or cortisol administration. Splanchnic extraction of aldosterone ($92 \pm 1\%$) is also not altered (Zipser et al., 1976). It is proposed that a fraction of aldosterone bound to plasma protein is displaced by cortisol into the red cells. Since aldosterone in both plasma and red cells is extracted by the liver the blood clearance rate does not change (Zipser et al., 1976). These studies have been extended by Chavarri et al. (1977) who have shown that in addition to a redistribution of aldosterone by cortisol, in vitro changes in temperature may influence the red blood cell:plasma ratio of aldosterone leading to changes in plasma clearance rate.

In summary, ACTH is an important stimulus to aldosterone secretion in man. It acts directly on the adrenal (Honn and Chavin, 1977) at physiological concentrations and has its effect enhanced by Na restriction and K. The effect is not sustained on either a normal or Na restricted diet. Displacement of aldosterone by cortisol from plasma proteins leads to an increase in the plasma clearance rate of aldosterone.

9. Dexamethasone Suppression

Administration of dexamethasone to suppress ACTH and endogenous glucocorticoid secretion has been reported to have various effects on aldosterone production. Dexamethasone or glucocorticoids reduced the basal aldosterone secretion rate and decreased aldosterone during dietary Na restriction as well as reducing the response to angiotensin II (Newton and Laragh, 1968; Spark, Gordon, Dale and Melby, 1968). Tan and Mulrow (1975) found that dexamethasone reduced plasma aldosterone levels from 329 ± 15 to 221 ± 21 pg/ml (913 ± 42 to 613 ± 58 pmol/l) in Na depleted subjects. Katz, Romfh and Smith (1975) also found lower plasma aldosterone levels in dexamethasone-treated subjects on a normal Na intake. In asthmatic patients after chronic treatment with corticosteroids for 5–9 years, aldosterone secretion was in the normal range and responded to Na restriction to the same extent as control subjects (Thomas and El-Shaboury, 1971). In contrast to these reports it has been shown that with dexamethasone episodic fluctuations of aldosterone plasma levels (Katz et al., 1975; Weinberger et al., 1975; Lommer et al., 1976; James et al., 1976) are observed and the response to infused ACTH (Dluhy et al., 1974; Kem et al., 1975; Hata et al., 1976) is normal. The variability in observed responses is probably due to the differences in protocols which have been used, the varied dosages and duration of treatment and whether or not the effect is examined in the same patient before and after dexamethasone.

10. Prostaglandins

The E and A classes of prostaglandins (PGE, PGA) have been shown to play an important role in circulatory and fluid homeostasis. Their effects on aldosterone secretion have not been completely elucidated and it is not yet clear whether prostaglandins play a part in physiological control of aldosterone in the human. Levels of immunoreactive PGA_1 have been shown to be increased in Na restriction and to fall with Na loading (Zusman, Spector, Caldwell and Speroff, Schneider and Mulrow, 1973). PGE_1 has

been shown to reduce aldosterone secretion in the Na depleted sheep
(Blair-West, Coghlan, Denton, Funder, Scoggins and Wright, 1971) and
PGA_1 to increase aldosterone secretion in the Na replete animal (Funder,
Blair-West, Coghlan, Denton, Scoggins and Wright, 1969). Both prostaglandins exerted their effects when infused directly into the adrenal arterial
supply. Sub-pressor doses of PGA_1 increased plasma aldosterone (Fichman,
Littenberg, Brooker and Horton, 1972; Golub, Speckart, Zia and Horton,
1976; Speckart, Zia, Zipser and Horton, 1977) by increasing secretion since
the metabolic clearance rate is not changed (Fichman, Littenberg, Woo and
Horton, 1973). PGA_1 also increases plasma aldosterone in anephric man
(Fichman and Horton, 1973). In another study Carr (1973) found that a
vaso-depressor dose of PGA_1 reduced blood pressure without effect on either
plasma renin activity or aldosterone excretion.

Although in their original report Fichman *et al.* (1972) found no change
in plasma renin activity subsequent studies (Golub *et al.*, 1976; Speckart
et al., 1977) have shown a rise in renin. Both renin and aldosterone increase
in a dose related manner in response to PGA_1 infusion, aldosterone increasing from a value of 4.8 ± 0.4 to 20.7 ± 1.2 ng/100 ml (130 ± 11 to
574 ± 25 pmol/l) at a dose of 0.6 μg/kg min^{-1} (Golub *et al.*, 1976). Investigation of the interrelationship between the renin–angiotensin–aldosterone
system and PGA_1 has shown that PGA_1 will raise aldosterone and renin
levels on a low Na diet. Further, the prostaglandin synthetase inhibitor
indomethacin produces a fall in both aldosterone and renin on a low Na diet
without change in Na excretion (Speckart *et al.*, 1977). Although Golub
et al. (1976) stated that indomethacin did not modify the aldosterone response
to angiotensin II, Norbiato, Bevilacqua, Raggi, Micossi, Moroni and Fasoli
(1978) reanalysed their data and established a significant reduction in
response. Tan and Mulrow (1977) have also shown that indomethacin
blunted the plasma renin activity and plasma and urinary aldosterone
response to furosemide. Norbiato *et al.* (1978) have examined the effect of
two other prostaglandin synthetase inhibitors (acetyl-salicylic acid and
diclofenac Na) and reported effects on aldosterone independent of changes
in plasma renin.

The effect of prostaglandins on aldosterone biosynthesis by the human
adrenal *in vitro* has been examined (Honn and Chavin, 1976; Honn and
Chavin, 1977a, b). PGE_1 and E_2 increased aldosterone output while $PGF_{1\alpha}$
and $F_{2\alpha}$ decreased it (Honn and Chavin, 1977a, b). Indomethacin inhibited
the ACTH stimulation of *in vitro* aldosterone output (Honn and Chavin,
1976). Later studies also showed dose-dependent inhibition or stimulation
by PGA_1 and A_2 on aldosterone output and effects of PGB_1 and PGB_2
similar to those of the E type prostaglandin.

11. Vasopressin

Administration of vasopressin results in a fall in aldosterone excretion on a low Na diet if water retention occurs. However, there appears to be no simple relation between the fall in aldosterone and the change in plasma volume (Cox, Leonard and Singer, 1961). In another study Goodwin, Ledingham and Laragh (1970) concluded that in normal man, changes in circulating levels of vasopressin or oxytocin do not play a physiological role in the control of Na excretion. This conclusion was based on the lack of effect of vasopressin on aldosterone excretion or plasma renin in water restricted subjects and the unimpressive fall in over-hydrated individuals. Of interest with regard to control of aldosterone is the report by Fichman, Michelakis and Horton (1974) that in normal volunteers receiving exogenous vasopressin and an increased water intake the renin response to Na deprivation is suppressed while aldosterone production is increased.

12. Acid–Base Balance

Aldosterone is closely associated with acid-base homeostasis, and administration of mineralocorticoids is associated with metabolic alkalosis (Roth and Gamble, 1965). Similarly, aldosterone deficiency results in acidosis (Perez, Oster and Uaamonde, 1974). However, little is known of the effect of acidification on aldosterone. Administration of intravenous NH_4Cl—an acidifying salt—over 2 hr decreased blood pH and bicarbonate but had little effect on Na excretion in Na restricted subjects (Kisch, Dluhy and Williams, 1976; Perez, Oster, Uaamonde and Katz, 1977). A significant fall in plasma renin without change in plasma aldosterone levels was observed by Kisch et al. (1976) while Perez et al. (1977) found an increase in plasma [K] and renin activity. Although the mechanism of effect of ammonium ion is unknown a direct effect of the cation on aldosterone secretion has been observed in sheep with autotransplanted adrenal glands (Blair-West, Coghlan, Denton, Goding, Wintour and Wright, 1968). It would appear that a direct effect may not be involved in the clinical studies since in contrast to the sheep experiments, there was no increase in blood ammonia level (Perez et al., 1977).

The effect of metabolic alkalosis (produced by selective depletion of hydrochloric acid by gastric suction) on aldosterone secretion has been examined by Kassirer, Appleton, Chazań and Schwarz (1967). After seven days of gastric alkalosis in normal subjects on a low Na intake aldosterone secretion fell from 300–700 µg/day (0·8–1·9 µmol/day) to about 200 µg/day (0·6 µmol/day). This fall was associated with an 8 mmol/l increase in plasma bicarbonate and a fall of 1·2 mmol/l in plasma [K].

13. Other Cations (Calcium, Magnesium and Lithium)

Although the cations K and Na are directly involved in aldosterone regulation, little is known of the role of other cations. Infusion of calcium chloride (0·42 mmol/min) into subjects on a low Na intake produced only a small decrease in plasma renin activity and no effect on plasma aldosterone (Kisch et al., 1976). Magnesium sulphate in an equimolar infusion produced no change in renin and a fall in aldosterone associated with a reduction in plasma [K]. Although the fall in plasma aldosterone was similar to that produced by 0·42 mmol/min sodium chloride the saline infusion resulted in a 40% decrease in renin (Kisch et al., 1976).

There have been no short term studies on the effect of lithium chloride. However, in two longitudinal studies the effect of lithium administration has been examined in manic-depressive and depressed patients. Although initial administration may be associated with a water and Na diuresis and a rise in aldosterone excretion (Murphy, Goodwin and Bunney, 1969) plasma aldosterone levels were normal when measured after 14 days and after 1–3 months of treatment (Pedersen, Amdisen and Darling, 1977).

14. Diurnal Rhythm

A diurnal pattern of aldosterone excretion with greater excretion during the daytime (see Table 8) was first shown by Venning, Dyrenfurth and Giroud (1956), Luetscher and Lieberman (1958) and Bartter, Delea, Halberg (1962). However, two other early studies failed to show any consistent change in excretion when postural change was eliminated (Muller, Manning and Riondel, 1958; Wolfe, Gordon, Island and Liddle, 1966). Michelakis and Horton (1970) demonstrated a diurnal rhythm of plasma aldosterone in supine man on both a normal and low Na diet. Although only four samples were taken throughout the day the highest plasma aldosterone values were found at 06.00 hr and 12.00 hr. There was also a close correlation between plasma renin activity and plasma aldosterone. In a more detailed investigation Williams, Cain, Dluhy and Underwood (1972) studied the diurnal variation in plasma aldosterone, cortisol, renin activity and K on high and low Na intakes and while the subjects were supine or carrying out normal activity. Plasma aldosterone levels were highest in the early morning. A close association was seen between plasma renin activity and aldosterone on all occasions, with a close correlation between cortisol and aldosterone only being observed in supine subjects. From a number of studies it is now clear that while the plasma level of aldosterone usually rises during sleep and reaches a peak early in the morning the closeness of its correlation with

Table 8

The effect of postural change and age on plasma aldosterone concentration (pg/ml) in man (1 pg/ml = 2·775 pmol/l).

	Na/K intake (mmol)	Posture	Time 06·00	12·00	18·00	24·00	References
Diurnal	Na 150 K 82	Supine	98 ± 27	71 ± 39	56 ± 26	116 ± 64	Michelakis and Horton (1970)
	Na 10 K 82	Supine	241 ± 81	266 ± 118	117 ± 61	134 ± 52	
	Na 200 K 200	Supine	280 ± 30	160 ± 30	110 ± 20	60 ± 10	Williams et al. (1972)
	Na 10 K 100	Supine	880 ± 70	560 ± 50	410 ± 50	310 ± 50	
	Na 130 K 70	Supine	122	97	38		Katz et al. (1975)
	Na 130 K 70	Supine and dex	131	18	20		

	Na/K intake (mmol)	Posture	Age (yr)		References
Age	Na 120	Supine	20–30	42 ± 5	Weidman et al. (1975)
			60–70	31 ± 4	
	Na 120	Upright	20–30	125 ± 26	
			60–70	56 ± 8	
	Na 10	Supine	20–30	138 ± 27	
			60–70	64 ± 9	
	Na 10	Upright	20–30	597 ± 150	
			60–70	203 ± 37	

plasma renin activity, cortisol and K may depend on Na intake and posture (Katz, Romfh and Smith, 1972; Breuer, Karlhausen, Muhlbauer, Fritzsche and Vetter, 1974; Vagnucci, McDonald, Drash and Wong, 1974; Kowarski, Lacerda and Migeon, 1975; Katz, Romfh and Smith, 1975; Armbruster, Vetter, Beckerhoff, Nussberger, Vetter and Siegenthaler, 1975; Weinberger, Kem, Gomez-Sanchez, Kramer, Martin and Nugent, 1975; Lommer, Distler, Nast, Sinterhauf, Walter and Wolff, 1976; Rubin, Poland, Gouin and Tower, 1978). In general the correlation with plasma renin activity is closer on a low Na intake (Katz et al., 1975; Armbruster et al., 1975; Weinberger et al., 1975) and during the afternoon and evening (Katz et al., 1972c). Changes in either plasma Na or K would appear to play little role in the rhythm. Often aldosterone varies independently of the factors known to be involved in its control (James, Tunbridge and Wilson, 1976; Weinberger et al., 1975). The secretion of aldosterone like that of cortisol is episodic (Katz et al., 1972c; Breuer et al., 1974; Vagnucci et al., 1974; Weinberger et al., 1975; Kowarski et al., 1975; James et al., 1976; Rubin et al., 1978) and remains episodic even after suppression of endogenous ACTH with dexamethasone (Weinberger et al., 1975). Dexamethasone has been administered in a number of studies to eliminate the role of ACTH but the diurnal pattern of plasma aldosterone and its episodic fluctuations remain on both normal and low Na intakes (Katz et al., 1975; Armbruster et al., 1975; Weinberger et al., 1975; Lommer et al., 1976; James et al., 1976). Episodic secretion has also been observed in subjects with high cervical spinal cord transection and in hypophysectomised patients (James et al., 1976). Measurement of adrenal venous secretion of aldosterone, in patients with idiopathic hirsutism, also shows that aldosterone secretion may often be independent of cortisol secretion (Huq, Pfaff, Jespersen, Zucker and Kirschner, 1976). Prolonged bedrest (five days) produced higher plasma renin and aldosterone peaks during sleep than during control conditions in the same subjects (Chavari, Ganguly, Luetscher and Zager, 1977). The diurnal rhythm of aldosterone secretion and plasma renin activity have been suppressed in supine subjects receiving acute β-blockade (Cugini, Manconi, Serdoz, Mancini and Meucci, 1977).

   Although it is not yet absolutely clear what determines the diurnal or episodic nature of aldosterone secretion (Rubin, 1975) it may be related to the timing of Na ingestion since Kunita, Obara, Komatsu, Hata and Okamoto (1976) have shown that administration of the normal daily intake of Na at night will abolish the diurnal rhythm.

15. Posture

An increased aldosterone excretion rate in ambulant subjects compared with bed-rested individuals was first reported by Muller, Manning and Riondel (1958) (Table 6). Gowenlock, Mills and Thomas (1959) examined the effects of acute change in posture from supine to standing and established that the rise in aldosterone excretion could be blocked by prevention of venous pooling, by immersion to the neck. A close association between the observed changes in aldosterone excretion and plasma renin activity was established (Cohen, Conn and Rovner, 1967) and a role for the sympathetic nervous system demonstrated (Gordon, Kuchel, Liddle and Island, 1967). Urinary catecholamine excretion increased with the change to upright posture in normal individuals but it, together with renin and aldosterone, did not change in a patient with severe autonomic insufficiency unless catecholamines were infused (Gordon et al., 1967). Part of the increase in plasma aldosterone concentration upon standing is due to a fall in metabolic clearance rate of 23% but the majority of the 6 fold increase in plasma levels is due to increased aldosterone secretion (Balikian, Brodie, Dale, Melby and Tait, 1968). Sitting also increased plasma levels but did so without a fall in clearance rate (Balikian et al., 1968). Tilting to produce the postural stimulus produces much greater falls in clearance (Bougas, Flood, Little, Tait, Tait and Underwood, 1964).

A number of other studies have examined in detail the relationship between the changes in plasma aldosterone and plasma renin activity or angiotensin II during postural change in both normal and Na restricted diets (Luetscher, Weinberger, Dowdy, Nokes, Balikian, Brodie and Willoughby, 1969; Michelakis and Horton, 1970; Williams, Cain, Dluhy and Underwood, 1972; Katz, Romfh, Zimmering, Kelly, 1972; Ito, Hidaka, Kato and Yoshitoshi, 1973; Reck, Beckerhoff, Vetter, Armbruster, Siegenthaler, 1975; Tuck, Dluhy and Williams, 1975; Sassard, Vincent, Annat and Bizollon, 1976; Sancho, Re, Burton, Barger and Haber, 1976; Cugini, Manconi, Serdoz, Mancini and Meucci, 1977). In only one study (Viol, Smith and Fitzgerald, 1976) has an increase in plasma renin activity been observed in response to tilting without change in plasma aldosterone. Increments of either plasma renin or angiotensin II occur within 5–20 min and plasma aldosterone is significantly elevated by 30 min reaching a peak by 90 min (Tuck et al., 1975). A low Na diet has been shown to amplify the response of both renin and aldosterone to the postural stimulus in some studies (Katz et al., 1972a; Katz, Romfh and Smith, 1972b; Tuck et al., 1975). Although it has been suggested that small increases in plasma K or ACTH may also play a role in increasing aldosterone secretion during postural change (Reck et al., 1975) it is clear that the renin–angiotensin system plays a primary role. Additional evidence to support this conclusion is the failure of upright posture to increase aldosterone in anephric man (Balikian et al., 1968; Bayard, Cooke, Tiller, Beitins, Kowarski, Walker and Migeon, 1971). Also Sancho et al. (1976)

have shown that the aldosterone response to tilting can be abolished by prior administration of an angiotensin converting enzyme inhibitor in normal subjects on both normal and low Na diets. Prior stimulation of aldosterone secretion by standing markedly reduces the aldosterone response to infused angiotensin II and ACTH on both normal and low Na diets (Katz et al., 1972b).

After prolonged bed-rest (5–14 days) tilting or standing results in an exaggerated circulatory and plasma renin response. However, bed-rest had little effect on the 08.00 hr plasma aldosterone concentration and the 12.00 hr ambulant value after bed-rest was similar to that observed before bed-rest (Melada, Goldman, Leutscher and Zager, 1975).

Change in posture from upright to supine results in a fall in plasma renin activity, angiotensin II and aldosterone (Tuck et al., 1975; Sassard et al., 1976; Cugini et al., 1977). Tuck et al. (1975) found a close relationship between the fall in angiotensin II and aldosterone over 4 hr but others have shown either a fall in renin without change in aldosterone over 60 min (Sassard et al., 1976) or a fall in renin with a slower fall in aldosterone (Cugini et al., 1977).

16. Fasting and Refeeding

During the first week of fasting a profound natriuresis occurs in both lean and obese subjects on both a normal and restricted Na intake (Bloom and Mitchell, 1960). The period of natriuresis is followed by a period of urinary Na conservation if the fasting is prolonged. Subsequent carbohydrate refeeding rapidly produces an antinatriuresis with Na excretion falling to a very low level (Kolanowski, Pizarro, De Gasparo, Desmecht, Harvengt and Crabbe, 1970; Boulter, Hoffman and Arky, 1973).

Aldosterone excretion (Verdy and Champlain, 1968), secretion (Kolanowski et al., 1970; Boulter, Spark and Arky, 1974) and plasma levels (Chinn, Brown, Fraser, Heron, Lever, Murchison and Robertson, 1970) progressively increase. As the fast continues, aldosterone production returns towards normal levels (Boulter et al., 1974) as Na excretion falls. During fasting the changes in aldosterone are dissociated from plasma renin concentration changes (Chinn et al., 1970; Boulter et al., 1974) both before and after a period of Na depletion Chinn et al., 1970). Neither ACTH nor plasma K appear to be a stimulus to aldosterone secretion during fasting (Chinn et al., 1970). The existence of a natriuresis in the presence of elevated aldosterone secretion has led to the proposal that the nephron is insensitive to aldosterone (Kolanowski, Desmecht and Crabbe, 1974; Boulter et al., 1974). However, Kolanowski, Desmecht and Crabbe (1976) provide evidence that this may not be true and that the Na loss is probably due to a fall in proximal tubular

Na reabsorption. Further, since spironolactone during a fast produces an enhanced natriuresis (Boulter, Spark and Arky, 1973; Kolanowski et al., 1976) and the salivary Na concentration is low it would appear that aldosterone is exerting an effect.

Refeeding of carbohydrates following a fast is associated with a marked anti-natriuresis (Boulter et al., 1974) and is associated with a fall in plasma aldosterone (Chinn et al., 1970) and aldosterone secretion (Boulter et al., 1974). Plasma renin levels rise in subjects on a normal Na intake (Boulter et al., 1974) but fell towards pre-fast levels in those Na depleted prior to fasting (Chinn et al., 1970). It has been proposed that glucagon may play a role in regulation of Na balance during fasting and refeeding since glucagon levels are elevated during fasting, and infused glucagon can produce a natriuresis; also glucagon will block the antinatriuretic effect of fludro-cortisone and abolish the antinatriuresis of carbohydrate refeeding (O'Brian, Saudek and Spark, 1974; Spark, Arky, Boulter, Saudek and O'Brian, 1975). Similarly, prevention of the refeeding antinatriuresis can be produced by massive amounts (1200 mg/day) of spironolactone (Boulter et al., 1973). Others have failed to show this effect of spironolactone (Hansen, Horlyck, Gronback and Iversen, 1967). It has been proposed that glucose may produce renal Na retention by mechanisms not involving aldosterone by influencing Na transport mechanisms proximal to the site of aldosterone action (Kolanowski et al., 1976). Evidence to support this hypothesis was obtained by production of an antinatriuresis with glucose during spirono-lactone treatment in the fasted individual.

The effect of feeding on the metabolic clearance rate of aldosterone in normal supine subjects has been examined (Akesode, Migeon and Kowarski, 1977). The clearance rate increased by 29% within 2 hr of eating, an increase consistent with the known effects of food intake on hepatic blood flow.

It has been suggested that carbohydrate feeding might produce Na retention by turning off glucagon or turning on insulin either of which might block or enhance the renal action of aldosterone (Laragh, 1973). Insulin produces hypokalemia and reduces aldosterone secretion in anephric man (Cooke, Horvath, Moore, Bledsoe and Walker, 1973). In contrast to the above study Hata, Kunita and Okamoto (1976) found that insulin-induced hypoglycemia increased plasma aldosterone in association with a rise in plasma renin activity and cortisol. Administration of propranolol or dexamethasone suppressed the renin or aldosterone levels respectively. They proposed that the increase in aldosterone was mediated by ACTH. In an earlier report James, Landon and Fraser (1968) found that although cortisol secretion was maximally stimulated by the insulin hypoglycemia plasma aldosterone levels were unchanged in subjects on a normal Na intake. Aldosterone increased on a low Na diet with insulin.

17. Immersion

Immersion to the neck for 4–6 hr results in a redistribution of extracellular fluid volume and leads to a relative increase in intrathoracic volume. ADH (Gauer, Henry and Behn, 1970) and plasma renin activity (Korz, Fishcher and Behn, 1969) are suppressed and Na, K and water excretion increased (Epstein, Duncan and Fishman, 1972). The physiological consequences of immersion were first studied as a model for weightlessness (Epstein and Saruta, 1971). Immersion to the neck results in a fall in urinary aldosterone excretion (Epstein and Saruta, 1971; Epstein, Fishman and Hale, 1971; Kulpmann, Wolfel, Skipka and Breuer, 1977) and plasma aldosterone levels (Crane and Harris, 1974; Epstein, Pins, Sancho and Haber, 1975a). Immersion reduces plasma aldosterone from 375 to 105 pg/ml (1041 to 291 pmol/l) by 210 min on a low Na intake (Epstein, Pins, Arrington, Denunzio and Engstrom, 1975b) and from 137 to 31 pg/ml (380 to 86 pmol/l) by 240 min in ambulant subjects on an unrestricted Na intake (Crane and Harris, 1974). The fall in aldosterone was accentuated in younger subjects (20–45 yr) compared with the aged since the latter group have lower pre-immersion aldosterone levels (Crane and Harris, 1974). Immersion to the waist only reduces plasma renin without effect on aldosterone excretion (Epstein and Saruta, 1971). The suppression of plasma aldosterone is closely correlated with the fall in plasma renin activity (Crane and Harris, 1974; Epstein *et al.*, 1975a) and there are no changes in plasma Na or K (Epstein *et al.*, 1975b) or plasma 17-hydroxycorticosteroid levels (Epstein *et al.*, 1971). The natriuresis and fall in aldosterone occurs on both normal (Epstein *et al.*, 1972; Crane and Harris, 1974) and low Na diets (Epstein *et al.*, 1975b). However, it is clear that the natriuresis is not only due to a fall in aldosterone but is due also to a fall in proximal fractional Na reabsorption (Epstein *et al.*, 1972; Epstein, Katsikas and Duncan, 1973). Recovery from immersion is accompanied by rapid rises in both plasma aldosterone and plasma renin activity (Crane and Harris, 1974; Epstein *et al.*, 1975b).

It has been proposed that immersion may be a more useful suppressive manoeuvre for aldosterone than intravenous saline loading since it produces a natriuresis without change in blood volume and an increase in body weight (Epstein *et al.*, 1975a).

18. Thermal Stress

Thermal stress produces an increase in plasma aldosterone on both normal and low Na intakes (Bailey, Bartos, Bartos, Castro, Dobson, Grettie, Kramer, Macfarlane and Sato, 1972). The increase in aldosterone is usually associated with an increase in plasma renin activity (Bailey *et al.*, 1972; Kosunen, Pakarinen, Kuoppasalmi and Adlercreutz, 1976) or angiotensin II (Kosunen *et al.*, 1976). Elevation in aldosterone may also occur without increase in plasma renin (Finberg and Berlyne, 1976) and without production of a Na deficit or dehydration (Kosunen *et al.*, 1976; Finberg and Berlyne, 1977). The rise in both aldosterone and renin can be reduced by acclimatisation (Finberg and Berlyne, 1977). While reduction in clearance rate of aldosterone may be involved in the increase in plasma level (Collins, Few and Finberg, 1977), changes in plasma K or Na or ACTH would appear unlikely to be involved (Collins, Few, Forward and Giec, 1969; Finberg and Berlyne, 1977; Finberg, Katz, Gazit and Berlyne, 1974). Exercise during exposure to heat results in an elevation of both plasma renin activity and aldosterone which can be reduced by administration of K-rich electrolyte solution to offset weight loss (Francis and McGregor, 1978). Earlier studies had also shown that the increase in urinary aldosterone excretion associated with thermal stress could be prevented by replacement of the Na deficit produced by the heat stress (Smiles and Robinson, 1971).

19. Exercise

Exercise either on a bicycle ergometer (Maher, Jones, Hartley, Williams and Rose, 1975; Bonelli, Waldhausl, Magometschnigg, Schwarzmeier, Korn and Hitzenberger, 1977) or running (Sundsfjord, Stromme, Refsum and Aakvaag, 1973; Kosunen and Pakarinen, 1976; Newmark, Himathongkam, Martin, Cooper and Rose, 1976) results in an increase in plasma aldosterone. This increase is associated with an elevation in plasma renin or angiotensin II (Maher *et al.*, 1975; Bonelli *et al.*, 1977; Kosunen and Pakarinen, 1976) due to increased sympathetic activity. While propranolol blocked the rise in plasma renin an increase in aldosterone was still observed (Bonelli *et al.*, 1977; Rose, Carroll, Lowe, Peterson and Cooper, 1970) and ACTH (Newmark *et al.*, 1976) may also be involved.

20. High Altitude

Acclimatisation to high altitude produces a decrease in aldosterone secretion (Slater, Tuffley, Williams, Beresford, Sonksen, Edwards, Ekins and McLaughlin (1969), excretion (Ayres, 1961; Hogan, Kotchen, Boyd and Hartley, 1973; Sutton, Viol, Gray, McFadden and Keane, 1977; Pines, Slater and Jowett, 1977) and plasma concentration (Jung, Dill, Horton and Horvath, 1971; Maher, Jones, Hartley, Williams and Rose, 1975; Sutton *et al.*, 1977). The effect is due to hypoxia or hypocapnia rather than the reduction in barometric pressure (Epstein and Saruta, 1972; Epstein and Saruta, 1973). Associated with the fall in aldosterone a decrease in K excretion (Slater, Williams, Edwards, Ekins, Sonksen, Beresford and McLaughlin, 1969; Frayser, Rennie, Gray and Houston, 1975; Sutton et al., 1977) and a rise in plasma [K] (Slater et al., 1969; Frayser et al., 1975) have been observed. The change in K excretion is thought to be a homoestatic mechanism to reduce K loss as a result of respiratory alkalosis (Slater et al., 1969). Plasma volume is also reduced (Jung et al., 1971). Changes in the renin–angiotensin are contradictory. Elevations in plasma renin activity were seen in response to high altitude by Tuffley, Rubenstein, Slater and Williams (1970). Hogan et al. (1973) and Maher et al. (1975) both reported a fall in plasma renin activity in response to high altitude, while Sutton et al. (1977) found no change. Cortisol secretion and plasma levels are usually increased (Slater et al., 1969; Sutton et al., 1977). The effect on the renin–aldosterone system may depend on altitude since Frayser et al. (1975) found little change at 10,000 ft but an increase in both plasma renin and aldosterone at 17,500 ft. Age may also modulate the response with little or no fall in aldosterone being seen in young subjects compared to those over 40 years (Jung et al., 1971). An increase in plasma aldosterone in response to exercise was seen during either acute (one day) or chronic (11 days) exposure to high altitude (Maler et al., 1975). Adaptation appeared to occur during chronic exposure and the response of aldosterone, renin and angiotensin II to exercise at this time were similar to those at sea level.

In studies aimed to simulate the conditions of space flight (hyperoxia at reduced barometric pressure) the response of the renin–aldosterone system to Na restriction was similar to that observed in controls (Epstein and Saruta, 1973). In actual space flight aldosterone excretion has been reported to increase (Lutwak, Whedon, Lachance, Reid and Lipscomb, 1969; Leach, Alexander and Johnson, 1972).

21. Prolactin

The dopaminergic agonist—bromocriptine—reduces prolactin secretion and has also been reported to inhibit the rise in plasma aldosterone which follows administration of frusemide (Edwards, Miall, Hanker, Thorner, Al-Dujaili and Besser, 1975). It did not inhibit release of renin or alter plasma [K]. In contrast to this study, bromocriptine had no effect on plasma aldosterone levels in either anephric or non-nephrectomised dialysis patients (Olgaard, Hagen, Madsen and Hummer, 1976) or patients with primary aldosteronism (Marek and Horky, 1976). The anti-dopaminergic drug—metoclopramide—increases plasma prolactin levels and has been reported to increase plasma aldosterone without change in serum electrolytes, renin or cortisol (Norbiato, Bevilacqua, Raggi, Micossi and Moroni, 1977). It is proposed that this may be due to a direct effect of the drug since a response was seen in hypophysectomised subjects. In contrast, Ohihara, Matsumana, Onishi, Miyai, Uozumi and Kumahara (1977) found that metoclopramide, at a lower dose, had no effect on aldosterone whilst increasing plasma prolactin. In a detailed study in normals Holland, Gomez-Sanchez, Kem, Weinberger, Krämer and Higgins (1978) found no relationship between plasma aldosterone and prolactin levels. Additional work is required to establish whether prolactin plays a physiological role in aldosterone secretion and in Na and water homeostasis in man.

22. Age

Aldosterone secretion rate and serum or plasma aldosterone concentrations are elevated in the new-born infant (Table 7) (Weldon, Kowarski and Migeon, 1967; Siegel, Fisher and Oh, 1974; Dillon, Gillin, Ryness and de Swiet, 1976) compared to values at six days or older. Although Weldon et al. (1967) found the aldosterone secretion rate of infants (11 days to 1 yr) to be similar to that of older children or of adults, a more recent study (Kowarski, Katz and Migeon, 1974) showed that plasma aldosterone during the first year of life is higher than at any other age.

Elderly subjects (70-yr-old group) were first shown to have a lower aldosterone secretion, clearance rate and hence plasma concentration by Flood, Gherondache, Pincus, Tait, Tait and Willoughby (1967). Other studies have examined in detail the relationship of the renin–angiotensin system to either aldosterone secretion (Tuck, Williams, Cain, Sullivan and Dluhy, 1973), excretion (Crane and Harris, 1976; Noth, Lassman, Tan, Fernandez-Cruz and Mulrow, 1977) or plasma aldosterone (Craine and Harris, 1974; Weidman, De Myttenaere-Bursztein, Maxwell and de Lima, 1975; Weidman, de Chatel, Schiffman, Bachmann, Beratta-Piccoli, Reubi, Ziegler and Vetter, 1977). Age-related decreases in both plasma renin activity or concentration and aldosterone were reported in all studies except that of Noth et al. (1977) who found a reduction in ambulatory plasma renin in elderly subjects without change in aldosterone. In the most detailed study (Weidman et al., 1977) found significant correlations between renin and aldosterone with an age-dependent progressive reduction in basal levels and in response to postural change. Others have shown that the renin–aldosterone response to Na restriction is also less in the aged (Crane and Harris, 1976; Weidman et al., 1975).

These changes do not appear to be related to either K or Na intakes or levels of plasma renin substrate (Crane and Harris, 1976). Further, aldosterone and cortisol responses to ACTH are not altered in the elderly (Weidmann, 1977).

23. Menstrual Cycle and Oral Contraceptives

The excretion rate, secretion rate, and peripheral plasma concentration of aldosterone is higher in the luteal phase than in the follicular phase of the menstrual cycle (Reich, 1962; Sundsfjord and Aakvaag, 1970, 1972, 1973; Katz and Rompfh, 1972; Schwartz and Abraham, 1975; Michelakis, Yoshida and Dormois, 1975; Frolich, Brand and van Hall, 1976), provided ovulation occurs. If there is no ovulation, or luteal failure, there is no rise in plasma aldosterone concentration (Sundsfjord and Aakvaag, 1972; Michelakis *et al.*, 1975). This would suggest that the rise in aldosterone is secondary to an increased concentration of progesterone and/or oestrogen. The situation here is analogous to that in pregnancy (discussed in Section D.2.4), in that whereas in general a correlation can be found between plasma aldosterone, progesterone, and renin activity, situations can arise in which the various parameters are dissociated. Plasma aldosterone values start to rise before ovulation and increased plasma progesterone (Frolich *et al.*, 1976). One subject on treatment with a β-blocker had increased plasma aldosterone concentration without increased plasma renin activity, and one woman who became pregnant during the study showed higher renin activity and aldosterone but no change in progesterone (Sundsfjord and Aakvaag, 1973). Women taking combination oestrogen/progestagen oral contraceptives show increases in plasma renin activity (Katz and Beck, 1974; Katz, Rompfh, Smith, Roper and Barnes, 1975) and sometimes plasma aldosterone (Beckeroff, Armbruster, Vetter, Leutscher and Siegenthaler, 1973; Katz *et al.*, 1975). Oestrogen-containing pills cause an elevation in renin–substrate concentration (Katz and Kappas, 1967; Katz and Beck, 1974) which may contribute to the increased plasma renin activity noted above. Thus variation in the blood concentration of oestrogen or progesterone may be associated with altered aldosterone secretion.

24. Pregnancy (Pre-eclampsia)

In women, higher than normal urinary excretion rates of free aldosterone or of its 18-glucuronide derivative have been reported in the third trimester of pregnancy (Martin and Mills, 1956; Rinsler and Rigby, 1957; Venning, Primrose, Caligaris and Dyrenfurth, 1957; Wolff, Koczorek and Buchborn, 1958). Jones, Lloyd-Jones, Riondel, Tait, Tait, Bulbrook and Greenwood (1959) found high normal to very high aldosterone secretion rates in six women between 32–38 weeks of gestation. In 15 pregnant women on normal sodium intake, the mean aldosterone secretion rate was 1000 µg/day (2·8 µmol/day) during the third trimester compared with a normal range of

85–216 µg/day (0·2–0·6 µmol/day) in the follicular phase (Watanabe, Meeker, Gray, Sims and Solomon, 1963). There appeared to be an increase by the fifteenth week; by the twentieth week the mean output was 892 µg/day (2·5 µmol/day) and in weeks 36–37 and 38–39, mean secretion rates were 1321 and 1586 µg/day (3·7 and 4·4 µmol/day) respectively. At each stage the variation between subjects was very large, with evidence of a correlation between sodium intake and aldosterone secretion, at least during the third trimester. In three subjects the mean secretion rate was 7843 µg/day (2·18 µmol/day) after 14 days on a sodium diet of 10 mEq/day.

Meyer *et al.* (1961) have shown that there is little or no alteration of binding of aldosterone to plasma protein during pregnancy and the studies of Tait *et al.* (1962) demonstrate that the metabolic clearance rates for aldosterone in normal and pregnant women do not differ significantly.

Tait and Little (1968) did find that the hepatic metabolism of aldosterone was altered such that while the splanchnic extraction actually decreased from 90% in non-pregnant subjects to 77% in pregnant women, more 18-glucuronide metabolite was formed in the splanchnic circulation and increased tetrahydroaldosterone glucuronide in extrasplanchnic sites, perhaps the foeto-placental unit. Pasqualini (1971) showed that when labelled aldosterone was injected into the human foeto-placental unit at 18–21 weeks of gestation a significant percentage was transformed by the foetal liver into tetrahydroaldosterone. Pasqualini *et al.* (1976) also found that 69–82% of aldosterone injected into the foetal guinea-pig was metabolised to tetrahydroaldosterone by the placenta, at 35–45 days (term $\simeq$ 67 days).

Peripheral plasma aldosterone has now been measured in various stages of human pregnancy by a number of groups (Weir, Paintin, Brown, Fraser, Lever, Morton, Robertson and Young, 1971; Weir, Brown, Fraser, Lever, Logan, McIlwaine, Morton, Robertson and Tree, 1975; Ledoux, Genest, Nowacynski, Küchel and Lebel, 1975; Weinberger, Kramer, Petersen, Cleary and Young, 1976; Smeaton, Anderson and Fulton, 1977; Wintour, Coghlan, Oddie, Scoggins and Walters, 1978). The values determined vary but all agree that peripheral plasma aldosterone is elevated after mid-gestation. Individual subjects vary, some showing very little change, others very marked increases, and varying at the time at which aldosterone starts to rise, but by 24 weeks of gestation the mean of group data is significantly increased above non-pregnant values.. One difficulty is that normal range values vary, another is that most of the studies have been done on out-patients on an uncontrolled salt intake, and in some series each patient has been bled only once. In one series in which the same women were bled sequentially throughout pregnancy the blood aldosterone of 11·8 ± 6·4 ng/100 ml (327 ± 178 pmol/l) (n = 6) (combined follicular and luteal values) rose to 27·3 ± 15·5 (758 ± 430) (n = 11) at 24 weeks, and reached a plateau at 52·4 ± 22·9 ng/100 ml (1454 ± 627 pmol/l) (n = 11) by 32 weeks (Wintour et al., 1978).

In other species the picture is different. Peripheral blood aldosterone concentration is not increased by pregnancy in the sheep (Wintour, Blair-West, Brown, Coghlan, Denton, Nelson, Oddie, Scoggins, Whipp and Wright, 1976) or monkey (Wintour, Knobil, Scoggins, Skinner and Coghlan, 1974). Whipp, Wintour, Coghlan and Scoggins (1976) measured peripheral blood concentration of aldosterone at three stages throughout pregnancy in conscious, unstressed guinea-pigs and found values not elevated at 20 days or 60 days but approximately double the non-pregnant values at 40 days (term = 68 days). Giry and Delost (1977) measured plasma aldosterone concentrations of 22·4 ± 3·9 ng/100 ml (622 ± 108 pmol/l) in guinea-pigs on day 62 of gestation, which was not significantly different from their values in non-pregnant females (24·1 ± 1·6 ng/100 ml) (669 ± 44 pmol/l) and found no increase until 48 hr before parturition at which time the values increased by 70%. Pregnancy in the rat is a time of rapid sodium accumulation as weight gain of approximately 45% of the original maternal body weight is made, 60% of this occurring during the last third of gestation. During pregnancy in the rat peripheral blood aldosterone concentration is increased (Whipp et al., 1978). The rise is modest—there being an approximate doubling of peripheral blood aldosterone concentration from 15·2 ± 7·8 ng/100 ml (422 ± 216 pmol/l), which is the peak non-pregnant value at oestrus, to 38·9 ± 19·0 ng/100 ml (1079 ± 527 pmol/l) at day 18 of a 22-day gestation period. The rise is evident by day 12. This elevation of aldosterone concentration in peripheral blood in pregnant rats is small compared with the 60 fold increase invoked by 72-hr sodium depletion (Bojesen, 1966) or the 200 fold increment induced by two weeks of sodium restriction (Hilfenhaus, 1977). When aldosterone production rate was determined by incubating maternal adrenals from term rats the values were double those of adrenals from non-pregnant rats, but sodium deficiency did not further increase the production rate in pregnant rats (Schneider and Mulrow, 1973).

The secretion rate of aldosterone in pregnant bitches late in gestation was elevated in nine of 19 animals studied (Robb, Davis, Johnson, Blaine, Schneider and Baumber, 1970) and as the removal rate of aldosterone is similar in pregnant and non-pregnant bitches (Johnson, Davis, Taylor and Shade, 1974) it is likely that the peripheral level would reflect the secretion rate. Thus there is considerable variation in the aldosterone levels in blood during pregnancy in the species so far studied. The next questions to be considered are is the high circulating aldosterone concentration in man an important physiological requirement, and what is the stimulus to the elevated secretion rate?

Based on the fact that when aldosterone excretion rate was lowered by administration of the heparinoid ROI-8307 natriuresis ensued in pregnant women, Ehrlich (1971) proposed that there were potent sodium-losing factors circulating in normal human pregnancy which required an increased aldosterone secretion rate for antagonism. This proposal was strengthened by the demonstration that aldosterone excretion rate fell when sodium retention was induced in pregnant women in the third trimester by the administration of synthetic mineralocorticoids (Ehrlich and Lindheimer, 1972). It has been suggested that the elevated concentration of progesterone which circulates in the pregnant women (Johansson, 1969) may act to cause sodium loss both by competitive inhibition with aldosterone (Landau and Lugibihl, 1958) and by a direct inhibition of sodium reabsorption at the proximal tubule (Oparil, Ehrlich and Lindheimer, 1975). The effect of aldosterone on the composition of parotid and submixillary saliva, however, appears not to be blocked as the sodium concentration is lower, and the potassium concentration higher, in the saliva of pregnant women than of non-pregnant women (Marder, Wotman and Mandel, 1972). There seems to be good agreement that when progesterone is administered to men for some days urinary sodium excretion increases as does urinary aldosterone excretion (Sundsfjord, 1971; Oelkers, Schöneshöfer and Blümel, 1974). As plasma renin activity and plasma angiotensin II concentration were also elevated by progesterone treatment (Oelkers *et al.*, 1974) the question arises as to whether in normal pregnancy the rise in renin–angiotensin is the primary stimulus to increased aldosterone secretion. Attempts have been made to correlate circulating concentrations of aldosterone and progesterone (Ledoux *et al.*, 1975; Weinberger *et al.*, 1976; Smeaton *et al.*, 1977) or plasma aldosterone and components of the renin–angiotensin system (Chesley, 1974; Weir *et al.*, 1975; Ledoux *et al.*, 1975; Weinberger *et al.*, 1976) in normal pregnant women. Although some correlation between plasma aldosterone and progesterone can be shown when data are grouped, there is no apparent correlation in the values in individual subjects. In toxaemia of pregnancy the aldosterone secretion rate and peripheral concentration are significantly decreased (Watanabe, Meeker, Gray, Sims and Solomon, 1965; Weinberger *et al.*, 1976) whereas plasma progesterone is normal (Weinberger *et al.*, 1976). Similarly, no strong correlation could be found between plasma aldosterone and plasma renin activity in normal pregnant women. However, some 65% of the renin routinely measured in pregnancy plasma by a method involving an acidification step is "inactive" renin of chorionic origin (Skinner, Cran, Gibson, Taylor, Walters and Catt, 1975). It has been suggested (Becker, Jayashi, Franks and Speroff, 1978) that if plasma renin activity is measured without the acidification step there is a better, though not perfect, correlation with plasma aldosterone concentration. As previously discussed, aldosterone secretion decreases in toxaemia, whereas plasma angiotensin II and plasma renin activity may remain in the normal pregnant range (Gordon, Symonds, Wilmshurst and Pawsey, 1973). It is of interest to note that in one case report of a woman who was toxaemic during an abdominal pregnancy both plasma renin activity and plasma aldosterone were greatly elevated over the values found in normal pregnant women by these authors (Baehler, Copeland, Stein and Ferris, 1975). Plasma sodium concentration is lower in the pregnant than in the non-pregnant woman (MacDonald and Good, 1972; Weir et al., 1975) and the urinary excretion of sodium following saline infusion was significantly lower in pregnant than in non-pregnant women (Weinberger et al., 1977) suggesting that a physiological need for sodium conservation exists. It is not possible at the present time to give one precise cause for the elevated aldosterone secretion seen in human pregnancy; a complex interplay of the factors discussed undoubtedly is involved, and there may yet be other important relationships to be discovered.

25. Foetal

In man information about aldosterone production by the foetus has been obtained from in vitro studies (Dufau and Villee, 1969), from experiments on previable foetuses aborted at mid-term (Pasqualini, Wiqvist and Diczfalusy, 1966), or from cord blood samples obtained at term (Bayard et al., 1970; Beitins et al., 1972; Katz, Beck and Makowski, 1974; Godard, Gaillard and Vallotton, 1976).

Dufau and Villee (1969) found that foetal adrenals, incubated in vitro would produce aldosterone from 16 weeks of gestation. Pasqualini et al. (1966) demonstrated that corticosterone infused into the foetal-placental unit at mid-term was converted to aldosterone. At term the concentration of aldosterone in foetal plasma was equal to, or greater than, that in maternal blood (Bayard et al., 1970; Beitins et al., 1972; Katz et al., 1974; Godard et al., 1976). Aldosterone appeared to cross the human placenta freely in both directions but Bayard et al. (1970) estimated that 80% of the foetal plasma aldosterone originated in the foetus. At mid-term Pasqualini (1971) found, in two cases, that if ^{3}H-aldosterone were injected into the umbilical vein and 15 min later the foetus was delivered, 28% of the injected radioactivity could be recovered from the maternal urine over the subsequent three days.

The suggestion that foetal blood aldosterone is of foetal origin in man is also supported by the findings of Pakraven, Kenny, Depp and Allen, 1974, of zero values in the umbilical arterial and venous blood of a boy with congenital absence of the adrenal glands. More information on foetal adrenal aldosterone production has come from animal experiments. Giry and Delost (1977) showed that the guinea-pig foetal adrenal content of aldosterone increased from day 62 until term (67 days) as did foetal plasma aldosterone concentration, which was less than the concentrations in maternal samples obtained simultaneously.

In the mouse the foetal plasma aldosterone increased over the three days preceding birth and at birth were seven days times those in maternal plasma (Dalle, Giry, Gay and Delost, 1978). Incubation of adrenals from term rat foetuses yielded approximately 10 ng/mg adrenal/hr (28 pmol/mg adrenal/hr) of aldosterone, and the output was doubled if the mothers were sodium deficient (Schneider and Mulrow, 1973). The only species in which extensive studies of foetal aldosterone secretion have been made over an extended period of gestation is the sheep. It has been shown that the adrenal glands of the foetus can secrete aldosterone when incubated *in vitro* from as early as day 40 of a gestation period of 147 $\pm$ 5 days (Wintour, Brown, Denton, Hardy, McDougall, Oddie and Whipp, 1975). At this time the adrenal cortex contains only one cell type, which is also capable of secreting cortisol and corticosterone, and is unusual for a steroid-producing cell in that it contains almost no agranular endoplasmic reticulum (Wintour, Brown, Denton, Hardy, McDougall, Robinson, Rowe and Whipp, 1977).

During acute *in vivo* studies adrenal secretion rates of aldosterone of 115–238 ng/hr (319–660 pmol/hr) were recorded in foetuses 110–134 days gestation by Alexander, Britton, James, Nixon, Parker, Wintour and Wright (1967) which accord well with values of 36–320 ng/hr (100–880 pmol/hr) in foetuses 118–140 days gestation in a later study (Wintour *et al.*, 1975). Aldosterone has been measured in the peripheral blood of acutely killed ovine foetuses from 60 days until term in concentrations equal to or greater than that in maternal blood (Wintour *et al.*, 1975), but one-seventieth of that in foetal adrenal venous blood. The concentration of aldosterone in the peripheral blood of chronically cannulated ovine foetuses of 96 or more days gestation is comparable to that found in the acutely sacrificed animals (Brown, Coghlan, Hardy and Wintour, 1978). Thus it seems well established that the foetal adrenals of a number of species do secrete aldosterone. The factors which regulate the foetal aldosterone production have been investigated via a number of approaches. Established stimuli to aldosterone production in the adult of most species are: sodium deficiency, increased plasma $[K^+]$, increased activity of the renin–angiotensin system and an acute elevation of ACTH. In order to test these putative stimuli on the foetal adrenal two major approaches may be made.

In the first approach a wide range of gestational ages, beginning with the very young (one-quarter of the total duration of gestation) foetal adrenals may be removed and incubated *in vitro* with or without putative stimulus. The pregnant ewes providing the foetuses may be in a state of sodium balance or deficiency. The complication involved in this type of experiment is that associated with all *in vitro* experiments—the information gained concerns what the gland *can* do, not necessarily what it does do *in vivo*.

A second type of investigation makes use of chronically cannulated foetuses from which peripheral blood may be collected in a variety of circumstances in which one or more putative stimulus operates. There are a number of complications here:

(i) Only foetuses during the latter half of gestation can be studied.

(ii) Unless it can be established that a substantial fraction of the aldosterone in the foetal peripheral blood is of foetal adrenal origin, rather than arising via transplacental passage from the mother, this approach will not prove fruitful. Studies in progress would now suggest that, in the ovine foetus, more than 80% of the aldosterone in foetal peripheral blood is of maternal origin until approximately 130 days (term 147 ± 5 days).

(iii) It is not easy to manipulate the environment of the foetus, e.g. to induce sodium deficiency, as it is to alter the environment of the adult. When the urine was drained constantly to the exterior of a sheep foetus over a six-day period, resulting in the loss of 1·42 l fluid containing a total of 61 mol of sodium, which was greater than the total exchangeable sodium of the foetus at that period (106 days gestation), plasma sodium concentration was normal as was the blood aldosterone concentration of 1·6 ng/100 ml (63 pmol/l) (Wintour, personal observation). With these reservations in mind one can examine the results so far obtained.

(a) ACTH

In vitro ACTH was able to stimulate aldosterone production from ovine foetal adrenal glands from as early as day 40 of a 147 ± 5 day gestation period (Wintour *et al.*, 1975). The effect of a tripling of aldosterone production rates with ACTH was observed until about four weeks before term, at which time the magnitude of the effect was decreased but ACTH remained a potent stimulus to aldosterone production *in vitro*. *In vivo*, in chronically cannulated ovine foetuses, ACTH infused intravenously for 90 min into foetuses 90 days until term, did not produce a consistent change in the peripheral blood aldosterone concentration (Brown *et al.*, 1978).

It would now seem that this result was partly due to the previously mentioned complication of transplacental passage of aldosterone.

(b) Increased K^+

In vitro ovine foetal adrenal glands will not produce increased quantities of aldosterone when incubated in a medium in which $[K^+]$ has been elevated from 4 to 8 mmol/l until late in gestation (Wintour *et al.*, 1975). Elevation of plasma $[K^+]$ in the chronically cannulated foetus does not significantly increase blood aldosterone concentration at any stage, suggesting that the ability to respond to this stimulus is developed late in ontogeny, and perhaps not until after birth (Wintour, unpublished observations).

(c) Angiotensin II

To date angiotensin II has been investigated only with *in vitro* preparations. When adrenals of ovine foetuses of less than 100 days gestation (two-thirds of total) were incubated with angiotensin II (2·5 ng/ml), there was a significant increment in aldosterone production rate (Wintour *et al.*, 1977). The ability of the adrenal to respond to AII appeared to disappear as the gestation period increased, only to return just at term.

(d) Sodium deficiency

As stated previously, it is difficult to produce a state of sodium deficiency in a foetus with an intact placental circulation. In ewes which have been made extremely sodium deficient, with maternal blood aldosterone values of 77–280 ng/100 ml (2·2–7·7 pmol/l), and plasma $[Na^+]$ decreased from 147 ± 3 to 135 ± 5 mmol/l, the foetal plasma $[Na^+]$ was essentially unchanged, and the foetal adrenals when incubated *in vitro* produced no more aldosterone than control adrenals (Wintour *et al.*, 1977). Adrenals taken from normal foetuses and incubated in a medium of low sodium (130 mmol/l) for 2 hr did not produce more aldosterone than age matched adrenals incubated in a medium with a $[Na^+]$ of 140 mmol/l. The gestation of the foetuses supplying these adrenals was 125–127 days, and it would be interesting to see if similar results occurred in either much younger animals or those close to term.

The ability of the foetal adrenal to secrete aldosterone and the factors which might regulate it are of some interest because aldosterone may act to alter the composition of foetal urine *in utero*, and foetal urine is important in amniotic fluid production in the last half of gestation (Minei and Suzuki, 1976). Pasqualini, Sumida and Gelly (1972) showed that both cytosol and nuclear receptors for aldosterone were present in the kidneys of foetal guinea-pigs about halfway through gestation. In the near-term foetal rat kidney there is an increasing amount of a Na-K ATPase which can be abolished by maternal adrenalectomy combined with metopirone treatment, but restored by injection of aldosterone (Geloso and Basset, 1974), suggesting that there are receptors for aldosterone in the foetal rat kidney. In the chronically cannulated ovine foetus the sodium:potassium ratio of the urine can be reduced by the infusion of aldosterone from two-thirds of the way through gestation (Lingwood, Coghlan, Hardy and Wintour, 1978).

T

E. PATHOLOGICAL VARIATIONS

The clinical picture and the tissue pathology in the disease states described below are usually well known and these aspects have been reviewed frequently by others. The commentary will emphasise the nature of the adrenal response with particular reference to aldosterone, and the mechanism causing the variation from normal as far as this is known.

1. Diseases of the Adrenal Cortex

(a) Primary hyperaldosteronism

Primary hyperaldosteronism (Conn's Syndrome, Conn, 1955) is a syndrome characterised by hypertension, muscle weakness, hypokalemic alkalosis and excessive K excretion. It is associated with elevated aldosterone production and suppressed renin levels. Although estimates of the incidence of the disorder have varied from 1–20% of the hypertensive population, more recent estimates suggest it may be as low as 0·01% (Tucker and Labarthe, 1977). Although this disorder was first associated with an aldosterone-secreting adenoma it is now recognised that a high proportion of patients have a similar syndrome associated with bilateral hyperplasia (George, Wright, Bell and Bartter, 1970; Baer, Sommers, Krakoff, Newton and Laragh, 1970). The disorder appears to be less severe in this latter group and aldosterone levels are not as high nor renin levels as suppressed as those with an adenoma (Baer et al., 1970). A further sub-group of glucocorticoid suppressible aldosterone is described in the following section.

Evaluation and screening of patients with essential hypertension for Conn's syndrome led to the recognition of a larger group of patients (15–20%) who also had suppressed plasma renin levels in response to Na restriction or postural change. Assessment of aldosterone production in these patients for inappropriate hypersecretion has led to numerous studies into the control of aldosterone in primary hyperaldosteronism.

On normal Na intakes (100–180 mmol/day) aldosterone secretion (Biglieri, Slaton, Schambelan, Kronfield, 1968; Cain, Tuck, Williams, Dluhy and Rosenoff, 1972), excretion (Biglieri, Slaton, Kronfield and Schambelan, 1967; Baer et al., 1970; Deck, Champion and Conn, 1973) and plasma levels are elevated (Oddie, Coghlan and Scoggins, 1972; Cain et al., 1972) above those seen in essential hypertension or normotensive subjects. The low total body K status of the patients may produce plasma aldosterone levels which are only in the upper range of normal (Kem, Weinberger, Mayes and Nugent, 1971; Brown, Chinn, Davies, Dusterdieck, Fraser,

Lever, Robertson, Tree and Wiseman, 1968). However, correction of the K deficit by oral K loading increases aldosterone secretion above that observed in normals (Slaton, Schambelan and Biglieri, 1969; Cain *et al.*, 1972). Plasma cortisol levels are normal in the syndrome but a significant proportion of patients have elevated levels of corticosterone and of DOC (Biglieri *et al.*, 1968); Oddie *et al.*, 1972) presumably due to altered bio-synthetic pathways in the adenoma or hyperplastic adrenal.

Restriction of Na intake to 10 mmol/day produces an increase in aldosterone secretion (Cain *et al.*, 1972), excretion and plasma levels (Cain *et al.*, 1972). However, the response is somewhat less than that observed in normals. The suppressed, but usually detectable, levels of plasma renin or angiotensin II may also show small but significant increases in response to Na restriction and upright posture (Stockigt, Collins and Biglieri, 1971).

On a high Na intake aldosterone production may be suppressed but plasma levels will remain significantly above those in other types of hyper-tension (Cain *et al.*, 1972; Helber, Kauffman, Maurer, Steiner, Durr, Euchenhofer, Wurz and Streicher, 1973). Similarly, administration of an intravenous saline load results in incomplete suppression of aldosterone (Espiner, Christlieb, Amsterdam, Jagger, Dobrzinsky, Lauler and Hickler, 1971; Kem *et al.*, 1971; Weinberger and Donohue, 1973). In another study intravenous expansion of plasma volume has been used to evaluate aldosterone suppression (George, Wright, Bell, Bartter, Brown, 1970). Immersion to the neck, a manoeuvre which suppresses aldosterone in normals, has no effect in primary aldosteronism (Crane and Harris, 1973).

Exogenous mineralocorticoid administration has also been used as a suppressive manoeuvre and neither DOCA (Cain *et al.*, 1972; Biglieri, Stockigt and Schambelan, 1972) nor 9α-fluorohydrocortisone (Biglieri *et al.*, 1970; Padfield, Allison, Brown, Ferriss, Fraser, Lever, Luke and Robertson, 1975) reduce aldosterone production.

ACTH plays an important role in the regulation of aldosterone in Conn's Syndrome. As in normals there is a diurnal rhythm of plasma aldosterone in supine patients which is closely associated with changes in cortisol (Kem, Weinberger, Gomez-Sanchez, Kramer, Lerman, Furuyama and Nugent, 1973; Schambelan, Brust, Chang, Slater and Biglieri, 1976). Episodic secretory episodes of aldosterone are observed and are also usually in parallel to changes in cortisol (Vetter, Berger, Armbruster, Siegenthaler, Werning and Vetter, 1974; Kem, Weinberger, Gomez-Sanchez, Higgins and Kramer, 1976). Administration of ACTH increases aldosterone secretion in primary aldosteronism but as in normals the response is transient (Newton and Laragh, 1968; Cain *et al.*, 1972). A recent study by Kem, Weinberger, Higgins, Kramer, Gomez-Sanchez and Holland (1978) has shown an in-creased responsiveness to infused ACTH with the rise in aldosterone being similar to that observed in normals on a low Na diet. Observations were made in those with hyperplasia and adenoma after dexamethasone suppression. This increased responsiveness was not seen in patients with low renin essential hypertension.

Dexamethasone administration may result in a reduction of plasma aldosterone (Vetter *et al.*, 1974), suppression of its episodic fluctuations (Kem *et al.*, 1976) and loss of the diurnal rhythm (Kem *et al.*, 1973). This does not always occur and there is considerable variability between individual patients. Even in the face of dexamethasone suppression hypersecretion of aldosterone persists (Cain *et al.*, 1972). Two interesting features have been observed. In the first study it has been shown that the fall in plasma aldosterone of up to 50% with dexamethasone is not sustained beyond 24 hr (Ganguly, Chavarri, Luetscher and Dowdy, 1977). The mechanism of the increase in aldosterone which occurs cannot be explained and may be due to an intrinsic stimulus within the adrenal tissue. In the second study it has been possible by using the suppression with dexamethasone to differentiate a group of patients with adenoma who have "ACTH dependent" aldosteronism. In this group dexamethasone produces a pronounced and sustained fall in aldosterone. Further, this group do not respond to angiotensin II. The remainder showed the transient fall with dexamethasone and a good angiotensin II response (Wenting, Man, IntVeld, Derkx, Brummelau and Schalekamp, 1978). In both groups a good response to ACTH was seen. The dexamethasone suppressible group do not fit the criteria for glucocorticoid-remediable aldosteronism (Sutherland, Ruse and Laidlaw, 1966).

While supine, patients with hyperplasia and adenoma have a normal diurnal rhythm of plasma aldosterone; on standing a significant difference is observed between the two groups (Ganguly, Dowdy, Luetscher and Melada, 1973; Schambelan, Brust, Chang, Slater and Biglieri, 1976). In those with hyperplasia an increase was seen and this rise as in normals was associated with a small rise in renin. With an adenoma a paradoxical fall in aldosterone was observed.

While studies have shown that angiotensin II can stimulate aldosterone secretion in primary aldosteronism (Spark, Dale, Kahn and Melby, 1969; Wenting *et al.*, 1978) a number of reports have failed to find a reproducible response (Horton, 1969; Slatton *et al.*, 1969).

Overall these studies suggest a considerable degree of heterogeneity in the primary aldosterone population and this probably accounts for the variability in the response to stimulatory and suppressive manoeuvres. The patients with adenomas appear to be more under the control of ACTH compared with those with hyperplasia who may show correlations with plasma renin (Schambelan *et al.*, 1976). It is clear that the aldosterone secretion in this disorder is not autonomous with perhaps the exception of those in which an adrenal carcinoma is involved.

The pathogenesis of bilateral hyperplasia is still not known and it has been proposed that an unidentified extra-adrenal stimulus may be involved (Coghlan et al., 1972). The report by Nicholls, Espiner, Hughes, Ross and Stewart (1975) of an aldosterone-stimulating substance in the plasma of a patient with hyperplasia has not been confirmed.

Preoperative differentiation of patients with an adrenal adenoma from those with hyperplasia is important because of the poor blood pressure response to surgery in the latter group (Biglieri, Schambelan, Slaton and Stockigt, 1970; Baer et al., 1970). A number of approaches have been described and are useful in making the distinction. These include (i) correlation of renin suppression with that for aldosterone after DOCA administration (Stockigt, Collins and Biglieri, 1971; Biglieri, Stockigt and Schambelan, 1972), (ii) multifactorial quadratic analysis of aldosterone, renin, Na and K values (Ferriss, Brown, Fraser, Kay, Lever, Neville O'Muirchearthaigh, Robertson and Symington, 1970) and (iii) the paradoxical fall in plasma aldosterone with morning ambulation in those with an adenoma (Ganguly et al., 1973).

Measurement of aldosterone in adrenal venous effluent has been also applied to the identification of the site of aldosterone adenomas (Melby, Spark, Dale, Egdahl and Kahn, 1967; Scoggins, Oddie, Hare and Coghlan, 1972; Horton and Finck, 1972; Nicolis, Mitty, Modlinger and Gabrilove, 1972; Ganguly et al., 1973; Espiner, Jameson, Perry, Miles, 1976). Although it is preferable to obtain blood from both adrenal veins it is not always possible to cannulate the right adrenal vein. An approach using the gradient of left adrenal vein to inferior vena cava for both aldosterone and cortisol has been developed and successfully used (Scoggins et al., 1972). This method has the disadvantage that it is difficult but not impossible to differentiate bilateral adrenal hyperplasia from a unilateral adenoma. The use of renal vein samples rather than adrenal vein collections has been suggested by Fukuchi, Takenouchi, Nakajima and Watanabe (1975). However, this approach may lead to errors in diagnosis if the right adrenal vein has direct drainage into the vena cava. The application of adrenal arteriography and venography to localisation of the aldosteronomas has been described by Kahn, Kelleher, Egdahl and Melby (1971) and Lee, Lin and Sibala (1973) but as an approach it is limited because of the small size of many of the tumours. An alternative approach has been the use of ^{131}I-19-iodocholesterol scintigraphy of the adrenal (Conn, Morita, Cohen, Beirwaltes, McDonald and Herwig, 1972) and this technique has been successfully applied in primary aldosteronism by Hogan, McRae, Schambelan and Biglieri (1976). It may well have a role in separation of adenoma from hyperplasia (Nakamura, Sawai, Fukuchi, Nakajima, Abe and Hoshino, 1975).

After unilateral adrenalectomy aldosterone production from the remaining adrenal may remain suppressed for a considerable period of time (Diglieri, Slaton, Silen, Galente and Forsham, 1966; Schambelan, Stockigt and Biglieri, 1972). The suppressed renin levels sometimes take some weeks to recover but it has been suggested by Morimoto, Takeda and Murakami (1970) that pre-operative spironolactone treatment may hasten the recovery. Although this may be true, hypoaldosteronism may still persist and the response to Na deprivation may be blunted (Bravo, Dustan and Tarazi, 1975). It is possible that spironolactone is itself inhibiting aldosterone biosynthesis (Erbler, 1974). Inhibition of aldosterone in this syndrome has also been observed following heparin administration (Ford and Bailey, 1966).

(b) Glucocorticoid-suppressible hyperaldosteronism

Glucocorticoid-suppressible hyperaldosteronism was first described by Sutherland et al. (1966) and has been identified in members of five other families (Miura, Yoshinaga, Goto, Katsushima, Maebashi, Demura, Iino, Demura and Torikai, 1968; New, Siegal, Peterson, 1973; Giebink, Gotlin, Biglieri and Katz, 1973; Stockigt, Coghlan, Oddie and Scoggins, 1975; Grim, Weinberger and Anand, 1977). A familial connection has been observed in all cases except those of Miura et al. (1968) and Stockigt et al. (1977). The syndrome has identical features to that of primary hyper-aldosteronism except that the hyperaldosteronism and hypertension are corrected by dexamethasone and the patients are usually younger than those seen with Conn's syndrome.

Although the aetiology of the hyperaldosteronism is not well understood, the proposal by Grim et al. (1977) of increased adrenal responsiveness to ACTH requires confirmation. Although dexamethasone suppression has been widely evaluated in other types of hyperaldosteronism the treatment is usually short term (up to 48 hr) and this may be too short a time to correct the hypersecretion in this syndrome (Giebink et al., 1973). These patients can be contrasted to the group with ACTH-dependent primary aldosteronism described by Wenting et al. (1978) who have an adenoma rather than hyper-plasia as the adrenal lesion.

(c) Pseudohyperaldosteronism: Liddle's syndrome

This disorder, first described by Liddle, Bledsoe and Coppage (1963), is characterised by hypertension, hypokalemic alkalosis and suppressed renin activity. Aldosterone secretion is negligible. A total of seven families with this syndrome have been described and evidence of a familial disorder is apparent in four of them (Liddle *et al.*, 1963; Aarskog, Stoa, Thorsen and Wefring, 1967; Milora, Vagnucci and Goodman, 1967; Helbock and Reynolds, 1970; Gardner, Lapey, Simopoulos and Bravo, 1971; Ohno, Harada, Komatsu, Saijo and Miyoshi, 1975; Wang, Chan, Yeung, Coghlan, Oddie, Scoggins and Stockigt, 1978). Untreated, the patients show little aldosterone or plasma renin response to Na restriction or Na loading, posture, ACTH, dexamethasone suppression or short term treatment with triamterene or spironolactone (Wang *et al.*, 1978).

Treatment with triamterene—an inhibitor of renal tubular ion transport—and a low Na diet corrects the disorder in blood pressure, K balance and may produce an increase in aldosterone secretion (Aarskog *et al.*, 1967). Studies in one patient (Wang *et al.*, 1978) would suggest that reduction in Na intake is important if aldosterone secretion is to be restored.

(d) Addison's disease (primary hypoadrenalism)

In this condition there is a characteristic, generalised adrenal insufficiency which is well demonstrated by a failure to show a significant steroid response to administration of ACTH (Christy, Wallace and Jailer, 1955; Eik-Nes, Sandberg, Migeon, Tyler and Samuels, 1955). Plasma concentrations of ACTH (Bethune, Nelson and Thorn, 1957; Meakin, Nelson and Thorn, 1959) and renin (Brown, Davies, Lever, Robertson and Tree, 1964d; Peart, 1965b) are elevated which is consistent with feedback considerations for both glucocorticoid and aldosterone regulation. Plasma concentrations of aldosterone calculated from secretion rate and metabolic clearance rate were very much less than normal in three cases reported by Kono *et al.* (1966). The MCR was significantly increased. Aldosterone secretion rate and excretion are essentially zero (New *et al.*, 1966), whilst renal excretion of sodium, salivary Na/K ratio (Frawley and Thorn, 1951) and sweat sodium concentration demonstrate an inability to conserve sodium. The condition is characterised by a marked hypotension. High sodium supplements plus glucocorticoid therapy sustain life in humans but mineralocorticoid supplements are essential in other species. Administration of ACTH to patients with Addison's disease on a high Na intake resulted in an aldosterone secretion rate of $54 \pm 13\,\mu g/day$ ($150 \pm 36\,nmol/day$), a value much less than the $541 \pm 210\,\mu g/day$ ($1501 \pm 583\,nmol/day$) found in normals on a similar Na intake (Tucci *et al.*, 1967). In the study of a patient with isolated glucocorticoid deficiency a failure of aldosterone to respond to ACTH has been observed (Spark and Etzkorn, 1977). Responses to a low Na diet and upright posture were normal. It has been postulated that the defect may be at the site of adrenal ACTH receptor.

(e) *Pseudohypoaldosteronism*

This unusual congenital salt-losing disorder was first described by Cheek and Perry (1958) and is characterised by severe Na wasting, weakness, dehydration and hyperkalemia. Aldosterone and renin levels are very high but often show little response to dietary Na manipulation and exogenous mineralocorticoid administration (Proesmanns, Geussens, Corbeel, Eeckels, 1973; Postel-Vinay, Alberti, Ricour, Lamal, Rappaport and Royer, 1974). Even though baseline plasma aldosterone levels are very high they have been shown to respond to angiotensin II, KCl and ACTH in this disorder (Rosler, Theodor, Boichis, Gerty, Ulick, Alagem, Tabachnik, Cohen and Rabinowitz, 1977). Treatment with a high Na intake produces clinical improvement. However, in the majority of the children with increasing age a spontaneous improvement occurs. Under these circumstances aldosterone secretion remains very high (8–10 times normal) but with little renal Na loss even on a normal diet. It has been proposed that the defect is a distal tubular insensitivity to aldosterone. A variant of this disorder with salivary and sweat Na loss rather than renal loss has also been described (Anand, Froberg, Northway, Weinberg and Wright, 1976). The disorder may have an autosomal dominant mode of inheritance (Limal, Rappaport, Dechaux, Riffaud and Morin, 1978).

(f) *Congenital adrenal hyperplasia*

The major dysfunction is due to a deficiency in the enzyme systems responsible for hydroxylation (Eberlain and Bongiovanni, 1955, 1956; Ch. V). As a result there is reduced secretion of 21-hydroxylated steroids, notably cortisol, resulting in elevated ACTH release, and increased adrenal secretion of 17α-hydroxyprogesterone and other androgenic steroids causing virilism. Plasma renin levels are elevated. The condition has been classified for convenience into a Na-losing variety and a non-Na losing virilising form. While it is well recognised that aldosterone production is low in the Na-losers (New, Miller and Peterson, 1966) it is now thought that the aldosterone deficiency of the Na-losers is a more severe expression of the same defect that occurs in the non-Na-losers (Godard, Riondel, Veyrat, Megevand and Muller, 1968; Rosler, Levine, Schneider, Novogrodev and New, 1977). Others have failed to distinguish the two groups on the basis of plasma renin and aldosterone measurements and the response to Na depletion (Strickland and Kotchen, 1972). A number of studies have examined the control of aldosterone in these two groups of patients. In the untreated salt losers aldosterone production or plasma levels are low with the lowest values being found in those with the greatest tendency to lose Na

(Kowarski, Finkelstein, Spaulding, Holman and Migeon, 1965; Bryan, Kliman and Bartter, 1965; New *et al.*, 1966; Loras, Haour and Bertrand, 1970; Pham-Huu-Trung, Raux, Gourmelen, Baron and Girard, 1976). The response to ACTH is poor (Pham-Huu-Trung *et al.*, 1976; Limal, Rappaport and Bayard, 1977) in either treated or untreated subjects. In the non-salt losing form aldosterone secretion is high and usually responds to Na restriction. Secretion falls to the normal range with exogenous corticosteroid treatment (Dahl, Rivarola and Bergada, 1972). It is proposed that the high concentration of aldosterone may compensate for the excessive secretion of steroid metabolites with a Na-losing tendency (progesterone and 17-hydroxyprogesterone). After ACTH administration over three days to non-Na losers it was found that aldosterone plasma levels and secretion were significantly increased over pre-ACTH levels (Beitins, Bayard, Kowarski and Migeon, 1972). In normal subjects ACTH produced only a transient increase in aldosterone secretion and plasma levels.

In a number of older children and adults with the Na-losing defect the plasma aldosterone levels may be elevated after prolonged treatment with cortisol. This increase in aldosterone appeared to be age related and occurred during puberty (Limal, Rappaport and Bayard, 1977). Their ability to respond to Na-losing crises and to ACTH was still impaired. These authors proposed the use of 9α-fluorocortisol to control the Na-losing tendency in this group and to avoid high dosages of cortisol. 9α-Fluorocortisol blunted the aldosterone response to ACTH.

Recently it has been shown by Rosler *et al.* (1977) in a study of seven patients treated with either suppressive doses of dexamethasone or replacement doses of glucocorticoid, that there is no clear distinction between the two types of the disorder. Patients showed varying degrees of Na depletion which was expressed in their plasma renin activity measurement. In those with a Na-losing tendency, renin was inappropriately elevated compared with aldosterone. They propose that rigorously controlled mineralocorticoid replacement should be given to all patients with the disorder. This group has also shown an important interrelationship between Na balance, ACTH secretion and the renin-angiotensin system in this disorder. This was reflected in an increase in plasma ACTH levels which were correlated to plasma renin during Na depletion in patients on replacement levels of glucocorticoid. When in positive Na balance due to mineralocorticoid replacement ACTH and plasma renin levels were normal and aldosterone excretion fell to < 0.1 µg/day (< 0.3 nmol/day).

(g) Other enzymic defects

(1) 18-Hydroxylation. Biosynthetic defects in aldosterone production may

lead to hypoaldosteronism and the existence of a salt-wasting disorder. These defects usually occur in children and it may be difficult to define precisely the cause of Na wasting. Dillon and Ryness (1975) have proposed the use of the aldosterone–plasma renin profile to aid in diagnosis.

Ulick (1976) has described the two inborn errors which occur in the final stages of aldosterone biosynthesis. These are:

(i) Corticosterone methyl oxidase defect Type 1. This is a defect in the first stage of the conversion of corticosterone to aldosterone and is characterised by very high corticosterone production relative to that of either aldosterone or 18OH-corticosterone. Plasma renin levels are high. Individuals with this defect have been described by Visser and Cost (1964); Degenhart, Frankena, Visser, Cost and van Seters (1966); Jean, Legrand, Meylan, Rieu and Astruc (1969) and Priscu, Maiorescu and Sischitu (1972).

(ii) Corticosterone methyl oxidase defect Type 2. A defect in the latter stage of the biosynthetic pathways leads to over-production of both corticosterone and 18OH-corticosterone relative to aldosterone (Ulick, Gautier, Vetter, Markello, Yaffe and Lowe, 1964; Milla, Trompeter, Dillon, Robins and Shackleton, 1977; David, Golan and Drucker, 1968; Rappaport, Dray, Legrand and Royer, 1968). A defect in cortisol production has also been reported in one of these cases (David, Asnis and Drucker, 1972).

A familial salt wasting syndrome with high levels of renin associated with inappropriately low levels of aldosterone has been described in five Jewish families in Iran (Rosler, Theodos, Gazit, Biochis and Rabinowitz, 1973). Detailed biochemical studies have shown a Type 2 enzyme block. A detailed evaluation of these families and the nature of their disorder has been described (Rosler, Rabinowitz, Theodor, Ramirez and Ulick, 1977). The best diagnostic feature was the ratio of the major urinary metabolites of 18OH-corticosterone to aldosterone. This value, normally less than 3, is greater than 100 in affected individuals. The aldosterone response to infusions of KCl and ACTH was normal in these patients but angiotensin II failed to increase aldosterone. It is proposed that this disorder is transmitted by an autosomal recessive gene (Cohen, Theodor and Rosler, 1977).

Both types of 18-hydroxylation defects have been successfully treated with exogenous mineralocorticoid and a high sodium intake.

(2) *17-Hydroxylation.* The syndrome of 17-hydroxylase deficiency was first described by Biglieri, Herron and Brust (1966). It is characterised by hypertension, hypokalaemia and a deficiency of gonadal steroid due to impaired biosynthesis of cortisol, androgens and oestrogens resulting in high levels of ACTH and excessive DOC and corticosterone production. The lack of oestrogens and androgens results in hypogonadism in females (Biglieri *et al.*, 1966; Goldsmith, Solomon and Horton, 1967; Mills, Wilson, Tait and Copper, 1967; Mallin, 1969; Linquette, Dupont, Radadot, Lefebvre, May

and Cappoeun, 1971; De Lange, Weeke, Artz, Jansen and Doorenbos, 1972; Wang, Yeung, Coghlan, Oddie, Scoggins and Stockigt, 1978) and pseudo-hermaphroditism in males (New, 1970; Mantero, Busnardo, Riondel, Veyrat and Austoni, 1971; Bricaire, Luton, Laudat, Legrand, Turpin, Corvol and Lemmer, 1972; Alvarez, Cloutier, Hales, 1973; Kershnar, Borut and Kogut, 1973; Tournaire, Audi-Parera, Loras, Blum, Castelnovo and Forest, 1976). It is of interest that in this syndrome aldosterone levels are often low and plasma renin is suppressed (Wang et al., 1978). With reversal of renin suppression in a number of patients aldosterone levels have risen (Goldsmith et al., 1967; New, 1970), while in others the aldosterone remains low (Bricaire et al., 1972; Biglieri and Mantero, 1973). It has been suggested that an associated defect in 18-dehydrogenation may be involved (Bricaire et al., 1972). However, in our patient (Wang et al., 1978) after prolonged prednisolone treatment aldosterone returned to normal. A combined 17α- and 18-hydroxylase deficiency has been reported in a male and was associated with hypoaldosteronism and very low levels of 18-OHDOC and 18OH-corti-costerone production (Waldhausl, Herkner, Nowotny and Bratusch-Marrain, 1978).

(3) *11-Hydroxylation*. Patients with a defect of 11-hydroxylation are hypertensive and virilised and exhibit hypokalemic alkalosis (hypertensive virilising congenital hyperplasia). Aldosterone levels are low and the features of mineralocorticoid excess are probably due to excessive DOC production (New and Seaman, 1970). Cortisol and corticosterone secretion are very low and unlike the secretion of their precursors do not respond to ACTH. Aldosterone does not respond to Na deprivation. This is in contrast to patients with a 21-hydroxylase defect. After dexamethasone treatment has suppressed the excessive DOC production a normal aldosterone response to Na restriction may be observed (New and Seaman, 1970; Sizonenko, Riondel, Kohlberg and Paunier, 1972). It is possible that this may be due to existence of the 11-hydroxylation defect only in the zona fasciculata. Aldosterone can also be increased by ACTH after dexamethasone and Na restriction (Sizonenko et al., 1972). Other cases have been described by Loras, Dazord, Roux and Bertrand (1971).

2. Diseases of other Endocrine Glands

(a) Anterior pituitary

The major pituitary disorders affecting the adrenal cortex are due to a variable degree of: (i) impaired synthesis or release of ACTH—hypo-pituitarism, (ii) over-secretion of ACTH—Cushing's disease. These conditions result in chronic hyposecretion or hypersecretion of cortisol with

adrenal atrophy or hyperplasia, respectively. A separate causative circum-
stance might be increased adrenal sensitivity to ACTH (Christy, Longson
and Jailer, 1957) or a factor such as the adrenal weight-maintaining factor
(Jailer, Longson and Christy, 1957). The pituitary–adrenal system was
reviewed by Liddle et al. (1962) and is described in Ch. V.

In hypopituitarism, aldosterone secretion appears to be only slightly
impaired. Watanabe (personal communication) found normal aldosterone
secretion rates in patients with panhypopituitarism, selective ACTH
deficiency and in hypophysectomised patients on sodium intake of 100
mmol/day. Aldosterone secretion increased to 400–500 µg/day (1·1–1·4
µmol/day) when sodium intake was reduced to 10 mmol/day. This measure
of independence of zona glomerulosa function in man is consistent with the
relatively unimpaired secretory capacity for aldosterone seen in chronically
hypophysectomised animals (Blair-West et al., 1964c; Bartter et al., 1964a).

Severe mineralocorticoid excess is not a feature of Cushing's disease.
Ross, Marshall-Jones and Friedman (1966) reviewed the findings in 50 cases
of Cushing's syndrome. Forty-five patients had bilateral adrenocortical
hyperplasia, but whatever the cause, hypokalemic alkalosis was consistently
absent in all 50 patients. Aldosterone secretion was not elevated. Corticosterone secretion rate is not usually elevated in Cushing's syndrome,
excepting patients with adrenal carcinoma (Biglieri, Hane, Slaton and
Forsham, 1963) and deoxycorticosterone secretion is often normal (Crane
and Harris, 1966). One group has reported that the increased blood pressure
depends upon the renin-angiotensin system. This was demonstrated by the
use of 1-S,ar-8-Ala analogue of angiotensin II (Dalakos, Elias, Anderson,
Streeten and Schroeder, 1978). However, the plasma renin concentration
was reported as elevated which is in contrast to many reports of normal or
suppressed values.

(b) Carcinoma of endocrine and other organs

There are now a substantial number of cases demonstrating adrenocortical
hyperplasia associated with carcinoma of the thymus, mediastinum and
pancreas but most frequently of the bronchus. Hypokalaemic alkalosis with
hypertension is frequently associated with the condition, particularly when
the primary lesion is not located in the adrenal gland. In many cases, the
hyperplastic adrenal cortex appears to be due to high blood levels of ACTH
or an ACTH-like substance released from the malignant tissue (Meador,
Liddle, Island, Nicholson, Lucas, Nuckton and Luetscher, 1962; Liddle,
Island, Ney, Nicholson and Shimizu, 1963). The subject has been reviewed
recently by Cope (1964b), O'Riordan, Blanshard, Moxham and Nabarro
(1966) and Friedman, Marshall-Jones and Ross (1966) (see Ch. IV). The hypokalaemic alkalosis does not appear to be associated with increased aldosterone

secretion. There is a very high cortisol production and this has been held responsible for the hypokalaemia. Corticosterone secretion may be increased, based upon the single case of Biglieri *et al.* (1963). Crane and Harris (1966) have suggested that increased production of deoxycorticosterone is responsible. The high mineralocorticoid activity displayed may be due to the joint contributions of these three steroids. (See also section on primary reninism.)

(c) *Thyroid gland*

Early studies based on aldosterone excretion in patients with abnormalities of thyroid function indicated that this parameter was normal other than when sodium intake was low (Lieberman and Luetscher, 1960). Later studies, however, were more definitive (Luetscher, Cohn, Camargo, Dowdy and Callaghan, 1963). These findings are set out in Table 9 with normal values from Tait *et al.* (1961). Similar studies have been carried out by Kono *et al.* (1966) with similar results. The subjects in the study of Luetscher *et al.* (1963) were on unrestricted sodium diet. The data suggest that aldosterone secretion rate in myxoedema is below the mean normal value. After treatment these subjects showed a significant rise, not revealed by the mean values presented in Table 9. The metabolic clearance rate was also significantly reduced. The initial volume of distribution V^1 may be larger than normal. In the hyperthyroid group the value for $\bar{V}$ (intercept of second component of the disappearance curve) is reduced while the overall clearance rate is elevated though the secretion rate is not commensurately elevated. The euthyroid group were essentially normal. In sodium restricted hyperthyroid patients the aldosterone secretion was blunted compared with normals in that the peripheral concentration was very much lower 47 ± 4 ng/100 ml (1304 ± 111 pmol/l) *vs.* 96 ± 9 ng/100 ml (2664 ± 250 pmol/l). This occurred in the face of the fact that the plasma renin concentration was higher than normal. Treatment with propranolol resulted in a significant fall in plasma renin concentration but the fall in aldosterone secretion was not significant (Cain, Dluhy, Williams, Selenkow, Milick and Richmond, 1973). Similar findings in hypothyroidism following propranolol treatment have been reported by Ogihara, Yamamoto, Muyal and Kumahara (1973).

Because Myers, Brannon and Holland (1950) have shown that liver blood flow is not increased in hyperthyroidism, the increased metabolic clearance in the hyperthyroid cases above would have to be extra-hepatic (see Section B.3). Renal blood flow is also increased. Luetscher *et al.* (1963) did not find any significant alteration in the pattern of urinary metabolites between the three groups. This is rather unexpected if as a result of the increased clearance of aldosterone the normal ratio between the liver and kidney had been disturbed. This question was also raised by Kono (1966).

Table 9

Aldosterone in thyroid disease.

Classification	V^1	$\bar{V}$	MCR (1/day)	Secretion rate (μg/day)[b]	Calc. peripheral level (ng/100 ml)[c]	References
Normal (5)	27	80	1620	130	7·7	Tait et al. (1961)
Hypothyroid (3)	43	80	1000	67	6·7	Luetscher et al. (1963)
Hyperthyroid (4)	–	58	1920	108	5·6	Luetscher et al. (1963)
Euthyroid (7)[a]	31	81	1340	100	7·5	Luetscher et al. (1963)

[a] Same subjects after treatment.
[b] 1 μg/day = 2·775 nmol/day.
[c] 1 ng/100 ml = 27·75 pmol/l.

(d) Renal disease

The renin–angioetensin system has been reviewed (Ch. XI). The kidney and probably the juxtaglomerular cells are the major source of the enzyme renin under normal circumstances. Studies demonstrating a causal link between the kidney, the renin–angiotensin system and the adrenal glomerulosa zone pointed to the importance of an endocrine function of the kidney in renal disease and other conditions associated with hyperaldosteronism. There is a great number of reports of pathological states with elevated renin or angiotensin blood level but only conditions in which the kidney disease may be primary will be described here. At the outset it should be emphasised that significant variations of aldosterone secretion in these patients may be due to resting sodium balance and may be complicated by treatment with low sodium diet, diuretics, aldosterone antagonists and other drugs.

(1) Accelerated hypertension. The hyperaldosteronism found in patients with severe hypertension is usually associated with excessive renin and angiotensin produced presumably due to progressive renal ischemia (Hollenberg, Epstein, Basch, Couch, Hicker and Merrill, 1969). Control of blood pressure usually results in a fall in both renin and aldosterone (McAllister, Van Way, Dayani, Anderson, Temple, Michelakis, Coppage and Oates, 1971). On a number of occasions high levels of aldosterone may persist even after a fall in plasma renin and it has been postulated that either there is an additional factor stimulating aldosterone or aldosterone secretion has become "autonomous". Beevers, Brown, Ferriss, Fraser, Lever, Robertson and Tree (1976) felt it was unlikely that autonomous aldosterone-secreting adenomata arise as a consequence of prolonged secondary aldosteronism after reviewing 136 cases of primary aldosteronism.

(2) Renal hypertension. Experimental studies have shown that renin and aldosterone are only transiently elevated following unilateral renal clamping (Blair-West, Coghlan, Denton, Orchard, Scoggins and Wright, 1968). Subsequently, elevated levels of aldosterone are found if Na depletion occurs. This hyperaldosteronism is associated with increased plasma renin concentration. In patients with renal artery stenosis levels of both renin and aldosterone are very variable (Vaughan, Buhler, Laragh, Sealey, Baer and Bard, 1973). This probably reflects the differences in Na and volume status of the individual patients. If hyperaldosteronism does exist both DOCA (Biglieri, Schambelan and Stockigt, 1972) or saline infusion (Kem, Weinberger, Mayes and Nugent, 1971) will reduce production as in normal subjects.

(3) Primary reninism. This rare syndrome first described by Robertson, Klidjian, Harding, Walters, Lee and Robb-Smith (1967) is characterised by

high levels of renin unresponsive to changes in Na intake, hyper-aldosteronism and severe hypokalaemic alkalosis (Kihara, Kitamura, Hoshino, Seida and Watanabe, 1968, Chambelan, Howen, Stockigt, Nooker and Biglieri, 1973; Brown, Fraser, Lever, Morton, Robertson, Tree, Bell, Davidson and Ruthven, 1973). The hypertension can be cured by surgical removal of the tumour-containing kidney. Wilm's tumour (Mitchell, Baxter, Blair-West and McCredie, 1970) is also associated with excessive production of renin. A single case of hyperaldosteronism associated with increased plasma renin activity and an oat cell carcinoma of the lung has been reported (Hauger-Klevene, 1970). The plasma renin levels may be responsive to postural change and they show a diurnal rhythm (Conn, Cohen, Lucas, McDonald, Mayor, Blough, Eveland, Bookstein and Lapides, 1972).

(4) *Chronic renal failure.* As in many other renal disorders there is con-siderable variation in aldosterone levels in patients with chronic renal insufficiency. Aldosterone levels are closely correlated with renin levels (Brown, Dusterdieck, Fraser, Lever, Robertson, Tree and Weir, 1971; Weidmann, Maxwell, Lupu, 1973; Paton, Lever, Oliver, Medina, Briggs, Morton, Brown, Robertson, Fraser, Tree and Gavras, 1975). In a recent study, Weidmann, Maxwell, de Lima, Hirsch and Franklin (1975), on patients with terminal renal failure and on dialysis, found close correlations between plasma renin, plasma K and plasma aldosterone in response to upright posture or ACTH. The response to dialysis was variable but if aldosterone rose it was closely correlated with renin.

(5) *Renal transplantation.* Investigations of the interrelationships between the renin–angiotensin system and aldosterone have been carried out in renal transplant recipients to examine the role of renal denervation on the response to Na restriction and upright posture. Although there is con-siderable variation between studies in the blood pressure of patients and the period of time from transplantation to investigation a number of generalisations can be made.

In an early study, Greene, Vander and Kowalczyk (1968) found a normal aldosterone and plasma renin response to Na restriction. Increases in plasma aldosterone (Keogh, Kirdani, Sandberg, Mittleman and Murphy, 1976; Pedersen and Kornerup, 1976; Sufrin, Kirdani, Sandberg and Murphy, 1978) and urinary aldosterone excretion (Bennett, McDonald, Lawson and Porter, 1974) together with an increase in plasma renin activity in response to dietary Na restriction has been found by most investigators in both hypertensive and normotensive recipients. Aldosterone and renin levels are also suppressed normally after intravenous Na loading (Keogh *et al.*, 1976) or a high Na diet (Bennett *et al.*, 1974; Pedersen and Kornerup, 1976). Sampson, Kirdani, Sandberg and Murphy (1972) reported elevated aldosterone secretion with normal renin in 11 patients but have subsequently reported normal plasma levels with elevated secretion rates suggesting an abnormality in clearance (Sufrin *et al.*, 1978). In the first few days after transplantation renin and aldosterone are both elevated probably due to some renal ischemia (Beckerhoff, Uhlschmid, Vetter, Armbruster and Siegenthaler, 1974). Elevated levels of aldosterone excretion were also reported by Cooke *et al.* (1973). It is probable that elevated levels of plasma K contribute to the raised aldosterone production. The aldosterone response to postural change also appears to be normal in the majority of transplant patients (Greene *et al.*, 1968; Cooke *et al.*, 1973; Beckerhoff *et al.*, 1974; Pedersen and Kornerup, 1976). The circadian rhythm of aldosterone in non-steroid treated transplant patients is as found in normals (Olgaard, Madsen, Roosen and Hammer, 1977). Patients treated with prednisone have an inverse circadian rhythm of aldosterone as well as in urinary Na and K excretion (Olgaard *et al.*, 1977).

(6) *Juxtaglomerular hyperplasia (Bartter's syndrome).* This syndrome is characterised by hypokalemic alkalosis, hyperaldosteronism, elevated levels of renin and is associated with juxtaglomerular cell hyperplasia (Bartter, Pronove, Gill and McCardle, 1962). Blood pressure is normal and pressor response to infused angiotensin II or norepinephrine is reduced. The excessive aldosterone secretion can not be suppressed by Na loading or by volume expansion (Bartter *et al.*, 1962). Aldosterone secretion was not increased by infusion of human renin (Bryan, Kliman, Gill and Bartter, 1964). Increases in aldosterone may be seen after dietary Na restriction (Bryan, MacCardle and Bartter, 1966). The elevated renin secretion in the syndrome can be reduced with propranolol as occurs in hypertensives. Aldosterone levels also fell to within the normal range but the hypokalemia persisted (Modlinger, Nicolis, Krakoff and Gabrilove, 1973). A diurnal rhythm of renin was also seen in this patient when supine on a high Na diet. In other patients it has been possible to suppress aldosterone while hypokalemia is present. However, with restoration of plasma K by K loading a high Na intake will no longer suppress aldosterone to normals levels (Solomon and Brown, 1975). In two patients infused with the angiotensin analogue [Sar^1-Ile^8-AII] before treatment a decrease in plasma aldosterone and blood pressure was seen (Sasaki, Okumura, Ikeda, Kawasaki, Fukiyama, 1976; Sasaki, Okumura, Asano, Arakawa, Kawasaki, 1977). After indomethacin the analogue raised blood pressure but had no effect on the basal levels of aldosterone (Sasaki *et al.*, 1977).

Cases reported before 1968 were reviewed in detail by Cannon, Leeming, Sommers, Winters and Laragh (1968) who postulated that the disorder was a type of Na-losing nephritis leading to hypersecretion of renin and aldosterone rather than a resistance to the pressor action of angiotensin II as proposed by Bartter. Defects in both proximal and distal sites of Na reabsorption have been implicated (Tomko, Yeh and Falls, 1976). Alterations in erythrocyte Na transport in Bartter's syndrome have been reported and further suggested a defect in cation transport (Gull, Vaitukaitis, Haddow and Klein, 1971; Gardner, Simipoulos and Shibolet, 1972). Trans-epithelial ion transport is also altered in the parotid gland (Heidland, Kreusser, Henneman, Krauf and Wigand, 1972).

It has been established that elevated prostaglandin (PGE$_2$) excretion was associated with the syndrome, and that inhibition of prostaglandin synthetase would correct the abnormalities in K, renin and aldosterone (Bartter, Gill, Frolich, Bowden, Hollifield, Radfar, Keiser, Oates, Seyberth and Taylor, 1976). Within two or three days indomethacin decreased PGE excretion by 69% and resulted in a 79% fall in renin and a 52% fall in aldosterone excretion in the supine subject (Gill, Frolich, Bowden, Taylor, Keiser, Seyberth, Oates and Bartter, 1976). The pressor responsiveness of angiotensin II is also restored. From similar studies Fichmann, Telfer, Zia, Speckart, Golub and Rude (1976) using propranolol or indomethacin suggested that the syndrome was due to β-adrenergic and prostaglandin-mediated proximal tubular rejection of Na leading to increased distal Na–K exchange. Demonstration of hyperplasia of the interstitial medullary cells—the site of prostaglandin synthesis further supported a role for a primary defect in renal prostaglandin production (Verberckmoes, van Damme, Clement, Amery and Michielsen, 1976; Donker, de Jong, van Eps, Brentjens, Bakker and Doorenbos, 1977). It was proposed that increased prostaglandins led to decreased Na reabsorption, volume depletion and hyper-secretion of renin and aldosterone. While a number of studies have shown a fall in aldosterone with indomethacin, there are exceptions (Bowden, Gill, Radfar, Taylor and Keiser, 1978).

Two additional studies (Halushka, Wohltmann, Privitera, Hurwitz and Margolius, 1977; Vinci, Gill, Bowden, Pisano, Izzo, Radfar, Taylor, Zusman, Bartter and Keiser, 1978) have established a close relationship between the changes in prostaglandins and the kallikrein–kinin system in this syndrome. It is proposed that the high bradykinin levels may cause the decreased pressor response to angiotensin II. Studies in normal man have examined the interrelationships between bradykinin, renin–angiotensin and aldosterone (Mersey, Williams, Hollenberg and Dluhy, 1977). However, neither acute elevation of angiotensin II nor K-induced increases in aldosterone were associated with increases in plasma bradykinin.

(7) *Hypoaldosteronism with hyporeninism.* A disorder of adults characterised by hyperkalemia with absent or reduced aldosterone but with no evidence of a biosynthetic enzyme defect and now known to have subnormal levels of plasma renin was first described by Hudson, Chobanian, Relman (1957). A comprehensive evaluation of the syndrome has been published by Schambelan, Stockigt and Biglieri (1972). Other cases in which control of

aldosterone secretion has been investigated include those by Perez, Siegel and Schreiner (1972), Sparagana (1975), Brezis and Litvin (1977) and Rado, Simatupang, Boer and Dorhout-Mess (1977). A large number of the patients also have diabetes mellitus (Sparagana, 1975; Kuhlmann, Vetter, Fischer and Siegenthaler, 1978).

Aldosterone does not respond normally to Na depletion, ACTH or K and plasma renin also fails to show the expected increase in response to upright posture and Na depletion. A distinction from Addison's disease and other defects with hypoaldosteronism can be made on the basis of the renin levels. Infusion of angiotensin II results in a significant rise in plasma aldosterone (Brown, Chinn, Fraser, Lever, Morton, Robertson, Tree, Waite and Parke, 1973) and it is suggested that the primary defect is a deficiency of renin.

In a number of ways these patients resemble those with autonomic insufficiency since this disorder is also associated with subnormal and unresponsive aldosterone and renin (Gordon *et al.*, 1967; Slaton and Biglieri, 1967). Patients can be successfully treated with exogenous mineralocorticoid (9α-fludrocortisone) which augments renal hydrogen ion secretion, corrects the hyperkalemia, increases ammonia excretion, and subsequently reduces the metabolic acidosis (Sebastian, Schambelan, Lindenfeld and Morris, 1977).

(*8*) *Essential hypertension.* The role of the renin–angiotensin and aldosterone systems in essential hypertension has been intensively studied for the past 20 years. This alone would justify the classification under renal. It is beyond the scope of this chapter to review in depth the progress that has been made. However, it is appropriate to summarise the present status of a number of different aspects relating to the control of aldosterone secretion in patients with essential hypertension.

It is generally accepted that aldosterone secretion, excretion and plasma levels are normal in the majority of essential hypertensive subjects. There are exceptional reports of increased plasma aldosterone levels (Genest, Nowaczynski, Kuchel, Boucher and Rojo-Ortega, 1977). There are a number of abnormalities in the control system that are apparent when aldosterone secretion is either stimulated or suppressed. These will be discussed below. Examination of the control of secretion in patients with essential hypertension was prompted by the observation that 20–25% of them had either a blunted, or nil response in plasma renin activity to Na depletion or upright posture (Helmer and Judson, 1968; Coghlan, Doyle, Jerums and Scoggins, 1972). It soon became clear that these patients—low renin–essential hypertension—did not have primary aldosteronism because aldosterone levels were normal. It has been proposed that these patients have hypersecretion of an adrenal mineralocorticoid. This evidence has been reviewed by Melby and Dale (1975), Liddle and Sennett (1975) and Genest *et al.* (1977). Measurements of plasma K, total body sodium, plasma volume or ECFV support this contention.

Incomplete suppression of aldosterone following Na loading by either a high Na intake or by intravenous saline loading has been shown in hypertensive patients (Weinberger, Dowdy, Nokes and Luetscher, 1968; Luetscher, Weinberger, Dowdy, Nokes, Balikian, Brodie and Willoughby, 1969; Collins, Weinberger, Dowdy, Nokes, Gonzales and Luetscher, 1970; Re, Sancho, Klemen and Haber, 1977). The rate of fall of plasma aldosterone in response to saline loading is also much slower in hypertensive subjects and no significant fall in either aldosterone or renin was observed until 120–140 min after starting the infusion. In normotensive subjects aldosterone had fallen in 20–30 min (Tuck, Williams, Dluhy, Greenfield and Moore, 1976). A number of other groups have not found significant differences between normals and the varying groups of hypertensive patients in response to Na loading (Kem, Weinberger, Mayes and Nugent, 1971; Espiner *et al.*, 1971; Luft, Grim, Willis, Higgins and Weinberger, 1977). Kawasaki, Delea, Bartter and Smith (1978) were able to identify a group who were "salt sensitive". This group appeared to intrinsically retain salt without any evident abnormalities in renin or aldosterone.

The aldosterone response to acute haemorrhage and to diuretic-induced volume depletion has been shown to be blunted in hypertensive patients Williams, Rose, Dluhy, McCaughn, Jagger, Hickler and Lauler, 1970). This lack of responsiveness occurred in both "normal" and "low renin" hypertensive patients. No differences in the response to ACTH was observed. Others have shown a subnormal response to Na restriction in patients with low renin (Collins *et al.*, 1970), while others have found a poor aldosterone response in association with normal increases in renin (Christlieb, Hickler, Lauler and Williams, 1969; Streeten, Schletter and Clift, 1969).

The aldosterone response to angiotensin II was shown to be similar in both normotensive and hypertensive subjects on both high Na and Na restricted diets by Mendelsohn *et al.* (1972). However, in contrast to this study Kisch, Dluhy and Williams (1976) have shown an increase in sensitivity for the aldosterone response to angiotensin II in hypertensive patients on a high Na intake. This same group (Moore, Williams, Dluhy, Bauli, Himathongkam and Greenfield, 1977) found that on a low Na diet, a group of normal renin hypertensive patients who had decreased sensitivity to angiotensin II compared with normotensive subjects. Taken together, these data suggest that hypertensive patients show a different response to Na-induced changes in adrenal sensitivity to angiotensin II (Williams, Dluhy and Moore, 1977). It has also been established that in low renin essential hypertension there is an increased sensitivity to angiotensin II when dexamethasone suppressed on a high Na intake when compared with either normal renin hypertensive patients or normal subjects (Wisgerhof and Brown, 1978). It was felt this could explain the dissociation of the renin–angiotensin–aldosterone axis often seen in these patients.

Although it has been reported that there is altered aldosterone metabolism in some patients with essential hypertension (Genest *et al.*, 1977) this finding has not been confirmed (Brown *et al.*, 1976). In this latter study the metabolic clearance rate was similar in both normal and low renin hypertension to that found in control subjects.

The very large number of papers concerning the use of angiotensin inhibiting analogues or converting enzyme inhibitor are reviewed elsewhere (Ch. XI). A recent paper using converting enzyme inhibitor showed that aldosterone appeared to rise in patients in the erect position despite this blockade (Gavras, Gavras, Textor, Volicer, Brunner and Rucinska, 1977).

(9) *Miscellaneous renal disorders.* There are a number of other renal disorders associated with hyperaldosteronism. These include nephrotic syndrome (Luetscher, Johnson, Dowdy, Hanery, Lew and Poo, 1954; Laragh, 1962), renal tubular acidosis (Gill, Bell, Bartter, 1967; Sebastian, McSherry and Morris, 1971). (See also Coghlan and Blair-West, 1967, and Coghlan *et al.*, 1971.)

3. Diseases of Non-endocrine Organs

(a) Cardiac failure

Malignant hypertension, trauma, severe sodium-losing or oedematous conditions and other clinical states may lead to circulatory failure and effects on aldosterone secretion in these states have been discussed in relation to the primary condition. The changes seen in uncomplicated congestive cardiac failure will be described here. There is often an abnormal tendency to retain dietary sodium resulting in oedema along with a reduction of renal blood flow and glomerular filtration rate (Merrill, Morrison and Brannon, 1946; Mokotoff, Ross and Leiter, 1948). Since early studies of Deming and Luetscher (1950) demonstrating high levels of deoxycorticosterone-like material in the urine of patients with congestive cardiac failure, and the demonstration by Simpson *et al.* (1953) that this substance was aldosterone, there have been several reports of increased urinary aldosterone excretion in this condition (Luetscher and Johnson, 1954b; Muller, Riondel, Manning and Mach, 1956; Wolff, Koczorek and Buchborn, 1958). However, estimates of aldosterone secretion rate have shown wide variation in untreated subjects on normal electrolyte intake, with many cases within the normal range (Ulick *et al.*, 1958; Laragh, 1962; Sanders and Melby, 1964; Camargo *et al.*,

1965; Hickie and Lazarus, 1966). Several workers have claimed that the high secretion rates often seen are the result of treatment with diuretics and low salt diet (Stuart-Harris, Cox, Leonard and Singer, 1962; Cox, Davies-Jones and Leonard, 1964; Hickie and Lazarus, 1966). Although aldosterone secretion may be near normal in untreated patients, several recent studies have suggested that the peripheral concentration of aldosterone may be nonetheless elevated. Tait, Bougas, Little, Tait and Flood (1965) found clearance rate, 800 ± 65 (s.e.) l/day, and hepatic extraction 71 ± 5 (s.e.)% in seven subjects with severe cardiac dysfunction. These values were substantially less than the mean levels in normal subjects, 1630 l/day and 93% respectively. The metabolic clearance rate was 1330 ± 140 (s.e.) l/day and splanchnic extraction was 89 ± 3 (s.e.)% in nine subjects with minimal cardiac dysfunction. Camargo et al. (1965), Cheveille et al. (1966) and Vecsi, Dusterdiech, Jahnecke, Lommer and Wolff (1969) demonstrated that hepatic clearance and extraction of aldosterone were reduced in patients with severe congestive failure. Plasma clearance rate was reduced in three of eight patients with mild to moderate dysfunction. The lowered metabolic clearance rate may be due to either decreased extraction and/or hepatic blood flow. The volume of distribution V^1 was reduced to 4·5 l (27 l normal). Aldosterone secretion rate was slightly above the normal range in only four of 13 patients (Camargo et al., 1965). Hickie and Lazarus (1966) found normal secretion rates of aldosterone in eight of 11 subjects but usually reduced metabolic clearance rate. Even though the secretion rate of aldosterone may be within the normal range, plasma concentrations of aldosterone may be higher than normal in subjects with cardiac dysfunction. High peripheral levels were observed by Wolff et al. (1964) but only in patients with sodium retention and ascites.

Notwithstanding this early evidence more recent studies (Coghlan et al., 1972; Nicholls, Espiner, Donald and Hughes, 1974; Vandongen and Gordon, 1970) have demonstrated that in untreated congestive cardiac failure the aldosterone peripheral concentration is low, together with renin. After treatment with spironolactone or diuretics these parameters may even fall to lower values until "dry weight" is reached when they both rise sharply.

The inescapable conclusion from these studies is that the plasma aldosterone concentration, although normal, is a crucial element in the sodium retention of congestive cardiac failure. Certainly the condition is partly attributable to renal insufficiency but the importance of increased sensitivity to aldosterone may be of cardinal importance (see Section A.2).

(b) Liver disease

The metabolism of aldosterone is carried out mostly in the liver (see Section

B.3), so that impaired hepatic function due to disease or possibly inborn enzyme defects might modify the plasma concentration and urinary excretion of aldosterone and its metabolites. In the case of cortisol, the half-life in plasma is prolonged and the turnover rate is decreased in hepatitis and hepatic cirrhosis but the miscible pool and plasma concentration are normal demonstrating a reduction of cortisol secretion by a negative feedback system (Peterson, 1960).

In hepatic cirrhosis the proportions in the urine of free aldosterone and of the 18-glucuronide are increased and the tetrahydroaldosterone fraction is decreased (Hurter and Nabarro, 1960; Coppage et al., 1962). The half-life of aldosterone is prolonged from an average of about 30 min (Tait et al., 1961; Wolff et al., 1964) to 40–90 min (Coppage et al., 1962; Wolff et al., 1964). It has been shown that experimental hepatic venous congestion in the dog also increased the half-life of aldosterone (Ayers, Davis, Lieberman and Carpenter, 1960) and causes increased aldosterone secretion (Orloff, Ross, Baddeley, Nutting, Spitz, Sloop, Neesby and Halasz, 1964). Peterson (1964) reported peripheral concentrations of aldosterone of 88 and 56 ng/100 ml (2442 and 1554 pmol/l) in two patients with severe and moderate cirrhosis respectively, compared with a normal mean value of 6·6 ng/100 ml (183 pmol/l). Urinary excretion of aldosterone was also greatly increased. Wolff et al. (1964) found normal concentrations (60 ng/100 ml (1665 pmol/l) by their method) in two of four patients without ascites but elevated levels (90–550 ng/100 ml; 2·5–15·3 nmol/l) in all six subjects with ascites. The question arises whether the high plasma concentration of aldosterone in cirrhosis, particularly in cases with oedema and ascites, is due to aldosterone hypersecretion or to impaired degradation. Of course, whether the patients are on treatment or not, and what stage, may be an important consideration just as is the case with congestive cardiac failure. In a careful study, Rosoff, Zia, Reynolds and Horton (1975) showed that although the reduced clearance rate (Coghlan et al., 1972; Tait et al., 1965; Camargo et al., 1965) contributes to the elevated plasma concentration increased secretion rate was the major contributing factor.

Plasma renin shows a positive correlation with plasma aldosterone concentration in most studies, for example Rosoff et al. (1973); Epstein, Levinson, Sancho, Haber and Re (1977); Vetter, Vetter, Beckerhoff, Glanger, Furrer, Hahn, Kolloch, Kruck, Kutz, Siegenthaler and Witassek (1977); Schroeder, Anderson, Goldman and Streeten (1976). However, renin was dissociated from plasma aldosterone during β-adrenergic blockade (Wilkinson, Bernadi, Smith, Jowett, Slater and William, 1977). Wilkinson et al. (1977) also found a better association between sodium excretion and plasma aldosterone concentration than did other groups. The general consensus was that other factors were more important in renal sodium retention than aldosterone. Once again renal sensitivity may be the crucial factor (see Section B.2).

4. Diseases of Non-endocrine Organs

(a) *Idiopathic oedema*

The literature on idiopathic oedema was reviewed by Luetscher, Dowdy, Arnstein, Lucas and Murray (1964b) and Edwards and Bayliss (1976). Reduced excretion of sodium and increased output of aldosterone are typical. Luetscher *et al.* (1964b) found the mean excretion of aldosterone-18-glucuronide in 14 subjects was 23·4 μg/day (44 nmol/day) compared with 10·7 μg/day (20 nmol/day) in 10 normals from another study. Aldosterone secretion rate was elevated in some cases and an interesting feature of their results was that, in some patients on high sodium intake, aldosterone secretion was within the normal range. Others have found renin and aldosterone peripheral blood concentration to be normal (Streeten, Dalakos, Souma, Fillerman, Clift, Schletter, Stevenson and Spetter, 1973; Oelkers, Rawer, Wrecterholt, Schonshofer and Palicki, 1977; Katz, 1977; Oelkers, Mapen, Molyahn and Hammerstein, 1975). Low sodium diet, elevation of the legs, diuretics and aldosterone antagonists usually result in successful management but in severe cases subtotal or total adrenalectomy provide relief. Histologically the adrenal glands are usually normal (Streeten, Louis and Conn, 1960).

Certain features of the disorder are of particular interest. Many patients show persistent sodium retention and massive weight gain during mineralocorticoid administration in contrast with the "escape" phenomenon shown by normal subjects (August *et al.*, 1958). This difference may be attributable to an abnormally high activity in these patients of the "extra-adrenal factor essential for chronic sodium retention" described by Davis *et al.* (1964) or the "peripheral sensitising factor" described by Blair-West *et al.* (1963b) in sodium depleted animals. Some patients show cycles of oedema and diuresis not related to the menstrual cycle (Thorn, 1957) and this is similar to the recurrent "escape" of normal subjects during DOC administration (Lee, Nelson and Thorn, 1961). The activity of the "sensitising factor" referred to above fluctuates in proportion to the total body sodium balance and the possibility exists that in patients with cyclic sodium retention and excretion, during the retention phase, the sensitising factor is progressively inhibited leading to a natriuresis. This causes sufficient sodium loss to increase the activity of the sensitising factor initiating another retention period. The proposal suggests essentially a reset of the sodium status at which the sensitising factor is evoked or abolished. Failure to escape would not be supported by the studies of Edwards and Bayliss (1976).

Serum potassium concentration is normal in most patients with idiopathic oedema. Sodium retention is aggravated by the upright posture and strikingly relieved by prolonged recumbency. Luetscher *et al.* (1964b) suggested that the aetiology is an exaggeration of the circulatory changes which normal man makes on assuming the upright posture but that postural hypotension was not common in these patients. They pointed out that sympathomimetic agents are often useful in management and thought that this might be related to the observation that these drugs may depress aldosterone secretion (Laragh, Angers, Kelly and Lieberman, 1960c). Mechanisms governing aldosterone response to postural change have been described in Section D.15. If the controlling system is mediated by increased activity of the sympathetic nervous system and release of catecholamines (Gordon *et al.*, 1966a) effective management by catecholamine therapy would indicate that the aetiology is more complex than a simple exaggeration of the normal mechanism. The role of other factors such as ADH, which was implicated by the studies of Streeten, Louis and Conn (1960), or dopamine (Kuchel, Cuche, Bure, Guthrie, Ungar, Nowaczynski, Boucher and Genest, 1977) will have to be further experimentally and clinically assessed.

(b) Miscellaneous

As aldosterone methodology has become more generally available measurements have been made in a variety of syndromes. This has been especially so when disorders of fluid or electrolyte balance are a feature of the disorder.

In patients with the syndrome of inappropriate antidiuretic hormone secretion (SIADH) basal plasma aldosterone levels and the response to angiotensin II, ACTH, upright posture and Na deprivation are similar to those seen in normal subjects (Fichman *et al.*, 1974). However, a clear dissociation between plasma renin and aldosterone is seen after Na restriction in both SIADH and normal subjects given ADH and water. Water restriction in SIADH results in increased plasma renin and aldosterone. In another study dissociation between renin and aldosterone was observed following water restriction but in contrast to the earlier reports a fall in plasma aldosterone was observed (Fyhrquist, Holmberg, Perheentupa and Wallenius, 1977). A further example of a marked dissociation between renin and aldosterone has been observed in a case of diabetes insipidus with adipsia (Schalekamp, Bever-Donker, Jansen-Goemans, Fawzi and Muller, 1976).

Under a condition of hypernatremia associated with Na depletion high renin levels were associated with low to normal aldosterone values

Autonomic insufficiency is associated with low levels of aldosterone and renin which are not normally responsive to upright posture or Na deprivation (Slaton and Biglieri, 1967; Gordon *et al.*, 1967). Prevention of postural hypotension by catecholamine infusion resulted in an augmented aldosterone and renin response to postural change (Gordon *et al.*, 1967). Lowered aldosterone secretion rates have also been reported in patients with autonomic failure (Wilcox, Aminoff and Slater, 1977). Two similar patients with postural hypotension had adequate responses to sodium restriction and tilting (Hedeland, Dymling and Hokfelt, 1969). These variable responses may be related to the degree of autonomic impairment.

In familial dysautonomia (Riley-Day syndrome) there is a dissociation between renin and aldosterone and a paradoxical response is shown to postural change (Rabinowitz, Landau, Rosler, Moses, Rotem and Freier, 1971; Landau, Friedman, Rosler, Moses, Freier, Rotem and Rabinowitz, 1977).

In Parkinson's disease there are reports of low concentrations of renin and aldosterone (Barbeau, Gillo-Joffery, Boucher, Nowaczynski and Genest, 1969; Michelakis and Robertson, 1970). These findings have not been confirmed by Wilcox *et al.* (1977).

In acromegaly, changes similar to those reported in patients with essential hypertension have been published (Caine, Williams, Dluhy, 1972; Werning, Schwerkert, Stuel, Vetter and Siegenthaler, 1970). Others have found symptoms more like those of primary aldosteronism (Strauch, Vallotton, Touilou and Bricaire, 1972).

Aldosterone secretion or excretion has been reported as normal in cystic fibrosis (Montalvo, McCaa and Cole, 1968), Duchenne muscular dystrophy (Garst, Vignos, Hadadey and Matthews, 1977) and myosthenia gravis (Kimura, Nakamoto, Nakamura and Ota, 1966).

Pseudo hyper-aldosteronism can be caused by excessive liquorice ingestion (Epstein, Espiner, Donald and Hughes, 1977) or laxative abuse (Fleming, Genuth, Gould and Kamionkowski, 1975).

There have been a number of reports of derangements in Na metabolism in psychiatric illness. Aldosterone excretion has been found to be lower in depressed patients than those with mania (Murphy, Goodwin and Bunney, 1969). In a single patient, Jenner, Gjessing, Cox, Davies-Jones, Hullin and Hanna (1967) reported the opposite. Further studies on patients with bipolar manic-depressive psychosis have shown changes in aldosterone with mood changes (Allsopp, Levell, Stitch and Hullin, 1972). Levels of aldosterone appear to be inappropriate for the plasma renin activity (Hullin, Jerram, Lee, Levell and Tyrer, 1977).

REFERENCES

Aarskog, D., Stoa, K. F., Thorsen, T. and Wefring, K. W. (1967). *Pediatrics*, **39**, 884.

Abelson, D. and Bondy, P. K. (1955). *Arch. Biochem. Biophys.* **57**, 208.

Abelson, D. and Brooks, R. V. (1960). *In* "Quantitative Paper Chromatography of Steroids" (D. Abelson and R. V. Brooks, eds), 1st edition. Cambridge University Press, Cambridge.

Abraham, S. F., Blair-West, J. R., Coghlan, J. P., Denton, D. A., Mouw, D. R. and Scoggins, B. A. (1976). *Acta endocr., Copenh.* **81**, 120.

Abraham, R. and Staudinger, Hj. (1964). *Z. Clin. Chem.* **2**, 16.

Adam, W. R. and Funder, J. W. (1977). *Clin. Exp. Pharmacol. Physiol.* **4**, 283.

Adamson, A. R. and Jamieson, S. W. (1972). *J. Endocr.* **53**, 425.

Aguilera, G. and Catt, K. J. (1978). *Proc. nat. Acad. Sci. USA.* (In Press).

Aguilera, G., Hauger, R. L. and Catt, K. J. (1978). *Proc. nat. Acad. Sci. USA.* **75**, 975.

Akesode, A., Migeon, C. J. and Kowarski, A. A. (1977). *J. clin. Endocr. Metab.* **45**, 849.

Al Dujali, E. A. S. and Edwards, C. R. W. (1978). *J. clin. Endocr. Metab.* **48**, 105.

Alexander, D. P., Britton, G. H., James, V. H. T., Nixon, D. A., Parker, R. A., Wintour, E. M. and Wright, R. D. (1968). *J. Endocr.* **40**, 1.

Allsop, M. N. E., Levell, M. J., Stitch, S. R. and Hullin, R. P. (1972). *Br. J. Psychiat.* **120**, 399.

Alvarez, M. N., Cloutier, M. D. and Hayles, A. B. (1973). *Pediat. Res.* **7**, 325.

Ames, R. P., Borkowski, A. J., Sicinski, A. N. and Laragh, J. H. (1965). *J. clin. Invest.* **44**, 1171.

Anand, S. K., Froberg, L., Northway, J. N., Weinberger, M. and Wright, J. C. (1976). *Pediat. Res.* **10**, 677.

Anderson, N. S. and Fanestil, D. D. (1976). *Endocrinology,* **98**, 676.

Antunes, J. R., Dale, S. L. and Melby, J. C. (1976). *Steroids,* **28**, 621.

Aragones, A., Aros, E. G., Lantos, C. P. and Luciano, G. A. (1976). *J. Steroid Biochem.* **4**, 175.

Armbruster, H., Vetter, W., Beckerhoff, R., Nussberger, J., Vetter, H. and Siegenthaler, W. (1975). *Acta endocr., Copenh.* **80**, 95.

August, J. T., Nelson, D. A. and Thorn, G. W. (1958). *J. clin. Invest.* **37**, 1549.

Axelrad, B. J., Cates, J. E., Johnson, B. B. and Luetscher, J. A. (1955). *Br. med. J.* **i**, 196.

Ayers, C. R., Davis, J. O., Lieberman, F. and Carpenter, C. C. J. (1960). *Abst. endocr. Soc.* **42**, 17.

Ayers, C. R., Davis, J. O., Lieberman, F., Carpenter, C. C. J. and Berman, M. (1962). *J. clin. Invest.* **41**, 884.

Ayers, P. J. (1961). *Nature, Lond.* **191**, 79.

Ayres, P. J., Barlow, J., Garrod, O., Kellie, A. F., Tait, J. F., Tait, S. A. S. and Walker, G. (1958). *In* "An International Symposium on Aldosterone", p. 73. Churchill, London.

Ayres, P. J., Garrod, O., Simpson, S. A. and Tait, J. F. (1957a). *Biochem. J.* **65**, 639.

Ayres, P. J., Gould, R. P., Simpson, S. A. and Tait, J. F. (1956). *Proc. biochem. Soc.* **63**, 19.

Ayres, P. J., Simpson, S. A. and Tait, J. F. (1957b). *Biochem. J.* **65**, 647.

Baehler, R. W., Copeland, W. E., Stein, J. H. and Ferris, T. F. (1975). *Am. J. Obstet. Gynec.* **122**, 545.

Baer, L., Sommers, S. C., Krakoff, L. R., Newton, M. A., Laragh, J. H. (1970). *Circ. Res.* **26, 27** (Suppl. I), 203.

Bailey, R. E., Bartos, D., Bartos, F., Castro, A., Dobson, R. L., Grettie, D. P., Kramer, R., Macfarlane, D. and Sato, K. (1972). *Experentia*, **28**, 159.

Bailey, R. E. and Ford, H. C. (1969). *Acta endocr., Copenh.* **60**, 249.

Balikian, H. M., Brodie, A. H., Dale, S. L., Melby, J. C. and Tait, J. F. (1968). *J. clin. Endocr. Metab.* **28**, 1630.

Baniukiewicz, S., Brodie, A., Flood, C., Motta, M., Okamoto, M:, Tait, J. F., Tait, S. A. S., Blair-West, J. R., Coghlan, J. P., Denton, D. A., Goding, J. R., Scoggins, B. A., Wintour, E. M. and Wright, R. D. (1967). *In* "Functions of the Adrenal Cortex" (K. W. McKerns, ed.). Appleton-Century-Crofts, New York.

Barbeau, A., Gillo-Joffery, L., Boucher, R., Nowaczynski, W. and Genest, J. (1969). *Science,* **165**, 291.

Barger, A. C., Berlin, R. D. and Tulenko, J. F. (1958). *Endocrinology*, **62**, 804.

Bartter, F. C., Delea, C. S., Halberg, F. (1962). *Ann. N.Y. Acad. Sci.* **98**, 969.

Bartter, F. C., Gill, J. R., Frolich, J. C., Bowden, R. E., Hollifield, J. W., Radfar, N., Keiser, H. R., Oates, J. A., Seyberth, H. and Taylor, A. A. (1976). *Trans. Assoc. Am. Physic.* **89**, 77.

Bartter, F. C., Pronove, P., Gill Jr., J. R. and MacCardle, R. C. (1962). *Am. J. Med.* **33**, 811.

Baulieu, E. E., Vigan, M. de, Bricaire, H. and Jayle, M. F. (1957). *J. clin. Endocr. Metab.* **17**, 1478.

Bayard, F., Ances, I. G., Tapper, A. J., Weldon, V. W., Kowarski, A. and Migeon, C. J. (1970). *J. clin. Invest.* **49**, 1389.

Bayard, F., Beitins, I., Kowarski, A. and Migeon, C. J. (1970). *J. clin. Endocr. Metab.* **31**, 1.

Bayard, F., Cooke, C. R., Tiller, D. J., Beitins, I. Z., Kowarski, A., Walker, W. G. and Migeon, C. J. (1971). *J. clin. Invest.* **50**, 1585.

Becker, R. A., Hayashi, R. H., Franks, R. C. and Speroll, L. (1978). *J. clin. Endocr. Metab.* **46**, 467.

Beckerhoff, R., Armbruster, H., Vetter, W., Luetscher, J. A. and Siegenthaler, W. (1973). *Lancet,* **i**, 1218.

Beckerhoff, R., Uhlschmid, G., Vetter, W., Armbruster, H. and Siegenthaler, W. (1974). *Kidney Int.* **5**, 39.

Beevers, D. G., Brown, J. J., Ferriss, J. B., Fraser, R., Lever, A. F., Robertson, J. I. S. and Tree, M. (1976). *Q. J. Med.* **XLV**, 401.

Beiser, S. M., Erlanger, B. F., Agate, F. J. and Lieberman, S. (1959). *Science,* **129**, 564.

Beitins, I. Z., Bayard, F., Kowarski, A. and Migeon, C. J. (1972a). *J. clin. Endocr.* **35**, 595.

Beitins, I. Z., Bayard, F., Levitsky, L., Anees, I. G., Kowarski, A. and Migeon, C. J. (1972b). *J. clin. Invest.* **51**, 386.

Bennett, W. M., McDonald, W. J., Lawson, R. K. and Porter, G. A. (1974). *Kidney Int.* **6**, 99.

Benraad, Th. J. and Kloppenberg, P. W. C. (1970). *J. clin. Endocr. Metab.* **31**, 581.

Best, J. B., Bett, J. H. N., Coghlan, J. P., Cran, E. J. and Scoggins, B. A. (1971). *Lancet,* **i**, 1353.

Bethune, J. E., Nelson, D. H. and Thorn, G. W. (1957). *J. clin. Invest.* **36**, 1701.

Biglieri, E. G. and Forsham, P. H. (1961). *Am. J. Med.* **30**, 564.

Biglieri, E. G. and Ganong, W. F. (1962). *Excerpta Med.* **51**, 223.

Biglieri, E. G., Hane, S., Slaton, P. E. and Forsham, P. E. (1963), *J. clin. Invest.* **42**,

516.

Biglieri, E. G., Herron, M. A. and Brust, N. (1966) *J. clin. Invest.* **45**, 1946.

Biglieri, E. G. and Mantero, F. (1973). *Res. Steroids,* **5**, 385.

Biglieri, E. G., Schambelan, M. and Slaton, P. E. (1969). *J. clin. Endocr. Metab.* **29**, 1090.

Biglieri, E. G., Schambelan, M., Slaton, P. E. and Stockigt, J. R. (1970). *Circ. Res.* **26, 27** (Suppl. 1), 195.

Biglieri, E. G., Schambelan, M. and Stockigt, J. R. (1972). *Clin. Res.* **20**, 163.

Biglieri, E. G., Slaton, P. E. Jr., Silen, W. S., Galante, M. and Forsham, P. H. (1966). *J. clin. Endocr. Metab.* **26**, 553.

Biglieri, E. G., Slaton, P. E., Kronfield, S. J. and Schambelan, M. (1967). *J. Am. Med. Assoc.* **201**, 510.

Biglieri, E. G., Slaton, P. E., Schambelan, M. and Kronfield, S. J. (1968). *Am. J. Med.* **45**, 170.

Biglieri, E. G., Stockigt, J. R. and Schambelan, M. (1972). *Am. J. Med.* **52**, 623.

Birkhauser, M., Gaillard, R., Riondel, A. M., Scholer, D., Vallotton, M. B., Muller, A. F. (1973). *Eur. J. clin. Invest.* **3**, 307.

Birkhauser, M., Godard, C., Loirat, C. and Vallotton, M. B. (1974). *Acta endocr., Copenh.* **75**, 561.

Birmingham, M. K. and Kurlents, E. (1958). *Endocrinology,* **62**, 47.

Blair-West, J. R., Cain, M. D., Catt, K. J., Coghlan, J. P., Denton, D. A., Funder, J. W., Scoggins, B. A., Stockigt, J. R. and Wright, R. D. (1969a). *In* "Hormonal Steroids" (V. H. T. James and L. Martini, eds), p. 571. Excerpta Medica, Amsterdam.

Blair-West, J. R., Cain, M. D., Catt, K. J., Coghlan, J. P., Denton, D. A., Funder, J. W., Scoggins, B. A. and Wright, R. D. (1971a). *Acta endocr.* **66**, 229.

Blair-West, J. R., Cain, M. D., Catt, K. J., Coghlan, J. P., Denton, D. A., Funder, J. W., Scoggins, B. A., Wintour, E. M. and Wright, R. D. (1970). *In* "Fourth Int. Cong. Nephrol." (N. Alwall, F. Bergland and D. Josephson, eds), p. 33. Karger, Basel.

Blair-West, J. R., Coghlan, J. P., Cran, E. J., Denton, D. A., Funder, J. W. and Scoggins, B. A. (1973). *Am. J. Physiol.* **224**, 1409.

Blair-West, J. R., Coghlan, J. P., Denton, D. A., Funder, J. W., Oddie, C. J., and Scoggins, B. A. (1973). *In* "Proc. IVth Int. Cong. Endocr." (R. O. Scow, ed.), ICS 273, p. 768. Excerpta Medica, Amsterdam.

Blair-West, J. R., Coghlan, J. P., Denton, D. A., Funder, J. W. Scoggins, B. A. and Wright, R. D. (1971b). *Endocrinology,* **88**, 367.

Blair-West, J. R., Coghlan, J. P., Denton, D. A., Goding, J. R., Munro, J. A., Wintour, E. M. and Wright, R. D. (1962). *Endocrinology,* **71**, 990.

Blair-West, J. R., Coghlan, J. P., Denton, D. A., Goding, J. R., Orchard, E., Scoggins, B. A., Wintour, E. M. and Wright, R. D. (1967). *In* "Third Int. Cong. Nephrol." (G. E. Schriener, ed.), p. 201. Karger, Basel.

Blair-West, J. R., Coghlan, J. P., Denton, D. A., Goding, J. R., Wintour, E. M. and Wright, R. D. (1963a). *Rec. Prog. Horm. Res.* **19**, 311.

Blair-West, J. R., Coghlan, J. P., Denton, D. A., Goding, J. R., Wintour, E. M. and Wright, R. D. (1968a). *Aust. J. exp. Biol. med. Sci.* **46**, 371.

Blair-West, J. R., Coghlan, J. P., Denton, D. A., Goding, J. R., Wintour, E. M. and Wright, R. D. (1965). *Endocrinology,* **77**, 501.

Blair-West, J. R., Coghlan, J. P., Denton, D. A., Goding, J. R. and Wright, R. D. (1963b). *J. clin. Invest.* **42**, 484.

Blair-West, J. R., Coghlan, J. P., Denton, D. A., Nelson, J. F., Wright, R. D. and Yamauchi, A. (1969b). *J. Physiol.* **205**, 563.

Blair-West, J. R., Coghlan, J. P., Denton, D. A., Orchard, D., Scoggins, B. A. and Wright, R. D. (1968b). *Endocrinology,* **83**, 1199.

Blair-West, J. R., Coghlan, J. P., Denton, D. A. and Scoggins, B. A. (1973). *In* "Handbook of Experimental Pharmacology" (I. H. Page and F. M. Bumpus, eds), Vol. XXXVII. Springer Verlag, Berlin.

Blair-West, J. R., Coghlan, J. P., Denton, D. A., Scoggins, B. A., Wintour, E. M. and Wright, R. D. (1970). *Aust. J. exp. Biol. med. Sci.* **48**, 253.

Blair-West, J. R., Coghlan, J. P., Denton, D. A., Scott, D. and Wright, R. D. (1968a). *Aust. J. exp. Biol. med. Sci.* **46**, 525.

Blair-West, J. R., Coghlan, J. P., Denton, D. A. and Wright, R. D. (1967b). *In* "Handbook of Physiology", Section 6—Alimentary Canal, Vol. II, p. 633. Am. Physiol. Soc., Washington.

Bledsoe, T., Liddle, G. W., Riondel, A., Island, D. P., Bloomfield, D. and Sinclair Smith, B. (1966). *J. clin. Invest.* **45**, 264.

Bloom, W. L. and Mitchell, W. R. (1960). *Arch. int. Med.* **106**, 321.

Bojesen, E. (1962). *Folia Med. Neerlandica, Additamentum,* **1**, 16.

Bojesen, E. (1964). *In* "Aldosterone" (E. E. Baulieu and P. Robel, eds), p. 163. Blackwell Scientific Publications, Oxford.

Bojesen, E. (1966). *Eur. J. Steroids,* **1**, 145.

Bojesen, E. and Degn, H. (1961). *Acta endocr., Copenh.* **37**, 541.

Bojesen, E. and Thuneberg, L. (1967). *In* "Qualitative and Quantitative Analyses of Steroid Hormones". (H. Carstensen, ed.), Marcel Dekker, New York.

Bonelli, J., Waldhausl, W., Magometschnigg, D., Schwarzmeier, J., Korn, A. and Hitzenberger, G. (1977). *Eur. J. clin. Invest.* **7**, 337.

Bougas, J., Flood, C., Little, B., Tait, J. F., Tait, S. A. S. and Underwood, R. (1964). *In* "Aldosterone" (E. E. Baulieu and P. Robel, eds), p. 25. Blackwell Scientific Publications, Oxford.

Boulter, P. R., Hoffman, R. S. and Arky, R. A. (1973). *Metabolism,* **22**, 675.

Boulter, P. R., Spark, R. F. and Arky, R. A. (1973). *Am. J. clin. Nutr.* **26**, 397.

Boulter, P. R., Spark, R. F. and Arky, R. A. (1974). *J. clin. Endocr.* **38**, 248.

Bowden, R. E., Gill, J. R., Radfar, N., Taylor, A. A. and Keiser, H. R. (1978). *J. Am. Med. Assoc.* **239**, 117.

Boyd, G. W., Adamson, A. R., Arnold, M., James, V. H. T. and Peart, W. S. (1972). *Clin. Sci.* **42**, 91.

Bravo, E. L., Dustan, H. P. and Tarazi, R. D. (1975). *J. clin. Endocr. Metab.* **41**, 611.

Breuer, H., Kaulhausen, H., Muhlbauer, L. O., Fritzgche, G. and Vetter, H. (1974). *In* Chronobiological Aspects of Endocrinology" (J. Aschoff, ed.). Schattauer—Verlag, Stuttgart.

Brezis, M. and Litvin, Y. (1977). *Isr. J. med. Sci.* **13**, 1013.

Bricaire, H., Luton, J. P., Laudat, P., Legrand, J. C., Turpin, G., Corvol, P. and Lemmer, M. (1972). *J. clin. Endocr. Metab.* **35**, 67.

Brodie, A. E., Shimizu, N., Tait, S. A. S. and Tait, J. F. (1967). *J. clin. Endocr.* **27**, 997.

Brodie, A. and Tait, J. F. (1967). *In* "Methods in Hormone Research" (R. I. Dorfman, ed.), Vol. 1, 2nd edition. Academic Press, New York, and London.

Brown, J. J., Brown, W. C., Fraser, R., Lever, A. F., Morton, J. J., Robertson, J. I. S., Roser, E. A., Trust, P. M. (1976). *Aust. N. Z. J. Med.* **6** (Suppl. 3), 48.

Brown, J. J., Chinn, R. H., Fraser, R., Lever, A. F., Morton, J. J., Robertson, J. I. S.,

Tree, M., Waite, M. A. and Parke, D. M. (1973). *Br. med. J.* **1**, 650.

Brown, E. H., Coghlan, J. P., Hardy, K. J. and Wintour, E. M. (1978). *Acta endocr., Copenh.* **88**, 364.

Brown, J. J., Chinn, R. H., Davies, D. L., Dusterdieck, G., Fraser, R., Lever, A. F., Robertson, J. I. S., Tree, M. and Wiseman, A. (1968). *Lancet*, **ii**, 55.

Brown, J. J., Davies, D. L., Lever, A. F., Robertson, J. I. S. (1963). *Lancet*, **ii**, 278.

Brown, J. J., Davies, D. L., Lever, A. F., Robertson, J. I. S. and Tree, M. (1964). *Biochem. J.* **93**, 594.

Brown, J. J., Dusterdieck, G., Fraser, R., Lever, A. F., Robertson, J. I. S., Tree, M. and Weir, R. J. (1971). *Br. med. Bull.* **27**, 128.

Brown, J. J., Fraser, R., Lever, A. F., Love, D. R., Morton, J. J. and Robertson, J. I. S. (1972). *Lancet*, **ii**, 1106.

Brown, J. J., Fraser, R., Lever, A. F., Morton, J. J., Robertson, J. R., Tree, M., Bell, P. R., Davidson, J. K. and Ruthven, I. S. (1973). *Lancet*, **ii**, 1228.

Bruinvels, J. and Noordwijk, J. v. (1962). *Nature, Lond.* **193**, 1260.

Brunner, H. R., Baer, L., Sealey, J. E., Ledingham, J. G. G. and Laragh, J. H. (1970). *J. clin. Invest.* **49**, 2128.

Bryan, G. T., Kliman, B. and Bartter, F. C. (1965). *J. clin. Invest.* **44**, 957.

Bryan, G. T., Kliman, B., Gill, J. R. and Bartter, F. C. (1964). *J. clin. Endocr.* **24**, 729.

Bryan, G. T., MacCardle, R. C. and Bartter, F. C. (1966). *Pediatrics,* **37**, 43.

Bull, M. B., Hillman, R. S., Cannon, P. J. and Laragh, J. H. (1970). *Circ. Res.* **27**, 953.

Bush, I. E. (1954). *Br. med. Bull.* **10**, 229.

Bush, I. E. (1962). *In* "The Chromatography of Steroids", 1st edition. Pergamon Press, Oxford.

Butkus, A., Coghlan, J. P., Paterson, R. P., Scoggins, B. A., Robinson, J. A. and Funder, J. W. (1976). *Clin. Exp. Pharmacol. Physiol.* **3**, 557.

Cahn, R. S., Ingold, C. K. and Prelog, V. (1966). *Angew. Chem.* **5**, 385.

Cain, J. P., Dluhy, R. G., Williams, G. H., Selenkow, H. A., Milech, A. and Richmond, S. (1973). *J. clin. Endocr. Metab.* **36**, 365.

Cain, J. P., Tuck, M. L., Williams, G. H., Dluhy, R. G. and Rosenoff, S. H. (1972). *Am. J. Med.* **53**, 627.

Cain, J. P., Williams, G. H. and Dluhy, R. G. (1972). *J. clin. Endocr.* **34**, 73.

Camargo, C. A., Dowdy, A. J., Hancock, E. W. and Luetscher, J. A. (1965). *J. clin. Invest.* **44**, 356.

Cannon, P. J., Ames, R. P. and Laragh, J. H. (1966). *J. clin. Invest.* **45**, 865.

Cannon, P. J., Leeming, J. M., Sommers, S. C., Winters, R. W. and Laragh, J. H. (1968). *Medicine,* **47**, 107.

Carey, R. M., Vaughan, E., Peach, M. J. and Ayers, C. R. (1978). *J. clin. Invest.* **61**, 20.

Carr, A. A. (1973). *Prostaglandins,* **3**, 621.

Carr, H. F. and Reddy, W. J. (1961). *Anal. Biochem.* **2**, 152.

Cartland, S. F. and Kuizenga, M. H. (1939). *Endocrinology,* **24**, 526.

Cassia, B., Felito, F. and Pittera, A. (1963). Inst. Pathol. Spec. Med. Metabol. Clin. Dell'Univ. Catina, p. 243.

Catt, K. J., Cain, M. D., Zimmet, P. Z. and Cran, E. (1969). *Br. med. J.* **1**, 819.

Chavarri, M., Ganguly, A., Luetscher, J. A. and Zager, P. G. (1977). *Aviation Space Environ. Med.* **48**, 633.

Chavarri, M., Luetscher, J. A., Dowdy, A. J. and Ganguly, A. (1977). *J. clin. Endocr. Metab.* **44**, 752.

Check, D. B. and Perry, J. W. (1958). *Arch. Dis. Childh.* **33**, 252.

Chesley, L. C. (1974). "Obstet. Gynecol. Ann." (R. M. Wynn, ed.), Vol. 3, p. 235.

Appleton-Century-Crofts, New York.

Cheville, R. A., Luetscher, J. A., Hancock, E. W., Dowdy, A. J. and Nokes, G. W. (1966). *J. clin. Invest.* **45**, 1302.

Chinn, R. H., Brown, J. J., Fraser, R., Heron, S. M., Lever, A. F., Murchison, L. and Robertson, J. I. S. (1970). *Clin. Sci.* **39**, 437.

Christlieb, A. R., Hickler, R. B., Lauler, D. P. and Williams, H. H.(1969). *New Engl. J. Med.* **281**, 128.

Christy, N. P., Wallace, E. Z. and Jailer, J. W. (1955). *J. clin. Invest.* **34**, 899.

Christy, N. P., Longson, D. and Jailer, J. W. (1957). *Am. J. Med.* **23**, 910.

Coghlan, J. P. and Blair-West, J. R. (1967). *In* "Hormones in Blood" (C. H. Gray and A. L. Bacharach, eds), Vol. II, p. 391, 2nd edition. Academic Press, London and New York.

Coghlan, J. P., Blair-West, J. R., Denton, D. A., Scoggins, B. A. and Wright, R. D. (1971). *Aust. N.Z. J. Med.* **1**, 178.

Coghlan, J. P., Denton, D. A., Goding, J. P. and Wright, R. D. (1960). *Postgrad. Med. J.* **36**, 76.

Coghlan, J. P., Doyle, A. E., Jerums, G. and Scoggins, B. A. (1972). *Clin. Sci.* **42**, 15.

Coghlan, J. P. and Scoggins, B. A. (1967). *J. clin. Endocr. Metab.* **27**, 1470.

Coghlan, J. P., Scoggins, B. A., Stockigt, J. R., Meerkin, M. and Hudson, B. (1971). *Bull. Postgrad. Comm. Med. (Univ. Sydney)*, **26**, 17.

Coghlan, J. P., Wintour, E. M. and Scoggins, B. A. (1966). *Aust. J. exp. Biol. med. Sci.* **44**, 639.

Cohen, T., Theodor, R. and Rosler, A. (1977). *Clin. Genet.* **11**, 25.

Cohen, E. L., Conn, J. W. and Rovner, D. R. (1967). *J. clin. Invest.* **46**, 418.

Collins, K. J., Few, J. D., Finberg, J. P. M. (1977). *J. Physiol.* **268**, 7P.

Collins, K. J., Few, J. D., Forward, T. J. and Giec, L. A. (1969). *J. Physiol.* **202**, 645.

Collins, R. D., Weinberger, M. H., Dowdy, A. J., Nokes, G. W., Gonzales, C. M. and Luetscher, J. A. (1970). *J. clin. Invest.* **49**, 1415.

Conn, J. W. (1955). *J. Lab. clin. Med.* **45**, 3.

Conn, J. W., Cohen, E. L., Lucas, C. P., McDonald, W. J., Mayor, G. H., Blough, W. M., Eveland, W. C., Boostein, J. J. and Lapides, J. (1972). *Arch. int. Med.* **130**, 682.

Conn, J. W., Morita, R., Cohen, E. L., Beirwaltes, W. H., McDonald, W. J. and Herwig, K. R. (1972). *Arch. int. Med.* **129**, 417.

Cooke, C. R., Horvath, J. S., Moore, M. A., Bledsoe, T. and Walker, W. G. (1973). *J. clin. Invest.* **52**, 3028.

Cooke, C. R., Ruiz-Maza, F., Kowarski, A., Migeon, C. J. and Walker, W. G. (1973). *Kidney Int.* **3**, 160.

Cope, C. L., Nicolis, G. and Fraser, B. (1961). *Clin. Sci.* **21**, 367.

Cope, C. L. (1964). "Adrenal Steroids and Disease", 1st edition. Pitman Medical Publishing Co., London.

Coppage Jr., W. S., Island, D., Smith, M. and Liddle, G. W. (1959). *J. clin. Invest.* **38**, 2101.

Coppage, W. S., Island, D. P., Cooner, A. E. and Liddle, G. W. (1962). *J. clin. Invest.* **41**, 1672.

Cortés, J. M., Péron, F. G. and Dorfman, R. I. (1963). *Endocrinology,* **73**, 713.

Corvol, P., Bertagna, X and Bedrossian, J. (1974). *Acta endocr., Copenh.* **75**, 756.

Cox, J. R., Leonard, P. J., Singer, B. (1961). *Clin. Sci.* **21**, 205.

Cox, J. R., Platts, M. M., Horn, M. E., Adams, R. and Miller, H. E. (1966). *J. Endocr.* **36**, 103.

Crabbe, J. (1961). *J. clin. Invest.* **40**, 2103.

Crane, M. G. and Harris, J. J. (1969a). *J. clin. Endocr. Metab.* **29**, 550.

Crane, M. G. and Harris, J. J. (1969b). *J. clin. Endocr. Metab.* **29**, 558.

Cranc, M. G. and Harris, J. J. (1973). *J. clin. Endocr. Metab.* **37**, 790.

Crane, M. G. and Harris, J. J. (1974). *Metabolism,* **23**, 359.

Crane, M. G. and Harris, J. J. (1976). *J. Lab. Clin. Med.* **87**, 947.

Cugini, P., Manconi, R., Serdoz, R., Mancini, A. and Meucci, T. (1977a). *Boll. Soc. H. Biol. Sper.* **53**, 263.

Cugini, P., Manconi, R. Serdoz, R., Mancini, A. and Meucci, T. (1977b). *Boll. Soc. H. Biol. Sper.* **53**, 781.

Culbertson, J. W., Williams, R. W., Ingelfinger, F. J. and Bradley, S. E. (1951). *J. Invest.* **30**, 305.

Dahl, V., Rivarola, M. A. and Bergada, C. (1972). *J. clin. Endocr. Metab.* **34**, 661.

Dalakos, T. G., Elias, A. N., Anderson, G. H., Streeten, D. H. P. and Schroeder, E. T. (1978). *J. clin. Endocr. Metab.* **46**, 114.

Dalakos, T. G. and Streeten, D. H. P. (1975). *Clin. Sci.* **48**, 161.

Dalle, M., Giry, J., Gay, M. and Delost, P. (1978). *J. Endocr.* **76**, 303.

David, R. R., Asnis, M. and Drucker, W. D. (1972). *J. clin. Endocr. Metab.* **35**, 604.

David, R., Golan, S. and Drucker, W. (1968). *Pediatrics,* **41**, 403.

Davis, J. O., Kliman, B., Yankopoulos, N. and Peterson, R. E. (1958). *J. clin. Invest.* **37**, 1783.

Davis, J. O., Holman, J. E., Carpenter, C. C. J., Urquhart, J. and Higgins, J. T. (1964). *Circulation Res.* **14**, 17.

Davis, J. O., Olichney, M. J., Brown, T. C. and Binnion, P. F. (1965). *J. clin. Invest.* **44**, 1433.

Deck, K. A., Champion, P. K. and Conn, J. W. (1973). *J. clin. Endocr. Metab.* **36**, 756.

Degenhart, H. J., Frankena, L., Visser, H. K., Cost, W. S. and Van Seters, A. P. (1966). *Acta physiol. pharmac. neerl.* **14**, 88.

Deheneffe, J., Cuesta, V., Briggs, J. D., Brown, J. J., Fraser, R., Lever, A. F., Morton, J. J., Robertson, J. I. S. and Tree, M. (1976). *Circ. Res.* **39**, 183.

De Lange, W. E., Weeke, A., Artz, W., Jansen, W., Doorenbos, H. (1972). *Acta med. scand.* **193**, 565.

Deming, Q. B. and Luetscher, J. A. (1950). *Proc. Soc. exp. Biol. Med.* **73**, 171.

Denton, D. A., Goding, J. R. and Wright, R. D. (1959). *Br. med. J.* **ii**, 447.

De Vries, C. P., Popp-Snijders, C., De Kieviet, W. and Akkerman-Faber, A. C. (1977). *J. Chrom.* **143**, 624.

Dillon, M. J., Gillin, M. E. A., Ryness, J. M. and de Swiet, M. (1976). *Arch. Dis. Childh.* **51**, 537.

Dillon, M. J. and Ryness, J. M. (1975). *Br. med. J.* **4**, 316.

Dluhy, R. G., Axelrod, L., Underwood, R. H. and Williams, G. H. (1972). *J. clin. Invest.* **51**, 1950.

Dluhy, R. G., Cain, J. P., Williams, G. H. (1974). *J. Lab. clin. Med.* **83**, 249.

Dluhy, R. G., Greenfield, M. and Williams, G. H. (1977). *J. clin. Endocr. Metab.* **45**, 141.

Dluhy, R. G., Himathongkam, T. and Greenfield, M. (1974). *Ann. int. Med.* **80**, 693.

Doe, R. P. and Seal, U. S. (1963). *J. clin. Invest.* **42**, 929.

Donker, A. J. M., de Jong, P. E., Statius van Eps, L. W., Brentjens, J. R. H., Bakker, K., Doorenbos, H. (1977). *Nephron,* **19**, 200.

Dufau, M. and Villee, D. B. (1969). *Biochim. biophys. Acta,* **176**, 637.

Dyrenfurth, I. and Venning, E. H. (1959). *Endocrinology,* **64**, 648.

Eberlein, W. R. and Bongiovanni, A. M. (1955). *J. clin. Endocr. Metab.* **15**, 1531.
Eberlein, W. R. and Bongiovanni, A. M. (1956). *J. biol. Chem.* **223**, 85.
Edelman, I. S. (1975). *J. Steroid Biochem.* **6**, 147.
Edelman, I. S., Bogoroch, R. and Porter, G. A. (1963). *Proc. natn. Acad. Sci. USA,* **50**, 1169.
Edelman, I. S. and Fanestil, D. D. (1970). *In* "Biochemical Actions of Hormones" (G. Litwick, ed.), Vol. 1. Academic Press, New York and London.
Edwards, C. R., Miall, P. A., Hanker, J. P., Thorner, M. D., Al-Dujaili, E. A., Besser, G. M. (1975). *Lancet,* **ii**, 903.
Edwards, O. M. and Bayliss, R. I. (1976). *Q. J. Med.* **477**, 425.
Efstratopoulos, A. D., Peart, W. S., and Wilson, G. A. (1974). *Clin. Sci. Mol. Med.* **46**, 489.
Ehrlich, E. N. (1971). *Am. J. Obstet. Gynec.* **109**, 963.
Ehrlich, E. N., Domiquez, O. V., Samuels, L. T., Lynch, D., Oberhelman, H. and Warner, N. E. (1963). *J. clin. Endocr. Metab.* **23**, 358.
Eherlich, E. W. and Lindheimer, M. D. (1972). *J. clin. Invest.* **51**, 1301.
Eik-Nes, K., Sandberg, A. A., Migeon, C. J., Tyler, F. H. and Samuels, L. T. (1955). *J. clin. Endocr. Metab.* **15**, 13.
Engel, L. L. and Carter, P. (1963). *In* "Physical Properties of the Steroid Hormones" (R. I. Dorfman, ed.), p. 1. Pergamon Press, Oxford.
Epstein, M., Duncan, D. C. and Fishman, L. M. (1972). *Clin. Sci.* **43**, 275.
Epstein, M., Epstein, E. A., Donald, R. and Hughes, H. (1977a). *Br. med. J.* **1**, 488.
Epstein, M., Fishman, L. M. and Hale, H. B. (1971). *Proc. Soc. exp. Biol. Med.* **138**, 939.
Epstein, M., Katsikas, J. C. and Duncan, D. C. (1973). *Circ. Res.* **32**, 228.
Epstein, M., Levinson, R., Sancho, J., Haber, E. and Re, R. (1977b). *Circ. Res.* **41**, 181.
Epstein, M., Pins, D. S., Arrington, R., Denunzio, A. G. and Engstrom, R. (1975a). *J. appl. Physiol.* **39**, 66.
Epstein, M., Pins, D. S., Sancho, J. and Haber, E. (1975b). *J. clin. Endocr. Metab.* **41**, 618.
Epstein, M., Sancho, J., Perez, G., Haber, E., Re, R. and Loutzenhiser, R. (1978). *J. clin. Endocr. Metab.* **46**, 309.
Epstein, M. and Saruta, T. (1971). *J. appl. Physiol.* **31**, 368.
Epstein, M. and Saruta, T. (1972). *J. appl. Physiol.* **33**, 204.
Epstein, M. and Saruta, T. (1973). *J. appl. Physiol.* **34**, 49.
Erbler, H. C. (1974). *Naunym—Schmiedebergs Arch. Pharmakol.* **286**, 145.
Erlanger, B., Borek, F., Berser, S. and Lieberman, S. (1957). *J. biol. Chem.* **228**, 713.
Esmesch, A. and Rahle, H. J. (1978). *Brain Res.* **147**, 154.
Espiner, E. A., Tucci, J. R., Jagger, P. I., Pauk, G. L. and Lauler, D. P. (1967). *Clin. Sci.* **33**, 125.
Espiner, E. A., Christlieb, A. R., Amsterdam, E. A., Jagger, P. I., Dobrzinsky, S. J., Lauler, D. P. and Hickler, R. S. (1971). *Am. J. Cardiol.* **27**, 585.
Espiner, E. A., Jamieson, J. B., Perry, E. G. and Miles, K. (1976). *N.Z. J. Med.* **83**, 313.
Espiner, E. A., Tucci, J. R., Jagger, P. I. and Lauler, D. P. (1967). *New Engl. J. Med.* **277**, 1.
Falbriard, R., Muller, A. F., Neher, R. and Mach, R. S. (1955). *Schweiz. med. Wschr.* **85**, 1218.
Fanestil, D. D. and Edelman, I. S. (1966). *Proc. natn. Acad. Sci. USA,* **56**, 872.

Farmer, R. W., Roup, W. G., Pellizzari, E. D. and Fabre, L. F. (1972). *J. clin. Endocr. Metab.* **34**, 18.

Farrell, G. L. (1954). *Proc. Soc. exp. Biol. Med.* **87**, 587.

Farrell, G. L. and Richards, J. B. (1953). *Proc. Soc. exp. Biol. Med.* **83**, 628.

Fieser, L. F. and Fieser, M. (1959). *In* "Steroids", p. 701, 1st edition. Reinhold Publishing Co., New York.

Feldman, D., Funder, J. W. and Edelman, I. S. (1972). *Am. J. Med.* **53**, 545.

Ferris, J. B., Brown, J. J., Fraser, R., Kay, A. W., Lever, A. F., Neville, A. M., O'Muirchcarthaigh, I. G., Robertson, J. I. S. and Symington, T. (1970). *Lancet,* **ii**, 995.

Fichman, M. and Horton, R. (1973). *Prostaglandins,* **3**, 629.

Fichman, M. P., Littenberg, G., Brooker, G. and Horton, R. (1972). *Circ. Res.* **30/31** (Suppl. 2), 19.

Fichman, M., Littenberg, G., Woo, J. and Horton, R. (1973). *Adv. Biosci.* **9**, 313.

Fichman, M. P., Michelakis, A. M. and Horton, R. (1974). *J. clin. Endocr. Metab.* **39**, 136.

Fichman, M. P., Telfer, N., Zia, P., Speckart, P., Golub, M. and Rude, R. (1976). *Am. J. Med.* **60**, 785.

Finberg, J. P. M. and Berlyne, G. M. (1976). *Isr. J. med. Sci.* **12**, 844.

Finberg, J. P. M. and Berlyne, G. M. (1977). *J. appl. Physiol.* **42**, 554.

Finberg, J. P., Katz, M., Gazit, H., Berlyne, G. M. (1974). *J. appl. Physiol.* **36**, 519.

Flanagan, M. J. and McDonald, J. H. (1967). *J. Urol.* **98**, 133.

Fleming, B. J., Genuth, G. M., Gould, A. B. and Kamionkowski, M. D. (1975). *Ann. int. Med.* **83**, 60.

Flood, C., Gherondache, C., Pincus, G., Tait, J. F., Tait, S. A. and Willoughby, S. (1967). *J. clin. Invest.* **46**, 960.

Flood, C., Layne, D., Ramcharan, S., Rossipal, E., Tait, J. F. and Tait, S. A. S. (1961). *Acta endocr., Copenh.* **36**, 237.

Flood, C., Pincus, G., Tait, J. F., Tait, S. A. S. and Willoughby, S. (1967b). *J. clin. Invest.* **46**, 717.

Ford, H. C. and Bailey, R. E. (1966). *Steroids,* **7**, 30.

Ford, H. C., Pieters, H. P. and Bailey, R. E. (1968). *J. clin. Endocr. Metab.* **28**, 451.

Francis, K. T. and MacGregor, R. (1978). *Aviation–Space Environ. Med.* **49**, 461.

Fraser, R., James, V. H. T., Brown, J. J., Isaac, P., Lever, A. F. and Robertson, J. I. S. (1965). *Lancet,* **ii**, 989.

Frawley, T. F. and Thorn, G. W. (1951). *In* "Proceedings 2nd Clinical ACTH Conference" (J. R. Mote, ed.), p. 115. Churchill, London.

Frayser, R., Rennie, I. D., Gray, G. W. and Houston, C. S. (1975). *J. appl. Physiol.* **38**, 636.

Fredland, P., Sallman, S. and Catt, K. J. (1975). *Endocrinology,* **97**, 1577.

Friedman, S. M., Gustafson, B. and Hamilton, D. (1966a). *Can. J. Physiol. Pharmac.* **44**, 409.

Friedman, S. M., Gustafson, B. and Hamilton, D. (1966b). *Can. J. Physiol. Pharmac.* **44**, 417.

Friedman, S. M., Gustafson, B., Hamilton, D. and Friedman, C. L. (1966c). *Can. J. Physiol. Pharmac.* **44**, 429.

Friedman, S. M., Marshall-Jones, P. and Ross, E. J. (1966d). *Q. J. Med.* **35**, 193.

Frölich, M., Brand, E. C. and van Hall, E. V. (1976). *Acta endocr., Copenh.* **81**, 548.

Fukuchi, S., Takenouchi, T., Nakajima, K., Watanabe, H. and Sugita, A. (1975). *Clin. Sci. mol. Med.* **49**, 187.

Funder, J. W., Blair-West, J. R., Coghlan, J. P., Denton, D. A., Scoggins, B. A. and Wright, R. D. (1969). *Proc. Aust. Endocr. Soc.*

Fyhrqulst, F., Holmberg, E., Perheentupa, J. and Wallenius, M. (1977). *J. clin. Metab.* **45**, 691.

Gall, G., Vaitukaitis, J., Haddow, J. E. and Klein, R. (1971). *J. clin. Endocr. Metab.* **32**, 562.

Ganguly, A., Chavarri, M., Luetscher, J. A. and Dowdy, A. J. (1977). *J. clin. Endocr. Metab.* **44**, 775.

Ganguly, A., Melada, G. A., Luetscher, J. A. and Dowdy, A. J. (1973). *J. clin. Endocr. Metab.* **37**, 765.

Gann, D. S., Delea, C. S., Gill Jr., J. R., Thomas, J. P. and Bartter, F. C. (1964). *Am. J. Physiol.* **207**, 104.

Gardner, J. D., Lapey, A., Simopoulous, A. P. and Bravo, E. L. (1971). *J. clin. Invest.* **50**, 2253.

Gardner, J. D., Simopoulos, A. P. and Shibolet, S. (1972). *J. clin. Invest.* **51**, 1565.

Garst, J., Vignos, P., Hadadey, M. and Matthews, D. N. (1977). *J. clin. Endocr. Metab.* **44**, 185.

Gavras, H., Gavras, I., Texton, S., Voleur, L., Brunner, H. and Rucinska, E. J. (1977). *J. clin. Endocr. Metab.* **46**, 220.

Gauer, O. H., Henry, J. P. and Behn, C. (1970). *Ann. Rev. Physiol.* **32**, 547.

Geloso, J-P. and Basset, J-C. (1974). *Pflugers Arch.* **348**, 105.

Genard, P., Palem-Vliers, M., Denoil, J., Van Cauwenberge, H. and Euchante, W. (1975). *J. Steroid Biochem.* **6**, 201.

Genest, J., De Champlain, J., Veyrat, R., Boncher, R., Tremblay, G. Y., Strong, C. G., Koiw, E. and Marc-Aurele, J. (1965). *Union Med. Canada* **94**, 1113.

Genest, J., Boucher, R., Nowaczynski, W., Koiw, E., de Champlain, J., Biron, P., Chrétien, M. and Marc-Aurèle, J. (1964). *In* "Aldosterone" (E. E. Baulieu and P. Robel, eds), p. 393. Blackwell Scientific Publications, Oxford.

Genest, J., Nowaczynski, W., Kuchel, O., Boucher, R. and Rojo-Ortega, J. M. (1977). *Mayo Clin. Proc.* **52**, 291.

George, E. P., Lazarus, L., Hickie, J. B., Freeman, A. and Kinnane, J. (1964). *Proc. Aust. Physiol. Soc.* **23**.

George, J. M., Wright, L., Bell, N. H., Bartter, F. C. (1970a). *Am. J. Med.* **48**, 343.

George, J. M., Wright, L., Bell, N. H., Bartter, F. C., and Brown, R. (1970b). *Am. J. Med.* **41**, 855.

Gfeller, J. and Siegenthaler, W. (1965). *Acta endocr., Copenh.* **49**, 510.

Giebink, G. S., Gottlin, R. W., Biglieri, E. G. and Katz, F. A. (1973). *J. clin. Endocr. Metab.* **36**, 715.

Gill, J. R., Bell, N. H. and Bartter, R. C. (1967). *Clin. Sci.* **33**, 577.

Gill, J. R., Frolich, J. C., Bowden, R. E., Taylor, A. H., Keiser, H. R., Seyberth, H. W., Oates, J. A. and Bartter, F. C. (1976). *Am. J. Med.* **61**, 43.

Giroud, C. J., Stachenko, J. and Venning, E. H. (1956). *Proc. Soc. exp. Biol. Med.* **92**, 855.

Giry, J. and Delost (1977). *Acta endocr., Copenh.* **84**, 133.

Gocke, D. J., Gerten, J., Sherwood, L. M. and Laragh, J. H. (1969). *Circ. Res.* **24**, Suppl. 131.

Gocke, D. J., Gerten, J., Sherwood, L. M., Oppenhoff, I. and Laragh, J. R. (1968). *Circ. Res.* **24**, Suppl. 1, 131.

Godard, C., Gaillard, R. and Vallotton, M. B. (1976). *Nephron,* **17**, 353.

Godard, C., Riondel, A. M., Veyrat, R., Megevand, A. and Muller, A. F. (1968).

Pediatrics, **41**, 883.

Godecke, W. and Gerike, U. (1971). *Steroids,* **17**, 59.

Goding, J. R. and Wright, R. D. (1964). *Aust. J. exp. Biol. med. Sci.* **42**, 443.

Goldsmith, O., Solomon, D. H. and Horton, R. (1967). *New Engl. J. Med.* **277**, 673.

Goldzieher, J. W. (1963). *In* "Physical Properties of the Steroid Hormones" (L. L. Engel, ed.), p. 288. Pergamon Press, Oxford.

Golub, M. S., Speckart, P. F., Zia, P. K. and Horton, R. (1976). *Circ. Res.* **39**, 574.

Gomez-Sanchez, C., Kem, D. C. and Kaplan, N. M. (1973). *J. clin. Endocr. Metab.* **36**, 795.

Gomez-Sanchez, C., Milewich, L and Holland, O. B. (1977). *J. Lab. clin. Med.* **89**, 902.

Goodfriend, T. and Levine, L. (1964). *Science,* **144**, 1344.

Goodfriend, T. L. and Peach, M. J. (1975). *Circ. Res.,* **36**/**37**, Suppl. 138.

Goodwin, F. J., Ledingham, J. G. and Laragh, J. A. (1970). *Clin. Sci.* **39**, 641.

Goodwin, T. J., James, V. H. T. and Peart, W. S. (1974). *Clin. Sci.* **47**, 235.

Gordon, R. D., Kuchel, O., Liddle, G. W. and Island, D. P. (1967). *J. clin. Invest.* **46**, 599.

Gordon, R. D., Kuchel, O., Island, D. P. and Liddle, G. W. (1966). *J. clin. Invest.* **45**, 1016.

Gordon, R. D., Symonds, E. M., Wilmshurst, E. G. and Pawsey, C. G. K. (1973). *Clin. Sci. mol. Med.* **45**, 115.

Gornall, A. G. and MacDonald, M. P., (1953). *J. biol. Chem.* **201**, 279.

Gornall, A. G. and Gwilliam, C. (1957). *Can. J. Biochem. Physiol.* **35**, 71.

Gosztonyi, T., Marton, I., Kemeny, V. and Vecsei-Weisz, P. (1962). *J. Chromat.* **10**, 29.

Gowenlock, A. H., Mills, J. N. and Thomas, S. (1959). *J. Physiol.* **146**, 133.

Greene, J. A., Vander, A. J. and Kowalczyk, R. S. (1968). *J. Lab. clin. Med.* **71**, 586.

Grim, C. E., Weinberger, M. H. and Anand, C. (1977). *In* "Juvenile Hypertension" (M. I. New L. S. Levine, eds), p. 109, Raven Press, New York.

Halushka, P. V., Wohltmann, H., Privitera, P. J., Hurwitz, G. and Margolius, H. S. (1977). *Ann. int. Med.* **87**, 281.

Haning, R., McCracken, J., St. Cyr, M., Underwood, R., Williams, G. and Abraham, G. (1972). *Steroids,* **20**, 73.

Haning, R., Tait, S. A. S. and Tait, J. F. (1970). *Endocrinology,* **87**, 1147.

Hansen, E. L., Horlyck, E., Gronback, P. and Iversen, M. (1967). *Acta med. scand.* **182**, 65.

Hartrodt, W., (1966). Excerpta Medica Int. Cong. Ser. 111, p. 236, Abst. 418.

Hata, S., Kunita, H. and Okamoto, M. (1976). *J. clin. Endocr. Metab.* **43**, 173.

Hauger, R. L., Aguilera, G. and Catt, K. J. (1978). *Nature, Lond.* **271**, 176.

Hauger, R. L. and Klevene, J. H. (1970). *Cancer,* **26**, 1112.

Hedeland, H., Dyuling, J. F. and Hökfelt, (1969). *Acta endocr., Copenh.* **42**, 399.

Heidland, A., Kreusser, W., Henneman, H., Knauf, H. and Wigand, M. E. (1972). *Klin. Wschr.* **50**, 959.

Helber, A., Kauffman, W., Meurer, K. A., Steiner, B., Durr, F., Euchenhofer, M., Wurz, H. and Streicher, E. (1973). *Klin. Wschr.* **51**, 404.

Helbock, H. J. and Reynolds, J. W. (1970). *Pediatr. Res.* **4**, 455.

Helmer, O. M. and Judson, W. E. (1968). *Circulation,* **38**, 865.

Hickie, J. B. and Lazarus, L. (1966). *Aust. Ann. Med.* **15**, 289.

Hilfenhaus, M. (1977). *J. Steroid Biochem.* **8**, 847.

Himathongkam, T., Dluhy, R. G. and Williams, G. H. (1975). *J. clin. Endocr. Metab.*

41, 153.

Ho, T., Hidaka, H., Kato, T., Yoshitoshi, Y. (1973). *Jap. Heart J.* **14**, 518.

Hogan, M. J., McRae, J., Schambelan, M. and Biglieri, E. G. (1976). *New Engl. J. Med.* **294**, 410.

Hogan, R. P., Kotchen, T. A., Boyd, A. E. and Hartley, L. H. (1973). *J. Appl. Physiol.* **35**, 385.

Holland, O. B., Gomez-Sanchez, C. E., Kem, D. C., Weinberger, M. H., Kramer, N. J. and Higgins, J. R. (1978). *J. clin. Endocr. Metab.* **45**, 1064.

Hollander, W., Kransch, D. M., Chobanian, A. V. and Melby, J. C. (1966). *Circ. Res.* Suppl. I, 1.

Hollenberg, N. K., Chenitz, W. R., Adams, D. F. and Williams, G. H. (1974). *J. clin. Invest.* **54**, 34.

Hollenberg, N. K., Epstein, M., Basch, R. I., Couch, N. B., Hickler, R. B. and Merrill, J. P. (1969). *Am. J. Med.* **47**, 855.

Hollenberg, N. K., William, G. H., Burger, B. and Hooshmand, I. (1975). *Clin. Sci. mol. Med.* **49**, 527.

Hollenberg, N. K., Williams, G., Burger, B., Ishikawa, I. and Adams, D. (1976). *J. clin. Invest.* **57**, 39.

Honn, K. V. and Chavin, W. (1976). *Biochem. Biophys. Res. Comm.* **72**, 1319.

Honn, K. V. and Chavin, W. (1977a). *Biochem. Biophys. Res. Comm.* **76**, 977.

Honn, K. V. and Chavin, W. (1977b). *Experientia,* **33**, 398.

Honn, K. V. and Chavin, W. (1977c). *Experientia,* **33**, 1237.

Horning, E. C. and Mauna, B. F. (1969). *J. Chromat. Sci.* **7**, 411.

Horton, R. (1969). *J. clin. Invest.* **48**, 1230.

Horton, R. and Finck, E. (1972). *Ann. int. Med.* **76**, 885.

Hudson, J. B., Chobanian, A. V. and Relman, A. S. (1957). *New Engl. J. Med.* **257**, 529.

Hullin, R. P., Jerram, T. C., Lee, M. R., Levell, M. J. and Tyrer, S. P. (1977). *Br. J. Psychiat.* **131**, 575.

Hume, D. M. (1962). *In* "Proceedings International Congress on Hormonal Steroids", p. 20. Excerpta Medica Int. Congr. Ser. 51. Excerpta Medica, Amsterdam, London, Milan, New York.

Hume, D. M. and Nelson, D. H. (1954). *Surg. Forum,* **5**, 568.

Huq, M. S., Pfaff, M., Jespersen, D., Zucker, I. R. and Kirschner, M. A. (1976). *J. clin. Endocr. Metab.* **42**, 230.

Hurter, R. and Nabarro, J. D. M. (1960). *Acta endocr., Copenh.* **33**, 168.

Hyatt, P., Bill, J., Gould, R. P., Tait, J. F. and Tait, S. A. S. (1976). *J. Endocr.* **71**, 71.

Ito, T., Hidaka, H., Kato, T. and Yoshitoshi, Y. (1973). *Jap. Heart J.* **14**, 518.

Ito, I., Woo, J., Haning, R. and Horton, R. (1972). *J. clin. Endocr. Metab.* **34**, 106.

Jailer, J. W., Longson, D. and Christy, N. P. (1957). *J. clin. Invest.* **36**, 1608.

James, V. H., Landon, J. and Fraser, R. (1968). *Mem. Soc. Endocr.* **17**, 141.

James, V. H. T., Tunbridge, R. D. G. and Wilson, G. A. (1976). *J. Steroid Biochem.* **7**, 941.

Jean, R., Legrand, J. C., Meylan, F., Rieu, D. and Astruc, J. (1969). *Arch. Franc. Pediat.* **26**, 769.

Jenner, F., Gjessing, L., Cox, J., Davies-Jones, A., Hullin, R. P. and Hanna, S. (1967). *Br. J. Psychiat.* **113**, 895.

Johansson, E. D. B. (1969). *Acta endocr., Copenh.* **61**, 607.

Johnson, B. B., Lieberman, A. H. and Mulrow, P. J. (1957). *J. clin. Invest.* **36**, 757.

Johnson, J. A., Davis, J. O., Taylor, A. A. and Shade, R. E. (1974). *Endocrinology,*

94, 580.

Johnston, C. O., Mendelsohn, F. A. O. and Doyle, A. E. (1972). *Circ. Res.* **30/31**, Suppl. 2, 203.

Jones, K. M., Lloyd-Jones, R., Riondel, A., Tait, J. F., Tait, S. A. S., Bulbrook, R. D. and Greenwood, F. C. (1959). *Acta endocr., Copenh.* **30**, 321.

Jung, R. C., Dill, D. B., Horton, R. and Horvath, S. M. (1971). *J. appl. Physiol.* **31**, 593.

Kahn, P. C., Kelleher, D., Egdahl, R. E. and Melby, J. C. (1971). *Radiology,* **101**, 71.

Kalant, H. (1958a). *Biochem. J.* **69**, 70.

Kalant, H. (1958b). *Biochem. J.* **69**, 93.

Kassirer, J. P., Appleton, F. M., Chazan, J. A. and Schwartz, W. B. (1967). *J. clin. Invest.* **46**, 1558.

Katz, F. H. (1977). *J. clin. Endocr. Metab.* **45**, 419.

Katz, F. H. and Beck, P. (1974). *J. clin. Endocr.* **39**, 1001.

Katz, F. H., Beck, P. and Makowski, E. L. (1974). *Am. J. Obstet. Gynec.* **118**, 51.

Katz, F. H. and Kappas, A. (1967). *J. clin. Invest.* **46**, 1768.

Katz, F. H. and Rompfh, P. (1972a). *J. clin. Endocr. Metab.* **34**, 819.

Katz, F. H., Romfh, P. and Smith, J. A. (1972b). *J. clin. Endocr. Metab.* **35**, 178.

Katz, F. H., Romfh, P. and Smith, J. A. (1972c). *Acta endocr., Copenh.* **71**, 153.

Katz, F. H., Romfh, P. and Smith, J. A. (1975a). *J. clin. Endocr. Metab.* **40**, 125.

Katz, F. H., Romfh, P., Smith, J. A., Roper, E. F. and Barnes, J. S. (1975b). *Acta endocr., Copenh.* **79**, 295.

Katz, F. H., Romfh, P., Zimmering, P. E. and Kelly, W. G. (1972d). *Steroids Lipids Res.* **3**, 90.

Kawasaki, T., Delea, C. S., Bartter, F. C. and Smith, H. (1978). *Am. J. Med.* **64**, 193.

Kelly, W. G., Bandi, L. and Lieberman, S. (1962a). *Biochemistry,* **1**, 792.

Kelly, W. G., Bandi, L., Shoolery, J. N. and Lieberman, S. (1962b). *Biochemistry,* **1**, 172.

Kelly, W. G., Bandi, L. and Lieberman, S. (1963a). *Biochemistry,* **2**, 1243.

Kelly, W. G., Bandi, L. and Lieberman, S. (1963b). *Biochemistry,* **2**, 1249.

Kelly, W. G. and Lieberman, S. (1964). *In* "Aldosterone" (E. E. Baulieu and P. Robel, eds), p. 103. Blackwell Scientific Publications, Oxford.

Kem, D. C., Gomez-Sanchez, C., Kramer, N. J., Holland, O. B. and Higgins, J. R. (1975). *J. clin. Endocr. Metab.* **40**, 116.

Kem, D. C. Weinberger, M. H., Gomez-Sanchez, C., Higgins, J. R. and Kramer, N. J. (1976). *J. Lab. clin. Med.* **88**, 261.

Kem, D. C., Weinberger, M. H., Gomez-Sanchez, C., Kramer, N. J., Lerman, R., Furuyama, S. and Nugent, C. A. (1973). *J. clin. Invest.* **52**, 2272.

Kem, D. C., Weinberger, M. H., Higgins, J. R., Kramer, N. J., Gomez-Sanchez, C. and Holland, O. B. (1978). *J. clin. Endocr. Metab.* **46**, 552.

Kem, D. C., Weinberger, M. H., Mayes, D. M. and Nugent, C. (1971). *Arch. int. Med.* **128**, 380.

Keogh, B., Kirdani, R., Sandberg, A. A., Mittleman, A. and Murphy, G. P. (1976). *Urology,* **7**, 248.

Kershnan, A. K., Borut, D. and Kogut, M. D. (1973). *Pediat. Res.* **7**, 329.

Kihara, I., Kitamura, S., Hoshino, T., Seida, H. and Watanabe, T. (1968). *Acta path. jap.* **18**, 197.

Kimura, T., Nakamoto, M., Nakamura and Ota, M. (1966). *J. clin. Endocr. Metab.* **26**, 1093.

Kisch, E. S., Dluhy, R. G. and Williams, G. H. (1976a). *Circ. Res.* **38**, 502.

Kisch, E. S., Dluhy, R. G., Williams, G. H. (1976b). *J. clin. Endocr. Metab.* **43**, 1343.

Kittinger, G. (1964). *Steroids,* **3**, 21.

Kliman, B. (1965). *Adv. Tracer Method,* **2**, 213.

Kliman, B. and Foster, D. W. (1962). *Analyt. Biochem.* **3**, 403.

Kolanowski, J., Desmecht, P. and Crabbe, J. (1974). *Eur. J. clin. Invest.* **4**, 375.

Kolanowski, J., Desmecht, P. and Crabbe, J. (1976). *Eur. J. clin. Invest.* **6**, 75.

Kolanowski, J., Pizarro, M. A., De Gasparo, M., Desmecht, P., Harvengt, C. and Crabbe, J. (1970). *Eur. J. clin. Invest.* **1**, 25.

Kondo, E., Mitsugi, T. and Tori, K. (1965). *J. Am. Chem. Soc.* **87**, 4655.

Kono, T. (1966) *In* "Steroid Dynamics" (G. Pincus, T. Nakao and J. F. Tait, eds), p. 427. Academic Press, New York and London.

Kono, T., Ikeda, F., Oseko, F., Nanno, M., Imura, H. and Endo, J. (1978). *Acta endocr., Copenh.* **87**, 359.

Kono, T., Oseko, F., Ikeda, F., Nanno, M. and Endo, J. (1977). *Acta endocr., Copenh.* **86**, 156.

Kono, T., Oseko, F., Shimpo, S., Nanno, M. and Endo, J. (1975). *J. clin. Endocr. Metab.* **41**, 1174.

Kono, T., Yoshimi, T. and Miyake, T. (1966). *In* "Steroid Dynamics" (G. Pincus, T. Nakao and J. F. Tait, eds), p. 429. Academic Press, New York and London.

Korz, R., Fishcher, F. and Behn, C. (1969). *Klin. Wschr.* **23**, 1263.

Kosunen, K. J., Pakarinen, A. J. (1976). *J. appl. Physiol.* **41**, 26.

Kosunen, K. J., Pakarinen, A. J., Kuoppasalmi, K. and Adlercreutz, H. (1976). *J. appl. Physiol.* **41**, 323.

Kowarski, A., Finkelstein, J., Loras, B. and Migeon, C. J. (1964). *Steroids,* **3**, 95.

Kowarski, A., Finkelstein, J. W., Spaulding, J. S., Holman, G. H. and Migeon, C. J. (1965). *J. clin. Invest.* **44**, 1505.

Kowarski, A., Katz, H. and Migeon, C. J. (1974). *J. clin. Endocr. Metab.* **38**, 489.

Kowarski, A., de Lacerda, L. and Migeon, C. J. (1975). *J. clin. Endocr.* **40**, 205.

Kuchel, O., Cuche, J. L., Bure, N. T., Guthrie, G. P., Ungar, T., Nowaczynski, W., Boucher, R. and Genest, J. (1977). *J. clin. Endocr. Metab.* **44**, 639.

Kuhlmann, U., Vetter, W., Fischer, E. and Siegenthaler, W. (1978). *Klin. Wschr.* **56**, 229.

Kuizenga, M. H. (1944). *In* "The Chemistry and Physiology of Hormones" (F. R. Moulton, ed.), p. 57. American Association of Advanced Science, Washington.

Kulpmann, W. R., Wolfel, M., Skipka, W. and Breuer, H. (1977). *J. clin. Chem. clin. Biochem.* **15**, 307.

Kunita, H., Obara, T., Komatsu, T., Hata, S., Okamoto, M. (1976). *J. clin. Endocr. Metab.* **43**, 756.

Kurtz, A. B. and Bartter, F. C. (1976). *Steroids,* **28**, 133.

Laidlaw, J. C., Cohen, M. and Gornall, A. G. (1958). *J. clin. Endocr. Metab.* **18**, 222.

Landau, H., Friedman, J., Rosler, A., Moses, G. W., Freier, S., Rotem, Y. and Rabinowitz, D. (1977). *Isr. J. med. Sci.* **13**, 278.

Landau, R. L. and Lugibihl, K. (1958). *J. clin. Endocr. Metab.* **18**, 1237.

Laragh, J. H. (1962). *Circulation,* **25**, 1015.

Laragh, J. H. (1973). *New Engl. J. Med.* **289**, 745.

Laragh, J. H., Angers, M., Kelly, W. G. and Lieberman, S. (1960a). *J. Am. med. Assoc.* **174**, 234.

Laragh, J. H., Cannon, P. J. and Ames, R. P. (1966). *Excerpta Med.* ICS **112**, 267.

Laragh, J. H., Ulick, S., Januszewicz, V., Deming, Q. B., Kelly, W. G. and Lieberman, S. (1960b). *J. clin. Invest.* **39**, 1091.

Leach, C. S., Alexander, W. C. and Johnson, P. C. (1972). *J. clin. Endocr. Metab.* **35**, 642.

Lebel, M., Schalekamp, M. A., Beevers, D. G., Brown, J. J., Davies, D. L., Fraser, R., Kremer, D., Lever, A. F., Morton, J. J., Robertson, J. F., Tree, M. and Wilson, A. (1974). *Lancet*, **ii**, 308.

Ledoux, F., Genest, J., Nowacynski, W., Kuchel, O. and Lebel, M. (1975). *J. Can. Med. Assoc.* **112**, 943.

Lee, K. R., Lin, F. and Sibala, J. (1973). *Am. J. Roentgenol.* **119**, 796.

Lee, J. B., Nelson, D. H. and Thorn, G. W. (1961). *J. clin. Endocr.* **21**, 1426.

Lewbart, M. L. and Mattox, V. R. (1961). *Analyt. Chem.* **33**, 559.

Liddle, G. W. (1964). *In* "Aldosterone" (E. E. Baulieu and R. Robel, eds), p. 519. Blackwell Scientific Publications, Oxford.

Liddle, G. W., Bledsoe, T. and Coppage, W. S. (1963). *Trans. Assoc. Am. Physic.* **76**, 199.

Liddle, G. W., Duncan, L. E. and Bartter, F. C. (1956). *Am. J. Med.* **21**, 380.

Liddle, G. W., Island, D. and Meador, C. K. (1962). *Rec. Prog. Horm. Res.* **18**, 125.

Liddle, G. W., Island, D., Ney, R. L., Nicholson, W. E. and Shimizu, N. (1963). *Arch. int. Med.* **111**, 471.

Liddle, G. W., Sennett, J. A. (1975). *J. Steroid Biochem.* **6**, 751.

Lieberman, A. H. and Luetscher, J. A. (1960). *J. clin. Endocr. Metab.* **20**, 1004.

Limal, J., Rappaport, R. and Bayard, F. (1977). *J. clin. Endocr. Metab.* **45**, 551.

Limal, J. M., Rappaport, R., Dechaux, M., Riffaud, C. and Morin, C. (1978). *Lancet*, **i**, 51.

Lingwood, B., Hardy, K. T., Coghlan, J. P. and Wintour, E. M. (1978). *J. Endocr.* **76**, 553.

Linquette, M., Dupont, A., Racadot, A., Lefebvre, J., May, J. P. and Cappoeun, J. P. (1971). *Ann. Endocr. (Paris)*, **32**, 574.

Lipschity, M. D., Schrier, R. W. and Edelman, I. S. (1973). *Am. J. Physiol.* **224**, 576.

Lommer, D., Distler, A., Nast, H. P., Sinterhauf, K., Walter, U. and Wolff, H. P. (1976). *Klin. Wschr.* **54**, 123.

Loras, B., Dazord, A., Roux, H. and Bertrand, J. (1971). *Rev. Eur. Etudes. Clin. Biol.* **16**, 585.

Loras, B., Haour, F. and Bertrand, J. (1970). *Pediat. Res.* **4**, 145.

Lowenstein, J. and Steele, J. M. (1977). *Kidney Int.* **11**, 128.

Lucis, O. J., Dyrenfurth, I. and Venning, E. H. (1961). *Can. J. Biochem. Physiol.* **39**, 901.

Lucis, O. J., Carballeira, A. and Venning, E. H. (1965). *Steroids*, **6**, 737.

Luetscher, J. A. and Axelrad, B. J. (1954a), *J. clin. Endocr. Metab.* **14**, 1986.

Luetscher, J. A. and Axelrad, B. J. (1954b). *Proc. Soc. exp. Biol. Med.* **87**, 650.

Luetscher, J. A., Camargo, C. A., Hancock, E. W., Dowdy, A. J. and Nokes, G. W. (1964a). *Trans Assoc. Am. Phys.* **77**, 224.

Luetscher, J. A., Camargo, C. A., Cheville, R. A., Hancock, E. W., Dowdy, A. J. and Nokes, G. W. (1966). *In* "Steroid Dynamics" (G. Pincus, T. Nakao and J. F. Tait, eds), p. 341. Academic Press, New York and London.

Luetscher, J. A., Cohn, A. P., Camargo, C. A., Dowdy, A. J. and Callaghan, A. M. (1963). *J. clin. Endocr. Metab.* **23**, 873.

Luetscher, J. A., Dowdy, A. J., Arnstein, A. R., Lucas, C. P. and Murray, C. L. (1964b). *In* "Aldosterone" (E. E. Baulieu and P. Robel, eds), p. 487. Blackwell Scientific Publications, Oxford.

Luetscher, J. A., Dowdy, A., Harvie, J., Neher, R. and Wettstein, A. (1955). *J. biol.*

Chem. **217**, 505.

Luetscher, J. A., Hancock, E. W., Camargo, C. A., Dowdy, A. J. and Nokes, G. W. (1965). *J. clin. Endocr. Metab.* **25**, 628.

Luetscher, J. A. and Johnson, B. B. (1954a). *J. clin. Invest.* **33**, 276.

Luetscher, J. A. and Johnson, B. B. (1954b). *J. clin. Invest.* **33**, 1441.

Luetscher, J. A. and Lieberman, A. H. (1958). *Arch. int. Med.* **102**, 314.

Luetscher, J. A., Weinberger, M. H., Dowdy, A. J., Nokes, G. W., Balikian, H. M., Brodie, A. H. and Willoughby, S. (1969). *J. clin. Endocr. Metab.* **29**, 1310.

Luft, F. C., Grim, C. E., Higgins, J. T. and Weinberger, M. H. (1977). *J. Lab. clin. Med.* **90**, 555.

Luft, F. C., Grim, C. E., Willis, L. R., Higgins, J. T. and Weinberger, M. H. (1977). *Circulatia*, **55**, 779.

Lund-Johansen, P., Thorsen, T. and Stoa, K. F. (1966). *Acta endocr., Copenh.* **53**, 177.

Lutwak, L., Whedon, G. D., Lachance, P. A., Reid, J. M. and Lipscomb, H. S. (1969). *J. clin. Endocr. Metab.* **29**, 1140.

MacDonald, H. N. and Good, W. (1972). *J. Obstet. Gynaec. Br. Commonw.* **79**, 441.

Maher, J. T., Jones, L. G., Hartley, L. H., Williams, G. H. and Rose, L. I. (1975). *J. appl. Physiol.* **39**, 18.

Mallin, S. R. (1969). *Ann. int. Med.* **70**, 69.

Mantero, F., Busnardo, B., Riondel, A., Veyrat, R. and Austoni, M. (1971). *Schweiz Med. Wschr.* **101**, 38.

Marder, M. Z., Wotman, S. and Mandel, I. D. (1972). *Am. J. Obstet. Gynec.* **112**, 233.

Marek, J. and Horky, K. (1976). *Lancet,* **ii**, 1409.

Martin, J. D. and Mills, I. H. (1956). *Br. med. J.* **ii**, 571.

Marusic, E. T. and Mulrow, P. J. (1967). *Endocrinology*, **80**, 214.

Mason, H. L. (1955). *Rec. Prog. Horm. Res.* **11**, 216.

Mason, P. A., Fraser, R., Morton, J. J., Semple, P. F. and Wilson, A. (1977). *J. Steroid Biochem.* **8**, 799.

Mattox, V. R., Mason, H. L., Albert, A. and Code, C. F. (1953). *J. Am. Chem. Soc.* **75**, 4869.

Mayes, D., Furuyama, S., Kem, D. C. and Nugent, C. A. (1970). *J. clin. Endocr. Metab.* **30**, 682.

McAllister, R. G., Vanway, C. W., Dayani, K., Anderson, W. J., Temple, E., Michelakis, A. M., Coppage, W. S. and Oates, J. A. (1971). *Circ. Res.* **28/29**, Suppl. 2, 160.

McCaa, R. E., Bower, J. D. and McCaa, C. S. (1973a). *Circ. Res.* **33**, 555.

McCaa, R. E., McCaa, C. S. and Guyton, A. C. (1975). *Circ. Res.* **36/37**, Suppl. 57.

McCaa, R. E., McCaa, C. S., Reid, D. G., Bower, J. D. and Guyton, A. C. (1972). *Circ. Res.* **31**, 473.

McCaa, R. E., Read, V. H., Cowley, A. W., Bower, J. D., Smith, G. V. and McCaa, C. S. (1973b). *Circ. Res.* **33**, 313.

McDonald, I. R., Goding, J. R. and Wright, R. D. (1958). *Aust. J. exp. Biol. med. Sci.* **36**, 83.

McDougall, J. R., Coghlan, J. P., Robinson, P. R. and Scoggins, B. A. (1978). Unpublished observations.

McKenzie, J. K. and Clements, J. A. (1974). *J. clin. Endocr. Metab.* **38**, 622.

Meador, C. K., Liddle, G. W., Island, D. P., Nicholson, W. E., Lucas, C. P., Nuckton, J. G. and Luetscher, J. A. (1962). *J. clin. Endocr. Metab.* **22**, 693.

Meakin, J. M., Nelson, D. H. and Thorn, G. W. (1959). *J. clin. Endocr. Metab.* **19**, 726.

Melada, G. A., Goldman, R. H., Luetscher, J. A. and Zager, P. G. (1975). *Aviat.*

Space Environ. Med. **46**, 1049.

Melby, J. C., and Dale, S. L. (1975). *J. Steroid Biochem.* **6**, 761.

Melby, J. C., Spark, R. F., Dale, S. L., Egdahl, R. H. and Kahn, P. C. (1967). *New Engl. J. Med.* **277**, 1050.

Melby, J. C., Wilson, T. E. and Dale, S. L. (1965). Quoted by A. Brodie and J. F. Tait in "Methods of Hormone Assay" (R. I. Dorfman, ed.), 2nd edition. Academic Press, New York and London.

Mendelsohn, F. A. O., Johnston, C. I., Doyle, A. E., Scoggins, B. A., Denton, D. A. and Coghlan, J. P. (1972). *Circ. Res.* **31**, 728.

Mendelsohn, F. A. and Mackie, C. (1975). *Clin. Sci. mol. Med.* **49**, 13.

Merrill, A. J., Morrison, J. L. and Brannon, E. S. (1946). *Am. J. Med.* **1**, 468.

Mersey, J. H., Williams, G. H., Hollenberg, W. K. and Dluhy, R. G. (1977). *Circ. Res.* **40**, Suppl. 1, 84.

Messerlie, F. H., Nowaczynski, W., Honda, M., Genest, J. and Kuchel, O. (1976). *J. clin. Endocr. Metab.* **42**, 1074.

Meyer, C. J., Layne, D. S., Tait, J. F. and Pincus, G. (1961). *J. clin. Invest.* **40**, 1663.

Michelakis, A. M. and Horton, R. (1970a). *Circ. Res.* **26/27**, 185.

Michelakis, A. M. and Robertson, D. (1970b). *J. Am. Med. Assoc.* **213**, 83.

Michelakis, A. M., Yoshida, H. and Dormois, J. C. (1975). *Am. J. Obstet. Gynec.* **123**, 724.

Mill, J. S. (1843). "A System of Logic", p. 505. Longmans, London.

Milla, R. G., Trompeter, R., Dillon, M. J., Robins, D. and Shackeleton, C. (1977). *Arch. Dis. Childh.* **52**, 580.

Mills, I. H., Wilson, R. J., Tait, A. D. and Copper, H. R. (1967). *J. Endocr.* **38**, XIX.

Milora, R., Vagnucci, A. and Goodman, A. D. (1967). *Clin. Res.* **15**, 482.

Minei, L. J. and Suzuki, R. (1976). *Obstet. Gynecol.* **48**, 177.

Mitchell, J. P., Baxter, T. J., Blair-West, J. R. and McCredie, D. A. (1970). *Arch. Dis. Childh.* **45**, 376.

Mitra, S., Genuth, S. M., Berman, L. B. and Vertes, V. (1972). *New Engl. J. Med.* **286**, 61.

Miura, K., Yoshingaga, K., Goto, K., Katsushima, I., Maebashi, M., Demura, H., Iino, M., Demura, R. and Torikai, T. (1968). *J. clin. Endocr. Metab.* **28**, 1807.

Modlinger, R. S., Nicolis, G. L., Krakoff, L. R. and Gabrilove, J. C. (1973). *New Engl. J. Med.* **289**, 1022.

Mokotoff, R., Ross, G. and Leiter, L. (1948). *J. clin. Invest.* **27**, 1.

Moolinaar, A. J. (1957). *Acta endocr., Copenh.* **25**, 161.

Montaloo, J. M., McCaa, C. S. and Cole, W. O. (1968). *J. clin. Endocr. Metab.* **28**, 582.

Moore-Ede, M. C., Meguid, M. M., Fitzpatrick, G. F., Boyden, C. M. and Ball, M. R. (1978). *Clin. Pharmacol. Ther.* **23**, 218.

Moore, T. J., Williams, G. H., Dluhy, R. G., Bavli, S. Z., Himathongkam, T. and Greenfield, M. (1977). *Circ. Res.* **41**, 167.

Morimoto, S., Takeda, R. and Murakami, M. (1970). *J. clin. Endocr. Metab.* **31**, 659.

Morris, D. J. and Davis, R. P. (1974). *Metabolism*, **23**, 473.

Muller, A. F., Manning, E. L. and Riondel, A. M. (1958a). *In* "International Symposium on Aldosterone" (A. F. Muller and C. M. O'Connor, eds), p. 111. J. and A. Churchill, London.

Muller, A. F., Manning, E. L. and Riondel, A. M. (1958b). *J. clin. Invest.* **37**, 918.

Muller, A. F., Riondel, A. M. and Manning, E. L. (1956a). *Helv. Med. Acta.* **4/5**, 572.

Muller, A. F., Riondel, A. M., Manning, E. L. and Mach, R. S. (1956b). *Schweiz. med. Wschr.* **86**, 1335.

Muller, J. (1971). *In* "Regulation of Aldosterone Biosynthesis" (J. Muller, ed.), Vol. 5, Monograph-Endocrinology. Stringer-Verlag. Berlin.

Murphy, D. L., Goodwin, F. G. and Bunney, W. E. (1969). *Lancet,* ii, 458.

Myers, J. D., Brannon, E. S. and Holland, B. C. (1950). *J. clin. Invest.* 29, 1069.

Nakamura, M., Sawai, Y., Fukuchi, S. Nakajima, K., Abe, M. and Hoshino, F. (1975). *Tohoku J. exp. Med.* 116, 191.

Neher, R. (1958). *In* "An International Symposium on Aldosterone" (A. F. Muller and C. M. O'Connor, eds), p. 11, 1st edition. J. and A. Churchill, London.

Neher, R. (1964). "Steroid Chromatography", 2nd English edition. Elsevier, Amsterdam.

Neher, R. and Wettstein, A. (1951). *Helv. chim. Acta,* 34, 2278.

Neher, R. and Wettstein, A. (1960). *Helv. chim. Acta,* 43, 623.

Neri, R., Tolksdorf, S., Beiser, S. M., Erlanger, B. F., Agate, F. J. and Lieberman, S. (1964). *Endocrinology,* 74, 593.

New, M. I. (1970). *J. clin. Invest.* 49, 1930.

New, M. I., Miller, B. and Peterson, R. E. (1966). *J. clin. Invest.* 45, 412.

New, M. I. and Seaman, M. P. (1970). *J. clin. Endocr. Metab.* 31, 361.

New, M. I., Siegal, E. J. and Peterson, R. E. (1973). *J. clin. Endocr. Metab.* 37, 93.

Newmark, S. R., Himathongbam, T., Martin, R. P., Cooper, K. H. and Rose, L. I. (1976). *J. clin. Endocr. Metab.* 42, 393.

Newton, M. A. and Laragh, J. H. (1968a). *J. clin. Endocr. Metab.* 28, 1006.

Newton, M. A. and Laragh, J. H. (1968b). *J. clin. Endocr. Metab.* 28, 1014.

Nicholls, M. G., Arius, A. A. and Espiner, E. A. (1975a). *Proc. Univ. Otago. Med. Sch.* 53, 24.

Nicholls, M. G., Espiner, E. A. and Donald, R. D. (1975b). *J. clin. Endocr. Metab.* 41, 186.

Nicholls, M. G., Espiner, E. A., Donald, R. A. and Hughes, H. (1974). *Clin. Sci. mol. Med.* 47, 301.

Nicholls, M. G., Espiner, E. A., Hughes, H., Ross, J. and Stewart, D. T. (1975c). *Am. J. Med.* 59, 334.

Nicolis, G. L., Mitty, H. A., Modlinger, R. S. and Gabrilove, J. L. (1972). *Ann. int. Med.* 76, 899.

Norbiato, G., Bevilacqua, M., Raggi, U., Micossi, P. and Moroni, C. (1977). *J. clin. Endocr. Metab.* 45, 1313.

Norbiato, G., Bevilacqua, M., Raggi, U., Micossi, P., Moroni, C. and Fasoli, A. (1978). *Acta endocr., Copenh.* 87, 577.

Noth, R. H., Lassman, N., Tan, S. Y., Fernandez-Cruz, A. and Mulrow, P. J. (1977a). *Arch int. Med.* 137, 1414.

Noth, R. H., Tan, S. Y. and Mulrow, P. J. (1977b). *J. clin. Endocr. Metab.* 45, 10.

Nowaczynski, W. J., Goldner, M. and Genest, J. (1955). *J. lab. clin. Med.* 45, 818.

Nowaczynski, W. J. and Steyermark, P. R. (1956). *Can. J. Biochem. Physiol.* 34, 592.

Nowotny, E., Abraham, R. and Staudinger, Hj. (1965). *Z. klin. Chem.* 3, 8.

Nowotny, E. and Staudinger, H. (1966). *Z. klin. Chem.* 4, 203.

O'Brian, J. T., Saudek, C. D. and Spark, R. F. (1974). *J. clin. Endocr. Metab.* 38, 1147.

O'Connor, W. J. (1962). "Renal Function." Edward Arnold, London.

Oddie, C. J., Coghlan, J. P. and Scoggins, B. A. (1972). *J. clin. Endocr. Metab.* 34, 1039.

Oelkers, W., Brown, J. J., Fraser, R., Lever, A. F., Morton, J. J. and Robertson, J. I. S. (1974a). *Circ. Res.* 34, 69.

Oelkers, W., Mapen, B., Molyahn, M. and Hammerstein, J. (1975a). *Klin. Wschr.*

53, 509.

Oelkers, W., Rawer, C., Wrecterholt, M., Schoneshofer, M. and Palicki, H. (1977). *Klin. Wschr.* **55**, 495.

Oelkers, W., Schoneshofer, M. J. and Blumel, A. (1974b). *J. clin. Endocr. Metab.* **39**, 882.

Oelkers, W., Schoneshofer, M., Schultze, G., Brown, J. J., Fraser, R., Morton, J. J., Lever, A. F. and Robertson, J. I. S. (1975b). *Circ. Res.* **36/37**, Suppl. 1, 49.

Oelkers, W., Schoneshofer, M., Schultze, G., Wenzler, M., Bauer, B., L'Age, M. and Fchm, H. L. (1978). *J. clin. Endocr. Metab.* **46**, 402.

Ogihara, T., Iinuma, K., Nishi, K., Arakawa, Y., Takagi, A., Kurata, K., Miyai, K. and Kumahara, Y. (1977a). *J. clin. Endocr. Metab.* **45**, 726.

Ogihara, T., Matsumana, S., Onishi, T., Miyai, K., Uozumi, T. and Kumahara, Y. (1977b). *Life Sci.* **20**, 523.

Ogihara, T., Yamarmaoto, T., Miyal, K. and Kumahara, Y. (1973). *Endocr. Japan,* **20**, 433.

Ohno, F., Harada, H., Komatsu, K., Saijo, K. and Miyoshi, K. (1975). *Endocr. Japan,* **22**, 163.

Olgaard, K. (1975). *Scand. J. clin. Lab. Invest.* **35**, 31.

Olgaard, K., Hagen, S., Madsen, S. and Hummer, L. (1976). *Lancet,* **ii**, 959.

Olgaard, K. and Madsen, S. (1977a). *Acta med. scand.* **201**, 77.

Olgaard, K., Madsen, S., Ladefoged, J. and Regeur, L. (1977b). *Eur. J. clin. Invest.* **7**, 61.

Olgaard, K., Madsen, S., Roosen, J. and Hammer, M. (1977c). *Scand. J. clin. Lab. Invest.* **37**, 431.

Oliver, W. J., Cohen, E. L. and Neel, J. V. (1975). *Circulation,* **52**, 146.

Oparil, S., Ehrlich, E. N. and Lindheimer, M. D. (1975). *Clin. Sci. mol. Med.* **49**, 139.

O'Riodan, J. L., Blanshard, S. P., Moxham, A. and Nabarro, J. D. (1966). *Q. J. Med.* **35**, 137.

Orloff, M. J., Ross, T. H., Baddeley, R. M., Nutting, R. O., Spitz, B. R., Sloop, R. D., Neesby, T. and Halasz, N. A. (1964). *Surgery,* **56**, 83.

Padfield, P. L., Allison, M. E. M., Brown, J. J., Ferriss, J. B., Fraser, R., Lever, A. F., Luke, R. G. and Robertson, J. I. S. (1975). *Clin. Endocr.* **4**, 493.

Pakravan, P., Kenny, F. M., Depp, R., and Allen, A. C. (1974). *J. Pediat.* **84**, 74.

Pasqualini, J. R. (1964a). *Nature, Lond.* **201**, 502.

Pasqualini, J. R. (1964b). *In* "Aldosterone" (E. E. Baulieu and P. Robel, eds), p. 131. Blackwell Scientific Publications, Oxford.

Pasqualini, J. R. (1964c). *In* "Structure and Metabolism of Corticosteroids" (J. R. Pasqualini and M. F. Jayle, eds), p. 77. Academic Press, London and New York.

Pasqualini, J. R. (1971). *Excerpta Med. Found. Int. Cong. Ser.* **219**, 487.

Pasqualini, J. R., Bedin, M. and Cogneville, A. M. (1976). *Acta Endocr.* **82**, 831.

Pasqualini, J. R., Uhrich, F. and Jayle, M. F. (1965). *Biochim. biophys. Acta,* **104**, 515.

Pasqualini, J. R., Sumida, C. and Gelly, C. (1972). *J. Steroid Biochem.* **3**, 543.

Pasqualini, J. R., Wiqvist, N. and Diczfalusy, E. (1966). *Biochim. biophys. Acta,* **121**, 430.

Paton, A. M., Level, A. F., Oliver, N. W., Medina, A., Briggs, J. D., Morton, J. J., Brown, J. J., Robertson, J. I. S., Fraser, R., Tree, M. and Gavras, H. (1975). *Clin. Nephrol.* **3**, 18.

Peach, M. J. and Chiu, A. T. (1974). *Circ. Res.* Suppl. 1, 7.

Peart, W. S. (1965b). *Pharmac. Rev.* **17**, 143.

Pechet, M. M., Hesse, R. M. and Kohler, H. (1960). *J. Am. chem. Soc.* **82**, 5251.

Pedersen, E. B., Amdisen, A. and Darling, S. (1977). *Int. Pharmacopsychiat.* **12**, 80.
Pedersen, E. B. and Kornerup, H. J. (1976). *Acta med. scand.* **200**, 501.
Pelletier, M., Ludens, J. H. and Fancsill, D. D. (1972). *Ji ch. hm. Med.* **130, 213.**
Perez, G. O., Oster, J. R. and Uaamonde, C. A. (1974). *Am. J. Med.* **57**, 809.
Perez, G. O., Oster, J. R., Uaamonde, C. A. and Katz, F. H. (1977). *J. clin. Endocr. Metab.* **45**, 762.
Perez, G., Siegal, L. and Schreiner, G. E. (1972). *Ann. int. Med.* **76**, 757.
Peron, F. G. (1961). *Endocrinology,* **69**, 39.
Peterson, R. E. (1960). *J. clin. Invest.* **39**, 320.
Peterson, R. E. (1964). *In* "Aldosterone" (E. E. Baulieu and P. Robel, eds), p. 145. Blackwell Scientific Publications, Oxford.
Pham-Huu-Trung, M. T. and Corvol, P. (1974). *Steroids,* **24**, 587.
Pham-Huu-Trung, M. T., Raux, M. C., Gourmelen, M., Baron, M. C. and Girard, F. (1976). *Acta endocr. Copenh.* **82**, 572.
Pines, A., Slats, J. D. H., Jowett, T. P. (1977). *Br. J. Dis. Chest,* **71**, 203.
Pittera, A., Cassia, B. and Felito, F. (1963a). *Bull. Soc. Ital. Biol. Sper.* **39**, 1503.
Pittera, A., Cassia, B. and Felito, F. (1963b). *Bull. Soc. Ital. Biol. Sper.* **39**, 1509.
Plouin, P. F., Corvol, P. and Menard, J. (1977). *Biomedicine,* **27**, 233.
Porter, C. C. and Silber, R. H. (1950). *J. biol. Chem.* **185**, 201.
Porter, S. A., Bogoroch, R. and Edelman, I. S. (1964). *Proc. natn. Acad. Sci. USA,* **52**, 1326.
Postel-Vinay, M., Alberti, G., Ricour, C., Lamal, J., Rappaport, R. and Royer, P. (1974). *J. clin. Endocr. Metab.* **39**, 1038.
Pratt, J. H., Dale, S. L. and Melby J. C. (1976). *J. clin. Endocr. Metab.* **42**, 355.
Priscu, R., Maiorescu, M. and Sischitiu, S. (1972). *Klin. Pad.* **184**, 408.
Proesmanns, W., Geussens, H., Corbeel, L. and Eeckels, R. (1973). *Am. J. Dis. Child.* **126**, 510.
Rabinowitz, D., Landau, H., Rosler, A., Moses, S., Rotern, Y. and Freier, S. (1974). *Metabolism,* **23**, 1.
Rado, J. P., Simatupang, T., Boer, P., Dorhout Mees, E. J. (1977). *Biomedicine,* **27**, 209.
Rapp, J. R. and Eik-Nes, K. B. (1966). *Anal. Biochem.* **15**, 386.
Rayfield, E. J., Rose, L. I., Dluhy, R. G. and Williams, G. H. (1973). *J. clin. Endocr. Metab.* **36**, 30.
Rappaport, R., Dray, F., Legrand, J. C. and Royer, P. (1968). *Pediatr. Res.* **2**, 456.
Rayyis, S. S. and Horton, R. (1971). *J. clin. Endocr. Metab.* **32**, 539.
Re, R. N., Sancho, J., Kliman, B. and Haber, E. (1977). *J. clin. Endocr. Metab.* **46**, 189.
Read, V. H., McCaa, C. S., Bower, J. D. and McCaa, R. E. (1973). *J. clin. Endocr. Metab.* **36**, 773.
Reck, G., Beckerhoff, R., Vetter, W., Armbruster, H. and Siegenthaler, W. (1975). *Klin. Wschr.* **53**, 955.
Reich, M. (1962). *Aust. Ann. Med.* **11**, 42.
Reichstein, T. and von Euw, J. V. (1938). *Helv. chim. Acta,* **21**, 1197.
Rinsler, M. G. and Rigby, B. (1957). *Br. med. J.* **ii**, 966.
Robb, C. A., Davis, J. O., Johnson, J. A., Blaine, E. H., Schneider, E. G. and Baumber, J. S. (1970). *J. clin. Invest.* **49**, 871.
Robertson, P. W., Klidjian, A., Harding, L. K., Walters, G., Lee, M. R. and Robb-Smith, A. H. T. (1967). *Am. J. Med.* **43**, 963.
Rose, L. I., Carroll, D. R., Lowe, S. L., Peterson, E. W. and Cooper, (1970). *J. appl. Physiol.* **29**, 449.

Rosler, A., Levine, L. S., Schneider, B., Novogroder, M. and New, M. I. (1977a). *J. clin. Endocr. Metab.* **45**, 500.

Rosler, A., Rabinowitz, D., Theodor, R., Ramirez, L. C. and Ulick, S. (1977b). *J. clin. Endocr.* **44**, 279.

Rosler, A., Theodor, R., Biochis, H., Gerty, R., Ulick, S., Alagem, M., Tabachnik, E., Cohen, B., Robinowitz, D. (1977c). *J. clin. Endocr. Metab.* **44**, 292.

Rosler, A., Theodos, R., Gazit, E., Biochis, H., and Rabinowitz, D. (1973). *Lancet,* i, 959.

Rosoff, L., Zia, P., Reynolds, T. and Horton, R. (1975). *Gastroenterology,* **69**, 705.

Ross, E. J., Marshall-Jones, P. and Friedman, M. (1966). *Q. J. Med.* **35**, 149.

Rossler, R. and Gaiser, H. (1974). *Dt. med. Wschr.* **99**, 685.

Roth, D. G. and Gamble, J. L. (1965). *J. Physiol.* **208**, 90.

Rovner, D. R., Conn, J. W., Knopf, R. F., Cohen, E. L. and Hsuem, M. T. Y. (1965). *J. clin. Endocr. Metab.* **25**, 53.

Roy, A. K., Ramirez, L. C. and Ulick, S. (1976). *J. Steroid Biochem.* **7**, 81.

Rubin, R. T. (1975). *Prog. Brain Res.* **42**, 73.

Rubin, R. T., Poland, R. E., Gouin, P. R. and Tower, B. B. (1978). *Psychosom. Med.* **40**, 44.

Sampson, D., Kirdani, R. Y., Sandberg, A. A. and Murphy, G. P. (1972). *Invest. Urol.* **10**, 66.

Sancho, J., Re, R., Burton, J., Barger, A. C. and Haber, E. (1976). *Circulation,* **53**, 400.

Sandberg, A. and Slaunwhite, W. R. (1971). *In* "The Human Adrenal Cortex" (N. P. Christy, ed.), p. 69. Harper-Row, New York.

Sandor, T. and Lanthier, A. (1962). *Acta endocr., Copenh.* **39**, 87.

Sandor, T. and Lanthier, A. (1963). *Acta endocr., Copenh.* **42**, 355.

Sasaki, H., Okumura, M., Ikeda, M., Kawasaki, T. and Fukiyama, K. (1976). *New Engl. J. Med.* **294**, 612.

Sasaki, H., Okumara, M., Asano, T., Arakawa, K. and Kawasaki, T. (1977). *Br. med. J.* **2**, 995.

Sassard, J., Vincent, M., Annat, G. and Bizollon, C. A. (1976). *J. clin. Endocr. Metab.* **42**, 20.

Schalekamp, M. A. D. H., Bever-Donker, S. C., Jansen-Goemans, A., Fawzi, T. D. and Muller, A. (1976). *J. clin. Endocr. Metab.* **43**, 287.

Schambelan, M., Stockigt, J. R. and Biglieri, E. G. (1972a). *New Engl. J. Med.* **287**, 573.

Schambelan, M., Howes, E. L., Stockigt, J. R., Noakes, C. A. and Biglieri, E. G. (1973). *Am. J. Med.* **55**, 86.

Schambelan, M., Brust, N. L., Chang, B. C. F., Slater, K. L. and Biglieri, E. G. (1976). *J. clin. Endocr. Metab.* **43**, 115.

Schambelan, M., Stockigt, J. R. and Biglieri, E. G. (1972b). *New Engl. J. Med.* **287**, 573.

Schmidlin, J. Anner, G., Billeter, J. R. and Wettstein, A. (1955). *Experientia,* **11**, 365.

Schmidlin, J., Anner, G., Billeter, J. R., Hensler, K., Ueberwasser, H., Wieland, P. and Wettstein, A. (1957). *Helv. chim. Acta,* **40**, 2291.

Schneider, G. and Mulrow, P. J. (1973). *Endocrinology,* **92**, 1208.

Scholer, D., Birkhauser, M., Peytremann, A., Riondel, A. M., Vallotton, M. B. and Muller, A. F. (1973). *Acta endocr., Copenh.* **72**, 293.

Scholer, D., Riondel, A. M. and Manning, E. L. (1972). *Acta endocr., Copenh.* **70**, 552.

Schroeder, E. T., Anderson, G. H., Goldman, S. H. and Streeten, D. H. (1976). *Kidney Int.* **9**, 511.

604   J. P. COGHLAN, B. A. SCOGGINS AND E. M. WINTOUR

Schwartz, U. D. and Abraham, G. E. (1975). *Obstet. Gynecol.* **45**, 339.

Scoggins, B. A., Coghlan, J. P. and Blair-West, J. R. (1966). *Proc. Aust. Phys. Soc.* **33**.

Scoggins, B. A., Oddie, C. J., Hare, W. S. C. and Coghlan, J. P. (1972). *Ann. int. Med.* **76**, 891.

Scoggins, B. A., Coghlan, J. P., Denton, D. A., Fan, J. S., McDougall, J. G., Oddie, C. S. and Shulkes, A. S. (1974). *Am. J. Physiol.* **226**, 198.

Sealey, J. E., Buhler, E. R., Laragh, J. H., Manning, E. L. and Brunner, H. R. (1972). *Circ. Res.* **31**, 367.

Sebastian, A., McSherry, E. and Morris, R. C., (1971). *J. clin. Invest.* **50**, 667.

Sebastian, A., Schambelan, M., Lindenfield, S. and Morris, R. C. (1977). *New Engl. J. Med.* **297**, 576.

Shade, R. E. and Grim, C. E. (1975). *J. clin. Endocr. Metab.* **40**, 652.

Sharp, G. W. S. and Leaf, A. (1966). *Physiol. Rev.* **46**, 593.

Sheppard, H., Mowles, T. F., Chart, J. J., Renzi, A. A. and Howie, N. (1964). *Endocrinology,* **74**, 762.

Sheppard, H., Swenson, R. and Mowles, T. F. (1963). *Endocrinology,* **73**, 819.

Siegal, S. R., Fisher, D. A. and Oh, W. (1974). *Pediatrics,* **53**, 410.

Siegenthaler, W. E., Dowdy, A. and Luetscher, J. A. (1962). *J. clin. Endocr. Metab.* **22**, 172.

Siegenthaler, W. E., Peterson, R. E. and Frimpter, G. W. (1964) *In* "Aldosterone" (E. E. Baulieu and P. Robel, eds), p. 51. Blackwell Scientific Publications, Oxford.

Silber, R. H. (1966). *Meth. biochem. Anal.* **14**, 63.

Simpson, S. A. and Tait, J. F. (1952). *Endocrinology,* **50**, 150.

Simpson, S. A. and Tait, J. F. (1955). *Rec. Prog. Horm. Res.* **11**, 183.

Simpson, S. A., Tait, J. F. and Bush, I. E. (1952). *Lancet,* **263**, 226.

Simpson, S. A., Tait, J. F., Wettstein, A., Neher, R., von Euw, J. and Reichstein, R. (1953). *Experientia,* **9**, 333.

Simpson, S. A., Tait, J. F., Wettstein, A., Neher, R., von Euw, J., Schindler, O. and Reichstein, T. (1954a). *Experientia,* **10**, 132.

Simpson, S. A., Tait, J. F., Wettstein, A., Neher, R., von Euw, J., Schindler, O. and Reichstein, R. (1954b). *Helv. chim. Acta,* **37**, 1163.

Simpson, S. A., Tait, J. F., Wettstein, A., Neher, R., von Euw, J., Schindler, O. and Reichstein, T. (1954c). *Helv. chim. Acta,* **37**, 1200.

Sizonenko, P. C., Riondel, A., Kohlberg, I. J. and Paunier, L. (1972). *J. clin. Endocr. Metab.* **35**, 281.

Skinner, S. L., Cran, E. J., Gibson, R., Taylor, R., Walters, W. A. W. and Catt, K. J. (1975). *Am. J. Obstet. Gynec.* **121**, 626.

Skrabul, F., Aubock, J., Edwards, C. R. and Braunsteiner, H. (1978). *Lancet,* **i**, 298.

Slater, J. D. H., Williams, E. S., Edwards, R. H. I., Ekins, R. P., Sonksen, P. H., Beresford, C. H., and McLaughlin, M. (1969a). *Clin. Sci.* **37**, 311.

Slater, J. D. H., Tuffley, R. E., Williams, E. S., Beresford, C. H., Sonksen, P. H., Edwards, R. H. T., Ekins, R. P. and McLaughlin, M. (1969b). *Clin. Sci.* **37**, 327.

Slaton, P. E. and Biglieri, E. G. (1967). *J. clin. Endocr. Metab.* **27**, 37.

Slaton, P. E., Schambelan, M. and Biglieri, E. G. (1969). *J. clin. Endocr. Metab.* **29**, 239.

Smeaton, T. C., Anderson, G. J. and Fulton, I. S. (1977). *J. clin. Endocr. Metab.* **44**, 1.

Smiles, K. A. and Robinson, S. (1971). *J. appl. Physiol.* **31**, 63.

Smith, L. L. and Bernstein, S. (1963). *In* "Physical Properties of the Steroid Hormones" (L. L. Engel, ed.), p. 321. Pergamon Press, Oxford.

Solomon, S., Bird, C. E., Wilson, R., Wiqvist, N. and Diczfalusy, E. (1964). *In*

"Proceedings 2nd International Congress of Endocrinology, London", p. 721. Excerpta Medica, Amsterdam.

Solomon, R. J. and Brown, R. S. (1975). *Am. J. Med.* **59**, 575.

Sonnenblick, E. H., Cannon, P. J. and Laragh, J. H. (1961). *J. clin. Invest.* **40**, 903.

Sparagana, M. (1975). *Biochem. Med.* **14**, 93.

Spark, R. F., Gordon, S. J., Dales, S. L. and Melby, J. C. (1968). *Arch. int. Med.* **122**, 394.

Spark, R. F., Arky, R. A., Boulter, P. R., Saudek, C. D. and O'Brian, J. T. (1975). *New Engl. J. Med.* **292**, 1335.

Spark, R. F. and Etzkorn, J. R. (1977). *New Engl. J. Med.* **297**, 917.

Spark, R. F., Dale, S. L., Kahn, P. C. and Melby, J. C. (1969). *J. clin. Invest.* **48**, 96.

Speckart, P., Zia, P., Zipser, R. and Horton, R. (1977). *J. clin. Endocr. Metab.* **44**, 832.

Stachenko, J. and Giroud, C. J. P. (1959). *Endocrinology*, **64**, 730.

Staub, M. C. and Dingman, J. F. (1961). *J. clin. Endocr. Metab.* **21**, 148.

Steele, J. M. and Lowenstein, J. (1974). *Circ. Res.* **35**, 592.

Steiger, M. and Reichstein, T. (1937). *Helv. chim. Acta*, **20**, 1164.

Stockigt, J. R., Coghlan, J. P., Oddie, C. J. and Scoggins, B. A. (1975). *Proc Aust. Endocr. Soc.* **18**, 33.

Stockigt, J. R., Collins, R. D., Biglieri, E. G. (1971). *Circ. Res.* **28**, 29 II 175.

Strauch, G., Vallolton, M. B., Tourton, Y., and Bicaire, H. (1972). *New Engl. J. Med.* **287**, 795.

Streeten, D. H. P., Dalakos, T. G., Souma, M., Fellerman, H., Clift, G. V., Schletter, F. E., Stevenson, C. T. and Speller, P. J. (1973). *Clin. Sci. mol. Med.* **45**, 347.

Streeten, D. H. P., Louis, L. H. and Conn, J. W. (1960). *Trans. Assoc. Am. Phys.* **73**, 227.

Streeten, D. H. P., Rapoport, A., and Conn, J. W. (1963). *J. clin. Metab.* **23**, 928.

Streeten, D. H. P., Schletter, F. E. and Clift, G. V. (1969). *Am. J. Med.* **46**, 844.

Strickland, A. L. and Kotchen, R. A. (1972). *J. Pediatr.* **81**, 962.

Sufrin, G., Kirdani, R., Sandberg, A. A. and Murphy, G. P. (1978). *Urology*, **11**, 46.

Sulya, L. L., McCaa, C. S., Read, V. H. and Bomer, D. (1963). *Nature, Lond.* **200**, 788.

Sundsfjord, J. A. (1971). *Acta endocr., Copenh.* **67**, 483.

Sundsfjord, J. A. and Aakvaag, A. (1970). *Acta endocr., Copenh.* **64**, 452.

Sundsfjord, J. A. and Aakvaag, A. (1971). *Obstet. Gynec. Surv.* **26**, 166.

Sundsfjord, J. A. and Aakvaag, A. (1972). *Acta endocr., Copenh.* **71**, 519.

Sundsfjord, J. A. and Aakvaag, A. (1973a). *Acta endocr., Copenh.* **73**, 499.

Sundsfjord, J. A., Stromme, S. B., Refsum, H. E. and Aakvaag, A. (1973b). *Acta endocr., Copenh.* Suppl. **177**, 184.

Sutherland, D. J. A., Ruse, J. C. and Laidlaw, J. C. (1966). *J. Assoc. Med. Can.* **95**, 1109.

Sutton, J. R., Viol, G. W., Gray, G. W., McFadden, M., and Keane, P. M. (1977). *J. appl. Physiol.* **43**, 421.

Swallow, R. L. and Sayers, G. (1969). *Proc. Soc. exp. Biol. Med.* **131**, 1.

Swann, H. G. (1940). *Physiol. Rev.* **20**, 493.

Tait, J. F. (1963). *J. clin. Endocr. Metab.* **23**, 1285.

Tait, J. F. and Burstein, S. (1964). "The Hormones", Vol. 5, p. 441. Academic Press, New York and London.

Tait, J. F. and Little, B. (1968). *J. clin. Invest.* **47**, 2423.

Tait, J. F., Little, B., Tait, S. A. S. and Flood, C. (1962). *J. clin. Invest.* **41**, 2093.

Tait, J. F. and Tait, S. A. S. (1976). *J. Steroid Biochem.* **7**, 687.

Tait, J. F., Tait, S. A. S., Albano, J. D., Brown, B. L., and Mendelsohn, F. A. (1975).

In "Research on Steroids" (H. Breuer *et al.*, eds) Vol. VI, p. 19. North Holland Publishing Co., Amsterdam and Oxford.

Tait, J. F., Tait, S. A. S., Gould, R. P. and Mee, M. S. (1973). *Proc. R. Soc. (Lond.)*, **185**, 375.

Tait, J. F., Tait, S. A. S., Little, B. and Laumas, K. (1961). *J. clin. Invest.* **40**, 72.

Tait, S. A. S. and Tait, J. F. (1962). *In* "Methods in Hormone Research" (R. I. Dorfman, ed.), Vol. I, p. 265. Academic Press, New York and London.

Tan, S. Y. and Mulrow, P. J. (1975). *J. clin. Endocr. Metab.* **41**, 126.

Tarazi, R. C., Dustan, H. D., Frohlich, E. D., Gifford, R. W., and Hoffman, A. C. (1970). *Arch. int. Med.* **125**, 835.

Thomas, J. P. and El-Shaboury, A. H. (1971). *Lancet*, **i**, 623.

Thorn, G. W. (1957). *Am. J. Med.* **23**, 507.

Todesco, S., Mantero, F., Terribile, V., Guarnieri, G. F. and Borsatti, A. (1973). *Lancet*, **ii**, 443.

Tomko, D. J., Yen, B. P. and Falls, W. F. (1976). *Am. J. Med.* **61**, 111.

Touchstone, J. C., Greene, J. W. and Kukovetz, W. R. (1959). *Anal. Chem.* **31**, 1693.

Tournaire, J., Audi-Parera, L., Loras, B., Blum, J., Castelnovo, P. and Forest, M. G. (1976). *Clin. Endocr.* **5**, 53.

Tucci, J. R., Espiner, E. A., Jagger, P. I., Pauk, G. L. and Lauler, D. P. (1967). *J. clin. Endocr. Metab.* **27**, 568.

Tuck, M. L., Dluhy, R. G. and Williams, G. H. (1974). *J. clin. Invest.* **53**, 988.

Tuck, M. L., Dluhy, R. G. and Williams, G. H. (1975). *J. Lab. clin. Med.* **86**, 754.

Tuck, M. L., Williams, G. H., Cain, J. P., Sullivan, J. M. and Dluhy, R. G. (1973). *Am. J. Cardiol.* **32**, 637.

Tuck, M. L., Williams, G. H., Dluhy, R. G., Greenfield, M. and Moore, T. J. (1976). *Circ. Res.* **39**, 711.

Tucker, R. M. and Labarthe, D. R. (1977). *Mayo Clin. Proc.* **52**, 549.

Tuffley, R., Rubenstein, D., Slater, J. D. H. and Williams, E. S. (1970). *Endocrinology*, **48**, 497.

Udenfriend, S. (1962). *In* "Florescence Assay in Biology and Medicine", p. 349. Academic Press, New York and London.

Ulick, S. (1976). *J. clin. Endocr.* **43**, 92.

Ulick, S., Gautier, E., Vetter, K., Markello, J. R., Yaffe, S. and Lowe, C. U. (1964). *J. clin. Endocr. Metab.* **24**, 669.

Ulick, S., Laragh, J. H. and Lieberman, S. (1958). *Trans. Assoc. Am. Phys.* **71**, 225.

Ulick, S., Kusch, K. and August, J. T. (1961). *J. Am. chem. Soc.* **83**, 4482.

Ulick, S., Nicolis, G. L. and Vetter, K. K. (1963). *In* "Aldosterone" (E. E. Baulieu and P. Robel, eds). Blackwell Scientific Publications, Oxford.

Ulick, S. and Lieberman, S. (1957). *J. Am. chem. Soc.* **79**, 6567.

Ulick, S. and Vetter, K. K. (1962). *J. biol. Chem.* **237**, 3364.

Ulick, S. and Vetter, K. K. (1965). *J. clin. Endocr. Metab.* **25**, 1015.

Underwood, R. H. and Tait, J. F. (1964). *J. clin. Endocr. Metab.* **24**, 1110.

Urquhart, J., Davis, J. O. and Higgins, J. T. Jr. (1964). *J. clin. Invest.* **43**, 1355.

Vagnucci, A. H., McDonald, R. H., Drash, A. C. and Wong. A. K. C. (1974). *J. clin. Endocr. Metab.* **38**, 761.

Vandongen, R. and Gordan, R. D. (1970). *Med. J. Aust.* **1**, 215.

Varsano-Aharon, N. and Ulick, S. (1973). *J. clin. Endocr. Metab.* **37**, 372.

Vaughan, E. D., Buhler, F. R., Laragh, J. H., Sealey, J. E., Baer, L. and Bard, R. H. (1973). *Am. J. Med.* **55**, 402.

Vecsei, D., Dusterdieck, A., Jahnecke, J., Lommer, D. and Wolff, H. P. (1969). *Clin.*

Sci. **36**, 241.

Venning, E. H., Dyrenfurth, I., and Giroud, C. J. (1956). *J. clin. Endocr. Metab.* **16**, 1326.

Venning, E. H., Primrose, T., Caligaris, L. C. S. and Dyrenfurth, I. (1957c). *J. clin. Endocr. Metab.* **17**, 473.

Verberckmoes, R., Van Damme, B., Clement, J., Amery, A. and Michielsen, P. (1976). *Kidney Int.* **9**, 302.

Verdy, M. and deChamplain, J. (1969). *Can. Med. Assoc. J.* **98**, 1034.

Vetter, W., Armbruster, H., Tschudi, B. and Vetter, H. (1974). *Steroids,* **23**, 741.

Vetter, W., Freedlender, E. and Haber, E. (1974). *Clin. Immunol. Immunopathol.* **2**, 361.

Vetter, H., Berger, M., Armbruster, H., Siegenthaler, W., Werning, C. and Vetter, W. (1974). *Clin. Endocr.* **3**, 41.

Vetter, H. and Vetter, W. (1974). *J. Ster. Biochem.* **5**, 197.

Vetter, H., Vetter, W., Beckeroff, R., Glonzer, K., Furrer, J., Hahn, C. L., Kollock, R., Kruck, F., Kutz, K., Siegenthaler, W. and Witasser, F. (1973). *Schweiz med. Wschr.* **107**, 1755.

Vetter, W., Zaruba, K., Armbruster, H., Beckerhoff, R., Reck, G. and Siegenthaler, W. (1974). *Clin. Endocr.* **3**, 411.

Vetter, W., Zaruba, K., Armbruster, H., Beckerhoff, R., Uhlschmid, G., Furrer, J. and Siegenthaler, W. (1976). *Clin. Nephrol.* **6**, 433.

Vinci, J. M., Gill, J. R., Bowden, R. E., Pisano, J. J., Izzo, J. L., Radfar, N., Taylor, A. A., Zusman, R. M., Bartter, F. C. and Keiser, H. R. (1978). *J. clin. Invest.* **61**, 1671.

Viol, G. W., Smith, E. K. and Fitzgerald, J. D. (1976). *Clin. Sci. mol. Med.* **51**, 553S.

Vischer, E., Schmidlin, J. and Wettstein, A. (1956). *Experientia,* **12**, 50.

Visser, H. K. A. and Cost, W. S. (1964). *Acta endocr., Copenh.* **47**, 589.

Wahlen, J. D., Tyler, F. D. and West, C. D. (1970). *Clin. Res.* **18**, 172.

Waldhausl, W., Herkener, K., Nowotny, P., and Bratusch-Marrain, P. (1978). *J. clin. Endocr. Metab.* **46**, 236.

Walker, W. G., Moore, M. A., Horvath, J. S. and Whelton, P. K. (1976). *Circ. Res.* **38**, 477.

Wang, C., Chan, R. K., Yeung, R., Coghlan, J. P., Oddie, C. J., Scoggins, B. A. and Stockigt, J. R. (1978). *Proc. Aust. Endocr. Soc.* **21**, 67.

Watanabe, M., Meeker, C. I., Gray, M. J., Sims, E. A. H. and Solomon, S. (1963). *J. clin. Invest.* **42**, 1619.

Watanabe, M., Meeker, C. I., Gray, M. J., Sims, E. A. H. and Solomon, S. (1965). *J. clin. Endocr. Metab.* **25**, 1665.

Wiedman, P., de Chatel, R., Schiffman, A., Bachmann, E., Beratta-Piccoli, C., Reubi, F. C., Ziegler, W. H., Vetter, W. (1977). *Klin. Wschr.* **55**, 725.

Weidman, P., De Myttenaere-Bursztein, S., Maxwell, M. H. and de Lima, J. (1975a). *Kidney Int.* **8**, 325.

Weidman, P., Horton, R., Maxwell, M. H., Franklin, S. S. and Fichman, M. (1973a). *Kidney Int.* **4**, 289.

Weidman, P., Maxwell, M. H., deLima, J., Hirsch, D. and Franklin, S. S. (1975b). *Kidney Int.* **7**, 351.

Weidman, P., Maxwell, M. H. and Lupu, A. N. (1973b). *Ann. int. Med.* **78**, 13.

Weinberger, M. H. and Donohue, J. P. (1973). *J. Urol.* **110**, 1.

Weinberger, M. H., Dowdy, A. J., Nokes, G. W. and Luetscher, J. A. (1968). *J. clin. Endocr. Metab.* **28**, 359.

Weinberger, M. H., Kramer, N. J., Grim, C. E. and Petersen, L. P. (1977). *J. clin. Endocr. Metab.* **44**, 69.

Weinberger, M. H., Kramer, D. C., Gomez Sanchez, C. E., Kramer, N. J., Martin B. T. and Nugent, C. A. (1975). *J. lab. Clin. Med.* **85**, 957.

Weinberger, M. H., Kramer, N. J., Petersen, L. P., Cleary, R. E. and Young, C. M. (1976). *In* "Hypertension in Pregnancy" (M. D. Lindheimer, A. I. Katz, J. F. P. Zuspan, eds), p. 263. John Wiley, New York.

Weir, R. J., Brown, J. J., Fraser, R., Lever, A. F., Lever, A. F., Logan, R. W., McIlwaine, G. M., Morton, J. J., Robertson, J. I. S. and Tree, M. (1975). *J. clin. Metab.* **40**, 108.

Weir, R. J., Paintin, D. B., Brown, J. J., Fraser, R., Lever, A. F., Morton, J. J., Robertson, J. I. S. and Young, J. (1971). *J. Obstet. Gynaecol. Br. Commonw.* **78**, 580.

Weldon, V. V., Kowarski, A. and Migeon, C. J. (1967). *Pediatrics,* **39**, 713.

Wenting, G. J., Man In't Veld, A. J., Derkx, F. H., Brummelen, P. W. and Schalekamp, M. A. D. H. (1978). *J. clin. Endocr. Metab.* **46**, 326.

Werning, C., Schwerkert, H. H., Steel, D., Vetter, W. and Siegenthaler, W. (1970). *Klin. Wschr.* **48**, 1365.

Wettstein, A. (1954). *Experientia,* **10**, 397.

Whipp, G. T., Coghlan, J. P., Shulkes, A., Skinner, S. L. and Wintour, E. M. (1978). *Aust. J. exp. Biol. med. Sci.* **56**, 545.

Whipp, G. T., Wintour, E. M., Coghlan, J. P. and Scoggins, B. A. (1976). *Aust. J. exp. Biol. med. Sci.* **54**, 71.

Wilcox, C. S., Amenoff, M. W. and Slater, J. D. (1977). *Clin. Sci. mol. Med.* **53**, 321.

Wilkinson, S. P., Bernade, M., Smith, I. K., Jowett, T. P., Slater, J. D. and Williams, R. (1977). *Gastroeterology,* **73**, 659.

Williams, G. H., Bailey, G. L., Hampers, C. L., Lauler, D. P., Merrill, J. P., Underwood, R. H., Blair-West, J. R., Coghlan, J. P., Denton, D. A., Scoggins, B. A. and Wright, R. D. (1973). *Kidney Int.* **4**, 280.

Williams, G. H., Braley, L. M. and Underwood, R. H. (1976). *J. clin. Invest.* **58**, 221.

Williams, G. H., Cain, J. P., Dluhy, R. G. and Underwood, R. H. (1972a). *J. clin. Invest.* **51**, 1731.

Williams, G. H., Dluhy, R. G. and Moore, J. J. (1977). *Mayo Clin. Proc.* **52**, 312.

Williams, G. H., Dluhy, R. G. and Underwood, R. H. (1970a). *Clin. Sci.* **39**, 489.

Williams, G. H., Rose, L. I., Dluhy, R. G., McCaughn, D., Jagger, P. I., Hickler, R. G. and Lauler, D. P. (1970b). *Ann. int. Med.* **72**, 317.

Williams, G. H., Tuck, M. L., Rose, L. I. Dluhy, R. G., Underwood, R. H. (1972b). *J. clin. Invest.* **51**, 2645.

Williamson, H. E. (1963). *Biochem. Pharmac.* **12**, 1449.

Wintour, E. M., Blair-West, J. R., Brown, E. H., Coghlan, J. P., Denton, D. A., Nelson, J., Oddie, C. J., Scoggins, B. A., Whipp, G. T. and Wright, R. D. (1976). *Clin. Exp. Pharmacol. Physiol.* **3**, 331.

Wintour, E. M., Brown, E. H., Denton, D. A., Hardy, K. J., McDougall, J. G., Oddie, C. J. and Whipp, G. T. (1975). *Acta endocr., Copenh.* **79**, 301.

Wintour, E. M., Brown, E. H., Denton, D. A., Hardy, K. J., McDougall, J. G., Robinson, P. M., Rowe, E. J. and Whipp, G. T. (1977). *In* "Research on Steroids VII" (C. Conti, ed.), p. 475. Elsevier, North Holland Biomedical Press, Amsterdam.

Wintour, E. M., Coghlan, J. P., Oddie, C. J., Scoggins, B. A., and Walters, W. A. W. (1978). *Clin. Exp. Pharmacol. Physiol.* **5**, 399.

Wintour, E. M., Knobil, E., Scoggins, B. A., Skinner, S. L. and Coghlan, J. P. (1974). *Clin. Exp. Pharmacol. Physiol.* **1**, 167.

Wisgerhof, M. and Brown, R. D. (1978). *J. clin. Invest.* **61**, 1456.

Wolfe, L. K., Gordon, R. D., Island, D. P. and Liddle, G. W. (1966). *J. clin. Endocr. Metab.* **26**, 1261.

Wolff, H. P., Koczorek, K. R. and Buchborn, E. (1958). *In* "An International Symposium on Aldosterone" (A. F. Muller and C. M. O'Connor, eds), p. 193. J. and A. Churchill, London.

Wolff, H. P., Lommer, D., Jahnecke, J. and Torbica, M. (1964). *In* "Aldosterone" (E. E. Baulieu and P. Robel, eds), p. 471. Blackwell Scientific Publications, Oxford.

Wong, P. Y., Talamo, R. C., Williams, G. H. and Colman, R. W. (1975). *J. clin. Invest.* **55**, 691.

Woods, T. J., McCaa, R. E., Bower, J. D. and McCaa, C. S. (1974). *Trans. Am. Soc. Ant. Int. Organs,* **20**, 154.

Yamamoto, T., Doi, K., Ogihara, T., Ichihara, K., Hatta, T. and Kumahara, Y. (1976). *Prog. Biochem. Pharmacol.* **12**, 174.

Yoroi, T. and Bentley, D. J. (1978). *Nature, Lond.* **271**, 79.

Yu, R., Anderton, J., Skinner, S. L. and Best, J. B. (1972). *Am. J. Med.* **52**, 707.

Zager, P. G., Burtis, W. J., Luetscher, J. A., Dowdy, A. J. and Sood, S. (1976). *J. clin. Endocr. Metab.* **42**, 207.

Zipser, R. D., Speckart, P. F., Zia, P. K., Edmiston, W. A., Lau, F. Y. K. and Horton, R. (1976). *J. clin. Endocr. Metab.* **43**, 1101.

Zusman, R. M., Spector, D., Caldwell, B. V., Speroff, L., Schneider, G. and Mulrow, P. (1973). *J. clin. Invest.* **52**, 1093.

XI. The Renin–Angiotensin System

BRENDA J. LECKIE, J. A. MILLAR, J. J. MORTON and P. F. SEMPLE

INTRODUCTION

Renin is a proteolytic enzyme which cleaves a decapeptide angiotensin I from its circulating substrate angiotensinogen. The biologically active octapeptide angiotensin II is formed by removal of the C-terminal histidyl-leucine residue from angiotensin I, by a peptidyldipeptide hydrolase or converting enzyme.

Major advances in our understanding of the role of the renin–angiotensin system in blood pressure control and salt and water homeostasis have been made as a result of the identification and synthesis of specific inhibitors of renin, converting enzyme and angiotensin II. Considerable progress in renin purification has been achieved using the renin-inhibitor pepstatin in affinity chromatography systems. It has recently been recognised that there exist inactive forms of the enzyme renin in blood and tissues. The precise chemical nature of these has been the subject of intense investigation.

Methods of measurement of renin and angiotensin II continue to be a subject of interest. The availability of a reference preparation of renin has permitted standardisation of renin assays. The development of antibody-trapping of angiotensin I as an alternative to chemical inhibition of angio-tensinases has simplified the measurement of the concentration of renin in small volumes of plasma.

There may be a renin–angiotensin system in the brain. Many components of the system have been identified in neural tissue and there is increasing interest in the central actions of angiotensin II.

A. RENIN

Renin is a member of the acid protease group of enzymes which also includes pepsin, chymosin, cathepsin D and various microbial enzymes. There are similarities in structure and catalytic action between the enzymes of this group (Foltmann and Pedersen, 1977). Renin is synthesised mainly in the juxta-glomerular cells of the afferent arteriole of the kidney where it is stored in granules (Cook, 1968). These sediment during ultracentrifugation in the "mitochondrial–lysosomal" fractions (Nustad and Rubin, 1970; Morimoto, Yamamoto and Ueda, 1972; Gross and Barajas, 1975; Morris and Johnston, 1976a, b). Renal renin is secreted into the blood. Thus renal vein plasma renin concentration is 10–20% higher than concurrent arterial values (Hosie, Brown, Lever, MacAdam, MacGregor and Robertson, 1970; Millar, Leckie, Semple, Morton, Sonkodi and Robertson, 1978). Bilateral nephrectomy causes a prompt fall in circulating renin levels (Devaux, Menard, Alexandre, Idatte, Meyer and Milliez, 1968; Amery and Hannon, 1969; Derkx, Wenting, Man In't Veld, Verhoeven and Schalekamp, 1978), and plasma renin concen-tration correlates with plasma levels of angiotensin I and angiotensin II (Morton, Semple, Waite, Brown, Lever and Robertson, 1976; Leckie, Brown, Lever, McConnell, Morton, Robertson and Tree, 1976). Renin-like enzymes have been detected in other tissues besides the kidney (Ganten, Hutchinson, Haebara, Schelling, Fischer and Ganten, 1976). Extrarenal sites of renin synthesis must exist in man since renin is detectable in the plasma of anephric patients (Weinberger, Wade, Aoi, Usa, Dentino, Luft and Grim, 1977; Leckie, McConnell, Grant, Morton, Tree and Brown, 1977).

1. Purification

Kidney renin has been purified to homogeneity by Inagami and Murakami (1977a). Their 133,000 fold purification was achieved by including an affinity chromatography step on pepstatin-agarose gel (Murakami and Inagami, 1975) and they also treated the kidney extract with protease inhibitors to eliminate proteases which could destroy the renin during purification. Care was taken to carry out the purification at a relatively neutral pH, compared with earlier procedures. Partial purifications of renin have been described by many groups as reviewed by Haber and Slater (1977). Some references are: pig renin—Haas, Lamfrom and Goldblatt (1953); Peart, Lloyd, Thatcher, Lever, Payne and Stone (1966); Skeggs, Lentz, Kahn and Hochstrasser (1967); Murakami and Inagami (1975) and Corvol, Devaux, Ito, Sicard, Ducloux and Menard (1977). Human renin—Haas, Goldblatt, Gipson and Lewis (1966); Lubash and Peart (1966); Lucas, Fukuchi, Conn, Berlinger, Waldhausl, Cohen and Rovner (1970); Overturf, Leonard and Kirkendall (1974); Slater, Burton and Haber (1975); Murakami, Inagami and Haas (1977). Rat renin—Auzan, Ducloux and Menard (1973); Lauritzen, Damsgaard, Rubin and Lauritzen (1976). Dog renin—Haas, Goldblatt, Lewis and Gipson (1972) and ox—Newsome (1969).

2. Properties

The purified pig enzyme is a glycoprotein of molecular weight (35,000–42,000 depending on the method of estimation. The pI is 5·2 (Inagami and Murakami, 1977a). Earlier reports (Skeggs et al., 1967; Newsome, 1969; Rubin, 1972) had suggested that there might be at least four forms of the enzyme differing in charge, but these findings are probably due to exposure of the renin to low pH during purification (Skeggs et al., 1967; Inagami and Murakami, 1977a). The pig enzyme, and also human renin and renin from mouse salivary glands can be inactivated by diazo-acetyl-D,L-norleucine methyl ester in the presence of cupric ion (Inagami, Murakami, Misono, Workman, Cohen and Suketa, 1977; McKown and Gregerman, 1975). This indicates that the active site of renin contains reactive carboxyl groups similar to those found at the active site of other acid proteases (Rajagopalan, Stein and Moore, 1966; Chen and Tang, 1972).

3. Renin–Substrate Reaction

Compared with other acid proteases renin shows a restricted substrate specificity. It cleaves a leucyl-leucyl bond in an α-globulin substrate to produce the decapeptide angiotensin I. Peptide renin substrates have been prepared and the minimum sequence required for substrate activity appears to be the octapeptide Pro–Phe–His–Leu–Leu–Val–Tyr–Ser (Skeggs, Lentz, Kahn and Hochstrasser, 1968; Reinharz and Roth, 1969). Competitive inhibitors of renin have been made by synthesising substrate analogues

(Skeggs *et al.*, 1968; Kokubu, Ueda, Fujimoto, Hiwada, Akatsu, Yamamura, Saito and Mizoguchi, 1968; Poulsen, Burton and Haber, 1973; Kokubu, Hiwada, Ito, Ueda, Yamamura, Mizoguchi and Shigezane, 1973; Burton Poulsen and Haber, 1975). Renin is inhibited by pepstatin (Morishima, Takita, Aoyagi, Takeuchi and Umezawa, 1973) which also inhibits pepsin and cathepsin. Renin is not affected by agents which inhibit serine proteases (Pickens, Bumpus, Lloyd, Smeby and Page, 1965; Ryan, McKenzie and Lee, 1968) nor by inhibitors of cysteine proteases or metallo-proteases (Pickens *et al.*, 1965; Rubin, 1972). The various classes of renin inhibitor are listed in Table 1. The pH optimum of the purified pig enzyme on pig substrate and on octapeptide substrate is between 6 and 7. The specific activity with pig substrate is 267 µg/hr/µg enzyme (Inagami and Murakami, 1977a).

4. Inactive Renin

Before 1970 there were suggestions that an inactive precursor of renin might exist although direct evidence was lacking (Meyer, Kruh, Biron, Milliez, Chevillard, Lorain and Pasquier, 1965; Skeggs *et al.*, 1967; de Vito, Cabrera and Fasciolo, 1970). Lumbers (1971) showed that amniotic fluid dialysed to pH 3·3 and then back to pH 7·4 had a higher renin concentration than amniotic fluid dialysed to pH 4·0 or above and suggested that this was due to acid-activation of an inactive renin. Since then, high-molecular-weight forms of renin that can be activated by acid, by proteolytic enzyme and by low temperature have been detected in the kidneys and plasma of several species (Reid, Morris and Ganong, 1978). The material activated by such treatments has been given different names by different groups of workers, e.g. "inactive renin" (Lumbers, 1971; Leckie and McConnell, 1975a; Derkx, van Gool, Wenting, Verhoeven, Man In't Veld and Schalekamp, 1976): "big renin" (Day and Leutscher, 1974) and "prorenin" (Sealey, Moon, Laragh and Alderman, 1976; Sealey, Moon, Laragh and Atlas, 1977). It is not yet clear if all these terms refer to the same substance.

(a) Kidney extracts

The renin concentration in extracts of pig kidney (Rubin, 1972; Boyd, 1972, 1974) and rabbit kidney (Leckie, 1973) was increased by exposure to a pH of 2·5–3·5. When pig or rabbit kidney extracts were submitted to gel filtration, a slow-acting or inactive form of renin with a molecular weight of around 55,000–60,000 was detected. The pig slow-acting renin was irreversibly activated by exposure to low (3·0) or high (10·5) pH and reversibly activated by a high concentration of sodium chloride. It appeared to be a protein–renin complex (Boyd, 1974). Rabbit inactive renin was irreversibly activated

Table 1

Inhibition of the renin–substrate reaction.

Type	Example	References
Irreversible	Diazo-acetyl-D,L norleucine methyl ester	McKown and Gregerman (1975)
	1,2 epoxy-3-phenoxy-propane	Inagami et al. (1977)
Reversible	Pepstatin	Gross et al. (1972)
	Substrate analogues e.g. Leu–Leu–Val–Phe–OMe[a]	Kokubu et al. (1968, 1973)
	H–Pro–His–Pro–Phe–His–Leu–Leu–Val–Tyr (and others)	Burton et al. (1975)
Uncharacterised	α–1 Trypsin inhibitor	Scharpé et al. (1976)
	"Rat plasma"	Schaechtelin et al. (1968)
		Barrett, Eggena and Sambhi (1973)
	"Plasma lipids"	Kotchen, Talwalker, Miller and Welch (1976)
		Kotchen, Talwalker and Welch (1977)
	"Renal cortex"	Levine et al. (1978)
		Boyd (1972)
		Leckie (1975)
	"Phospholipid"	Smeby, Sen and Bumpus (1967)
		Osmond, Ross and Holub (1973)

[a] Methyl ester.

by dialysis to pH 2·5, and dissociated into active renin plus a renin inhibitor when chromatographed on DEAE cellulose (Leckie and McConnell, 1975a). Acidification destroyed the inhibitor. Levine, Lentz, Kahn, Dorer and Skeggs (1976, 1978) studied the activation of a renin of molecular weight 60,000 in pig kidneys. Inactive renins of molecular weight 140,000 and 60,000 were isolated from pig kidney by Murakami, Matoba and Inagami (1976), but it was necessary to include protease inhibitors in the buffer, otherwise active renin was recovered. High-molecular-weight renins appeared to be the native form in the kidney and could be converted to active renin by proteolysis (Inagami et al., 1977; Leckie, 1973; Hirose, Matoba and Inagami, 1976; Levine et al., 1978). Human kidneys may contain inactive renin. Day and Leutscher (1974, 1975) and Day, Leutscher and Gonzales (1975) found a "big renin" of molecular weight 60,000 in the kidney and plasma of patients with Wilm's tumour, renal carcinoma and diabetic nephropathy. Evidence for an inactive renin in normal human kidney is conflicting (Day and Leutscher, 1974; Eggena, Chu, Barrett and Sambhi, 1977) but Slater and Haber (1976) isolated a high-molecular weight renin (mw 63,000) from normal human kidney. Morris and Johnston (1976b) showed that inactive renin was present in granules from rat kidney cortex, although Lauritzen et al. (1976) were unable to isolate high molecular weight renin from rat kidney.

(b) Plasma and amniotic fluid

Renin in human plasma can be activated by acidification (Skinner, Lumbers and Symonds, 1972; Derkx, van Gool, Wenting, Verhoeven, Man In't Veld and Schalekamp, 1976; Boyd, 1977; Leckie et al., 1977) by trypsin (Cooper, Osmond, Scaiff and Ross, 1974; Day et al., 1975; Leckie, McConnell and Jordan, 1977) and by exposure to cold (Osmond, Ross and Scaiff, 1973; Sealey et al., 1977). Acid and trypsin appear to act on the same material since they both increase plasma renin concentration to the same extent (Leckie et al., 1977). Cold-activation is slow (Sealey et al., 1976) or undetectable (Leckie et al., 1977b) at 4° but takes place over four days at $-5°$. Since cold-activation can be inhibited by Trasylol, Osmond and Loh (1978) and Atlas, Sealey and Laragh (1977) suggested that it involved the action of a proteolytic enzyme on inactive renin. Earlier, Morris and Lumbers (1972) had shown that an endogenous enzyme activator appeared to be responsible for the acid-activation of amniotic fluid inactive renin. The acid-activation of plasma inactive renin is prevented by inhibitors of serine proteases and since these inhibitors have no effect on the renin-substrate reaction in either untreated or acidified plasma, they must be acting on an enzyme that is responsible for acid-activation: Acid $\rightarrow$ activating protease $\rightarrow$ inactive renin $\rightarrow$ active renin. Day and Leutscher (1975) and Day, Leutscher and Zager (1976) detected a "big renin" of molecular weight 60,000 in the plasma of certain patients. (The molecular weight did not change after acidification.) Boyd (1977) reported the presence of inactive renin of molecular weight 46,000 in normal plasma and Leckie *et al.* (1977a) showed inactive renin of molecular weight 55,000 in plasma from a patient with renal hypertension. There is some argument as to whether plasma inactive renin is derived from the kidney, particularly as plasma from anephric patients can show normal (Leckie *et al.*, 1977) or high (Weinberger *et al.*, 1977) inactive renin levels. However, the concentration of inactive renin falls after bilateral nephrectomy (Derkx, Wenting, Man In't Veld, Verhoeven and Schalekamp, 1978). The half-life is 150–165 min as against 50–80 min for active renin and this may account for the biphasic disappearance curves found for "total renin" by Amery and Hannon (1969). Also, a positive venous-arterial difference in inactive renin has been observed in the human (Millar *et al.*, 1978) and some patients with renal artery stenosis show high inactive renin levels on the affected side (Derkx *et al.*, 1978).

Acute stimulation of the renin-angiotensin system in man may not alter or may increase or decrease plasma inactive renin concentration. Derkx *et al.* (1976) noted a fall in plasma inactive renin, and a rise in plasma active renin concentration after administration of diazoxide, or on tilting. Millar *et al.* (1978), and Weinberger, Aoi and Grim (1977), noted an increase in concentration of both active and inactive renin after administration of frusemide. Dietary sodium depletion did not alter (Millar *et al.*, 1978), or increased (Sealey, Moon, Laragh and Atlas, 1977), plasma inactive renin levels; while sodium depletion caused by administration of spironolactone to normal people resulted in a rise of plasma inactive renin concentration (Millar, Cumming, Fraser, Mason, Leckie, Morton, Ramsay and Robertson, 1978). The administration of fludrocortisone to normal subjects suppressed both active and inactive renin concentration in plasma (Millar *et al.*, 1978b).

Plasma levels of inactive renin are raised during pregnancy (Skinner *et al.*, 1972; Skinner, Cran, Gibson, Taylor, Walters and Catt, 1975; Leckie *et al.*, 1977) and in some patients with hypertension or renal tumour (Day *et al.*, 1976; De Leiva, Christlieb, Melby, Graham, Day, Leutscher and Zager, 1976; Derkx *et al.*, 1978; Atlas, Laragh, Sealey and Moon, 1977; Leckie *et al.*, 1977).

In rabbits, plasma inactive renin remained a constant proportion of the total after haemorrhage but the concentration fell during sodium depletion (Grace, Munday, Noble and Richards, 1977a, 1977b).

The biochemical nature and function of inactive renin is still unknown.

To summarise; in hog, rabbit and human kidneys, renin of molecular weight around 60,000 has been detected and renins of even higher molecular weight (150,000) may be present. These high-molecular-weight renins are relatively inactive and their enzymatic activity can be increased by the action of acid and proteases. Activation by acid involves the participation of a protease. Activation is sometimes, but not invariably, associated with a fall in molecular weight. However, some workers are unable to detect high-molecular-weight renin or report that it cannot be activated. Inactive renin is also present in human plasma and may be derived from the kidney, although it is not known whether plasma inactive renin is identical with the material detected in kidneys. Evidence for the function of inactive renin as a storage form of the enzyme was obtained by de Senarclens, Pricam, Banichahi and Vallotton (1977). They showed that the amounts of acid-activable renin in the kidney and the granulation of the juxtaglomerular cell as assessed by electron microscopy increased when renin synthesis was stimulated then abruptly suppressed.

5. Iso-renin

Renin-like enzymes exist in many tissues beside the kidney (Carretero, Bujak and Houle, 1971; Ganten, Schelling, Vecsei and Ganten, 1976; Bing, Eskildsen, Faarup and Frederikson, 1967). Table 2 summarises some properties of those enzymes that have been studied most extensively.

(a) Salivary gland renin

Salivary gland renin (Werle, Vogel and Göldel, 1957; Hackenthal, Koch, Bergemann and Gross, 1972; Gutman, Levy and Shorr, 1973) has been purified from male mouse tissue by Cohen, Taylor, Murakami, Michelakis and Inagami (1972). The amino acid composition of the mouse enzyme is similar to that of renal renin (Michelakis, Cohen, Taylor, Murakami and Inagami, 1974). The salivary enzyme may be released into the blood (Bing and Poulsen, 1976; Weinberger et al., 1977) and its genetic regulation has been studied (Wilson, Erdös, Dunn and Wilson, 1977).

(b) Brain iso-renin

(Ganten, Minnich, Granger, Hayduk, Brecht, Barbeau, Boucher and Genest, 1971; Fischer-Ferraro, Nahmod, Goldstein and Finkielman, 1971; Haulica, Branisteanu, Rosca, Stratone, Berbeleu, Balan and Ionescu, 1975). The dog and human brain enzyme acts more readily on tetradecapeptide (TDP) substrate than on dog, hog or human angiotensinogen and its pH optimum on both TDP and angiotensinogen is lower than that of renal renin. It is inhibited by antibodies to partially purified renal renin but to a lesser extent than the renal enzyme (Ganten, Marquez-Julio, Granger, Hayduk, Karsunky, Boucher and Genest, 1971; Husain and Jones, 1977; Daul, Heath and Garey, 1975). Day and Reid (1976) showed that the dog brain enzyme is similar to cathepsin D. It seems probable that brain tissue contains both cathepsin D

Table 2

Iso-renins.

Enzyme	Species	Substrate and pH optimum		References
Salivary gland renin	Mouse	TDP[a]	6·5	Cohen et al. (1972)
				Michelakis et al. (1974)
				Inagami et al. (1977)
		Rat	8·0–8·5	Bing and Poulsen (1976)
	Rat	Rat	6·0	Hackenthal (1972)
Brain renin	Dog	Dog	5·0	Ganten et al. (1971)
	Dog	Dog	4·5	Day and Reid (1976)
	Human	Hog	4·5–5·5	Daul et al. (1975)
		Human	Inactive	
	Dog	Dog	7·0	Fischer-Ferraro et al. (1971)
	Rat	Dog	4·4–4·8	Husain et al. (1977)
Pseudorenin	Hog	TDP	4·5	Skeggs et al. (1969)
		Hog	5·0	
Uterus	Rabbit	Rabbit	6·0	Anderson et al. (1968)
				Ryan and Johnson (1969)
	Dog	Dog	7·1	Carretero et al. (1970)
	Dog	Dog	7·0	Potter et al. (1977)
	Rat	Rat	4·0	Gutman (1976)
Blood vessel	Hog	Hog	6·7–7·5	Gould (1964)

[a]Tetradecapeptide.

and a renin-like enzyme. The possible physiological importance of the renin-like enzyme from brain is discussed by Ganten et al., (1976) and Reid (1977).

The pseudorenin found by Skeggs, Lentz, Kahn, Dorer and Levine (1969) in pig kidney and rat tissues also has a low pH optimum, acts readily on TDP and may be a cathepsin-like enzyme.

(c) Uterine renin

(Gross, Schaechtelin, Ziegler and Berger, 1964; Bing and Faarup, 1966; Ryan and Johnson, 1969; Geelhoed, Vander and Carlson, 1970; Ryan, 1970; Jorgensen, 1974; Hodani, Carretero and Hodgkinson, 1969; Gordon, Ferris and Mulrow, 1967). Uterine renin is similar to renal renin in pH optimum, molecular weight and electrophoretic mobility but differences in Km have been noted (Carretero and Houle, 1970; Anderson, Herbert and Mulrow, 1968; Potter, McDonald, Metcalfe and Porter, 1977). The rabbit uterine enzyme is neutralised by antibodies to partially purified hog renal renin (Bing and Faarup, 1966). The rat enzyme of Gutman and Mazur-Ruder (1976) shows a lower pH optimum, is activated by K^+ and is probably different from the dog and rabbit uterine enzymes described above. Renin is produced by human chorion and uterus in tissue culture (Symonds, Stanley and Skinner, 1968). Placenta (Stakemann, 1960; Ziegler, Riniker and Gross, 1967) and human amniotic fluid (Brown, Davis, Doak, Lever and Robertson, 1964) also contain renin.

(d) Blood vessel walls

The enzyme found by Gould, Skeggs and Kahn (1964) in blood vessel walls is similar to renin. The authors concluded that it might either be absorbed from the blood or synthesised in situ. The concentration of the enzyme in arterial walls is altered by changes in dietary sodium (Hayduk, Brecht, Vladutiu, Rojo-Ortega, Boucher and Genest, 1970) and the administration of aldosterone and sodium chloride (Rosenthal, 1976).

(e) Adrenal

Renin-like enzymes are present in the adrenals of rabbit (Ryan, 1967), rat (Ganten, Ganten, Kubo, Granger, Nowaczynski, Boucher and Genest, 1974), dog (Hayduk, Boucher and Genest, 1970) and ox (Ryan, 1972).

6. Renin Assay

Many renin assay techniques have been reported but in this section comments will be restricted to those which we believe are of general applicability to modern renin assays. There are three main methods of renin assay: measurement of the rate of production of angiotensin I (AI) from either homologous or heterologous angiotensinogen, measurement of the rate of cleavage of a synthetic substrate and measurement of the amount of renin using antibodies to purified renin.

(a) With natural angiotensinogen

Most assays measure AI generated in a defined incubation mixture. "Plasma renin activity" (PRA) methods involve the inhibition of angiotensinase in plasma, generally by chemical inhibitors, followed by determination of the velocity of the reaction when plasma reacts with endogenous angiotensinogen. The AI produced is measured by radioimmunoassay which has almost completely superseded the previous bioassay methods. PRA methods have been described by Gould, Skeggs and Kahn (1966); Skinner (1967); Haber, Koerner, Page, Kliman and Purnode (1969); Boucher, Veyrat, de Champlain and Genest (1964); Boyd, Adamson, Fitz and Peart (1969); Poulsen and Jorgenson (1974). The method of Poulsen (1971, 1973) is particularly interesting since the need for chemical inhibition of angiotensinase activity is eliminated. The AI generated during the assay is trapped by an excess of antibody to AI and is thus protected from the action of angiotensinases. The trapped angiotensin can then be measured by radioimmunoassay.

PRA methods have some disadvantages. The concentration of substrate in plasma varies within limits that could affect the velocity of the renin reaction (Gould and Green, 1971). Thus the rate of AI generation can depend on the amount of endogenous substrate as well as the amount of renin present. Since these methods depend on endogenous angiotensinogen they cannot be used to measure renin in fractionated plasma, e.g. after column chromatography. Also, they are more difficult to calibrate against standard renin, although internal calibration methods have been described (Haas, Gould and Goldblatt, 1968; Giese, Jorgensen, Nielsen, Lund and Munck, 1970). If such an internal calibration is used variations in velocity of AI generation due to variations in substrate concentration can be accounted for and a measure of the renin concentration in the plasma is obtained.

"Plasma renin concentration" (PRC) methods involve the incubation of renin plasma or tissue extracts with exogenous renin substrate. Ideally, human angiotensinogen should be used for human renin but the difficulty of preparing sufficient amounts of renin-free and angiotensinase-free human angiotensinogen has led to the use of angiotensinogen from nephrectomised animals, e.g. sheep (Skinner, 1967) or ox (Brown et al., 1964). Human plasma is freed from angiotensinase by the addition of inhibitors or by extraction and is incubated with a known amount of added angiotensinogen. The rate of production of AI is measured. The use of antibody-trapping (Poulsen and Jorgensen, 1974; Millar et al., 1978) is a useful alternative to chemical inhibition or extraction. The use of exogenous substrate overcomes some of the disadvantages of the PRA method. However some of the older PRC methods that involve extraction and acidification of plasma measure total rather than active renin since inactive renin is activated by these procedures (Leckie et al., 1976; Skinner et al., 1972).

A comparison of several renin assay methods has been described by Bangham, Robertson, Robertson, Robinson and Tree (1975) and an International Reference Preparation of human renin is available as a standard to calibrate renin assays. If such a standard was generally used, the results of the renin assays from different laboratories would be comparable.

W

(b) With artificial substrates

An interesting development in renin assay is the use of synthetic substrates, such as the substrates described by Skeggs et al. (1968) and Levine, Dorer, Kahn, Lentz and Skeggs (1970) and the octapeptide of Reinharz and Roth (1969).

However these substrates are more readily attacked by peptidases and by proteases than is the natural angiotensinogen. Production of AI from tetradecapeptide substrate by proteases other than renin can occur, particularly at acid pH. Peptide substrates have not been widely used for the assay of renin in plasma. The development of synthetic substrates for radiochemical (Mendelsohn and Johnston, 1971), fluorimetric or spectrophotometric methods of renin assay, could be useful in the study of the purified enzyme.

(c) Direct assay

Renin assays based on the immunoassay of the enzyme molecule rather than its enzymatic activity have been described for mouse renin (Malling and Poulsen, 1977) and hog renin (Hirose, Inagami and Workman, 1977). A sufficiently pure antibody for the direct immunoassay of human renin has not yet been prepared.

The discovery of cryoactivation at $4°$ has potential implications for sampling techniques, as pointed out by Sealey et al. (1977). However, activation at this temperature (in contradistinction to that at $-5°$) is very slow and we find that over a period of 2 hr is unmeasurable except in those rare plasma samples where the proportion of inactive renin is abnormally increased (Millar et al., 1978). We consider that the requirement for low blank values for AI outweighs possible cryoactivation, and recommend cooling of blood samples to $4°$ immediately after sampling, with separation and freezing of plasma within 2 hr. This procedure will give undetectable levels of AI in the zero time sample without measurable activation of inactive renin.

(d) Inactive renin

The concentration of inactive renin can be estimated by finding the difference between the concentration of total renin and active renin in a sample of plasma, amniotic fluid or kidney extract; where total renin = renin concentration after treatment with acid or trypsin and active renin = renin concentration of untreated plasma (Lumbers, 1970; Leckie et al., 1977). Sealey et al. (1976) describe a method of measuring "prorenin" by assaying plasma before and after cryoactivation. Since inactive renin concentration is a derived value it is subject to a larger error than measurements of total or active renin concentration alone. While this is not important in detecting large variations of inactive renin such as those that can occur in the plasma of patients with renal tumours (Day *et al.*, 1976; Leckie *et al.*, 1978) measurements of small differences, such as those between renal arteries and veins, can be hampered (Millar *et al.*, 1978).

7. Renin Release

Davis and Freeman (1976) have comprehensively reviewed the mechanisms involved in the release of renin. Three main factors determine the rate of renin release:

(i)   the sympathetic nervous system and an adrenergic (probably beta-adrenergic) receptor;

(ii)   a renal vascular stretch receptor and the macula densa;

(iii) various humoral agents: sodium, potassium and calcium ions, angiotensin II and arginine vasopressin.

Recent studies suggest that prostaglandins may have an important role (Dew and Michelakis, 1974; Romero and Strong, 1977; Gill, Frolich, Bowden, Taylor, Keiser, Seyberth, Oates and Bartter, 1976).

There is now much evidence that the adrenergic nervous system and a beta-adrenergic receptor increase renin synthesis and secretion. The juxtaglomerular apparatus is richly innervated (Barajas, 1964; Wagermark, Ungerstedt and Ljungqvist, 1968; Muller and Barajas, 1972; Hartroft, 1966). Electrical stimulation of the renal nerves results in renin release (Vander, 1963) and the renin content of the rat kidney diminishes substantially after denervation (Taquini, Blaquier and Taquini, 1964). The renal nerves are involved in the renin response to tilting, upright posture, exercise and cold (Zanchetti and Stella, 1975; Assaykeen, Castellino, Love and Stamey, 1971; Brown, Davies, Lever, McPherson and Robertson, 1966; Fasola, Martz and Helmer, 1968; Gordon, Kuchel, Liddle and Island, 1967; Stella and Zanchetti, 1977): a nervous reflex may be involved. In the dog, blood angiotensin II concentration is increased by bilateral surgical interruption of the vagi (Hodge, Lowe and Vane, 1966). Vagal cooling results in a marked increase in the rate of renin release which is prevented by renal denervation (Mancia, Romero and Shepard, 1975). The neural effect on renin is probably mediated by beta-adrenergic receptors (Ganong, 1973); isoprenaline-stimulated secretion of renin is suppressed by DL-propranolol (Assaykeen, Tanigawa and Allison, 1974; Vandongen, Peart and Boyd, 1973). Plasma renin activity (PRA) is reduced by oral propranolol in patients with essential hypertension (Buhler, Laragh, Baer, Vaughan and Brunner, 1972). Increases in renin secretion induced by diuretics are at least partially dependent on the sympathetic nervous system (Vander and Luciano, 1967; Naughton,

Bertoncello and Skinner, 1975; Winer, Chokshi, Myung and Freedman, 1969; Stella and Zanchetti, 1977). However, a component of the effect may be independent (Johns and Singer, 1973).

Since 1959 it has been recognised that a baroreceptor is involved in the control of renin release (Tobian, Tomboulian and Janecek, 1959). The non-filtering kidney preparation developed by Blain, Davis and Witty (1970) has proved a useful tool in the investigation of the vascular stretch mechanism: in this model the macula densa does not function. Studies with the non-filtering kidney have confirmed that the renin response to haemorrhage and lowered perfusion pressure is independent of the renal nerves and the macula densa (Blaine et al. 1970; Blaine, Davis and Prewitt, 1971). The stretch receptor appears to respond to changes in afferent arteriolar wall tension and factors altering this tension, the sympathetic nervous system and hormones which affect vascular tone, may act through this mechanism. The responses to heart failure, renal artery stenosis, sodium depletion, volume expansion, haemorrhage and high blood pressure may all be explained on this basis (Davis and Freeman, 1976).

The hypothesis that the macula densa exerts an important effect on renin has been difficult to examine. The available evidence suggests the stimulus is a decreased sodium or chloride load in the renal tubule (Vander and Carlson, 1969; Freeman, Davis, Gotshall, Johnson and Spielman, 1974).

Angiotensin II probably exerts a negative feedback on renin (Vander and Geelhoed, 1965; Davis, 1975; Millar, Samuels, Haber and Barger, 1975). Antidiuretic hormone (ADH) also inhibits the release of renin (Shade, Davis, Johnson, Gotshall and Spielman, 1973). Other humoral factors may also have a role: the plasma concentrations of sodium potassium and calcium may be important.

B. ANGIOTENSINOGEN

1. Purification and Properties

Human angiotensinogen has been purified by Tewksbury, Premau, Dumas and Frome (1977). Their preparation was homogenous on ultracentrifugation. Two N-terminal amino acids were identified as alanine, and aspartic acid or asparagine. This suggested that either two polypeptide chains were present or that a mixture of angiotensinogen and molecules that had lost a portion of the N-terminal polypeptide chain had been isolated. Since leucine was not detected as an N-terminal amino acid this suggests that there was no des-angiotensin I angiotensinogen in the preparation. Another purification procedure for human angiotensinogen is that of Eggena et al. (1976) who obtained a homogenous preparation in the presence of 1% sodium dodecyl sulphate on polyacrylamide gel electrophoresis. The molecular weight was 110,000 by gel filtration. In contrast, angiotensinogen purified by Printz, Printz and Dworschack (1977) had a molecular weight of 66,000. Multiple forms of angiotensinogen in human plasma may be detected after polyacrylamide gel electrophoresis (Eggena, Barrett, Hidaka, Thananopavarn, Golub and Sambhi, 1977) or isoelectric focusing (Printz, Printz, Lewicki and Gregory, 1977).

Hog angiotensinogen was studied by Skeggs, Lentz, Hochstrasser and Kahn (1963) and multiple forms were detected on DEAE cellulose chromatography. The molecular weight of all the forms was around 57,000. A comparison of human and animal angiotensinogen has been made by Printz et al. (1977).

2. Measurement

Most methods of angiotensinogen estimation depend on the incubation of angiotensinogen with excess renin in the presence of angiotensinase inhibitors and measurement of the maximum amount of angiotensin I produced (Gould et al., 1966; Tree, 1973; Rosset and Veyrat, 1971; Poulsen, 1967, 1971; Skinner et al., 1972; Johnstone et al., 1977). The preparation of pure human angiotensinogen has resulted in the development of a direct assay for plasma angiotensinogen (Eggena et al., 1977).

Plasma angiotensinogen concentration is increased during pregnancy (Weir, Paintin, Robertson, Tree, Fraser and Young, 1970; Skinner et al., 1972) and oral contraceptive administration (Skinner, Lumbers and Symonds, 1969; Helmer and Judson, 1967; Tree, 1973). The effect of steroids on plasma angiotensinogen concentration has been studied in rats (Krakoff and Eisenfeld, 1977). Plasma angiotensinogen concentration is lowered in some cases of liver disease (Ayers, 1967), nephrotic syndrome and untreated Addison's disease (Tree, 1973).

The kinetic constants of the human renin and human angiotensinogen reaction have been studied by Haas and Goldblatt (1967), Gould and Green (1971), Rosenthal, Wolff, Weber and Dahlheim (1971), Printz et al. (1977) and Hackenthal, Hackenthal, and Hofbauer (1977). Rosenthal et al. (1971) calculated that the concentration of renin substrate in normal plasma is sufficient to permit angiotensin I formation at around 85% of the maximum possible velocity but Gould and Green (1971) calculated that the normal substrate concentration only allowed 44% of the maximum possible. It appears that the renin substrate concentration in normal plasma may be within a range capable of affecting the rate of angiotensin I production and thus the concentration of angiotensin II in plasma. However, plasma angiotensin II concentration correlates closely with plasma renin concentration (Morton *et al*, 1976) and renin concentration is likely to be more important than substrate concentration in determining the "in vivo" angiotensin II level.

C. THE ANGIOTENSINS

1. Angiotensin I

The immediate product of the renin–angiotensinogen reaction is the decapeptide angiotensin I (Figs 1 and 2) which probably has no biological activity. There is one report suggesting that angiotensin I has an effect on renal blood flow which is not due to conversion to angiotensin II (Itskovitz and McGiff, 1974). Radioimmunoassay methods have been described for the measurement of angiotensin I in blood (Waite, 1973; Barrett, Eggena and Sambhi, 1977). In man, Semple (1977) reported that the plasma concentrations of angiotensin I were on average 33% lower in the left ventricle than in the main pulmonary artery. This probably reflects conversion of angiotensin I to II within the vasculature of the lung.

2. Conversion of Angiotensin I to II

The enzyme responsible for the conversion of angiotensin I to the biologically active octapeptide angiotensin II is a peptidyldipeptide hydrolase which splits a histidyl-leucine dipeptide from the C-terminal end of the decapeptide (Fig. 2). The enzyme is identical with kininase II which cleaves bradykinin. The subject has been reviewed by Vane (1974), Erdös (1975, 1976, and Oparil (1977).

(a) Site

Although the enzyme was first identified in plasma (Skeggs, Marsh, Kahn and Shumway, 1954), it is now clear that the vascular endothelium, particularly in the lung (Ng and Vane, 1967, 1968; Vane, 1974) is responsible for angiotensin II formation *in vivo*. Studies with an immunoperoxidase technique have demonstrated converting enzyme on the surface of the pulmonary endothelium (Ryan, Ryan, Schultz, Whitaker, Chung and Dover, 1975); it may be located on the pinocytic vesicles of the endothelial cells (Smith, Ryan and Smith, 1973). Although isolated pulmonary arteries convert angiotensin I more readily than systemic arteries (Aiken and Vane, 1970), Ody and Junod (1977) reported that collagenase-dispersed endothelial cells from the pig aorta had similar enzyme activity to cells from the pulmonary artery. Several studies have demonstrated some conversion in limb (Collier and Robinson, 1974), renal (Di Salvo, Peterson, Montefusco and Menta, 1971), splanchnic (Di Salvo, Britton, Galvas and Sanders, 1973) and coronary circulations (Britton and Di Salvo, 1973). Subjects on cardiopulmonary bypass have appreciable circulating levels of angiotensin II (Favré, Valloton and Muller, 1974). Although homogenates of lung have appreciable "angiotensinase" activity (Cushman and Cheung, 1971), the intact pulmonary vasculature, in contrast to that in other tissues, does not destroy angiotensin II (Vane, 1974). The close apposition of endothelial cells in the pulmonary capillaries may prevent blood angiotensin II from gaining access to tissue "angiotensinase" enzymes. In man, plasma levels of angiotensin II are higher in the left ventricle than in the pulmonary artery (Semple, 1977).

Amino acid position	1	2	3	4	5	6	7	8	9	10	11	12	13	14
Angiotensin I	Asp	Arg	Val	Tyr	$\begin{cases} Val \\ Ile \end{cases}$	His	Pro	Phe	His	Leu	—	—	—	—
Angiotensin II	Asp	Arg	Val	Tyr	$\begin{cases} Val \\ Ile \end{cases}$	His	Pro	Phe	–	—	—	—	—	—
Angiotensin III	-	Arg	Val	Tyr	Ile	His	Pro	Phe	–	—	—	—	—	—

Fig. 1. The amino acid sequence of the angiotensins. Angiotensin III is des-Asp[1]-angiotensin II.

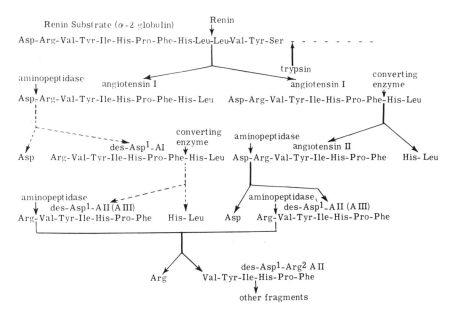

Fig. 2. Formation and metabolism of the angiotensins.

(b) Properties of the enzyme

Converting enzyme has been purified from lung, plasma and kidney of several species. The literature on purification has been reviewed by Erdös (1975). The enzyme from several sources has been purified to homogeneity but estimates of its molecular weight vary (Oparil, 1977): it requires a divalent cation cofactor and has an absolute requirement for halide. Rabbit pulmonary converting enzyme is a zinc-containing glycoprotein with a molecular weight of 129,000 (Das and Soffer, 1975). The human plasma enzyme is also an acidic glycoprotein of molecular weight 140,000 (Lanzillo and Fanburn, 1977): it may originate in the vascular endothelium. In patients with sarcoidosis the plasma concentration of converting enzyme is raised (Lieberman, 1974). Antisera to the enzyme have been raised but their use *in vivo* in animals is limited by pulmonary oedema, which is often lethal (Soffer and Case, 1978).

(c) Inhibitors

Bakhle (1968) first observed that bradykinin-potentiating factor, a mixture of peptides from the venom of the South American pit viper, *Bothrops jararaca*, inhibited the conversion of angiotensin I by particles of canine lung. Two such peptides which inhibited converting enzyme, a pentapeptide and a nonapeptide were isolated and synthesised (Ondetti, Williams, Sabo, Pluscec, Weaver and Kocy, 1971; Stewart, Ferreira and Greene, 1971; Cheung and Cushman, 1973). Both were effective *in vivo* (Stewart *et al.*, 1971) but most subsequent studies were carried out with the nonapeptide, which has a longer duration of action (Greene, Camargo, Krieger, Stewart and Ferreira, 1972). The structure of these peptides is shown in Table 3. The nonapeptide inhibits

Table 3

Angiotensin inhibitors and bradykinin.

Angiotensin analogues
  [Sar^1, Ala^8]–angiotensin II: Sar–Arg–Val–Tyr–Ile–His–Pro–Ala
  [Sar^1, Thr^8]–angiotensin II: Sar–Arg–Val–Tyr–Ile–His–Pro–Thr
  [Sar^1, Ile^8]–angiotensin II: Sar–Arg–Val–Tyr–Ile–His–Pro–Ile
  des-Asp^1 [–Ile^8]–angiotensin II: Arg–Val–Tyr–Ile–His–Pro–Ile

Converting enzyme inhibitors
  Nonapeptide: Pyr–Trp–Pro–Arg–Pro–Glu–Ile–Pro–Pro
  Pentapeptide: Pyr–Lys–Trp–Ala–Pro
  Proline derivative (orally active): D–2–methyl–3–mercapto propranoyl–L–proline

Bradykinin
  Arg–Pro–Pro–Gly–Phe–Ser–Pro–Phe–Arg

---

the pressor action of injected angiotensin I in man (Collier, Robinson and Vane, 1973) and prevents the conversion of endogenous angiotensin I in the dog (Morton, Semple, Ledingham, Stewart, Tehrani, Garcia and McGarrity, 1977). It has been used to delineate the role of angiotensin II in the control of blood pressure, renal blood flow, salt and water homeostasis and aldosterone secretion. As a result of a systematic search, an orally active derivative of proline (D-2-methyl-3-mercapto-propanoyl-L-proline, SQ14225 or Captopril) has been synthesised. It is an effective competitive inhibitor of converting enzyme (Ondetti, Rubin, Cushman, 1977). It inhibits the pressor action of injected angiotensin I in man (Ferguson, Brunner, Turini, Gavras and McKinstry, 1977), and the conversion of endogenous angiotensin I in the dog (Morton, Casals-Stenzel, Lever, Millar, Riegger and Tree, 1978): the duration of action in normal subjects is between two and four hours.

3. Angiotensin II

(a) Structure

Two forms of naturally occurring angiotensin II have been identified (Fig. 1). Isoleucine is the amino acid in position 5 in angiotensin derived from horse (Lentz, Skeggs, Woods, Kahn and Shumway, 1956; Skeggs, Kahn and Shumway, 1956), pig (Bumpus, Schwarz and Page, 1957; Bumpus, Schwarz and Page, 1958) or man (Arakawa, Nakatani, Minohara and Nakamura, 1967; Arakawa, Minohara, Yamada and Nakamura, 1968). There is also indirect evidence that this is the natural form of angiotensin II in the rabbit (Macdonald, Louis, Renzini, Boyd and Peart, 1970), dog (Caravaggi, Bianchi, Brown, Lever, Morton, Powell-Jackson, Robertson and Semple, 1976) and rat (Powell-Jackson, Brown, Lever, MacGregor, Macadam, Titterington, Robertson and Waite, 1972). Valine is found in position 5 in ox renin (Elliot and Peart, 1957) and probably also sheep renin (Cain, Catt, Coghlan and Blair-West, 1970).

(b) Catabolism

The circulating half-life of angiotensin II is less than 30 sec: blood contains "angiotensinase" enzymes but the circulating hormone is mainly destroyed in passage across the splanchnic, limb, kidney and cerebral vascular beds (Ryan, 1974; Ledingham and Leary, 1974). The rate of blood flow may be important: in the kidney, reduction of renal blood flow results in an increase in the extraction of labelled angiotensin II (Baillie and Oparil, 1977). The principal enzyme involved in the catabolism of circulating angiotensin II may be an aminopeptidase but this remains uncertain (Ryan, 1974). Early reports that venous blood of man contains substantial amounts of des-Asp^1, Arg^2-angiotensin II (Cain, Catt and Coghlan, 1969a, b) have not been confirmed (Semple, Boyd, Dawes and Morton, 1976). Plasma from human limb blood, and mixed venous plasma also contain only low concentrations of des-Asp^1-angiotensin II and des-Asp^1,Arg^2-angiotensin II (Semple *et al.*, 1976; Semple, 1977).

(c) Des-Asp^1-angiotensin II

In mammals, the stimulation of aldosterone secretion by depletion of sodium is principally mediated by the renin–angiotensin system (review, Brown, Fraser, Lever, Morton and Robertson, 1977). Adrenal and vascular receptors for angiotensin II have different characteristics (Bravo, Khosla and Bumpus, 1975a): it has been suggested that the C-terminal heptapeptide des-Aspartyl-angiotensin II, so-called angiotensin III (Figs 1 and 2) may be the effector hormone (Goodfriend and Peach, 1975; Davis and Freeman, 1977). There are reports that the heptapeptide is at least equipotent with angiotensin II in stimulating aldosterone in man (Kono, Oseko, Shimpo, Nanno and Endo, 1975), rat (Campbell, Brooks and Pettinger, 1974), sheep (Blair-West, Coghlan, Denton, Funder, Scoggins and Wright, 1971), dog (Freeman, Davis, Lohmeier and Spielman, 1976; Bravo, Khosla and Bumpus, 1976) and rabbit (Steele, Neusy and Lowenstein, 1976). Other studies have suggested that this peptide is less potent than angiotensin II in man (Carey, Vaughan, Peach and Ayers, 1978), rat (Campbell, Schmitz and Itskovitz, 1977a and b) and dog (McCaa, 1977). Some of these differences may be explained by different rates of metabolism or volumes of distribution of the two peptides (Semple, Nicholls, Tree and Fraser, 1978). As shown in Fig. 2, des-Asp^1-angiotensin II may also be formed by the action of converting enzyme on des-Asp^1-angiotensin I (Tsai, Peach, Khosla and Bumpus, 1975; Chiu, Ryan, Stewart and Dorer, 1976; Ackerly, Tsai and Peach, 1977; Larner, Vaughan, Tsai and Peach, 1976). The concentration of des-Asp^1-angiotensin II in plasma from man and the dog is small relative to the octapeptide (Semple *et al.*, 1976; Caravaggi *et al.*, 1976). In contrast, the arterial concentration of des-Asp^1-angiotensin II in the rat is similar to that of angiotensin II (Semple and Morton, 1976). The nonapeptide des-Asp^1-angiotensin I has yet to be demonstrated in the circulation. It has only weak pressor and aldosterone stimulating properties in conscious rats (Campbell *et al.*, 1977b).

(d) Structure–activity relationships

The Merrifield solid phase procedure has permitted the synthesis of large numbers of analogues of angiotensin II. This has led to the synthesis of competitive inhibitors of the biological action of the hormone and has given information about structure-activity relationships within the molecule. The subject is reviewed by Khosla, Smeby and Bumpus (1974) and Bumpus (1977). The phenyl group in position 8 seems vital for biological activity: substitution or removal greatly reduces the myotropic and vasopressor activity of the peptide. The phenylalanine carboxyl group in position 8 is necessary for binding to the receptor. The distance of the C-terminal carboxyl from phenyl-alanine in angiotensin I probably accounts for its lack of biological activity. Other groups which are important for receptor binding are the aromatic residues in positions 4 and 6 and the guanido group in position 2. The N-terminus of the peptide appears less important since substitution of the carboxyl group with an amide does not affect biological activity. Des-Asp^1 angiotensin II has between 15 and 50% of the pressor activity of the parent peptide (Bumpus, Khairallah, Arakawa, Page and Smeby, 1961; Schwyzer, 1963). As mentioned before there is uncertainty about the potency of this heptapeptide relative to angiotensin II in stimulating aldosterone secretion. Further removal of amino acids from the N-terminal position results in smaller metabolites which have no biological activity.

(e) Inhibitory analogues (Table 3)

The recognition of the critical importance of position 8 in the biological activity of angiotensin II was a key step in the development of angiotensin II blocking agents (Khairallah, Toth and Bumpus, 1970). Khairallah *et al.* (1970) demonstrated that [Ala^8]-angiotensin II could inhibit the effect of angiotensin II on isolated guinea-pig ileum. Several analogues with sub-stitutions in position 8 have some inhibitory properties. The introduction of sarcosine into position 1 together with alanine in position 8 created a much more effective inhibitory peptide (Fessler, Sipos, Denning, Pals and Masucci, 1972). Aminopeptidase A, specific for aspartic and glutamic acid residues, is probably an important enzyme in the catabolism of circulating angiotensin II (Khairallah, Page, Bumpus and Smeby, 1962). Substitution of sarcosine in position 1 prevents the degradation by aminopeptidase A which results in a substantial increase in the half-life (Bumpus, 1977). [Sar^1,Ile^8]- and [Sar^1,Thr^8]-angiotensin II are both potent inhibitors of angiotensin II: the Ile^8 analogue probably has more agonist activity than the Ala^8 analogue (Saltman, Fredlund and Catt, 1976) the Thr^8 analogue has less (Bumpus, 1977).

An analogue of des-Asp^1-angiotensin II, des-Asp^1[Ile^8]-angiotensin II has been used to examine the hypothesis that the heptapeptide mediates the effect of angiotensin II on aldosterone. The heptapeptide analogue has been reported to be more effective than [Sar^1,Ile^8]-angiotensin II in preventing the increase in aldosterone secretion induced by angiotensin II in the dog

(Bravo, Khosla and Bumpus, 1975b) and restriction of sodium intake in the rat (Peach, Sarstedt and Vaughan, 1976). In contrast, it has been found less effective than [Sar^1,Ile^8]-angiotension II in blocking the stimulation of aldosterone by angiotensin II and des-Asp^1-angiotensin II in canine glomerulosa cells (Saltman *et al.*, 1976).

[Sar^1,Ala^8]-angiotensin II has been extensively used in man and animals. A hypotensive effect has been consistently observed in hypertensive patients with raised plasma levels of renin and angiotensin II (Soffer and Case, 1978; Brown, Brown, Fraser, Lever, Morton, Robertson and Rosei, 1976; Brunner, Gavras, Laragh and Keenan, 1973; Streeton, Anderson and Dalakos, 1976). Patients with low plasma renin values may exhibit a mild pressor response to the analogue, a result of its partial agonist properties (Case, Wallace, Keim, Weber, Drayer, White, Sealey and Laragh, 1976). In addition, [Sar^1,Ala^8]-angiotensin II produces an initial transient pressor response which is associated with a rise in the plasma concentration of noradrenaline (McGrath, Ledingham and Benedict, 1977) and may be due to increased adrenergic neurone activity. The hope that the analogue might provide a cheap and effective screening test for surgically curable renovascular hypertension has not been realised. The blood pressure response to the peptide is closely correlated with the circulating plasma concentration of renin or angiotensin II.

(*f*) Measurement (*angiotensins I and II*)

Methods of measuring circulating angiotensin by the rat blood pressure method were insensitive and have been superseded by radioimmunoassay methods. The historical development of these methods has been reviewed (Morton *et al.*, 1976). The following comments refer mainly to the methods used in our laboratory (Waite, 1973; Dusterdieck and McElwee, 1971a).

(*1*) *Antisera.* Both angiotensins are small molecules (mw 1295 and 1046) and are weakly antigenic. If the peptides are conjugated with bovine or rabbit serum albumin (Goodfriend, Levine and Farman, 1964) this antigen will usually produce antibodies with a high titre. Other successful methods used to enhance the antigenicity of the peptide include absorption to carbon particles (Boyd and Peart, 1968) or injection in Freund's adjuvant (Dietrich, 1966; Hefferman, Gilliland and Prout, 1967; Pierach, 1969).

The C-terminal end of the peptide appears to determine immunological specificity (Dietrich, 1967). Antisera to angiotensin II usually cross-react to a small extent with angiotensin I (0·5–2%) and to a high degree with metabolites of angiotensin II containing the C-terminal five amino acids. There is usually a 100% cross-reaction between [Asn^1,Val^5]-angiotension II (Hypertensin, Ciba) and the naturally occurring [Ile^5]-angiotensin II.

The lack of specificity of angiotensin II antisera would be a problem if plasma contained appreciable concentrations of immunoreactive metabolites. Human and dog plasma contains only small concentrations of these fragments (Semple *et al.*, 1976; Caravaggi *et al.*, 1976) and for practical purposes the metabolites may be disregarded. Angiotensin I does not usually interfere in the assay. If large concentrations of angiotensin I are present in plasma containing small concentrations of angiotensin II then this cross-reaction may become important. This may occur after administration of inhibitors of converting enzyme to man or animals (Morton *et al.*, 1977; Morton *et al.*, 1978). The accumulation of angiotensin I is increased by the stimulation of renin secretion by these enzyme inhibitors.

[Sar^1,Ala^8]-angiotensin II (Saralasin) may also cross-react with angiotensin II antisera although the cross-reaction with our angiotensin II antiserum is only 0·0045%. Plasma concentrations of the analogue may exceed 300 ng/ml (306 nmol/l) (Pettinger, Keeton and Tanaka, 1975): this is equivalent to between 15 and 20 pg of angiotensin II/ml plasma (Agabiti-Rosei, Brown, Brown, Fraser, Trust, Lever, Morton and Robertson, 1978).

(2) *Labelled angiotensin.* Both peptides contain a tyrosine residue in position 4 and are readily iodinated with ^{125}I using the chloramine T method of Greenwood, Hunter and Glover (1963). Some damage to the labelled hormone is usual with this technique, probably due to the formation of diiodinated angiotensin. Purification is necessary using column chromatography on DEAE Sephadex at 7·5 (Dusterdieck and McElwee, 1971b). Both angiotensins can be purified by this technique: the further advantage is the removal of unlabelled peptide resulting in a labelled angiotensin of higher specific activity.

We and others (Stockigt, Collins and Biglieri, 1971) have observed that labelled angiotensin I deteriorates more rapidly on storage than labelled angiotensin II.

(3) *Standard preparations.* Bangham and Cotes (1974) have reviewed the standardisation of radioimmunoassay methods. A reference preparation of [Ile^5]-angiotensin II is available from the National Institute for Biological Standards and Control, Holly Hill, London. The commercially available synthetic analogue [Asn^1,Val^5]-angiotensin II (Hypertensin, Ciba) has a consistent composition and gives standard curves identical with those obtained using the reference preparation. If [Asn^1,Val^5]-angiotensin II is used as the standard it is important that the antiserum has an equal affinity for both peptides.

Angiotensin I and II are readily adsorbed on to glass surfaces, especially in dilution. Standard preparations should be stored in a relatively concentrated form and protein should be included in all buffers used in the assay procedure.

(4) *Extraction from plasma.* Correct sampling procedures are essential for

the accurate measurement of circulating levels of the angiotensins. For angiotensin II it is essential to inhibit both the conversion of angiotensin I to II and blood angiotensinase enzymes. EDTA is an effective inhibitor of angiotensin conversion (Skeggs et al., 1956; Gocke, Gerten, Sherwood and Laragh, 1969). Further inhibitors are necessary to completely inhibit angiotensinase activity. This may be achieved by drawing the blood directly into methanol (Catt, Cain and Coghlan, 1967) or into a mixture of 2,3-dimercapto-propanol (BAL) and EDTA (Boyd, Landon and Peart, 1967). We use a combination of EDTA and o-phenanthroline which effectively inhibits converting enzyme and angiotensinases in plasma for up to 6 hr at room temperature. To avoid accumulation of angiotensin I, it is preferable to draw the blood into a cooled syringe, centrifuge and separate the plasma at $+ 4°$. For angiotensin I measurements it is necessary to take the blood into iced ethanol (Waite, 1973).

Most angiotensin II immunoassay methods employ an extraction step. We extract angiotensin I from the purified ethanol extract using Dowex H^+ resin at pH 6·0: angiotensin II is extracted directly from plasma using Dowex H^+ resin. Batch extraction is simple to perform and large numbers of samples can be processed without difficulty. Other workers have used columns of ion exchange resins (Page, Haber, Kimura and Purnode, 1969; Hollemans, van der Meer and Kloosterziel, 1969; Sundsfjord, 1970) and Boyd et al. (1969, 1972) used Fuller's earth. Cain et al. (1972) used SE-Sephadex columns and Nicholls and Espiner (1976) used ethanol to precipitate plasma proteins. Methods have been described using unextracted plasma (Goodfriend, Ball and Farley, 1968; Gocke et al., 1969; Emanuel, Cain and Williams, 1973).

(5) Radioimmunoassay. A detailed account of the radioimmunoassay has been given by Morton et al. (1976). Bound and free hormone can readily be separated using either dextran- or plasma-coated charcoal (Herbert, Lau, Gottlieb and Bleicher, 1965; Morton et al., 1976).

(6) Normal range. Circulating plasma angiotensin II has been found to range from 10 pg/ml (pmol/l) to around 100 pg/ml (pmol/l). Values obtained by methods using extraction are generally lower than those using unextracted plasma. The normal range in our laboratory is 5–35 pg/ml (pmol/l) (Düsterdieck and McElwee, 1971). Plasma proteins may produce nonspecific interference. Circulating angiotensin I values are similar to those of angiotensin II (Semple, 1977).

(7) Measurement of des-Asp¹-angiotensin II. It has not proved possible to produce specific antisera to this peptide. Semple et al. (1976) used an initial paper chromatography step to separate this peptide from angiotension II and the two other immunoreactive metabolites, des-Asp¹,Arg²-angiotensin II and des-Asp¹,Arg²,Val³-angiotensin II. Only small concentrations of immunoreactive metabolites of angiotensin II were identified in human blood. In contrast, substantial circulating amounts of des-Asp¹-angiotensin

II were identified in arterial blood of the rat (Semple and Morton, 1976).

(g) Physiology

(1) Blood pressure and renal blood flow. Angiotensin II causes vasoconstriction in the skeletal, mesenteric and renal vascular beds. In addition, small concentrations of angiotensin II can produce a rise in blood pressure by mechanisms mediated by the central nervous system (Bickerton and Buckley, 1961; Severs, Daniels, Smookler, Kinnard and Buckley, 1966; Deuben and Buckley, 1970), without significant changes in heart rate or cardiac output (Buckley, Singh, Steenberg and Jandyhyala, 1977). Angiotensin II has several other central actions; these include stimulation of the secretion of antidiuretic hormone and thirst (Ferrario, Gildenberg and McCubbin, 1972; Fitzsimons, 1975). The evidence for and against a separate brain renin–angiotensin system has recently been reviewed (Reid, 1977).

In addition to its well known immediate pressor effect angiotensin II infused into animals for periods of days results in a further slow rise in blood pressure (Dickinson and Lawrence, 1963; Cowley and McCaa, 1976). The principal mechanism involved is probably baroreceptor resetting with smaller contributions from a rise in cardiac output (Cowley and Declue, 1976). There is increasing evidence for a primary pathogenetic role for renin and angiotensin II in renovascular hypertension in man and in the two-kidney model in the rat (Riegger, Lever, Millar, Morton and Slack, 1977; Review, Davis, 1977). The oral inhibitor of converting enzyme should be valuable in testing this hypothesis.

The renal vasculature is exquisitely sensitive to angiotensin II: increases in plasma concentration of as little as 3 pmol/1 reduce renal blood flow in man (Hollenberg, Solomon, Adams, Abrams and Merrill, 1972). In man, it seems likely that circulating angiotensin II has an important role in renal vascular homeostasis during restriction of sodium intake (Hollenberg, Williams, Taub, Ishikawa, Brown and Adams, 1977). Thurau has proposed that intrarenal angiotensin II may regulate renal function and blood flow (Thurau, 1964; Thurau, Schnerman, Nagel, Horster and Wahl, 1967). The brush border of the proximal tubule contains high concentration of converting enzyme (Ward, Gedney, Dowben and Erdos, 1975). Levels of angiotensin II, measured by immunoassay in the kidneys of salt-deficient rats are two to 14 fold greater than levels in arterial blood (Mendelsohn, 1976). A physiological role for intrarenal angiotensin II in glomerulo-tubular feedback remains to be established.

Angiotensin II stimulates the release of a prostaglandin E-like substance in the isolated perfused kidney (Needleman, Kauffman, Douglas, Johnson and Marshall, 1973; McGiff, Crowshaw, Terragno, Lonigro, Strand, Williamson, Lee and Ng, 1970; Blumberg, Nishikawa, Denny, Marshall and Needleman, 1977). Prostaglandins may modulate the action of angiotensin II on the renal vasculature.

(2) *Aldosterone, salt and water balance.* In man and most mammalian species changes in aldosterone secretion in response to manipulation of sodium balance are probably mediated by the renin–angiotensin system (review, Brown *et al.*, 1977). Studies with angiotensin II and converting enzyme blocking agents have confirmed that the rise in plasma concentrations of aldosterone which occurs in response to deprivation of sodium is mediated largely by circulating angiotensin II (Sancho, Re, Burton, Barger and Haber, 1976; Stephens, Davis, Freeman, Watkins and Khosla, 1077; McCaa, 1977). Depletion of sodium produces reciprocal changes in the sensitivity of the adrenal glomerulosa and vascular smooth muscle to angiotensin II (Oelkers, Brown, Fraser, Lever, Morton and Robertson, 1974; Hollenberg, Chenitz, Adams and Williams, 1974). The increased adrenal sensitivity is not solely due to a change in the properties of angiotensin II receptors (Williams, Hollenberg and Braley, 1976). In man, angiotensin II and sodium deprivation also result in marked increases in the plasma concentrations of a steroid which may be the immediate precursor of aldosterone, 18-hydroxycorticosterone (Mason, Fraser, Morton, Semple and Wilson, 1977).

In addition to its effect on aldosterone, angiotensin II directly stimulates renal sodium reabsorption (Vander, 1963; Waugh, 1972). This effect is independent of changes in glomerular filtration rate, renal plasma flow, filtration fraction or intracortical distribution of blood flow (Johnson and Malvin, 1977). Studies with the competitive antagonist [Sar^1,Ile^8]-angiotensin II in sodium-depleted dogs suggests that angiotensin may have a direct effect in regulating renal haemodynamics and electrolyte excretion, particularly in states of sodium depletion (Hall, Guyton, Trippodo, Lohmeier, McCaa and Cowley, 1977). The stimulation of aldosterone and the direct renal effect of angiotensin II in states of sodium deficiency probably act together as a means of conserving extracellular fluid volume.

REFERENCES

Ackerley, J. A., Tsai, B. S. and Peach, M. J. (1977). *Circ. Res.* **41**, 231.

Agabiti-Rosei, E., Brown, J. J., Brown, W. C. B., Fraser, R., Trust, P. M., Lever, A. F., Morton, J. J. and Robertson, J. I. S. (1978). *Clin. Endocr.* **10**, 227.

Aiken, J. W. and Vane, J. R. (1970). *Nature, Lond.* **228**, 30.

Amery, A. K. P. C. and Hannon, R. C. (1969). *Lancet*, **i**, 679.

Anderson, R. C., Herbert, P. M. and Mulrow, P. J. (1968). *Am. J. Physiol.* **215**, 774.

Arakawa, K., Minohara, A., Yamada, J. and Nakamura, M. (1968). *Biochim. biophys. Acta*, **168**, 106.

Arakawa, K., Nakatani, M., Minohara, A. and Nakamura, M. (1967). *Biochem. J.* **104**, 900.

Assaykeen, T. A., Castellino, R. A., Love, T. A. and Stamey, T. A. (1971). *Arch. int. Med.* **128**, 378.

Assaykeen, T. A., Tanigawa, H. and Allison, D. J. (1974). *Eur. J. Pharmacol.* **26**, 285.

Atlas, S. A., Laragh, J. H., Sealey, J. E. and Moon, C. (1977). *Lancet*, **ii**, 785.

Atlas, S. A., Sealey, J. E. and Laragh, J. H. (1977). *Kidney Int.* **12**, 495.

Auzan, C., Ducloux, J. and Menard, J. (1973). *C. r. Acad, Sci., Paris*, **277**, 2561.

Ayers, C. R. (1967). *Circ. Res.* **20**, 594.

Bailie, M. D. and Oparil, S. (1977). *Circ. Res.* **41**, 283.

Bakhle, Y. S. (1968). *Nature, Lond.* **220**, 919.

Bangham, D. R. and Cotes, P. M. (1974). *Br. med. Bull.* **30**, 12.

Bangham, D. R., Robertson, I., Robertson, J. I. S., Robinson, C. J. and Tree, M. (1975). *Clin. Sci. mol. Med.* **48**, 135s.

Barajas, L. (1964). *Lab. Invest.* **13**, 916.

Barrett, J. D., Eggena, P. and Sambhi, M. P. (1973). *In* "Mechanisms of Hypertension", p. 223. Elsevier, Amsterdam and New York.

Barrett, J. D., Eggena, P. and Sambhi, M. P. (1977). *Clin. Chem.* **23**, 464.

Bickerton, R. K. and Buckley, J. P. (1961). *Proc. Soc. exp. Biol.* New York **106**, 834.

Bing, J., Eskildsen, P. S., Faarup, P. and Frederiksen, O. (1967). *Circ. Res.* **20 and 21** (Suppl. II), 3.

Bing, J. and Faarup, P. (1966). *Acta path. microbiol. scand.* **67**, 169.

Bing, J. and Poulsen, K. (1976). *Acta path. microbiol. scand.* **84**, 285.

Blaine, E. H., Davis, J. O. and Prewitt, R. L. (1971). *Am. J. Physiol.* **220**, 1593.

Blaine, E. H., Davis, J. O. and Witty, R. T. (1970). *Circ. Res.* **27**, 1081.

Blair-West, J. R., Coghlan, J. P., Denton, D. A., Funder, J. W., Scoggins, B. A. and Wright, R. D. (1971). *J. clin. Endocr. Metab.* **32**, 575.

Blumberg, A. L., Nishikawa, K., Denny, S. E., Marshall, G. R. and Needleman, P. (1977). *Circ. Res.* **41**, 154.

Boucher, R., Veyrat, R., de Champlain, J. and Genest, J. (1964). *Can. Med. Assoc. J.* **90**, 194.

Boyd, G. W. (1972). *In* "Hypertension 1972" (J. Genest and E. Koiw, eds), p. 161. Springer, New York.

Boyd, G. W. (1974). *Circ. Res.* **35**, 426.

Boyd, G. W. (1977). *Lancet*, **i**, 215.

Boyd, G. W., Adamson, A. R., Fitz, A. E. and Peart, W. S. (1969). *Lancet*, **i**, 213.

Boyd, G. W., Landon, J. and Peart, W. S. (1967). *Lancet*, **ii**, 1002.

Boyd, G. W. and Peart, W. S. (1968). *Lancet*, **ii**, 129.

Boyd, G. W. and Peart, W. S. (1974). *In* "Angiotensin" (I. Page and F. M. Bumpus, eds), p. 211. Springer-Verlag, Berlin.

Bravo, E. L., Khosla, M. C. and Bumpus, F. M. (1975a). *Am. J. Physiol.* **228**, 110.

Bravo, E. L., Khosla, M. C. and Bumpus, F. M. (1975b). *J. clin. Endocr. Metab.* **40**, 530.

Bravo, E. L., Khosla, M. C. and Bumpus, F. M. (1976). *Circ. Res.* **38**, (Suppl. II), 11.

Britton, S. and Di Salvo, J. (1973). *Am. J. Physiol.* **225**, 1226.

Brown, J. J., Brown, W. C. B., Fraser, R., Lever, A. F., Morton, J. J., Robertson, J. I. S. and Rosei, E. A. (1976). *Aust. N.Z. J. Med.* (Suppl. 3) **6**, 48.

Brown, J. J., Davies, D. L., Doak, P. B., Lever, A. F., Robertson, J. I. S. and Tree, M. (1964). *Lancet*, **ii**, 64.

Brown, J. J., Davies, D. L., Lever, A. F., McPherson, D. and Robertson, J. I. S. (1966). *Clin. Sci.* **30**, 279.

Brown, J. J., Fraser, R., Lever, A. F., Morton, J. J., and Robertson, J. I. S. (1977). *In* "Hypertension" (J. Genest, E. Koiw and O. Kuchel, eds), p. 874. McGraw-Hill, New York.

Brunner, H. R., Gavras, H., Laragh, J. H. and Keenan, R. (1973). *Lancet*, **ii**, 1045.

Buckley, J. P., Singh, S., Steenberg, M. L. and Jandyhyala, B. S. (1977). *Circ. Res.* **40** (Suppl. 1), 52.

Bühler, F. R., Laragh, J. H., Baer, L., Vaughan, E. D. and Brunner, H. R. (1972). *New Engl. J. Med.* **287**, 1209.

Bumpus, F. M. (1977). *Fed. Proc.* **36**, 2128.

Bumpus, F. M., Khairallah, P. A., Arakawa, K., Page, I. H. and Smeby, R. (1961). *Biochim. biophys. Acta*, **46**, 38.

Bumpus, F. M., Schwarz, H. and Page, I. H. (1957). *Science*, **125**, 886.

Bumpus, F. M., Schwarz, H. and Page, I. H. (1958). *Circulation*, **17**, 664.

Burton, J., Poulsen, K. and Haber, E. (1975). *Biochemistry*, **14**, 3892.

Cain, M. D., Catt, K. J. and Coghlan, J. P. (1969a). *J. clin. Endocr.* **29**, 1639.

Cain, M. D., Catt, K. J. and Coghlan, J. P. (1969b). *Biochim. biophys. Acta*, **199**, 322.

Cain, M. D., Catt, K. J., Coghlan, J. P. and Blair-West, J. R. (1970). *Endocrinology*, **86**, 955.

Cain, M. D., Coghlan, J. P. and Catt, K. J. (1972). *Clin. chim. Acta*, **39**, 21.

Campbell, W. B., Brooks, S. N. and Pettinger, W. A. (1974). *Science*, **184**, 994.

Campbell, W. B., Schmitz, J. M. and Itskovitz, H. D. (1977a). *Life Sci.* **28**, 803.

Campbell, W. B., Schmitz, J. M. and Itskovitz, H. D. (1977b). *Endocrinology*, **100**, 46.

Caravaggi, A. M., Bianchi, G., Brown, J. J., Lever, A. F., Morton, J. J., Powell-Jackson, J. A., Robertson, J. I. S. and Semple, P. F. (1976). *Circ. Res.* **38**, 315.

Carey, R. M., Vaughan, E. D., Peach, M. J. and Ayers, C. R. (1978). *J. clin. Invest.* **61**, 20.

Carretero, O., Bujak, B. and Houle, J. A. (1971). *Am. J. Physiol.* **220**, 1468.

Carretero, O. and Houle, J. A. (1970). *Am. J. Physiol.* **218**, 689.

Case, D. M., Wallace, J. M., Keim, H. J., Weber, M. A., Drayer, J. I. M., White, R. P., Sealey, J. E. and Laragh, J. N. (1976). *Am. J. Med.* **61**, 790.

Catt, K. J., Cain, M. D., Coghlan, J. P. (1967). *Lancet*, **ii**, 1005.

Chen, K. C. S. and Tang, J. (1972). *J. biol. Chem.* **247**, 2566.

Cheung, H. S. and Cushman, D. W. (1973). *Biochim. biophys. Acta*, **293**, 451.

Chiu, A. T., Ryan, J. W., Stewart, J. M. and Dorer, F. E. (1976). *Biochem. J.* **155**, 189.

Cohen, S., Taylor, J. M., Murakami, K., Michelakis, A. M. and Inagami, T. (1972). *Biochemistry*, **11**, 4286.

Collier, J. G. and Robinson, B. F. (1974). *Clin. Sci. mol. Med.* **47**, 189.

Collier, J. G., Robinson, B. F. and Vane, J. R. (1973). *Lancet*, **i**, 72.

Cook, W. F. (1968). *J. Physiol.* **194**, 73.

Cooper, R. M., Osmond, D. H., Scaiff, K. D. and Ross, L. J. (1974). *Fed. Proc.* **33**, 584.

Corvol, P., Devaux, C., Ito, T., Sicard, P., Ducloux, J. and Menard, J. (1977). *Circ. Res.* **41**, 616.

Cowley, A. W. and Declue, J. W. (1976). *Circ. Res.* **39**, 779.

Cowley, A. W. and McCaa, R. E. (1976). *Circ. Res.* **39**, 788.

Cushman, D. W. and Cheung, H. S. (1971). *Biochim. biophys. Acta*, **250**, 261.

Cushman, D. W., Cheung, H. S. and Ondetti, M. A. (1977). *Biochemistry*, **16**, 5484.

Das, M. and Soffer, R. L. (1975). *J. biol. Chem.* **250**, 6762.

Daul, C. B., Heath, R. G. and Garey, R. E. (1975). *Neuropharmacology*, **14**, 75.

Davis, J. O. (1975). *Clin. Sci. mol. Med.* **48**, 35.

Davis, J. O. (1977). *Circ. Res.* **40**, 439.

Davis, J. O. and Freeman, R. H. (1976). *Physiol. Rev.* **56**, 1.

Davis, J. O. and Freeman, R. H. (1977). *Biochem. Pharmacol.* **26**, 93.

Day, R. P. and Leutscher, J. A. (1974). *J. clin. Endocr. Metab.* **38**, 923.

Day, R. P. and Leutscher, J. A. (1975). *J. clin. Endocr. Metab.* **40**, 1085.

Day, R. P., Leutscher, J. A. and Gonzales, C. M. (1975). *J. clin. Endocr. Metab.* **40**, 1078.

Day, R. P., Leutscher, J. A. and Zager, P. G. (1976). *Am. J. Cardiol.* **37**, 667.

Day, R. P. and Reid, I. A. (1976). *Endocrinology*, **99**, 93.

DeLeiva, A., Christlieb, A. R., Melby, J. C., Graham, C. A., Day, R. P., Leutscher, J. A. and Zager, P. G. (1976). *New Engl. J. Med.* **295**, 639.

Derkx, F. H. M., Gool, J. M. G., Wenting, G. J., Verhoeven, R. P., Man in't Veld, A. J. and Schalekamp, M. A. D. H. (1976). *Lancet*, **i**, 196.

Derkx, F. H. M., Wenting, G. J., Man In't Veld, A. J., Verhoeven, R. P. and Schalekamp, M. A. D. H. (1978). *Clin. Sci. mol. Med.* **54**, 529.

Deuben, R. R. and Buckley, J. P. (1970). *J. Pharm. exp. Ther.* **175**, 139.

Devaux, C., Menard, J., Alexandre, J. M., Idatte, J. M., Meyer, P. and Milliez, P. (1968). *Lancet*, **i**, 300.

Dew, M. E. and Michelakis, A. M. (1974). *Pharmacologist*, **16**, 198.

Dickinson, C. J. and Lawrence, J. R. (1963). *Lancet*, **i**, 1354.

Dietrich, F. M. (1966). *Int. Arch. Allergy*, **30**, 497.

DiSalvo, J., Britton, P., Galvas, P. and Sanders, T. W. (1973). *Circ. Res.* **32**, 85.

DiSalvo, J., Peterson, A., Montefusco, C. and Menta, M. (1971). *Circ. Res.* **29**, 398.

Dorer, F. E., Kahn, J. R. and Lentz, K. T. (1974). *Circ. Res.* **34**, 824.

Düsterdieck, G. O. and McElwee, G. (1971a). *Eur. J. clin. Invest.* **2**, 32.

Düsterdieck, G. D. and McElwee, G. (1971b). *In* "Radioimmunoassay Methods" (K. E. Kirkham and W. M. Hunter, eds), p. 24. Churchill, Livingstone, Edinburgh.

Eggena, P., Barrett, J. D., Hidaka, H., Chu, C. L., Thananopavarn, C., Golub, M. S. and Sambhi, M. P. (1977). *Circ. Res.* **41**, 34.

Eggena, P., Chu, C. L., Barrett, J. D. and Sambhi, M. P. (1976). *Biochim. biophys. Acta*, **427**, 208.

Elliot, D. F. and Peart, W. S. (1957). *Biochem. J.* **65**, 246.

Emanuel, R. L., Cain, J. P. and Williams, G. H. (1973). *J. lab. Clin. Med.* **81**, 632.

Erdös, E. G. (1975). *Circ. Res.* **36**, 247.

Erdös, E. G. (1976). *Am. J. Med.* **60**, 749.

Fasola, A. F., Martz, B. L. and Helmer, O. M. (1968). *J. Appl. Physiol.* **25**, 410.

Favré, L., Valloton, M. B. and Muller, A. F. (1947). *Eur. J. clin. Invest.* **4**, 135.

Ferguson, B. K., Turini, G. A., Brunner, H. R. and Gavras, H. (1977). *Lancet*, **i**, 775.

Ferrario, C. M., Gildenberg, P. L. and McCubbin, J. W. (1972). *Circ. Res.* **30**, 257.

Fessler, D. C., Sipos, F., Denning, G. S., Pals, D. T. and Masucci, F. D. (1972). *J. med. Chem.* **15**, 1015.

Fischer-Ferraro, C., Nahmood, V. E., Goldstein, D. J. and Finkielman, S. (1971). *J. exp. Med.* **133**, 353.

Fitzsimons, J. T. (1975). *In* "Control Mechanisms in Drinking" (G. Peters, J. T. Fitzsimons and Peters-Haefeli), p. 97. Springer-Verlag, Berlin.

Foltmann, B. and Pedersen, V. B. (1977). *In* "Advances in Experimental Medicine and Biology" (J. Tang, ed.), p. 3. Plenum Press, New York.

Freeman, R. H., Davis, J. O., Gotshall, R. W., Johnson, J. A. and Spielman, W. S.

(1974). *Circ. Res.* **35**, 307.

Freeman, R. H., Davis, J. O., Lohmeier, T. E. and Spielman, W. S. (1977). *Fed. Proc.* **36**, 1766.

Ganong, W. F. (1973). *Fed. Proc.* **32**, 1782.

Ganten, D., Ganten, U., Kubo, S., Granger, P., Nowaczynski, W., Boucher, R. and Genest, J. (1974). *Am. J. Physiol.* **227**, 224.

Ganten, D., Hutchinson, J. S., Haebara, H., Schelling, P., Fischer, H. and Ganten, U. (1976). *Clin. Sci. mol. Med.* **51**, 117s.

Ganten, D., Marquez-Julio, A., Granger, P., Hayduk, K., Karsunky, K. P., Boucher, R. and Genest, J. (1971). *Am. J. Physiol.* **221**, 1733.

Ganten, D., Minnich, J. L., Granger, P., Hayduk, K., Brecht, H. M., Barbeau, A., Boucher, R. and Genest, J. (1971). *Science,* **173**, 64.

Ganten, D., Schelling, P., Vecsei, P. and Ganten, U. (1976). *Am. J. Med.* **60**, 760.

Geelhoed, G. W., Vander, A. J. and Carlson, J. (1970). *Proc. Soc. exp. Biol. Med.* **133**, 479.

Giese, J., Jørgensen, M., Nielsen, M. D., Lund, J. O. and Munck, O. (1970). *Scand. J. clin. Lab. Invest.* **26**, 355.

Gill, J. R., Frolich, J. C., Bowden, R. E., Taylor, A. A., Keiser, H. R., Seyberth, H. W., Oates, J. A. and Bartter, F. C. (1976). *Am. J. Physiol.* **61**, 43.

Gocke, D. J., Gerten, J., Sherwood, L. M. and Laragh, J. H. (1969). *Circ. Res.* **24/25** (Suppl. 1), 131.

Goodfriend, T. L., Ball, D. L. and Farley, D. B. (1968). *J. lab. Clin. Med.* **72**, 648.

Goodfriend, T. L., Levine, L. and Farman, G. D. (1964). *Science,* **144**, 1344.

Goodfriend, T. L. and Peach, M. J. (1975). *Circ. Res.* **36**, (Suppl. 1), 937.

Gordon, P., Ferris, T. F. and Mulrow, P. J. (1967). *Am. J. Physiol.* **212**, 703.

Gordon, R. D., Kuchel, O., Liddle, G. W. and Island, D. P. (1967). *J. clin. Invest.* **46**, 599.

Gould, A. B. and Green, D. (1971). *Cardiovasc. Res.* **5**, 86.

Gould, A. B., Skeggs, L. T. and Kahn, J. R. (1964). *J. exp. Med.* **119**, 389.

Gould, A. B., Skeggs, L. T. and Kahn, M. D. (1966). *Lab. Invest.* **15**, 1802.

Grace, S., Munday, K. A., Noble, A. R. and Richards, H. K. (1977a). *J. Physiol.* **270**, 72.

Grace, S., Munday, K. A., Noble, A. R. and Richards, H. K. (1977b). *J. Physiol.* **273**, 85.

Greene, L. J. and Camargo, C. M., Krieger, E. M., Stewart, J. M. and Ferreira, S. H. (1972). *Circ. Res.* (Suppl. 11), **31**, 62.

Greenwood, F. C., Hunter, W. M. and Glover, J. S. (1963). *Biochem. J.* **89**, 114.

Gross, D. M. and Barajas, L. (1975). *J. lab. Clin. Med.* **85**, 467.

Gross, F., Lazar, J. and Orth, H. (1972). *Science,* **175**, 656.

Gross, F., Schaechtelin, G., Ziegler, M. and Berger, M. (1964). *Lancet,* i, 914.

Gutman, Y., Levy, M. and Shorr, J. (1973). *Br. J. Pharmacol.* **47**, 59.

Gutman, Y. and Mazur-Ruder, M. (1976). *Br. J. Pharmacol.* **56**, 285.

Haas, E. and Goltblatt, H. (1967). *Circ. Res.* **20**, 45.

Haas, E., Goldblatt, H., Gipson, E. C. and Lewis, L. (1966). *Circ. Res.* **19**, 739.

Haas, E., Gould, A. B. and Goldblatt, H. (1968). *Lancet,* i, 675.

Haas, E., Goldblatt, H., Lewis, L. and Gipson, E. C. (1972). *Circ. Res.* **31**, 65.

Haas, E., Lamfrom, H. and Goldblatt, H. (1953). *Arch. Biochem.* **42**, 368.

Haber, E., Koerner, T., Page, L. B., Kliman, B. and Purnode, A. (1969). *J. clin. Endocr. Metab.* **29**, 1349.

Haber, E. and Slater, E. E. (1977). *Circ. Res.* **41**, (Suppl. 1), 36.

Hackenthal, E., Hackenthal, R. and Hofbauer, K. G. (1977). *Circ. Res.* **41** (Suppl. 2), 49.

Hackenthal, E., Koch, C., Bergemann, T. and Gross, F. (1972). *Biochem. Pharmacol.* **21**, 2779.

Hall, J. E., Guyton, A. E., Trippodo, N. C., Lohmeier, T. E., McCaa, R. E. and Cowley, A. W. (1977). *Am. J. Physiol.* **232**, F538.

Hartroft, P. M. (1966). *Lab. Invest.* **15**, 1127.

Haulica, I., Branisteanu, D. D., Rosca, V., Stratone, A., Berbeleu, V., Balan, G. and Ionescu, L. (1975). *Endocrinology,* **96**, 508.

Hayduk, K., Boucher, R. and Genest, J. (1970). *Proc. Soc. exp. Biol. Med.* **134**, 252.

Hayduk, K., Brecht, H. M., Vladutiu, A., Rojo-Ortega, J. M., Boucher, R. and Genest, J. (1970). *Proc. Soc. exp. Biol. Med.* **135**, 271.

Hefferman, A. G. A., Gilliland, P. F. and Prout, T. E. (1967). *Irish J. Med. Sci.* Sixth series, no. 500, 343.

Helmer, O. M. and Judson, W. E. (1967). *Am. J. Obstet. Gynec.* **99**, 9.

Herbert, V., Lau, K. S., Gottlieb, C. W. and Bleicher, S. J. (1965). *J. clin. Endocr.* **25**, 1375.

Hirose, S., Inagami, T. and Workman, R. J. (1977). *Circulation,* **56**, 214.

Hirose, S., Matoba, T. and Inagami, T. (1976). *Circulation,* **53/54** (Suppl. II), 42.

Hodani, A. A., Carretero, O. A. and Hodgkinson, C. P. (1969). *Obstet. Gynaecol.* **34**, 358.

Hodge, R. L., Lowe, R. D. and Vane, J. R. (1966). *Nature, Lond.* **211**, 491.

Hollemans, H. J. G., van der Meer, J. and Kloosterziel, W. (1969). *Clin. chim. Acta,* **24**, 353.

Hollenberg, N. K., Chenitz, W. R., Adams, D. F. and Williams, G. H. (1974). *J. clin. Invest.* **54**, 34.

Hollenberg, N. K., Solomon, H. S., Adams, D. F., Abrams, H. L. and Merrill, J. P. (1972). *Circ. Res.* **31**, 750.

Hollenberg, N. K., Williams, G. H., Taub, K. J., Ishikawa, I., Brown, C. and Adams, D. F. (1977). *Kidney Int.* **12**, 285.

Hosie, K. F., Brown, J. J., Harper, A. M., Lever, A. F., MacAdam, R. D., McGregor, J. and Robertson, J. I. S. (1970). *Clin. Sci.* **38**, 157.

Husain, A. and Jones, C. W. (1977). *Br. J. Pharmacol.* **60**, 281p.

Inagami, T. and Murakami, K. (1977a). *J. biol. Chem.* **252**, 2978.

Inagami, T. and Murakami, K. (1977b). *Circ. Res.* **41** (Suppl. 11), 16.

Inagami, T., Murakami, K., Misono, K., Workman, R. J., Cohen, S. and Suketa, Y. (1977). *In* "Advances in Experimental Medicine and Biology" (J. Tang, ed.), Vol. 95, p. 225. Plenum Press, New York.

Itskovitz, H. D. and McGiff, J. C. (1974). *Circ. Res.* (Suppl. 1) **34**, 63.

Johns, E. J. and Singer, B. (1973). *Eur. J. Pharmacol.* **23**, 67.

Johnson, M. D. and Malvin, R. L. (1977). *Am. J. Physiol.* **232**, F298.

Jørgensen, J. (1974). *Acta path. microbiol. scand.* **82**, 742.

Kahn, J. R., Skeggs, L. T., Shumway, M. P. and Wisenbaugh, P. E. (1952). *J. exp. Med.* **95**, 523.

Khairallah, P. A., Page, I. H., Bumpus, F. M. and Smeby, R. R. (1962). *Science,* **138**, 523.

Khairallah, P. A., Toth, A. and Bumpus, F. M. (1970). *Med. Chem.* **13**, 181.

Khosla, M. C., Smeby, R. R. and Bumpus, F. M. (1974). *In* "Angiotensin" (I. H. Page and F. M. Bumpus, eds), p. 126. Springer-Verlag, Berlin.

Kokubu, T., Hiwada, K., Ito, T., Ueda, E., Yamura, Y., Mizoguchi, T. and Shigezane,

642   B. J. LECKIE ET AL.

K. (1973). *Biochem. Pharmacol.* **22**, 3217.

Kokubu, T., Ueda, E., Fujimoto, S., Hiwada, K., Kato, A., Akutsu, H., Yamamura, T., Daito, J. and Mizoguchi, T. (1968). *Nature, Lond.* **217**, 456.

Kotchen, T. A., Talwalker, R. T., Miller, M. C. and Welch, W. T. (1976). *J. clin. Endocr. Metab.* **43**, 971.

Kotchen, T., Talwalker, R. T. and Welch, W. J. (1977). *Circ. Res.* **41**, 46.

Kono, T., Oseko, F., Shimpo, S., Manno, M. and Endo, J. (1975). *J. clin. Endocr. Metab.* **41**, 1174.

Krakoff, L. R. and Eisenfeld, A. J. (1977). *Circ. Res.* **41** (Suppl. II), 43.

Lauritzen, M., Damsgaard, J. J., Rubin, I. and Lauritzen, E. (1976). *Biochem. J.* **155**, 317.

Lanzillo, J. J. and Fanbury, B. L. (1977). *Biochemistry,* **16**, 5491.

Larner, A., Vaughan, E. D., Tsai, B. S. and Peach, M. J. (1976). *Proc. Soc. exp. Biol. Med.* **152**, 631.

Leckie, B. (1973). *Clin. Sci.* **44**, 301.

Leckie, B., Brown, J. J., Lever, A. F., McConnell, A., Morton, J. J., Robertson, J. I. S. and Tree, M. (1976). *Lancet,* **ii**, 748.

Leckie, B. and McConnell, A. (1975a). *Circ. Res.* **36**, 513.

Leckie, B., McConnell, A. Grant, A., Morton, J. J., Tree, M. and Brown, J. J. (1977). *Circ. Res.* **40** (Suppl. 1), 46.

Leckie, B., McConnell, A. and Jordan, J. (1977). *In* "Advances in Experimental Medicine and Biology" (J. Tang, ed.), Vol. 95, p. 249. Plenum Press, New York.

Ledingham, J. G., and Leary, W. P. (1974). *In* "Angiotensin" (I. H. Page and F. M. Bumpus, eds), p. 111. Springer-Verlag, Berlin.

Lentz, K. E., Skeggs, L. T., Woods, K. R., Kahn, J. R. and Shumway, M. P. (1956). *J. exp. Med.* **104**, 183.

Levine, M., Dorer, F., Kahn, J., Lentz, K. and Skeggs, L. T. (1970). *Anal. Biochem.* **34**, 366.

Levine, M., Lentz, K. E., Kahn, J. R., Dorer, F. E. and Skeggs, L. T. (1976). *Circ. Res.* **38** (Suppl. 2), 90.

Levine, M., Lentz, K. E., Kahn, J. R., Dorer, F. E. and Skeggs, L. T. (1978). *Circ. Res.* **42**, 368.

Lieberman, J. (1974). *Ann. Rev. resp. Dis.* **109**, 743.

Lubash, G. D. and Peart, W. S. (1966). *Biochim. biophys. Acta,* **122**, 289.

Lucas, C. P., Fukuchi, S., Conn, J. W., Berlinger, F. G., Waldhausl, W. K., Cohen, E. L. and Rovner, D. R. (1970). *J. Lab. clin. Med.* **76**, 689.

Lumbers, E. R. (1971). *Enzymologia,* **40**, 329.

McCaa, R. (1977). *Circ. Res.* (Suppl. 1). **25**, 1.

MacDonald, G. J., Louis, W. J., Renzini, V., Boyd, G. W. and Peart, W. S. (1970). *Circ. Res.* **27**, 197.

McGiff, J. C., Crowshaw, K., Terragno, N. A., Lonigro, A. J., Strand, J. C., Williamson, M. A., Lee, J. B. and Ng, K. K. F. (1970). *Circ. Res.* **27**, 765.

McGrath, B. P., Ledingham, J. G. G. and Benedict, C. R. (1977). *Clin. Sci. mol. Med.* **53**, 341.

McKown, M. and Gregerman, R. I. (1975). *Life Sci.* **16**, 71.

Malling, C. and Poulsen, K. (1977). *Biochim. biophys. Acta,* **491**, 532.

Mancia, G., Romero, J. C. and Shepard, I. T. (1975). *Circ. Res.* **36**, 529.

Mason, P. A., Fraser, R., Morton, J. J., Semple, P. and Wilson, A. (1977). *J. Steroid Biochem.* **8**, 799.

Mendelsohn, F. A. O. (1976). *Clin. Sci. mol. Med.* **51**, 111.

Mendelsohn, F. A. O. and Johnston, C. I. (1971). *Biochem. J.* **121**, 241.

Meyer, P., Kruh, J., Biron, P., Milliez, P., Chevillard, C., Lorain, M. and Pasquier, R. (1965). *In* "Club International sur l'hypertension Arterielle" (P. Milliez and P. Tcherdakoff, eds), p. 57. L'Expansion Scientifique Francaise, Paris.

Michelakis, A. M., Cohen, S., Taylor, J., Murakami, K. and Inagami, T. (1974). *Proc. Soc. exp. Biol. Med.* **147**, 118.

Millar, J. A., Cumming, A., Fraser, R., Mason, P., Leckie, B. J., Morton, J. J., Ramsey, L. E. and Robertson, J. I. S. (1978). *In* "Proceedings of the Searle Symposium, Nice" (G. M. Addison, N. W. Asmussen, P. Corvol, P. W. C. Kloppenborg, N. Norman, R. Schroder and J. I. S. Robertson, eds), p. 412. Excerpta Medica, Amsterdam.

Millar, J. A., Leckie, B. J., Semple, P. F., Morton, J. J., Sonkodi, S. and Robertson, J. I. S. (1978). *Circ. Res.* **43** (Suppl. 1), 120.

Miller, E. D., Samuels, A. I., Haber, E. and Barger, A. C. (1975). *Am. J. Physiol.* **228**, 448.

Morimoto, S., Yamamoto, K. and Ueda, J. (1972). *J. appl. Physiol.* **33**, 306.

Morishima, H., Takita, T., Aoyagi, T., Takeuchi, T. and Umezawa, H. (1970). *J. Antibiotics,* **23**, 263.

Morris, B. J. and Johnston, C. I. (1976a). *Biochem. J.* **154**, 625.

Morris, B. J. and Johnston, C. I. (1976b). *Endocrinology,* **98**, 1466.

Morris, B. J. and Lumbers, E. R. (1972). *Biochim. biophys. Acta,* **289**, 385.

Morton, J. J., Casals-Stenzel, J., Lever, A. F., Millar, J. A., Riegger, A. J. G. and Tree, M. (1979). *Br. J. clin. Pharmacol.* **7** (Suppl. 2), 233.

Morton, J. J., Semple, P. F., Ledingham, I. McA., Stuart, B., Tehrani, M. A., Garcia, A. R. and McGarrity, G. (1977). *Circ. Res.* **41**, 301.

Morton, J. J., Semple, P. F., Waite, M. A., Brown, J. J., Lever, A. F. and Robertson, J. I. S. (1976). *In* "Hormones in Human Blood" (H. N. Antoniades, ed.), p. 607. Harvard University Press, Cambridge, MA.

Muller, J. and Barajas, L. (1972). *J. Ultrastruct. Res.* **41**, 533.

Murakami, K. and Inagami, T. (1975). *Biochem. biophys. Res. Commun.* **62**, 757.

Murakami, K., Inagami, T. and Haas, E. (1977). *Circ. Res.* **41** (Suppl. 11), 4.

Murakami, K., Matoba, T. and Inagami, T. (1976). *Fed. Proc.* **35**, 1355.

Naughton, R. J., Bertoncello, I. and Skinner, S. L. (1975). *Clin. Exp. Pharmacol. Physiol.* **2**, 213.

Needleman, P., Kauffman, A. H., Douglas, J. R., Johnson, E. M. and Marshall, G. R. (1973). *Am. J. Physiol.* **224**, 1415.

Newsome, H. H. (1969). *Biochim. biophys. Acta,* **185**, 247.

Ng. K. K. F. and Vane, J. R. (1967). *Nature, Lond.* **216**, 762.

Ng. K. K. F. and Vane, J. R. (1968). *Nature, Lond.* **218**, 144.

Nicholls, M. G. and Espiner, E. A. (1976). *New Z. Med. J.* **83**, 399.

Nustad. K. and Rubin, I. (1970). *Br. J. Pharmacol.* **40**, 326.

Ody, C. and Junod, A. F. (1977). *Am. J. Physiol.* **232**, C95.

Oelkers, W., Brown, J. J., Fraser, R., Lever, A. F., Morton, J. J. and Robertson, J. I. S. (1974). *Circ. Res.* **34**, 69.

Ondetti, M. A., Rubin, B. and Cushman, D. W. (1977). *Science,* **196**, 441.

Ondetti, M. A., Williams, N. J., Sabo, E. F., Pluscec, J., Weaver, E. R. and Kocy, O. (1971). *Biochemistry,* **10**, 4033.

Oparil, S. (1977). *In* "Hypertension" (J. Genest, E. Koiw and O. Kuchel, eds), p. 156. McGraw-Hill, New York.

Osmond, D. H. and Loh, A. Y. (1978). *Lancet,* **i**, 102.

Osmond, D. H., Ross, L. J. and Holub, B. J. (1973). *Can. J. Biochem.* **51**, 855.

Osmond, D. H., Ross, L. J. and Scaiff, K. D. (1973). *Can. J. Physiol. Pharmacol.* **51**, 105.

Overturf, M., Leonard, M. and Kirkendall, W. M. (1974). *Biochem. Pharmacol.* **23**, 671.

Page, L. B., Haber, E., Kimiera, A. Y. and Purnode, A. (1969). *J. clin. Endocr.* **29**, 200.

Peach, M. J., Sarstedt, C. A. and Vaughan, E. D. (1976). *Circ. Res.* (Suppl. 2) **38**, 117.

Peart, W. S., Lloyd, A. M., Thatcher, G. N., Lever, A. F., Payne, N. and Stone, N. (1966). *Biochem. J.* **99**, 708.

Pettinger, W. A., Keeton, L. and Tanaka, K. (1975). *Clin. Pharmacol. Ther.* **17**, 146.

Pickens, P. T., Bumpus, F. M., Lloyd, A. M., Smeby, R. R. and Page, I. H. (1965). *Circ. Res.* **17**, 438.

Pierach, C. A., Jacobson, M. E. and Carlson, K. L. (1969). *Verh. dtsch. Ges. inn. Med.* **75**, 191.

Potter, D. M., McDonald, W. J., Metcalfe, J. and Porter, G. A. (1977). *Am. J. Physiol.* **233**, E434.

Poulsen, K. (1967). *Acta path. microbiol. scand.* **69**, 19.

Poulsen, K. (1971). *J. lab. Clin. Med.* **78**, 309.

Poulsen, K. (1973). *Scand. J. clin. Lab. Invest.* **31** (Suppl.) 132.

Poulsen, K., Burton, J. and Haber, E. (1973). *Biochemistry,* **12**, 3877.

Poulsen, K., Burton, J. and Haber, E. (1975). *Biochim. biophys. Acta,* **400**, 258.

Poulsen, K. and Jørgensen, J. (1974). *J. clin. Endocr. Metab.* **39**, 816.

Powell-Jackson, J. D., Brown, J. J., Lever, A. F., MacGregor, J., Macadam, R. F., Titterington, D. M., Robertson, J. I. S. and Waite, M. A. (1972). *Lancet,* **i**, 774.

Printz, M. P., Printz, J. and Dworschack, R. T. (1977). *J. biol. Chem.* **252**, 1654.

Printz, M. P., Printz, J. M., Lewicki, I. J. A. and Gregory, T. (1977). *Circ. Res.* **41** (Suppl. 11), 37.

Rajagopalan, T. G., Stein, W. H. and Moore, S. (1966). *J. biol. Chem.* **241**, 4295.

Reid, I. A. (1977). *Circ. Res.* **41**, 147.

Reid, I. A., Morris, B. J. and Ganong, W. F. (1978). *Ann Rev. Physiol.* **40**, 377.

Reinharz, A. and Roth, M. (1969). *Eur. J. Bioch.* **7**, 334.

Riegger, A. J. G., Lever, A. F., Millar, J. A., Morton, J. J. and Slack, B. (1977). *Lancet,* **ii**, 1317.

Romero, J. C. and Strong, C. G. (1977). *Circ. Res.* **40**, 35.

Rosenthal, J. (1976). *Clin. Sci. mol. Med.* **51**, 121s.

Rosenthal, J., Wolff, H. P., Weber, P. and Dahleim, H. (1971). *Am. J. Physiol.* **221**, 1292.

Rosset, E. and Veyrat, R. (1971). *Eur. J. clin. Invest.* **1**, 328.

Rubin, I. (1972). *Scand. J. clin. Lab. Invest.* **28**, 51.

Ryan, J. W. (1970). *Biochem. J.* **116**, 159.

Ryan, J. W. (1967). *Science,* **158**, 1589.

Ryan, J. W. (1972). *Experientia,* **29**, 407.

Ryan, J. W. (1974). *In* "Angiotensin" (I. H. Page and F. M. Bumpus, eds), p. 81. Springer-Verlag, Berlin.

Ryan, J. W. and Johnson, D. C. (1969). *Biochim. biophys. Acta,* **191**, 386.

Ryan, J. W., McKenzie, J. K. and Lee, M. R. (1968). *Biochem. J.* **108**, 679.

Ryan, J. W., Ryan, U. S., Schultz, D. R., Whitaker, C., Chung, H. and Dorer, F. E. (1975). *Biochem. J.* **146**, 497.

Saltman, S., Fredlund, P. and Catt, K. J. (1976). *Endocrinology,* **98**, 894.

Sancho, J., Re, R., Burton, J., Barger, A. G. and Haber, E. (1976). *Circulation,* 53, 400.

Sarstedt, C. A., Vaughan, F. D. and Peach, M. J. (1975). *Circ. Res.* 37, 350.

Schaechtelin, G., Baechtold, N., Haefeli, L., Regoli, D., Gaudry-Parades, A. and Peters, G. (1968). *Am. J. Physiol.* 215, 632.

Scharpé, S., Eid, M., Cooreman, W. and Lauwers, A. (1976). *Biochem. J.* 153, 505.

Schwyzer, R. (1963). *Pure Appl. Chem.* 6, 265.

Sealey, J. E., Moon, C., Laragh, J. H. and Alderman, M. (1976). *Am. J. Med.* 61, 731.

Sealey, J. E., Moon, C., Laragh, J. and Atlas, S. (1977). *Circ. Res.* 40 (Suppl. 1), 41.

Semple, P. F. (1977). *J. clin. Endocr. Metab.* 44, 915.

Semple, P. F., Boyd, A. S., Dawes, P. M. and Morton, J. J. (1976). *Circ. Res.* 39, 671.

Semple, P. F. and Morton, J. J. (1976). *Circ. Res.* 38 (Suppl. 11), 122.

Semple, P. F., Nicholls, M. G., Tree, M. and Fraser, R. (1978). *Endocrinology,* 103, 1476.

de Senarclens, C. F., Pricam, C. E., Banichahi, F. D. and Vallotton, M. B. (1977). *Kidney Int.* 11, 161.

Severs, W. B., Daniels, A. E., Smoobler, H. H., Kinnard, W. S. and Buckley, J. P. (1966). *J. Pharm. exp. Ther.* 153, 530.

Shade, R. E., Davis, J. O., Johnson, J. A., Gotshall, R. W. and Spielman, W. S. (1973). *Am. J. Physiol.* 224, 926.

Skeggs, L. T., Kahn, J. R. and Shumway, H. P. (1956). *J. exp. Med.* 103, 295.

Skeggs, L. T., Lentz, K. E., Hochstrasser, H. and Kahn, J. R. (1963). *J. exp. Med.* 118, 73.

Skeggs, L. T., Lentz, K. E., Kahn, J. R., Dorer, F. E. and Levine, M. (1969). *Circ. Res.* 25, 451.

Skeggs, L. T., Lentz, K. E., Kahn, J. R. and Hochstrasser, H. (1967). *Circ. Res.* 20/21 (Suppl. II), 91.

Skeggs, L. T., Lentz, K. E., Kahn, J. R. and Hochstrasser, H. (1968). *J. exp. Med.* 128, 13.

Skeggs, L. T., Lentz, K. E., Kahn, J. R., Shumway, H. P. and Woods, K. R. (1956). *J. exp. Med.* 104, 193.

Skeggs, L. T., Marsh, W. H., Kahn, J. R. and Shumway, N. P. (1954). *J. exp. Med.* 99, 275.

Skinner, S. L. (1967). *Circ. Res.* 20, 391.

Skinner, S. L., Cran, E. J., Gibson, R., Taylor, R., Walters, W. A. W. and Catt, K. J. (1975). *Am. J. Obstet. Gynec.* 121, 626.

Skinner, S. L., Lumbers, E. R. and Symonds, E. M. (1969). *Clin. Sci.* 36, 67.

Skinner, S. L., Lumbers, E. R. and Symonds, E. M. (1972). *Clin. Sci.* 42, 479.

Slater, E. E., Burton, J. and Haber, E. (1975). *Circulation,* 52 (Suppl. II), 97.

Slater, E. E. and Haber, E. (1976). *Circulation,* 53/54 (Suppl. II), 143.

Smeby, R. R., Sen, S. and Bumpus, F. M. (1967). *Circ. Res.* 21 (Suppl. II), 129.

Smith, U., Ryan, J. W. and Smith, D. S. (1973). *J. cell. Biol.* 56, 492.

Soffer, R. L. and Case, D. B. (1978). *Am. J. Med.* 64, 147.

Stakemann, O. (1960). *Acta path. microbiol. scand.* 50, 350.

Steele, J. M., Neusy, A. J. and Lowenstein, J. (1976). *Circ. Res.* (Suppl. II), 38, 113.

Stella, A. and Zanchetti, A. (1977). *Am. J. Physiol.* 232, H500.

Stephens, G. A., Davis, J. O., Freeman, R. H., Watkins, B. E. and Khosla, M. C. (1977). *Endocrinology,* 101, 378.

Stewart, J. N., Ferreira, S. H. and Greene, L. J. (1971). *Biochem. Pharmacol.* 20, 1557.

Stockigt, J. R., Collins, R. D. and Biglieri, E. G. (1971). *Circ. Res.* 28, 29 (Suppl. 1), 175.

Y

Streeten, D. H., Anderson, G. H. and Dalakos, T. G. (1976). *Am. J. Med.* **60**, 817.

Sundsfjord, J. A. (1970). *Acta endocr., Copenh.* **64**, 181.

Symonds, E. M., Stanley, M. A. and Skinner, S. (1968). *Nature, Lond.* **217**, 1152.

Taquini, A. C., Blaquier, P. and Taquini (1964). *Can. Med. Assoc. J.* **90**, 210.

Tewksbury, D. A., Premau, M. R., Dumas, M. L. and Frome, W. L. (1977). *Circ. Res.* (Suppl. II) **41**, 29.

Thurau, K. (1964). *Am. J. Med.* **36**, 698.

Thurau, K., Schnermann, J., Nagel, W., Horster, M. and Wohl, M. (1967). *Circ. Res.* **20–21** (Suppl. II), 79.

Tree, M. (1973). *J. Endocr.* **56**, 159.

Tsai, B. S., Peach, M. J., Khosla, M. C. and Bumpus, F. M. (1975). *J. med. Chem.* **18**, 1180.

Tobian, L., Tomboulian, A. and Janecek, J. (1959). *J. clin. Invest.* **38**, 605.

Vander, A. J. (1963). *Am. J. Physiol.* **205**, 133.

Vander, A. J. and Carlson, J. (1969). *Circ. Res.* **25**, 145.

Vander, A. J. and Geelhoed, G. W. (1965). *Proc. Soc. exp. Biol. Med.* **120**, 399.

Vander, A. J. and Luciano, J. R. (1967). *Circ. Res.* (Suppl. II) **20 and 21**, 69.

Vandongen, R., Peart, W. S. and Boyd, G. W. (1973). *Circ. Res.* **32**, 290.

Vane, J. W. (1974). *In* "Angiotensin" (I. M. Page and F. M. Bumpus, eds), p. 31. Springer-Verlag, Berlin.

De Vito, E., Cabrera, R. R. and Fasciolo, J. C. (1970). *Am. J. Physiol.* **219**, 1042.

Wagermark, J., Ungerstedt, U. and Ljungqvist (1968). *Circ. Res.* **22**, 149.

Waite, M. A. (1973). *Clin. Sci. mol. Med.* **45**, 51.

Ward, P. E., Gedney, C. G., Dowben, R. M. and Erdös, E. G. (1975). *Biochem. J.* **151**, 755.

Waugh, W. H. (1972). *Can. J. Physiol. Pharmacol.* **50**, 711.

Weinberger, M., Aoi, W. and Grim, C. (1977). *Circ. Res.* **41** (Suppl. II), 21.

Weinberger, M., Wade, M. B., Aoi, W., Usa, T., Dentino, M., Luft, F. and Grim, C. E. (1977). *Circ. Res.* (Suppl. I) **40**, 1.

Weir, R. J., Paintin, D. B., Robertson, J. I. S., Tree, M., Fraser, R. and Young, J. (1970). *Proc. R. Soc. Med.* **63**, 1101.

Werle, E., Vogel, R. and Goldel, L. F. (1957). *Arch. exp. Path. Pharmacol.* **230**, 236.

Williams, G. H., Hollenberg, N. K., Breley, L. M. (1976). *Endocrinology,* **98**, 1343.

Wilson, C. M., Erdös, E. G., Dunn, J. F. and Wilson, J. D. (1977). *Proc. natn. Acad. Sci. USA,* **74**, 1185A.

Winer, N., Chokshi, D. S., Myung, S. Y. and Freedman, A. D. (1969). *J. clin. Endocr.* **29**, 1169.

Zanchetti, A. and Stella, A. (1975). *Clin. Sci. mol. Med.* **48**, 215s.

Ziegler, M., Riniker, B. and Gross, F. (1967). *Biochem. J.* **102**, 28.

XII. Endocrinology in Clinical Medicine

RAYMOND GREENE

Endocrinology began as a branch of physiology but has now progressed to be, if not a branch of medicine itself, at least a field of knowledge essential for every branch of medicine. The clinical specialist, whatever may be his chosen field of interest, needs a knowledge of endocrinology to arrive at a greater understanding of his subject. The cardiologist cannot neglect the effect of hyperthyroidism, of disorders of the renin–angiotensin–aldosterone system or of catecholamines and the sympathetic nervous system. The emergence of our knowledge of mechanisms of the hypothalamic control of the anterior pituitary emphasises the major role of endocrinology in neurology (pituitary tumours were first studied by the neurologist). The dermatologist must be aware of the numerous, often bizarre, changes of the skin and hair accompanying many disorders of the endocrine system. The integrated roles of parathyroid hormone, calcitonin and of vitamin D (the last as a prohormone) in bone disease, and those of growth hormone, insulin and other growth factors, of glucagon, adrenal cortical hormones and the prostaglandins in the metabolic response to injury are of fundamental importance in medicine and surgery.

An appreciation of the interactions of many hormones during pregnancy and in many women's diseases is now an essential part of obstetrics and gynaecocology. Endocrinology, more perhaps than other medical specialities, depends heavily on the basic sciences, chemistry, physiology and pharmacology, in the elucidation of its obscure problems, not only in diagnosis and treatment, but also in the search for a cause.

In clinical endocrinology, there has been remarkable development and application of specialised analytical techniques which held sway at the time of the earlier editions of this book. The techniques have much improved, but in addition they are now applied in kinetic tests (e.g. stimulation or inhibition tests of hormone secretion), tests to measure metabolic clearance rates, production and secretion rates, tests to determine the interaction of hormones, an example of the application of basic research to clinical diagnosis is the hypothalmic releasing and release inhibiting hormones so admirably described by Arimura and Schally. Increased knowledge of the detailed mode of action of hormones is also influencing clinical medicine, for example, of our increasing knowledge of receptors and the formation of antibodies to them. Synthetic antihormones are also playing their part in therapy.

The specialist in any branch of medicine or surgery will encounter a philosophical difficulty. He produces, or reproduces with amendments of his own, the description of "a disease", i.e. he describes a deviation from health of a fairly constant kind which is encountered in a number of patients, and the larger the number, the more convinced he is that he is describing what with conscious vagueness he calls "a disease". Measles is a disease or at worst is a concept asymptotic to that description. Whipple's "disease" is rare enough to be a doubtful entity. Endocrinological knowledge will help to avoid these problems. If in every case of disease "X" there is a constant endocrinological deviation from that found in healthy people, a deviation not found except in association with the symptoms and signs of "X" disease, one or two convenient hypotheses are possible. The endocrinological abnormality is the cause of the clinical abnormality or vice versa, but neither hypothesis may be correct and something hitherto unsuspected may have caused both clinical and endocrinological abnormalities or they may be chance coincidents. Correlations do not establish causal connections, though the probability of such connections increases with increased correlation.

An obvious example of the mistakes into which the unwary clinician may be led is afforded by a laboratory investigation that does not fall strictly within the purview of this book. When the thyroid uptake of radioactive iodine was introduced as a test of thyroid function many clinicians assumed that a high uptake always indicated excessive activity of the gland and a low uptake reduced activity. It soon emerged that in several disorders in which the thyroid function was obviously deficient the uptake was high, because the gland was capable of taking up radioactive iodine, but because of abnormality of the synthetic pathway was incapable of converting it into thyroxine. Moreover, the patient's thyroid could be utilising iodine maximally for thyroxine synthesis yet radioactive iodine uptake may be low because the thyroid already contained all the iodine it could store, perhaps because of a radiological investigation, possibly months or years before, with an iodine-containing radioopaque substance.

Mistakes may be made by laboratory workers and by clinicians, but for many years most physicians leaned to the view that if the laboratory findings and the clinical findings were inconsistent, the latter were more likely to be correct. This is perhaps acceptable in an emergency because one of the commonest causes is in the labelling in the ward of the specimen to be examined. Laboratory errors certainly still occur but with the present high standards of quality control are less likely than an error in the preparation of the report or a misunderstanding, either of which can be quickly elucidated by a telephone call. In the absence of any such explanation, the investigation should be repeated, sometimes quickly, and if the discrepancy between clinical and laboratory findings persists, then either the clinical diagnosis is wrong or a new form of the disease has been uncovered (e.g. the various forms of hypothyroidism); or the effect of some hitherto unsuspected factor may be interfering with the investigation (e.g. an effect of age, diet, recumbancy or drug).

When the last edition of this book was published, many of the complicated endocrinological investigations were usually unattainable except in a few specialised centres. This situation has changed and with some of the simplest techniques the smallest laboratory can provide a service using commercially available kits or centrally provided reagents. This in itself can lead to problems when laboratories carry out only occasional assays and underlines the supreme importance of appropriate quality control. With more complicated techniques there are many national systems (e.g. the supraregional assay service (SAS) in the United Kingdom) and international systems of laboratories which can provide them when essential for most parts of the world.

The chapter dealing with the catecholamine hormones, dopamine, adrenaline and noradrenaline may well be the one that will most deeply stir the imagination of the general physician. Adrenaline captured it as long ago as 1895, when it was discovered by Oliver and Schäfer who described the vasoconstrictor effects and its influence on blood pressure. The importance of adrenaline in clinical medicine is widespread but in few branches is exactly defined. Its influence, and that of its subsequently discovered partner, noradrenaline, is made manifest not only in cardiovascular disorders of many kinds but in respiratory disease, the wide range of the allergies, de-rangements of carbohydrate metabolism, even in psychiatry and throughout the study of functional and psychosomatic disorders. With the recognition of the importance of dopamine it cannot be doubted that the improved methods of measuring the levels of these three hormones in the blood is leading to a great increase in clinical knowledge, especially in relation to various secondary factors such as the effect of drugs, disease states and physiological environment. Much has already been added to our knowledge of essential hypertension, coronary disease, peripheral vascular disease, the response to burns and, naturally, to the diagnosis of phaeochromocytoma.

Perhaps the most important advance has been in the study of the thyroid-

stimulating substances TSH, thyroid stimulating globulins and the hypothalamic TSH releasing hormone (TSH-RH). Disturbances of the feedback
mechanism between thyroid and pituitary may now be more accurately
delineated especially since synthetic TSH-RH is now commercially available
and reliable radioimmunoassays are now available for measuring TSH,
thyroxine, triiodothyronine, reverse triiodothyronine and thyroid antibodies.
Certainly increased TSH blood levels are seldom the cause of hyperthyroidism except when arising from a TSH-secreting ectopic tumour.

We know now rather more than we did at the time of the previous edition
about the fourth thyroid hormone, calcitonin. Secreted by the C cells, it has
become clinically important by reason of its secretion in excess in medullary
carcinoma of the thyroid and of its effectiveness in the treatment of hitherto
intractable Paget's disease. It may well be important in other diseases of
bone. Since the last edition there has been a leap forward in our knowledge of
vitamin D which can now be regarded as a prohormone with origins in skin,
and with liver and kidney carrying out essential subsequent metabolic
steps. The advances in our knowledge of growth hormone have been spec-
tacular. Radioimmunological assays of growth hormone can now tell the
clinician whether acromegaly is active and therefore in need of drastic
treatment. Already the exact diagnosis of the various forms of growth
retardation has been made easier, but the influence of growth hormone is
far wider than was previously suspected. It antagonises insulin and influences
the metabolism of protein, fat, carbohydrate, minerals and electrolytes, but
so far there is no evidence that it is concerned with human diabetes except
perhaps in acromegaly. Growth hormone has no direct effect on the formation
of complex organic sulphates in cartilage which is necessary for skeletal
growth without a synergism with somatomedin which is synthesised in the
liver and perhaps the kidney. As discussed in Vol 1, Ch. V, low levels of
somatomedin are found in familial forms of growth retardation with high
growth hormone levels and high levels in acromegaly.

We have learned that growth hormone may arise from sources other than
the pituitary, for instance in some pulmonary carcinomata. We know far more
about its mechanisms of control, both hypothalamic and metabolic. The
plasma levels have been measured in such diverse conditions as malnutrition
and obesity. Bromocriptine may be useful in conditions in which the
secretion of growth hormone is excessive.

There have been important advances in the management of diabetes
mellitus in recent years, many of them made possible by biochemical dis-
coveries, including methods of assaying insulin, growth hormone and
glucagon in blood. Further development of these may eventually be of great
practical use.

The clinician has awaited with impatience the discovery of easily applicable routine methods of determining other pituitary and pituitary-like hormones, especially perhaps the gonadotrophins. These methods are now available. Information obtained in this way may help to solve the diagnostic and therapeutic problems set by toxaemia of pregnancy, habitual abortion, hydatidiform mole, choriocarcinoma, foetal death and disorders of menstruation and the climacteric. The diagnosis of the various types of hypogonadism in both sexes is made easier now that methods for determining plasma gonadotrophins are readily available. The management of patients with mammary carcinoma treated by hypophysectomy may be assisted by the measurement of gonadotrophins, the level of which helps to show the extent to which the operation has been complete.

The interest of clinicians in the determination of the gonadal hormones is not confined to gynaecologists and endocrinologists. It is now realised, perhaps a little belatedly, that the effects of oestrogens, progestogens and androgens on physiological processes are widespread. Indeed, it seems at least teleologically unlikely that any hormone of only local importance would be distributed wastefully to every cell of the body. But whereas the wide-spread activity of thyroxine was realised generations ago, that of the other hormones has not until lately been recognised. Oestrogens are linked with many of the body's biochemical reactions. They influence water metabolism, modify the actions of other hormones and affect the growth of tumours, the balance of the autonomic system and the function of the cerebral cortex.

The general importance of the androgens rests chiefly on their anabolic activity. They have been used extensively as promotors of growth in growth retardation and to increase the weight of wasted patients. In the past the metabolites of androgens were usually measured in the urine as 17-oxo-steroids but now the numerous androgens and their conjugates can be measured in blood. Studies of androgen metabolism may solve the problem of hypertrichosis in women, which causes greater misery than many more lethal diseases. If progesterone does not so far seem to have so wide a range of activity as oestradiol and testosterone, this is probably only because it has been studied less. In particular, we have had to rely on the excretion of pregnanediol in urine, knowing that this is less than ideal as an index of progesterone secretion. Only in recent years have determinations of progesterone in blood become commonplace, but even so, only a few of many disorders of menstruation and pregnancy have so far been explained by the simultaneous determination of gonadotrophins, progesterone and oestradiol in blood.

Oxytocin empties the mammary alveoli and causes vasodilation in the limbs, as well as exercising its well known function on the uterus. It seems inconceivable that it should not have other functions and that its determination in blood will grow in importance as the assay becomes easier to perform. Recent work, still insufficiently confirmed, suggests that vasopressin may be concerned with the function of memory.

One of the most exciting developments has been the discovery of enkephalin, natural transmitters with the pharmacological actions of morphine. Indeed, it would appear that the actions of morphine are explained by the presence of receptors for the compound in the brain, which are identical with those of the enkephalins, a fact that may explain the disastrous symptoms of withdrawal of morphine from the addict. So far, two distinct molecules have been identified, methionine and leucine enkephalins, both pentapeptides. In addition there exists a series of longer peptides found in highest concentration in the pituitary gland. That these facts are relevant to the problems of addiction and withdrawal can hardly be doubted but how they are relevant is still speculative.

In recent years much attention has been focused on the relationship of the prostaglandins to a wide range of physiological and pathological effects, especially inflammation. Salmon and Flower have admirably summarised the complexity of the prostaglandins with their precursors and metabolites and now synthetic antagonists and even inhibitors of their synthesis which can be of considerable pharmacological and therapeutic interest. Even the mechanism of action of the salicylates is now better understood.

The last edition of this book contained no chapter on the gastro-intestinal hormones. In this edition there are two chapters on the subject, the second dealing with three long-recognised hormones: gastrin, cholecystokinin and secretin. Radioimmunoassay has permitted investigation in disease in greater depth than ever before. The other chapter is an excellent overall review of the amine precursor uptake and decarboxylation or APUD system which has already changed our concepts of the control of gastro-intestinal function and clarified our ideas on many hitherto obscure tumours and the effects.

So much has been done. No one reading this book can fail in admiration for the imagination shown and the labour expended in applying endocrinology to medicine.

The contributors reveal no complacency about what has been written on current methods for determining hormones whether in blood or in any other biological material. Almost every chapter refers to desirable, and often to possible, developments for improving techniques, to give greater sensitivity, precision or accuracy. It is perhaps pertinent at the end of this book to pause for a moment and enquire what the attainment of these goals may mean.

The investigation of hormone levels in blood, and of many other body constituents, passes through a series of stages, as has already been stressed in the first chapter of this book. From qualitative physiological and pathological studies, research workers have passed to quantitative evaluation using biological, chemical or physiochemical procedures, or a combination of them. After this stage the endocrinologist has tried, with no small success, to correlate abnormal changes in plasma hormone levels with the degree of departure from the physiologically healthy, whether the departure be of endocrine origin or not. I shall here do no more than refer in passing to the basic problem of what the term "abnormal" signifies for any one hormone in any one individual, adding that some of the information collected in Roger J. Williams' "Biochemical Individuality" (1958) must make one think critically about the meaning of the term and its relation to that other abstract and mainly statistical concept, the average. However, assuming that there is such a thing as a norm, even though this be a range and not a precise value, current investigation has done much for its importance not only for each of the increasing number of hormones in the blood but also for the extent to which these ranges may be different in the sexes, different age groups, diet (whether in relation to amount, components of either vitamins, major minerals such as sodium and calcium, or trace metals, or the energy-producing foodstuffs). It is now appreciated that normal ranges can be altered by disease apparently unrelated to the endocrinopathy which would be indicated by these abnormal findings in a normal person.

Much recent work is concerned with how hormones work. Hormones produce a response in their target organs by combining with an appropriate receptor which is either at the cell surface as with protein hormones or, as with steroid hormones, in the cells into which the small molecule hormones can pass freely. Mutants occur in which the receptors are defective, e.g. in testicular feminisation (an unfortunate term), the receptors for androgens are abnormal or absent so that although the individual is chromosomally male and produces testosterone normally he remains somatically female. Although much is known of the "second messenger system" involving the adenylcyclase and related systems, with many hormones the transducer system translating hormone receptor interactions into the hormonal response remains obscure.

The role of receptors in tumour tissue in the mediation of tumour growth, the effect on these of hormone deprivation or administration of hormone antagonists or excess hormone treatment may assist in assessing the appropriateness or otherwise of various treatments of malignant tumours. The formation of antibodies to receptors may well provide a new treatment for hormone excess or of hormone dependent tumours. Indeed the recent upsurge of immunological science is already being applied extensively to endocrinology whether it is in the autoimmune diseases affecting one or more endocrine organs or indeed in our knowledge of thyroid stimulating immunoglobulin.

Nothing but basic biochemical and probably biophysical, studies can advance our knowledge, which is surely essential if the clinical assessments made from consideration of hormone levels in the blood are to have anything more than a purely empirical basis.

The third edition of "Hormones in Blood" must make it clear how endocrinology is a discipline which must be explored and developed by basic scientists and clinicians alike to their mutual advantage.

REFERENCE

Williams, R. J. (1958). "Biochemical Individuality." John Wiley, New York.

Subject Index